TEXTBOOK OF MICROBIOLOGY
for
BSc/MSc Nursing Students

TEXTBOOK OF MICROBIOLOGY
for
BSc/MSc Nursing Students

Prof. (Dr.) K. R. Aneja
MSc, PhD, FBS, FPSI, FMSI, FIMS, FSBA
Formerly Professor and Chairman,
Department of Microbiology
Kurukshetra University, Kurukshetra
Haryana, India

Dr. Sushma Aneja
Formerly Principal
Education Department
Government of Haryana

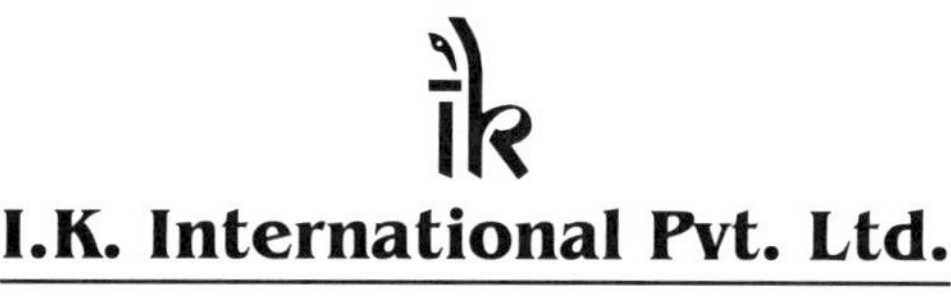

I.K. International Pvt. Ltd.
NEW DELHI

Published by
I.K. International Pvt. Ltd.
4435-36/7, Ansari Road, Daryaganj
New Delhi-110 002 (India)
E-mail: info@ikinternational.com
Website: www.ikbooks.com

ISBN 978-93-90620-59-3

Published by Krishan Makhijani for I.K. International Pvt. Ltd., 4435-36/7, Ansari Road, Daryaganj, New Delhi-110 002 and Printed by Rekha Printers Pvt. Ltd., Okhla Industrial Area, Phase II, New Delhi-110 020.

Dedicated to the Sweet Memories of
My Lovely Wife and Coauthor of the Book

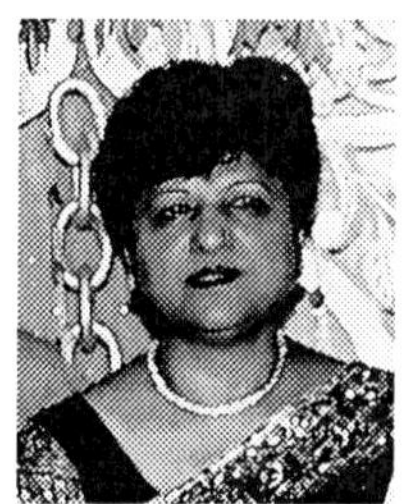

Dr. Sushma Aneja

Preface

Microbiology is the study of microorganisms (microbes): bacteria, archaea, fungi, algae, protozoa, helminths (cellular organisms), viruses, prions and viriods (acellular organisms) that are too small to be seen with the naked eye. The study of infectious diseases, called **medical microbiology** and the battle between the invading organisms and human's immune system, called **immunology**, are the two applied branches of microbiology. Microbiology has proven to be one of the most important disciplines in biology making it possible to identify how some of the organisms could cause disease, discover how to treat them with antibiotics and even use of some microbes for humans diets and industries.

Throughout human history communicable diseases such as leprosy, Black death, Spanish flu pandemic of 1918 and smallpox have severely affected humanity. Some of the historically important diseases occur even today such as TB, yellow fever, HIV/AIDS, influenza and malaria.

Microbes are everywhere and evolving to cause new diseases. The most important recent pandemic outbreaks of 21st century have been the 2003 SARS pandemic caused by the coronavirus (SARS-CoV-1) and the current ongoing COVID-19 pandemic caused by another coronavirus (SARS-CoV-2). COVID-19 has caused over 5 million deaths of the over 253 million cases/infections reported globally. Other than the loss of life and humans suffering from post-COVID effects, COVID-19 has significantly changed the world, as it paused economies and prevented social interaction, both of which inevitably impacted mental health and food security and much more for the global population.

Microbes are always one step ahead of us by developing mechanisms and creating new genes to resist means of control/eradication by antibiotics/vaccines developed by us.

21st century nursing is the glue that holds a patient's healthcare journey together. Nursing is the profession or practice within the healthcare system and the nurses or nursing practitioners form the backbones providing care for the patient. Study of microbiology is immensely important to the nursing profession. Knowledge of microbiology helps a nurse in every field of healthcare system. Most significant is in the specific control of spreads of infection, preventing infection to oneself, spreading infections from one to another and from the inanimate objects/environment, creating aseptic conditions, and collection of clinical specimen aseptically for diagnosis, treatment and research.

This textbook has been structured based on the curriculum of **Indian National Council (INC)** and keeping in mind the need and standards of BSc 1st year nursing students. It provides a solid background of the subject of microbiology written in a simple, lucid and understandable language. Fascinating images and conceptual diagrams have been used that support the text concisely and provide a clear insight into fundamental concepts and understanding of microbes. A unique feature of the book is that every chapter has key points, important questions and MCQs with answers for quick review, recapitulation and preparation for examination to enhance their performance. It contains up-to-date information about infectious diseases, their causative agents, treatment and preventive measures including vaccines.

This book contains a total of 80 chapters included under five Units covering all aspects of microbiology for BSc nursing students:

UNIT I : Introduction: Principles, historical development of microbiology, and its importance to nursing.

UNIT II : General characteristics, classification and identification of microorganisms.

UNIT III : Methods of infection control and role of a nurse in hospital-acquired infections/nosocomial control programme.

UNIT IV : Disease producing organisms: Bacteria, viruses, fungi, parasites and rodent vectors, and collection of clinical specimens for diagnosis.

UNIT V : Immunity: Concept, types/classification, serological tests, immunization, and immunization/vaccination schedule.

We sincerely hope that this textbook will serve as a vehicle for understanding the world of microbes, especially germs, related to nursing profession and treating patients in judicious ways under their care. It would prove to be invaluable for the nursing community, and others involved in the healthcare system.

Kurukshetra (India)

Prof. (Dr.) K. R. Aneja
Dr. Sushma Aneja

Acknowledgements

I am to start by acknowledging, the exceptionally beautiful, lovely, sweet, smiling every day, with impressive personality, the Coauthor of the book my wife Dr. Sushma Aneja, Principal, DIET, Kurukshetra, the inspirer and backbone of the book who originated the idea, helped and supported me till the completion of the manuscript last page but couldn't live to see the project underway. She was as important to the book as I am. Thank you so much Dearest.

I am extremely grateful to my family members: my sons (Dr. Raman and Dr. Ashish), my daughter-in-laws (Neha and Anu), my lovely grandchildren (Radha and Anish) and siblings (daughter-in-law's parents) for their help and valuable support. They all keep me going at every step during this venture. Without their cooperation this book would not have seen the dawn of the day.

I am especially grateful to one of my closest Dr. Vibha Bhardwaj, Director Environment Laboratories and National Technical Expert Member of Environment Sector in the Ministry of Industry and Advanced Technology, Government of UAE, for the encouragement and motivation, specifically after the sudden death of Mrs. Aneja to complete the pending proof reading to fulfil her dreams and release of the book at the earliest possible well advance of the beginning of the new Nursing course.

I am also thankful to my mentor Prof. R.S. Mehrotra & Mrs. Mehrotra for their encouragement. The authors are also thankful to Professor Raj Kumar Salar of Biotechnology Department, Chaudhary Devi Lal University, Sirsa and Dr. Vikas Kumar, Assistant Prof, Biotechnology Department, Maharishi Markandeshwar (Deemed to be University), Mullana (Ambala). I wish to thank EVERYBODY who ever said anything positive to me or taught me something, I heard it all, and it meant anything.

I am extremely thankful to Almighty God and Joy maa Guru Ji, most of all, because without their blessing, we would not have been able to do this wonderful work done for the nursing community.

Prof. (Dr.) K.R. Aneja
Dr. Sushma Aneja

Contents

UNIT V: FUNDAMENTALS OF IMMUNOLOGY

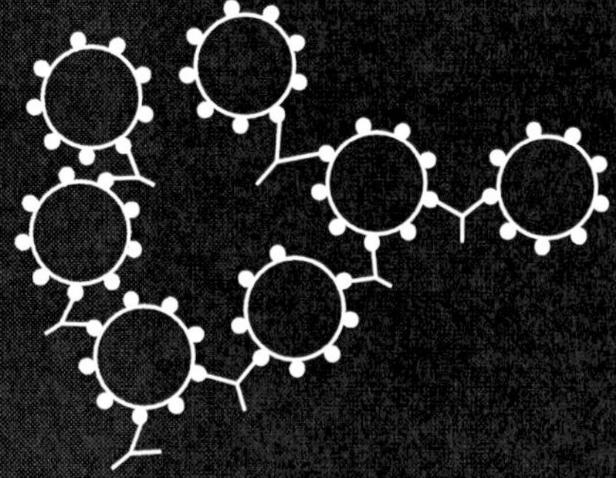

Unit I

INTRODUCTION TO MICROBIOLOGY

- Introduction, Importance and Relevance of Microbiology to Nursing
- Historical Development of Microbiology

1

Introduction, Importance and Relevance of Microbiology to Nursing

MICROBIOLOGY

Microbiology is the study of microorganisms. **Microorganisms** (also called **microbes**) are tiny organisms that cannot be seen with naked eyes, but can be seen only through the microscopes. These are of nine types which include cellular organisms (e.g., bacteria, archaea, protozoa, fungi, algae, parasitic worms) and acellular entities (viruses, viroids, prions). The term microbiology is derived from the Greek words: *mikros* = small, *bios* = life, *logos* = to study.

SUBDISCIPLINES OF MICROBIOLOGY

Branches or subdisciplines of microbiology are categorized into **pure** (based on the organisms studied) and **applied fields** (based on the applications of knowledge). These include:

- **Bacteriology** – the study of bacteria and archaea.
- **Mycology** – the study of fungi.
- **Virology** – the study of viruses.
- **Protozoology** – the study of protozoans.
- **Phycology** (or **algology**) – the study of algae.
- **Parasitology** – the study of parasites (protozoa and helminths).
- **Medical microbiology** – the study of microbes that infect humans, the diseases they cause, the way they cause, their diagnosis, prevention and treatment. There are five kinds of microorganisms that cause infectious diseases: bacteria, viruses, fungi, protozoa, helminths, and one type of infectious protein, called prions.
- **Immunology** – the study of host responses toward pathogens, i.e., immunity.

- **Pharmaceutical microbiology** – the science of manufacturing antibiotics, vaccines and other health products.
- **Nursing microbiology** – the science that deals with the application of knowledge in medical microbiology at the bedside of patients during nursing care. It provides nursing students in the skills and knowledge to prevent the transmission of germs in healthcare settings, to oneself, from inanimate objects and from one patient to another, in addition to the difference between pathogenic and nonpathogenic microbes.

WHY STUDY MICROBIOLOGY?

Microorganisms are ubiquitous – found in almost all natural elements on the planet. Scientists estimate that there are a nonillion (10^{30}) microbial cells currently in existence on the earth, and nearly 10 trillion (10^{13}) bacterial cells make up a human's microbiome. The lives of humans, plants and animals are all intrinsically linked to the microbes that continually recycle key nutrients such as carbon and nitrogen, degrade organic matter and shape our day-to-day existence and are essential for keeping the planet healthy. Microbes are the simple models to study the life processes.

Positive Impacts on Human Life

Microorganisms act as sources of food (e.g., edible mushrooms, single-cell proteins), as probiotics (yogurt, sauerkraut, pickles), producers of alcoholic beverages (wine, beer), antibiotics (e.g., penicillin, streptomycin, chloramphenicol, tetracycline, cephalosporin), and solvents to preservatives and pharmaceuticals, in agriculture (e.g., biofertilizers, biopesticides, biodegradation and in bioremediation) and for combating diseases (e.g., vaccines) and in biotechnology to manipulate microorganisms, plants and animals.

Negative Impacts on Human Life

Some microorganisms act as pathogens (disease causing agents) of humans, plants and animals; cause of food spoilage, corrosion, as allergens and the cause of bad smells, in addition to their misuse in bioterrorism.

SCOPE OF MICROBIOLOGY

There is vast scope in microbiology due to its involvement in many fields like medicine, pharmacy, dairy, industry, agriculture, environment, clinical research, chemical technology and nanotechnology. Knowledge of microbiology is indispensably linked with nursing practice.

The scientists who specialize in the field of microbiology are called **microbiologists**. A microbiologist can innovate new diagnostic kits and discover new drugs, develop and test antibiotics and vaccines.

Career Opportunities for Microbiologists

- Microbiologists can research and teach in colleges, universities, and clinical and industrial settings.
- Their work place can be in microbiology based industries, such as pharmacy, breweries, distilleries, dairy, enzyme, spawn, biofertilizer, biopesticide and food.
- They can work at or set up their own pathology/diagnostic labs.
- They can work to control infection, monitoring of indoor environment, protect public health and safeguard the environment.
- They can join nursing and health-related professions.

WHAT IS NURSING?

Nursing is a noble profession of providing care for the sick. It aims at promotion of health, prevention of illness and the care of the sick, disabled and dying people so that they may attain, maintain or recover optimal health and quality of life.

NURSE

Nurse is a person trained to care for the sick or infirm, especially in a hospital. Nursing staff is familiar with practices to prevent the occurrence and spread of infection in hospital, called nosocomial infection and maintain appropriate practices for all patients throughout their stay in hospital. Nurses play an important role in the field of preventive medicine and healthcare.

IMPORTANCE/RELEVANCE OF MICROBIOLOGY IN NURSING

The study of microbiology helps a nursing professional to understand the principles of sterilization and disinfection, diagnosis, prevention, control and treatment of infections and creation of aseptic environment thereby contributing to reduction of mortality and morbidity and duration of hospital stay for inpatients. Microbiology makes aware about new diseases and modern molecular identification methods.

- **Sterilization and disinfection.** Nursing students are taught the adequacy of **sterilization** (killing or removal of all microorganisms in a material or on an object) and **disinfection** (reducing the number of pathogenic organisms on objects or in materials) procedures in surgical and medical practice, in addition to test the efficacy of these procedures in the laboratory.

  The study helps to create and maintain sterile atmosphere in the operation theatres, insulators used in intensive care nurseries, in understanding the time and temperature required for sterilization of various instruments/tools used in clinical settings, the exact concentration and time required for antiseptics at the skin surface during injecting.

- **Diagnosis and treatment of infection.** The study helps in safe collection and handling of specimens/samples for microbiological examination for proper diagnosis of human pathogens involved in various infections assisting the physicians about the cause of the disease.

  Nursing students also learn to determine the susceptibility/ resistance of pathogenic microorganisms to antimicrobial agents for prescribing the proper antibiotics/drugs or prophylaxis of infection in monitoring antibiotics use and in reducing the bacterial resistance against antibiotics.

- **Prevention and control of nosocomial infection.** Microbial control practices like aseptic techniques, wound washing, hand washing or general hygiene which are based on the principles of microbiology helps in reducing the nosocomial (hospital-acquired) infections.

  Nosocomial infections are monitored/prevented/controlled by an infection control team of workers, which includes an infection control nurse and is headed by the infection control doctor. The major functions of this team include: surveillance and control of infections and monitoring of hygienic practices, advising the infection control committee on matters of policy concerned with the prevention of transmission of the infection to other patients, especially in communicable (infectious) disease wards.

- **Transmission of human pathogens.** The knowledge of microbiology helps a nurse to know the sources, and mode of transmission of pathogens and spread of infections from one person to another and to the communities, thereby suggesting the ways to prevent them.

It also helps in monitoring to prevent the infections of serving patients through foodborne pathogens and transmission of handborne (faecal) pathogens through proper handwashing.

- **Disposal of hospital wastes.** Hospital wastes sometimes have dangerous infectious agents which would contaminate the earth and/or air if disposed of without treatment. Study of microbiology helps in proper disposal of the waste to prevent the transmission of infectious diseases.

KEY POINTS

- **Microbiology** is the study of microscopic organisms that cannot be seen with the naked eyes.
- The organism that cannot be seen without the use of a microscope is called a **microorganism**.
- **Nursing** is a profession of providing care for the sick and elderly people.
- **Nurse** is a person trained to care for the sick.
- **Knowledge of microbiology helps a nursing student** to understand the infectious diseases, including their agents and routes of transmission, their prevention and medications used to treat them, to create sterile environment and the body's immune response.

IMPORTANT QUESTIONS

1. Describe briefly:
   (a) Subdisciplines/branches of microbiology.
   (b) Why should we study microbiology?
   (c) Relevance/importance of microbiology in nursing.
   (d) Career opportunities for microbiologists.
   (e) Negative impacts of microorganisms on humans.

MULTIPLE-CHOICE QUESTIONS

1. Life on the earth would be much better if all microorganisms were eradicated. True or false?
2. Microbiologists who study fungi are called
   (a) Phycologists (b) Mycologists
   (c) Parasitologists (d) Protozoologists.

3. Microorganisms
 (a) Include only bacteria and viruses
 (b) Are considered to be visible with the naked eyes
 (c) Are usually harmful to our well-being
 (d) Do not play an essential role in our environment
 (e) None of the above.

4. Knowledge of microbiology helps a nursing student in the
 (a) Creation of sterile environment
 (b) Prevention of infectious diseases
 (c) Routes of transmission of pathogens
 (d) The body's immune response
 (e) All of the above
 (f) None of the above.

5. Which of the following is not a branch of microbiology?
 (a) Zoology
 (b) Mycology
 (c) Phycology
 (d) Virology
 (e) Parasitology.

6. The study of medical microbiology is important in
 (a) Diagnosis (b) Bioremediation
 (c) Chemotherapy (d) Both (a) and (c).

7. The essential function performed by bacteria on the earth
 (a) Cause diseases
 (b) Produce antibiotics
 (c) Control pests
 (d) Decompose organic material and recycle elements.

8. Beneficial activity/activities of microorganisms
 (a) Are used to produce antibiotics
 (b) Provide nitrogen for plant growth
 (c) Are used as biopesticides
 (d) All of the above
 (e) None of the above.

ANSWERS TO MCQs

1. False	2. (b)	3. (e)	4. (e)	5. (a)
6. (d)	7. (d)	8. (d).		

2

Historical Development of Microbiology

The term microbiology was introduced by **Louis Pasteur**, who demonstrated that the fermentation was caused by the growth of bacteria and yeasts. Microbiology as a discipline is over 100 years old and has three distinct historical eras:

- *Early history of microbiology* (mid-17th century) – Discovery of microbial life.
- *Transition period* (late 17th and 18th century) – Theory of spontaneous generation.
- *The golden age of microbiology* (1857–1920) – Pasteur and Koch era.

DISCOVERY OF MICROBIAL LIFE

The existence of microorganisms was predicted many centuries before they were first observed, for example, by the **Jains** in India and **Marcus Terentius Varro** in ancient Rome.

Robert Hooke, a British scientist, is known to have made first microscopic observation in 1665 of the sporulating structures of molds (fungi) among the specimens of cells he viewed using a compound microscope (one in which light passes through two lenses). Eleven years later in 1676, a Dutch merchant named **Antonie van Leeuwenhoek** with the simple single-lens microscopes designed by himself made careful observation of microscopic organisms, which he called *animalcules.* Leeuwenhoek is considered the *Father of microbiology* since he is regarded as one of the first to provide accurate description of protozoa, yeasts and bacteria.

After the death of Leeuwenhoek in 1723, the study of microbiology did not develop rapidly because the interest in microorganisms was not high. In the 17th and 18th century, scientists debated the theory of **spontaneous generation** (also called ***abiogenesis***), which stated that *microorganisms arise from lifeless (nonliving) matter* such as beef broth. This theory was disputed by **Francesco Redi**, an Italian naturalist and physician, in 1668 who gave the doctorine of *omne vivum ex vivo,* that is, the living things arise from others of the same kind by his *three-jar experiment* (Fig. 2.1). He showed that fly maggots do not arise from the decaying meat, as others believed if the meat is covered to prevent the entry of flies into the jar.

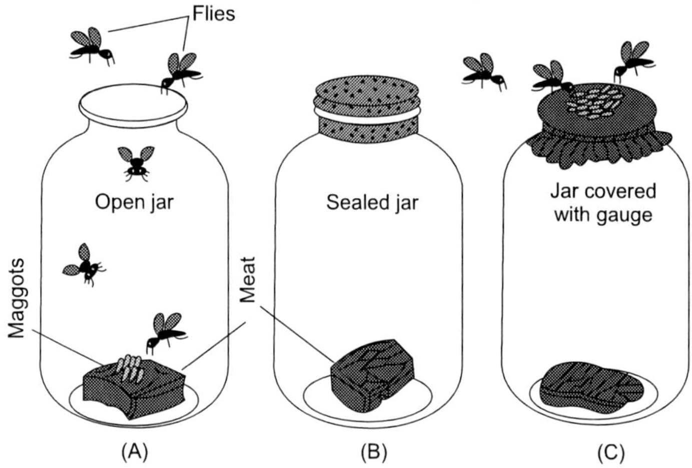

Fig. 2.1 Redi's three-jar experiment (1668) refuting the spontaneous generation of maggots in meat. When meat is exposed in an open jar: flies lay their eggs on it and the eggs hatch into maggots (fly larvae) (A). In a sealed jar, however, no maggots appear (B). If the jar is covered with gauze, maggots hatch from eggs that the flies lay on top of the gauze, but still no maggots appear in the meat (C).

An English cleric **John Needham** advanced spontaneous generation (SG) but **Lazzaro Spallanzani**, an Italian Catholic priest in 1768 disputed the theory showing that boiled broth would not give rise to microscopic forms of life. Spallanzani paved the way for **Louis Pasteur**, who finally disproved the theory of SG in the 1861 by his classic *swan-neck flask experiment,* in which air-borne microorganisms were prevented from entering the growth medium while allowing unadulterated air access to the bacterial culture. He devised a series of *swan-neck flasks* filled with broth (Fig. 2.2). He left the flasks open to the air, but the flasks had a curve in the neck so that microbes would fall into the neck, not the broth. The flasks did not become contaminated (as he predicted they would not), and Pasteur's experiment put to rest the notion of spontaneous generation. Pasteur applied in a very effective way two essential techniques used daily by the microbiologists; *sterilization* and the *aseptic technique*. Sterilization was required to ensure that the growth medium in the swan-neck flask contained no organisms at the beginning of his experiment.

He applied the aseptic technique by designing the swan-neck flask so that it prevented the entry of any **unwanted organisms** into his experiment and successfully disproved the theory of spontaneous generation of life.

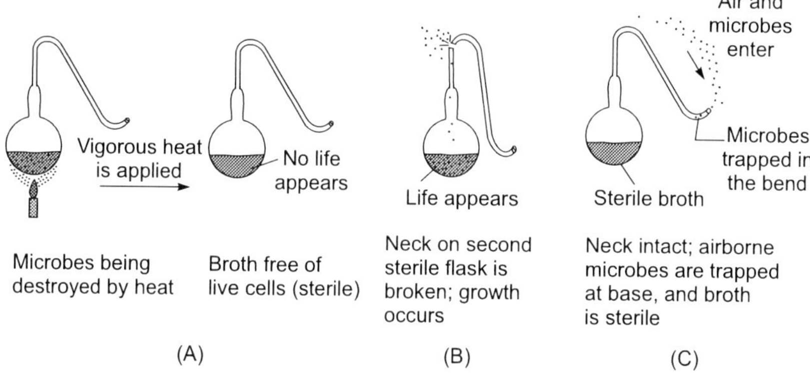

Fig. 2.2 Pasteur's swan-neck flasks experiment to disprove the spontaneous generation of life theory.

The **golden age of microbiology** blossomed through the work of a French microbiologist, **Louis Pasteur** (scientific microbiology) and a German microbiologist, **Robert Koch** (medical microbiology).

Pasteur worked in the middle and late 1800s and the laid the foundation of scientific microbiology. He is known as the *father of modern microbiology*. He discovered bacteria were involved in food spoilage and souring of wine and dairy products. He called attention to the importance of microbes in everyday life and stirred scientists to think that if bacteria could make the wine 'sick' then perhaps they could cause human illness and postulated the **germ theory of disease** *which states that microorganisms are the cause of many diseases.*

Robert Koch, the *father of medical microbiology*, in the 1880s developed a technique for isolating microorganisms and growing them in **pure culture** – a culture of microorganisms in which only one cell type is present, on a solid medium. **Agar**, suggested by **Angelina Hesse**, the American wife of **Koch's** assistant, was used for solidifying broths for bacterial growth instead of gelatin (potato slices were used before the introduction of gelatin). Agar is superior to gelatin due to: many fewer bacteria metabolize agar than gelatin, agar remains a gel at room temperature and firms at temperature as high as 65°C, and melts at 85-90°C, while gelatin liquefies at about 30°C. Isolated colonies that developed on the solid medium surface represented pure cultures of bacteria.

Pasteur's attempts to prove the germ theory, were unsuccessful. It was Robert Koch who in 1876 provided the proof by cultivating anthrax bacteria followed by injecting the pure cultures of the bacilli into mice and showed that the bacilli caused anthrax (*Bacillus anthracis*). The procedures used by Koch came to be known as **Koch's postulates**: a series of four rules or postulates or principles (Fig. 2.3) that aided in the definitive establishment of the germ theory of disease and remain even today the "gold standard" in medical microbiology. Moreover, these postulates provided definitive evidence for an organism to be the **causative agent of a disease**. In addition to anthrax, Koch identified the causative agent of tuberculosis (*Mycobacterium tuberculosis*).

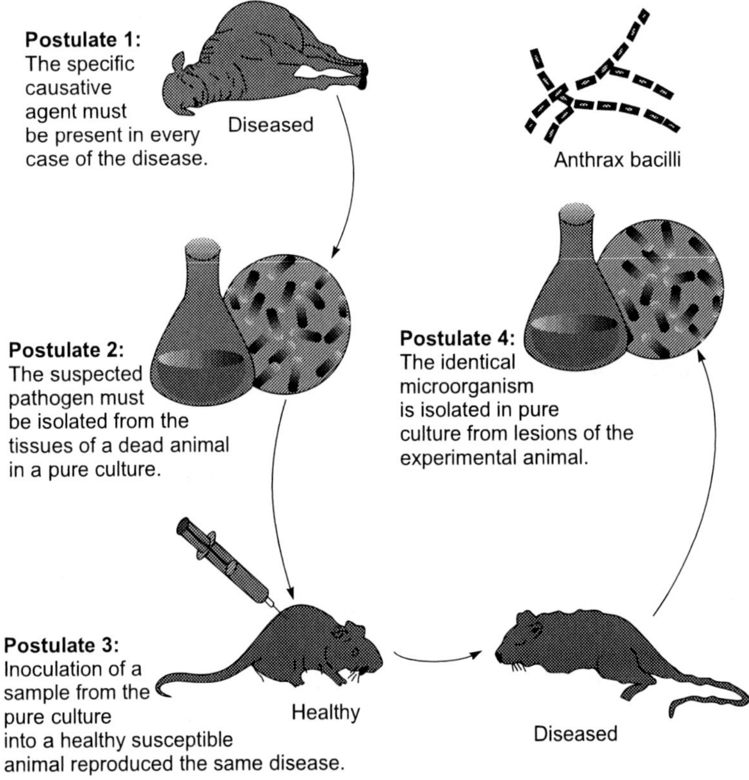

Fig. 2.3 Koch's postulates with their demonstration.

In addition to the development of sterilization, aseptic techniques, the germ theory of disease and the Koch's postulates, causative agents of several infectious diseases were identified during the golden age of microbiology, leading to the ability to halt epidemics by interrupting the spread of germs.

Despite the advances in microbiology, it was rarely possible to render life-saving therapy to an infected patient. Then, after World War II, the **antibiotics** (penicillin, the first antibiotic from the mold *Penicillium notatum* by Alexander Fleming) were introduced to medicine. The incidence of tuberculosis, pneumonia, meningitis, syphilis, and many other infectious diseases declined with the use of antibiotics.

Microbiology, being an active research field, it is impossible to present a complete history of notable contributions made by various scientists/workers in different areas of microbiology, hence are listed here in Table 2.1.

Table 2.1 Landmark discoveries in microbiology that occurred between 1665 and 1997

Year	Investigator	Landmark discovery
1665	Hooke	First observation of cells
1673	van Leeuwenhoek	First observation of live microorganisms
1735	Linnaeus	Binomial nomenclature for organisms
1798	Jenner	First vaccine
1835	Bassi	Silkworm fungus
1840	Semmelweis	Childbirth fever
1853	de Bary	Fungal plant disease
1857	Pasteur	Fermentation
1861	Pasteur	Proved that life did not arise spontaneously from nonliving matter
1864	Pasteur	Pasteurization
1867	Lister	Aseptic surgery
1876	Koch	Germ theory of disease
1879	Neisser	*Neisseria gonorrhoeae*
1881	Koch	Pure cultures
1881	Finley	Yellow fever
1882	Koch	*Mycobacterium tuberculosis*

Contd.

Table 2.1 Contd.

1882	Hesse	Agar (solid) media
1883	Koch	*Vibrio cholerae*
1884	Metchnikoff	Phagocytosis
1884	Gram	Gram-staining procedure
1884	Escherich	*Escherichia coli*
1887	Petri	Petri dish
1889	Kitasato	*Clostridium tetani*
1890	von Bering	Diphtheria antitoxin
1890	Ehrlich	Theory of immunity
1892	Winogradsky	Sulphur cycle
1898	Shiga	*Shigella dysenteriae*
1908	Ehrlich	Syphilis
1910	Chagas	*Trypanosoma cruzi*
1911	Rous	Tumour-causing virus (1966 Nobel Prize)
1929	Fleming	Penicillin
1929	Griffith	Transformation in bacteria
1934	Lancefield	Streptococcal antigens
1935	Stanley, Northrup, Summer	Crystallized virus
1941	Beadle and Tatum	Relationship between genes and enzymes
1943	Delbruck and Luria	Viral infection of bacteria
1944	Avery, MacLeod, McCarty	DNA as the genetic material
1944	Waksman, Schatz	Streptomycin
1946	Lederberg and Tatum	Bacterial conjugation
1953	Watson and Crick	DNA structure
1957	Jacob and Monod	Protein synthesis regulation

Contd.

Table 2.1 Contd.

1959	Stewart	Viral cause of human cancer
1962	Edelman and Porter	Antibodies
1964	Epstein, Achong, Barr	Epstein-Barr virus as cause of human cancer
1971	Nathans, Smith, Arber	Restriction enzymes (used for recombinant DNA technology)
1972	Berg	Genetic engineering
1975	Dulbecco, Temin, Baltimore	Reverse transcriptase
1978	Woese	Archaea
1978	Mitchell	Chemiosmotic mechanism
1981	Margulis	Origin of eukaryotic cells
1982	Klug	Structure of tobacco mosaic virus
1983	McClintock	Transposons
1988	Deisenheter, Huber, Michel	Bacterial photosynthesis pigments
1994	Cano	Reported to have cultured 40-million-year-old bacteria
1997	Prusiner	Prions

EMINENT MICROBIOLOGISTS WITH THEIR NOTABLE CONTRIBUTIONS

Antonie van Leeuwenhoek: Father of Microbiology

- Leeuwenhoek (24 October 1632–26 August 1723: aged 90 years) was a Dutch businessman and scientist of Delft, Holland (currently Netherlands).
- He did pioneering work in microscopy and discovered microorganisms (called animalcules) from diverse habitats in 1676.
- He was also the first person to describe spermatozoa, red blood cells and blood flow in capillaries in 1677.

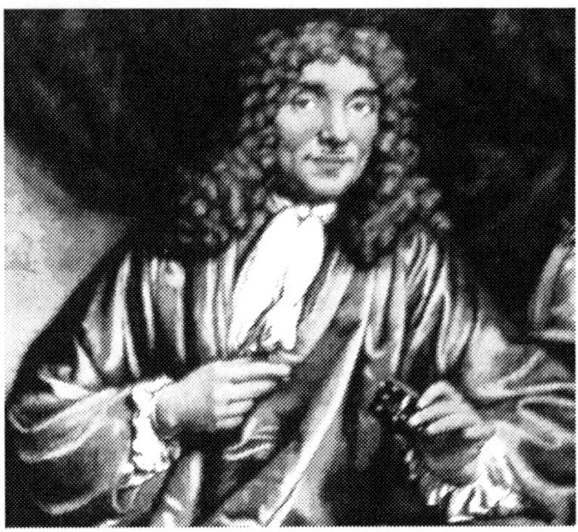

Fig. 2.4 Antonie van Leeuwenhoek.

Edward Jenner: Father of Modern Vaccination or Immunology

- Jenner (17 May 1749–26 January 1823: aged 73 years) was an English physician of Berkeley, England.
- He described the protective effectiveness of cowpox against smallpox on May 14, 1796.
- Jenner postulated that the pus in the blisters that milkmaids recovered from cowpox (a disease similar to smallpox, but much less virulent) protected them from smallpox.
- He pioneered the world's first vaccine: the smallpox vaccine in 1798.
- The terms vaccine and vaccination were devised by Jenner.
- He was the first person to describe the brood parasitism of cuckoo bird (known for laying their eggs in the nests of other birds).

Louis Pasteur: Father of Modern Microbiology

- Louis Pasteur (27 December 1822-28 September 1895: aged 72 years) was a French chemist and microbiologist of Dole, France and is regarded as one of the three main founders of bacteriology.
- Pasteur in 1861 disproved the doctorine of spontaneous generation of organisms by his famous **swan-neck flasks** (so on because of their S-shaped flasks resembling a swan's neck).
- He, in 1857, showed living organisms (yeasts) are involved in the fermentation process.

- The first person to report the existence of anaerobic organisms (yeasts) in 1857.
- He in 1857 reported that the fermentation process could be inhibited (arrested) by passing air (O_2) through the fermenting fluid, the process is called **Pasteur effect**.
- He in 1858 showed microbial growth was responsible for spoiling beverages (e.g., beer, wine and milk).
- He invented **pasteurization** in 1862 to kill harmful microorganisms by heating between 60°C and 100°C.
- He in 1865 reported that parasitic microbes are the cause of silkworms and saving the French silk industry through a method of prevention of contamination of healthy silkworm eggs.
- Pasteur developed vaccines for *anthrax* in 1881 and *rabies* (hydrophobia) in 1885.
- He demonstrated the relationship between germ and disease, and diseases are caused by microorganisms.
- He is regarded as one of the **Fathers of the Germ Theory of Disease** as well as the Father of Modern Microbiology.

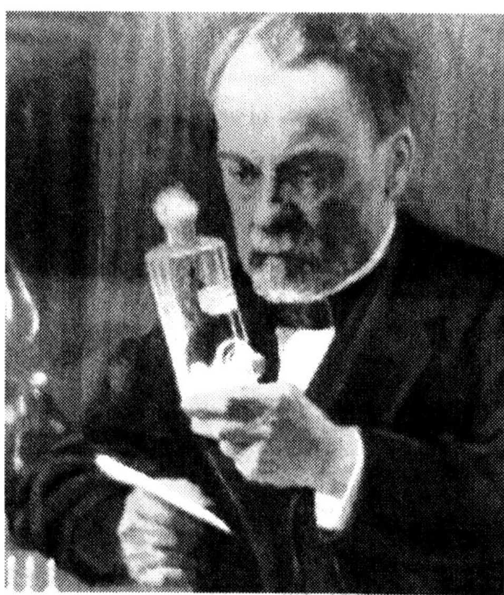

Fig. 2.5 Louis Pasteur.

Joseph Lister: Father of Modern Surgery

- Joseph Lister (5 April 1827–10 February 1912: aged 84 years) was a famous British surgeon, born at Upton Homes, West Ham, England.

- He was Professor of Surgery at the University of Glasgow and Edinburgh (Scotland) and King's College, London.
- He in 1867 developed a system of antiseptic surgery by using *carbolic acid* (later known as *phenol*) on the skin as an **antiseptic**.
- He also used carbolic acid to sterilize instruments (i.e., a **disinfectant**).
- Lister in 1878 demonstrated the specific cause of **milk souring**.
- He is known as the **Father of Antiseptic (or Modern) Surgery**.

Elie Metchnikoff: Father of Innate (Natural) Immunity

- Elie Metchnikoff (15 May 1845–15 July 1916: aged 71 years) a Nobel Prize winner of 1908, was a Ukrainian (Russian) zoologist born at Ivanovka, Russian umpire.
- He is credited with the discovery of phagocytes (macrophages) that engulf foreign bodies such as bacteria in 1882.
- He coined the term *phagocytosis* (*phage* = to eat and *cyte* = cell) means the eating of cells, i.e., a *cell-mediated immunity*.
- He reported that in human blood, leukocytes carry out *phagocytosis against invading bacteria.*
- He gave cellular (phagocytic) theory of immunity in 1892.
- He notably contributed on increasing human longevity by consuming lactic acid producing bacteria (i.e., **yogurt**). He wrote *"that a man will live to be a hundred if he eats enough yogurts"*.
- He in 1903 coined the term **geronotology** from the Greek *geron* = old man, i.e., the study of the phenomena of aging.
- **Metchnikoff** and **Paul Ehrlich** were jointly awarded the 1908 Nobel Prize in Physiology/Medicine.

Robert Koch: Father of Medical Microbiology

- Robert Koch (11 December 1843–27 May 1910: aged 66 years) a Noble Prize winner of 1905, was a German physician and microbiologist.
- He identified the specific causative agents of anthrax (1876), tuberculosis (1886) and cholera (1883).
- He developed pure culture techniques by isolating bacteria on solid culture media by using gelatin (1881) followed by agar-agar (1882) on the suggestion of **Fanny Hesse**.
- He verified the **Germ theory of disease** in 1883.

- He in 1884 gave **Koch's postulates**: a set of four principles to prove that a specific microbe causes a specific disease.
- He is popularly known as "**Father of Practical Bacteriology**" and "**Father of Medical (clinical) Microbiology**"

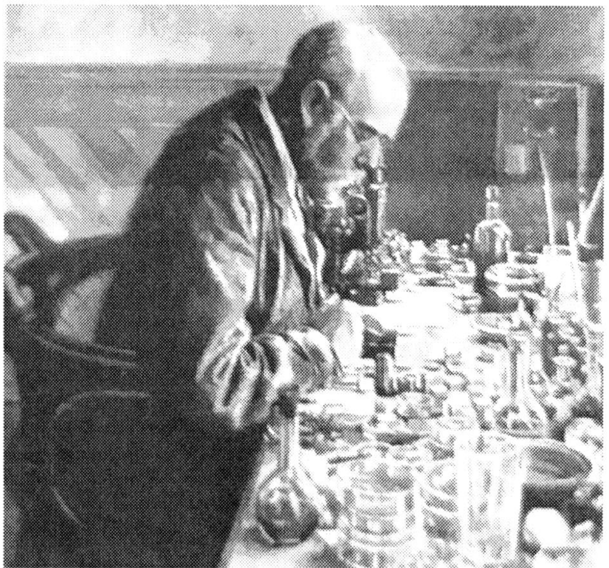

Fig. 2.6 Robert Koch.

Paul Ehrlich: Father of Chemotherapy

- Paul Ehrlich (14 March 1859–20 August 1915: aged 61 years) a Jewish by birth (Noble Prize winner of 1908), was a German Jewish physician.
- He revealed the chemical basis of stains in 1879 and invented the precursor technique to Gram staining.
- Acid fastness mechanism was revealed by him in 1882.
- He gave the **minimum lethal dose** concept.
- Discovery of the first synthetic drug **arsphenamine** (**salvarsan**) to treat syphilis called a magic bullet.
- He pioneered the concept of antimicrobial chemotherapy based on the fact that pathogens could selectively be killed with drugs without harming the host.
- He developed **antiserum** to combat diptheria and conceived a technique for standardizing therapeutic serums.
- He is popularly called the **"Father of Chemotherapy"** and **"Father of Immunochemistry"**.

Alexander Fleming: Discoverer of Penicillin

- Alexander Fleming (6 August 1818–11 March 1955: aged 75 years), a Nobel Prize winner of 1945, was a Scottish doctor who worked at St. Mary's Hospital in London.
- In 1923, Fleming discovered the antibacterial enzyme **lysozyme** from the *nasal secretion* (fluid from nose) that has the power to kill certain bacteria.
- In 1928, he discovered the world's first **antibotic** substance penicillin G (Benzylpenicillin) from the mold *Penicillium notatum*, which was an accidental discovery.
- Fleming shared the Noble Prize in 1945 in Physiology/Medicine with two other scientists **Howard Florey** and **Ernst Boris Chain** for the discovery of penicillin.

KEY POINTS

- **Robert Hooke** was the first person to see the sporulating structures of molds.
- With his simple microscope, **Leeuwenhoek** made detailed descriptions of living organisms, he called them **animalcules**.
- The theory of spontaneous generation or abiogenesis was abandoned for biogenesis by Redi, Spallanzani and Pasteur.
- Early microbiology blossomed with the conceptual developments of sterilization, aseptic techniques, growing of isolated colonies of bacteria (pure culture) on agar media, and the germ theory of disease.
- Germ theory of disease postulated by Pasteur was finally proved by Koch during the golden age of microbiology.
- A microorganism is accepted as the causative agent of a disease if it satisfies the Koch's postulates.

IMPORTANT QUESTIONS

1. Write a brief essay on the history of microbiology or bacteriology.
2. Write short notes on:
   (a) Spontaneous generation.
   (b) Redi's three-jar experiment.
   (c) Koch's postulates.
3. Describe the major contributions of the following scientists to the field of microbiology:
   (a) Antonie van Leeuwenhoek.
   (b) Robert Koch.

(c) Louis Pasteur.
(d) Edward Jenner.
(e) Joseph Lister.
(f) Alexander Fleming.
(g) Elie Metchnikoff.
(h) Paul Ehrlich.

MULTIPLE-CHOICE QUESTIONS

1. Louis Pasteur and Francesco Redi performed experiments disproving the spontaneous generation life theory.

   True or false?

2. Koch's postulates are the four criteria designed to assess whether a microorganism causes a disease is causative relationship between a microbe and a disease. True or false?

3. Spontaneous generation refers to the living cells arising only from other living cells. True or false?

4. Which of the following pioneers is credited with the discovery of microorganism using high quality magnifying lenses (early microscopes)?

   (a) Hooke (b) Koch
   (c) Leeuwenhoek (d) Semmelweis.

5. The purpose of the swan-neck flasks that Louis Pasteur designed to disprove spontaneous generation of life theory is to:

   (a) Pasteurize the meat broth
   (b) Prevent air from entering the flask
   (c) Allow the multiplication of microorganisms in the broth
   (d) Trap the microorganisms and prevent them from reaching the broth.

6. Aseptic technique and sterilization were used by ——— in their experiments to the development of microbiology:

   (a) Leeuwenhoek (b) Koch
   (c) Pasteur (d) All of the above.

7. The techniques of sterilization were introduced by:

   (a) Pasteur (b) Koch
   (c) Needham (d) Redi.

8. Robert Koch subsituted agar in place of gelatin as a solidifying agent in culture media at the suggestion of:

   (a) Loeffler (b) Petri
   (c) Kitasato (d) Hesse.

9. The term microbiology, "as the study of microscopic organisms" was coined by:
   (a) Jenner (b) Leeuwenhoek
   (c) Koch (d) Pasteur.

10. The germ theory of disease states that
   (a) Microorganisms do not cause infectious diseases
   (b) Not all microorganisms are harmful
   (c) Microorganisms that invade other organisms can cause disease in those organisms
   (d) Microorganisms can spontaneously arise in debilitated hosts
   (e) None of the above.

11. Which of the following scientists used carbolic acid (phenol) as an antiseptic and disinfectant and was popularly called the Father of antiseptic surgery?
   (a) Metchnikoff (b) Lister
   (c) Fleming (d) Ehrlich.

12. Which of the following scientists discovered *salvarsan*, the first synthetic drug to treat syphilis?
   (a) Fleming (b) Lister
   (c) Ehrlich (d) Metchnikoff.

ANSWERS TO MCQs

1. True	2. True	3. False	4. (a)	5. (d)
6. (c)	7. (a)	8. (d)	9. (d)	10. (c)
11. (b)	12. (c).			

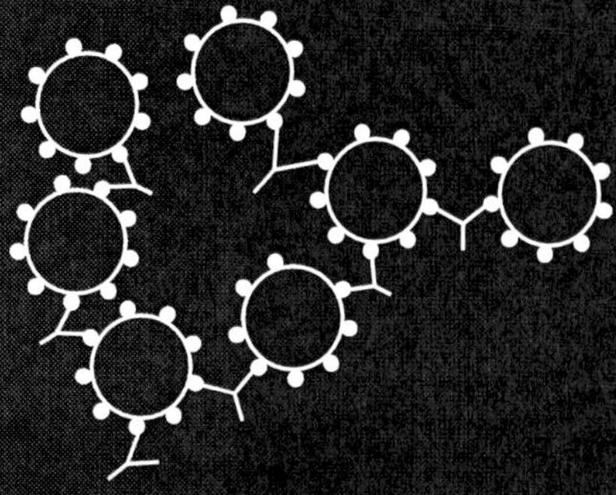

Unit II

GENERAL CHARACTERISTICS OF MICROORGANISMS

- Classification of Microorganisms
- Characteristics of Microorganisms
- Bacterial Morphology
- Structure and Functions of a Bacterial Cell
- Bacterial Motility and Locomotion
- Colonization of Pathogenic Bacteria
- Reproduction and Mode of Genetic Transfer in Bacteria
- Growth and Nutrition of Microorganisms
- Culture Media
- Culture Methods
- Microscope and Microscopy
- Staining and Hanging Drop Mount Techniques
- Bacterial Classification/Taxonomy
- Laboratory Methods for Identification of Bacteria

3

Classification of Microorganisms

The term **microbe** is short for **microorganism**, which means a small organism. Microbes are everywhere—a largely unseen world of living things that support life processes. They are very diverse and represent all the great kingdoms of life. In fact, in terms of numbers most of the diversity of life on the earth is represented by microbes.

CLASSIFICATION AND TAXONOMY

Classification is the grouping of living organisms based on their basic, distinguishing and shared characters.

Taxonomy (derived from Greek *taxis* = means arrangement and *nomos* = means name) is the science dealing with the description, identification, naming and classification of organisms. **Carl Linnaeus**, a *Swedish Botanist regarded as the Father of Taxonomy*, developed the system of *binomial nomenclature*, a two-name system for each living organism: the Genus name and the species name. These names are all written in Latin (italics), as *Escherichia coli*. Each species assigned to a genus is kept at a lower level of hierarchy of ranks (family, order, class, division/phylum, kingdom and domain). In simple words, rank-based classification of organisms is called *taxonomy*.

CLASSIFICATION OF MICROORGANISMS

Microbes are grouped or classified in various ways. Based on the cell type, microorganisms are categorized into three types: Eukaryotic microorganisms, prokaryotic microorganisms, and noncellular microorganisms (Fig. 3.1)

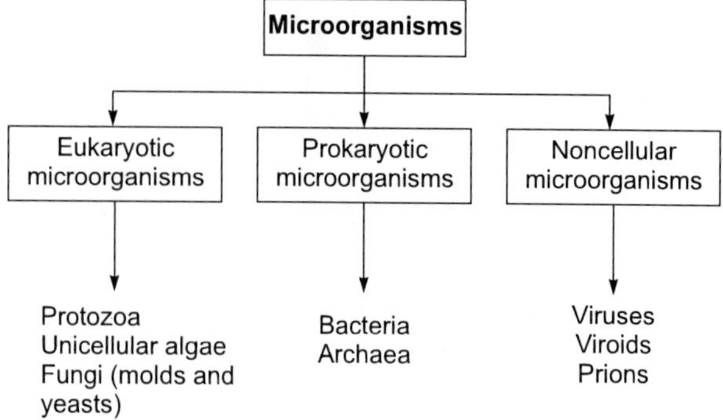

Fig. 3.1 Three categories of microorganisms with their examples.

A. Eukaryotic Microorganisms

Eukaryotic (Gr. *eu* = true + *karyon* = nucleus) *microorganisms* have a well-defined nucleus whose genomic DNA is contained in a nucleus surrounded by a membrane (i.e., membrane-enclosed organelle). Their cell structure is similar to those of humans and other animals. They are self-sufficient and capable of leading independent lives. Examples include:

- **Fungi:** Molds, yeasts and mushrooms
- **Protozoa:** *Plasmodium, Giardia*
- **Unicellular algae:** *Chlamydomonas*

B. Prokaryotic Microorganisms

Prokaryotic (Gr. *pro* = before, primitive + *karyon* = nucleus) *microorganisms* lack a defined nucleus and membrane-enclosed organelles. Examples include:

- **Bacteria:** *Escherichia coli, Mycobacterium tuberculosis, Spirullina.*
- **Archaea:** Methanogens, extreme halophiles.

C. Noncellular Microorganisms

Noncellular (also called *acellular*) *microorganisms* are without any cell forms. Examples include:

- **Viruses:** Poliovirus, HIV, Hepatitis virus.
- **Viroids:** Potato spindle tuberviroid.
- **Prions:** Creutzfeldt Jacob disease (CJD), mad - cow disease.

A summary of features distinguishing prokaryotes and eukaryotes are shown in Table 3.1 and Fig. 3.2.

Table 3.1 Differences of cell organization in prokaryotic and eukaryotic organisms

	Prokaryotes	Eukaryotes
1.	Cell wall is non-cellulosic made of peptidoglycan (murein)	Cell wall is cellulosic in plants and chitinous in fungi
2.	DNA is naked	DNA is combined with proteins
3.	Division is by amitosis	Division is by mitosis or meiosis
4.	Nuclear envelope is not present	Nuclear envelope is present
5.	Lack a nucleus and other membrane-enclosed organelles	Nucleus and other membrane-bound organelles are present
6.	Single chromosome present	Multiple chromosomes present
7.	70S ribosomes present (S-Svedberg unit)	80S ribosomes present
8.	Chloroplast absent	Chloroplast present
9.	Nucleolus is missing	Nucleolus is present
10.	Locomotor organ is flagellum	Locomotor organs are cilia and flagella
11.	Endoplasmic reticulum is absent	Endoplasmic reticulum is present
12.	Golgi apparatus is absent	Golgi apparatus is present
13.	Pili are present	Pili are absent
14.	Guanine: Cytosine ratio is 28 to 33	Guanine: Cytosine ratio is 40
15.	Examples include bacteria, archaea	Examples include algae, fungi, protozoa, plants and animals

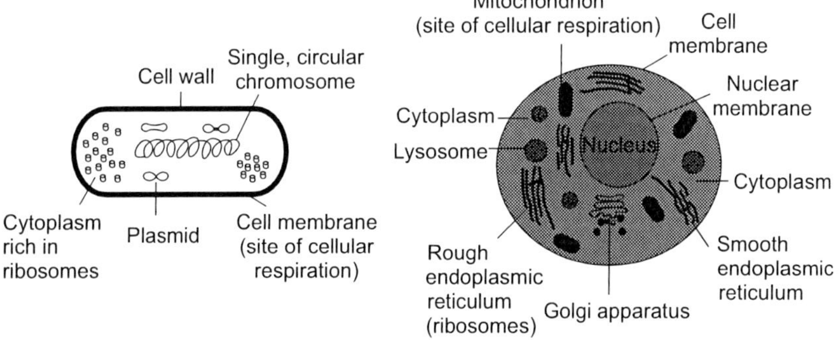

Fig. 3.2 Diagrammatic representation of the structure of prokaryote (bacterium) (A) and eukaryote (animal) (B) cells.

CLASSIFICATION OF MICROORGANISMS ACCORDING TO WHITTAKER

According to **five-kingdom system** proposed in 1969 by **Robert Harding Whittaker**, an American plant ecologist, the cellular microorganisms are classified into 3 kingdoms:

Kingdom	Characteristics	Examples
• Monera (Prokaroytae)	Prokaryotic unicellular organisms, nutrition mode variable	Eubacteria, Archaebacteria
• Fungi	Eukaryotic heterotrophic with absorptive mode of nutrition	Molds, yeasts, mushrooms, rusts, smuts
• Protista	Eukaryotic, heterotrophic, a few autotrophic	Protozoans, slime molds, some algae

WOESE'S THREE-DOMAIN CLASSIFICATION

Carl Woese, an American molecular biologist, in 1978 proposed the currently accepted three-domain classification system of life (i.e., all cellular living organisms). This classification is based on the sequences of nucleotides in ribosomal RNA (molecular level), that categorizes all living organisms into three **domains** (rank above the level of a kingdom, i.e., superkingdom):

Domain	Characteristics	Examples
• *Bacteria*	Unicellular prokaryotes with peptidoglycan in their cell walls	Eubacteria (= true bacteria)
• *Archaea*	Unicellular prokaryotes without peptidoglycan in their cell walls	Achaebacteria (= archaea)
• *Eukarya*	Unicellular and multicellular eukaryotes	Algae, fungi, protozoa, plants and animals

KEY POINTS

- **Classification** is the grouping of living organisms based on their basic, distinguishing shared characteristics.
- Naming of an organism by two names is called **binomial nomenclature**, a classification system devised by Linnaeus, a Swedish botanist.
- Based on the cell type, microbes are classed as **prokaryotic**, **eukaryotic** and **acellular organisms**.

- **Three-domain classification** of living organisms is based on sequences of nucleotides in ribosomal RNA (rRNA), a system devised by Carl Woese.
- **Domain** is a rank above the level of a kingdom (i.e., super-kingdom).

IMPORTANT QUESTIONS

1. Describe briefly:
   (a) An account of classification of microorganisms.
   (b) Differences between prokaryotes and eukaryotes.
   (c) Carl Woese's three-domain classification.
   (d) Categories of microorganisms based on the nature of cell.

MULTIPLE-CHOICE QUESTIONS

1. Which of the following organisms is not considered a microorganism?
   (a) Mushroom (b) Algae
   (c) Protozoa (d) Bacterium.
2. The science involved in the classification of organisms is:
   (a) Scientology (b) Taxonomy
   (c) Classificology (d) Microbiology.
3. Using binomial nomenclature, the first name designates the genus while the second name designates the:
   (a) Order (b) Family
   (c) Specific epithet (d) Variety.
4. Which of the following is/are prokaryotic organisms?
   (a) Bacteria (b) Archaea
   (c) Protists (d) Both (a) and (b).
5. Which of the following is/are acellular organisms?
   (a) Bacteria
   (b) Prions
   (c) Viruses
   (d) Both (b) and (c)
   (e) All of the above.
6. A prominent difference between prokaryotic and eukaryotic cell is the:
   (a) Lack of pigmentation in eukaryotes
   (b) Presence of a nucleus in eukaryotes

(c) Larger size of prokaryotes
(d) Presence of a cell wall in prokaryotes.

7. All are eukaryotic microorganisms EXCEPT:
(a) Mushrooms (b) Protozoans
(c) Archaea (d) Algae.

8. Five-kingdom system of classification of living organisms was proposed by:
(a) Carl Woese (b) Linnaeus
(c) Whittaker (d) Ainsworth.

ANSWERS TO MCQs

1. (a) 2. (b) 3. (c) 4. (d) 5. (d)
6. (b) 7. (c) 8. (c).

4

Characteristics of Microorganisms

Microorganisms or **microbes** (derived from Greek words: *mikros* = small + *bios* = life) are microscopic organisms that cannot be seen with the naked eye and exist as unicellular, multicellular or cell clusters. These are a largely unseen world of living things that occur everywhere supporting life processes on this beautiful planet – the earth. They range in size from ultramicroscopic viruses 20 nm diameter to large protozoans 50 μm or more in diameter. The large microbes are as much as 2,50,000 times the size of the smallest ones (Table 4.1). Single-celled microorganisms were the first forms of life to develop on the earth approximately 3-4 billion years ago.

Organisms that cause infectious diseases can be grouped into seven major categories: bacteria, fungi, protozoa, viruses, prions (micro organisms), helminths and arthropods (parasites). Knowing characteristics of these organisms is an important part of microbiology and essential for diagnosis, treatment and control of infectious diseases.

Health scientists and workers are concerned with just such microbes (bacteria, viruses, fungi, protozoa) and parasites (helminths) and with treating and preventing the diseases they cause. Major features of the infectious agents and the diseases they cause are summarized in Table 4.1.

CHARACTERISTICS OF VARIOUS TYPES OF MICROORGANISMS

BACTERIA

- **Bacteria** (sing: **bacterium**) are single-celled prokaryotes.
- Bacterial cells lack membrane-enclosed organelles (including a nucleus).
- They contain a long, double-stranded circular molecule of DNA, which is not contained within a defined nucleus.
- The DNA is tightly coiled into a region of the cell known as the **nucleoid** (see Fig. 3.1).

Table 4.1 Categories of human pathogens and parasites with their characteristics

Taxonomic category	Size	Propagation site(s)	Example(s)	Disease(s)
Prions	< 20 nm	Intracellular	Prion protein	Creutzfeldt-Jacob disease
Viruses	20-300 nm	Obligate intracellular	Poliovirus	Poliomyelitis
Bacteria	0.2-15 μm	Obligate intracellular Extracellular Facultative intracellular	*Chlamydia trachomatis* *Streptococcus pneumoniae* *Mycobacterium tuberculosis*	Trachoma, urethritis Pneumonia Tuberculosis
Fungi	2-200 μm	Extracellular Facultative intracellular	*Candida albicans* *Histoplasma capsulatum*	Thrush Histoplasmosis
Protozoa	1-50 μm	Extracellular Facultative intracellular Obligate intracellular	*Trypanosoma gambiense* *Trypanosama cruzi* *Leishmania donovani*	Sleeping sickness Chagas disease Kala azar
Helminths	3 mm-10 m	Extracellular Intracellular	*Wuchereia bancrofti* *Trichinella spiralis*	Filariasis Trichinosis

- They possess a rigid cell wall (except *Mycoplasma*) composed of **peptidoglycan** (a carbohydrate and protein complex).
- Many bacteria are motile, using a unique pattern of flagella.
- In bacteria, many of the metabolic functions are carried out by the plasma membrane (that are performed by the membrane-bound organelles in eukaryotes).
- They reproduce by *binary fission*.
- Most bacteria are *heterotrophic* and can utilize a range of substrates aerobically and anaerobically.
- They lack sexual reproduction but *genetic recombination* takes place by *conjugation*, *transformation* and *transduction*.

Examples: *Bacillus anthracis* (cause of anthrax).
Escherichia coli (cause of urinary tract infections).
Mycobacterium tuberculosis (cause of tuberculosis).

ARCHAEA

- **Archaea** (= **Archaebacteria**) (sing: **archaeon**) are single-celled prokaryotes similar to bacteria, (i.e., they lack membrane-bound nucleus and other membrane-bound organelles in their cells).
- They are the oldest organisms living on the earth.
- They are more closely related to eukaryotic cells than they are to bacteria.
- Their cell walls lack peptidoglycan found in bacteria.
- Arechaea membranes have ether bonds connecting fatty acids to molecules of glycerol.
- They have multiple RNA polymerases that contain multiple peptides (more than eight) similar to eukaryotic organisms.
- They are found under extreme environmental conditions and are called **extremophiles**.
- They include thermophiles, extreme halophiles, extreme thermo-acidophiles and methanogens.

Examples: *Pyrobolus fumari* (upper temperature limit for life at 113°C). *Picrophilus* genus is capable of growth at a pH of less than 0.5. *Methanococcus* (methanogen).

FUNGI

- **Fungi** (sing: **fungus**) are **eukaryotes**, but are quite distinct from plants and animals.

- They are single-celled (yeasts) and muticellular organisms which grow as thread-like filaments (hyphae) (Fig. 4.1).
- They have a thick cell wall composed of **chitin** (a biomolecule made up of two units of N-acetyl glucosamine).
- They have a distinct nucleus containing chromosomes surrounded by porous nuclear membrane.
- They lack chlorophyll hence are *heterotrophic* in their mode of nutrition. Some of them may be parasitic, saprophytic or symbiotic.
- The reserve food material in fungi is **glycogen**. Starch is absent.
- They obtain nutrients solely by **absorption** by releasing the enzymes into their surroundings, breaking the complex molecules into simple ones outside the cell (i.e., **extracellularly**).
- Reproduction takes place by formation of asexual spores (zoospores, sporangiospores, conidia) and sexual spores (ascospores, basidiospores, zygospores).

Examples: Molds (*Aspergillus, Penicillium, Mucor, Rhizopus, Histoplasma, Trichophyton*)
Yeasts (*Saccharomyces, Candida, Cryptococcus*)
Mushrooms (*Agaricus, Amanita, Morchella*)
Rusts (*Puccinia*).

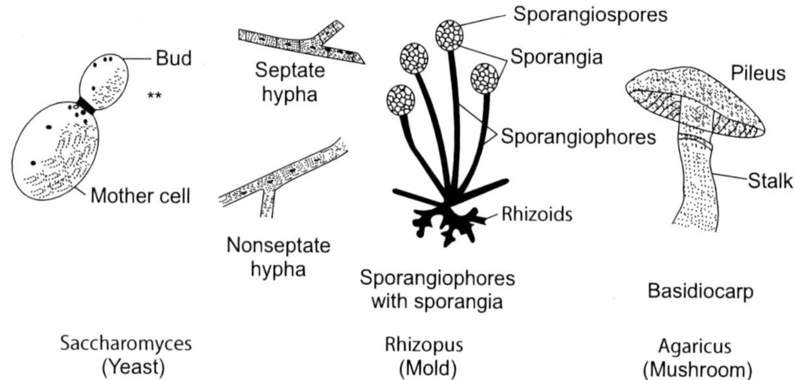

Fig. 4.1 Fungi: Morphological types in yeasts, molds and mushrooms.

ALGAE

- **Algae** (sing: **alga**) (Fig. 4.2) are eukaryotic, *thalloid organisms* that have no roots, stems or leaves.
- They have cholorophyll and other pigments to carry out photosynthesis, hence are ***autotrophic*** like plants.

- These are aquatic occurring either as unicellular or multicellular organisms.
- Population of free-floating unicellualr algae occurs in water as *phytoplankton.*
- Algae reproduce both by asexual and sexual means.
- Asexual reproduction takes place by fragmentation (colonial and filamentous algae), spore formation (as in fungi) and by binary fission (as in bacteria).
- Sexual reproduction occurs through the formation of differentiated sex cells.
- Life cycle of algae shows *alternation of generations*:

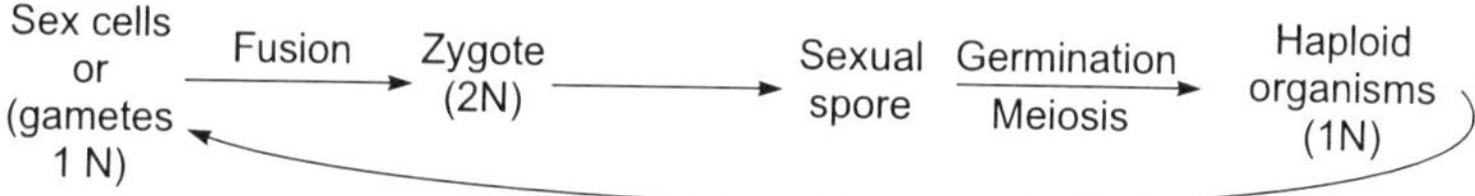

- Algae occur in water, moist soil, on the surface of moist rocks and wood. Some algae live in symbiotic association with fungi called **lichens**.

Examples: *Chlamydomonas, Volvox, Vaucheria.*

Prototheca, a green alga, causes **protothecosis,** a disease in dogs, cats or cattle (*Prototheca wickerhamii,* and P. *zopfii*) and humans (*P. wickerhamii*).

Cephaloeuros viriscens causes **red rust** and systemic disease in tea, coffee, mango, guava and citrus (except lime and lemon).

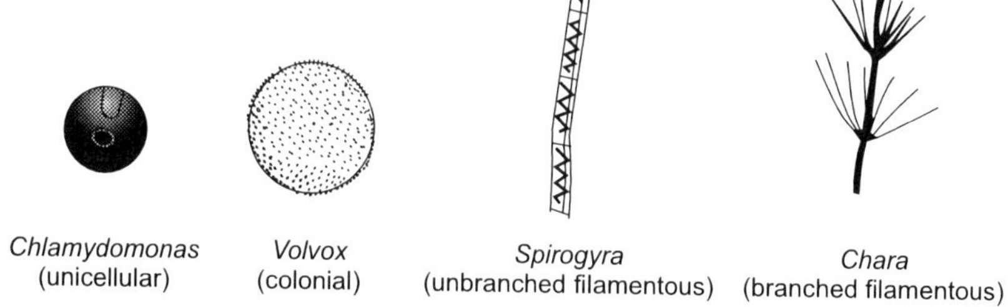

Fig. 4.2 Algal morphology. Flagellated unicellular (*Chlamydomonas*) and colonial (*Volvox*) algae. Multicellular filamentous–unbranched (*Spirogyra*) and branched (*Chara*) algae.

PROTOZOA

- **Protozoa** (sing: **protozoan**) (Greek for *first animals*) are single-celled, eukaryotic microscopic organisms (5 μm – 1 mm length/diameter).
- They are animal-like.
- They do not have cell wall, some, however, possess a flexible layer, called *pellicle*.
- They have the ability to move by pseudopodia, flagella or cilia.
- The have heterotrophic mode of nutrition, wherby the free-living forms ingest particulates (e.g., bacteria, yeasts, algae) while the parasitic forms derive nutrients from the body fluids of their hosts.
- They reproduce primarily by asexual means (such as fission, budding, schizogamy) and sexual means (by conjugation).
- During their life cycle, protozoa have a trophozoite (feeding stage), some form cysts during adverse conditions.
- Protozoa are found in water, soil, and as normal microbiota of animals.
- They are classified into four groups based on their mode of locomotion: Flagellates or Mastigophora (flagella), Sarcodina (pseudopodia), Ciliophora (cilia) and Sporozoa (lack motility) (Fig. 4.3).

Examples: *Amoeba, Paramecium*

Plasmodium spp. cause malaria in humans.

Entamoeba histolytia causes amebic dysentery in humans

Giardia lamblia causes giardiasis.

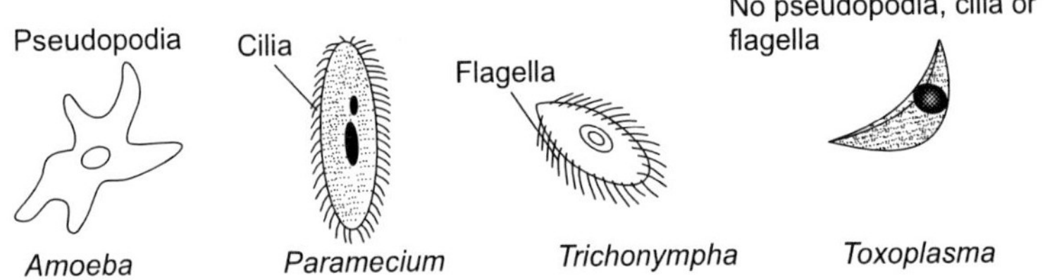

Fig. 4.3 Representative protozoan genera of four groups.

VIRUSES

- **Viruses** (Latin *virus* = poison or venum) (Fig. 4.4) are acellular and ultramicroscopic entities.
- They are neither prokaryotic nor eukaryotic.

- They are composed of a nucleic acid and a few proteins (i.e., **nucleoproteins**).
- The genetic material of a virus is either DNA or RNA, never both.
- They contain a protein coat called the **capsid**.
- The complete unit of nucleic acid and capsid is called **nucleocapsid**.
- They are obligate intracellular parasites of different hosts—bacteria (bacteriophages), protozoa, fungi, algae, plants and animals.
- They do not respire, do not metabolize, as they do not grow but do reproduce by using the cellular machinery of their hosts.
- Some viruses have **glycoprotein spikes**, called **peplomers**, which help them to attach to the host cell receptors.
- They are filterable and can be crystallized and stored in a container on a shelf for years, without losing the ability to invade their host.

Examples: Human immunodeficiency virus (HIV) that causes AIDS or HIV disease.
Poliovirus causes poliomyelitis (polio).
Smallpox virus causes smallpox.
Tobacco mosaic virus (TMV) causes leaf mosaic of tobacco.

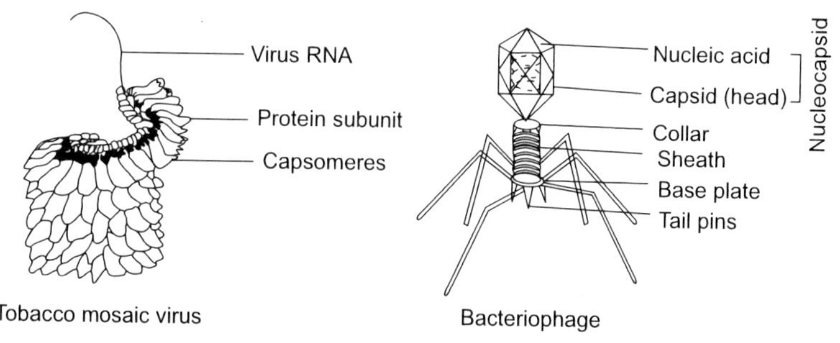

Fig. 4.4 Viruses. Tobacco mosaic virus (TMV), single-stranded RNA virus with a helical symmetry. Bacteriophages, viruses infecting prokaryotes (bacteria and archaea) having DNA as the genetic material.

VIROIDS

- **Viroids** are acellular ultramicroscopic infectious agents, solely composed of a small circular strand of single-stranded RNA, and cause diseases of plants.

- They do not have protein coating.
- They are composed solely of RNA.
- They are endowed with autonomous replication and evolution.
- They use host enzymes for nucleic acid synthesis.
- Some viroids are **ribozymes**, having catalytic properties.
- Hepatitis D virus (HDV) , a human pathogen, is a defective RNA virus similar to a viroid.
- Viroids are known to cause diseases of plants solely.

Examples: *Potato spindle tuber viroid* (PSTVd) causes potato spindle tuber disease.

PRIONS

- **Prions** are ultramicroscopic proteinaceous infectious particles (< 100 nm).
- They are host-derived proteins and lack a nucleic acid genome.
- Their protein can fold in multiple, structurally abstract ways.
- Prions may propagate by transmitting their misfolded protein state.
- They cause neurodegenerative diseases of humans and other animals characterized by microscopic holes in tissues leading to a "spongy" architecture in grain.
- They are extremely resistant to all the conventional forms of disinfection processes but can be inactivated by autoclaving at 134°C for 18 minutes.
- They are transmitted by ingestion of contaminated tissues (meat), but can occur via medical procedures.

Examples:

- Creutzfeldt - Jacob disease (CJD) of humans.
- Kuru of humans.
- Scrapie of sheep.
- Bovine spongiform encephalopathy (BSE), or mad cow disease of cattle.

HELMINTHS

- **Helminths** (Gr. *helmins* = an intestinal worm) are commonly called **parasitic worms**.

- These are large multicellular eukaryotic organisms (centimetres to metres in length) which can generally be seen with the naked eye when they are mature.
- They either live as parasites or free of a host in water and soil.
- Helminths include members of the following taxa. **cestodes** (tapeworms), **nematodes** (roundworms), **trematodes** (flukes) and **monogeneans**.
- They lack or have reduced means of locomotion because they are transmitted from one host to another.
- The helminths do not replicate within the body unlike pathogens (e.g., bacteria, viruses, fungi).
- All helminths produce eggs (also called ova) as a result of sexual reproduction which are released in faeces and act as the infective stage for causing the disease called **helminthiasis**.
- Helminths are either **hermaphrodites** (i.e., have both sexes ♂ and ♀) (e.g., tapeworms) or have their sexes differentiated (e.g., roundworms).
- Many parasitic helminths do not have a digestive system and instead absorb nutrients from the body fluids and tissues of their host.
- Helminth eggs (or ova) are a good **indicator organisms** to assess the safety of sanitation and reuse systems because they are the most environmentally resistant pathogens of all pathogens (viruses, bacteria and protozoa).
- The study of parasitic worms and their effects on their hosts is called **helminthology**.

Examples:
- *Ascaris lumbricoides* (giant roundworm) causes **ascariasis**.
- *Taenia solium* (pork tapeworm) causes **taeniasis**.
- *Schistosoma* spp. (blood flukes or schistosomes) cause **schistosomiasis**.

ARTHROPODS

- **Arthropods** (*arthros* = joint + *podos* = foot) are jointed legged animals that cause human diseases either directly or as vectors of pathogens.
- They are characterized by segmented bodies, hard chitinous exoskeleton, and jointed legs.
- They are found in all environments in fresh and salt water, and as parasites of animals and plants.

- They cause human diseases directly by their feeding on blood or body tissues (e.g., insects, ticks, mites, mosquitoes) and indirectly transmitting other infections, particularly viruses, bacteria and protozoa.
- Arthropods are not microbes themselves but can transmit microbial diseases, hence called **vectors**.
- The study of parasites (helminths and arthropods) is called **parasitology**.

Examples: Arthropod bite infections: tick paralysis scabies (sarcoptic mange), flea bites, pediculosis, chigger dermatitis, and myiasis.

Arthrod vectors: Dengue fever, yellow fever (by mosquitoes), plague (fleas), lyme disease (hard ticks), spotted fever (ticks), epidemic typhus (ticks, lice)

KEY POINTS

- **Microorganisms** are microscopic organisms that cannot be seen with naked eye.
- Organisms that cause infectious diseases can be grouped into seven major categories: prions, viruses, bacteria, fungi, protozoa, helminths and arthropods.
- Identification of pathogenic organisms is essential for correct diagnosis, treatment and control of infectious diseases.
- **Bacteria** are prokaryotes, their DNA (chromosome) is not contained within a nucleus and there are relatively few cytoplasmic organelles.
- **Viruses** are acellular particles also called **"virions"** made up of a nucleic acid (DNA or RNA) and proteins, called **nucleic proteins**.
- **Fungi** are achlorophyllous, heterotropic eukaryotes, have a thick *chitin* containing cell wall, and grow as filaments called hyphae or single-celled yeasts.
- **Protozoa** are single-celled animals, 2-100 µm, occurring both as free-living organisms and as parasites. Both can cause diseases in humans by infecting body tissues and organs.
- **Prions** are unusual proteinaceous infectious particles lacking a nucleic acid genome, cause diseases characterized by changes in the brain (spongiform encephalopathies) and motor disturbances.

- **Helminths** are multicellular worms (animals) that often parasitize gastrointestinal tract, majority of them do not replicate within the host.
- **Arthropods** are jointed legged parasites that cause human diseases either directly or as vectors of pathogens.
- **Viroids** are acellular organisms composed of RNA and cause diseases in plants only.
- **Algae** are chlorophyllous eukaryotic thalloid organisms.

IMPORTANT QUESTIONS

1. What are microorganisms? Give diagnostic features of bacteria. Name any two major human bacterial diseases with their causative agents.
2. Differentiate between:
   (a) Bacteria and viruses
   (b) Bacteria and fungi
   (c) Viruses and prions.
3. Describe the major differentiating features among viruses, viroids and prions.
4. What are the unique features of helminths.

MULTIPLE-CHOICE QUESTIONS

1. All are prokaryotic organisms EXCEPT:
   (a) Viruses (b) Bacteria
   (c) Archaea (d) All of the above.
2. All are eukaryotes EXCEPT:
   (a) Fungi
   (b) Algae
   (c) Protozoa
   (d) Blue green algae (cyanobacteria).
3. All are noncellular organisms EXCEPT:
   (a) Prions (b) Yeasts
   (c) Viroids (d) Viruses.
4. Parasitology is the study related to:
   (a) Pathogens (b) Bacteria and viruses
   (c) Nematodes (d) All of the above.

5. Which of the following is not associated with bacteria?
   (a) Cell wall composed of peptidoglycan
   (b) Prokaryotic organism
   (c) Flagella for motility
   (d) Presence of membrane-enclosed intracellular structures.
6. Which of the following is *not* associated with fungi?
   (a) Cellulosic cell wall
   (b) Heterotrophic
   (c) Membrane-bound organelles
   (d) Body composed of thread-like hyphae.
7. All of the following are true for viruses EXCEPT:
   (a) Are acellular
   (b) Obligate intracellular parasites
   (c) Only DNA as the genetic material
   (d) Virus particle is called a virion.
8. Prions are the infectious particles made up of:
   (a) DNA (b) RNA
   (c) Protein (d) All of the above.
9. All of the following belong to helminths EXCEPT:
   (a) *Shistosoma* (b) *Ascaris*
   (c) *Trypanosoma* (d) *Trichinella*.
10. All of the following are arthropod bite infections EXCEPT:
   (a) Tick paralysis (b) Scabies
   (c) Chigger dermatitis (d) Dengue fever.
11. All of the following are true for viroids EXCEPT:
   (a) Composed of DNA (b) Are acellular
   (c) Some are ribozymes (d) Cause diseases of plants.

ANSWERS TO MCQs

1. (a) 2. (d) 3. (b) 4. (c) 5. (d)
6. (a) 7. (c) 8. (c) 9. (c) 10. (d)
11. (a).

5
Bacterial Morphology

Bacteria (sing: **bacterium**) are **prokaryotes** (from the Greek meaning prenucleus) that lack membrane-enclosed organelles and a nucleus. Their DNA is usually a single circularly arranged chromosome not surrounded by a membrane, cell wall contains the polysaccharide peptidoglycan, and usually divide by binary fission (asexual mode of reproduction).

BACTERIAL MORPHOLOGY

Bacterial morphology deals with the size, shape and arrangement of bacterial cells. The shape of a bacterium is determined by heredity. Genetically, most bacteria are **monomorphic** (i.e., of single shape), however, shape is altered by environmental factors.

Genetically, a few bacteria are **pleomorphic** (i.e., have many shapes). *Rhizobium* and *Corynebacterium* are the common examples.

Bacterial cell morphology, especially shape and arrangenemts are key means for describing bacteria.

SIZE OF BACTERIA

Bacteria are microscopic organisms that range in size from those just barely visible with light microscopy (0.2 μm) to those measuring a thousand times that size.

Size of cocci ranges from 0.5 – 3.0 μm in diameter, bacilli ranges from 0.5 – 20 μm in length and 0.2 – 2.0 μm in width; vibrio and spirilla ranges from 0.5 – 100 μm in length and 0.2 – 2.0 μm in width; and spirochetes vary from 0.5 – 250 μm in length and 0.1 to 3.0 μm in width. Dimensions of interesting bacteria:

- *Escherichia coli*, a common rod-shaped bacterium (bacillus) is 2 – 6 μm (length) × 1.1 – 1.5 μm (width).
- *Mycoplasma galliceptium*, a wall-less bacterium, 200–300 nm (0.2 – 0.3 μm) is the **world's smallest bacterium**.
- *Thiomargarita namibiensis*, 100–300 μm (sometimes 750 μm), is the **world's largest bacterium**.

Bacteria are measured using a calibrated ocular micrometre under a compound microscope or using an electron microscope.

The metric unit **micrometre** (1/1,000,000 or 10^{-6} of a metre = 0.001 mm = one-millionth of a metre = 0.000039 inch), commonly called a **micron** (μm) is used to take dimensions of bacteria and other microorganisms.

SHAPES OF BACTERIA

Bacteria exist in three basic shapes: **coccus, bacillus** and **spiral** (Fig. 5.1).

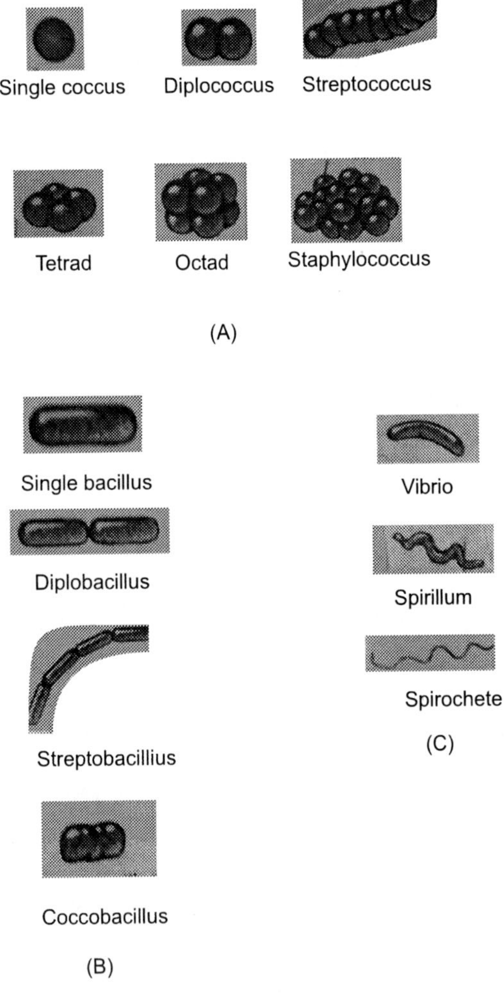

Fig. 5.1 Shapes and arrangements (group patterns) of bacteria. (A) Cocci, (B) Bacilli and (C) Spiral.

1. **Cocci** (sing: **coccus**) (from Gr. *kokkos* meaning berry) are bacterial cells that are spherical, round or oval, and resemble tiny balls. Strep throats which is caused by *Streptocccus* are tiny, spherical cells.
2. **Bacilli** (sing: **bacillus**) (from Latin *baculus* meaning small staff or rod) are bacterial cells that are rod-shaped and resemble a pill. Some bacilli are rounded ends while others have squared ends. *Bacillus anthracis,* the cause of anthrax, is rod-shaped (bacillus).

   "Bacillus" has two meanings in microbiology: bacillus in romans refers to a bacterial shape, and when capatalized and italicized (e.g., *Bacillus*), it refers to a specific genus.

   When a rod is short and plump and looks like a coccus, it is called a **coccobacillus** (plural: **coccobacilli**) (e.g., *Haemophilus influenzae*).
3. **Spiral bacteria** have twisted or helical morphology that resembles little cork screws. These bacteria appear in three forms (Fig. 5.1).
   - **Vibrio** (from Latin *vibrare* meaning to shake) – a curved or comma-shaped rod (e.g., *Vibrio cholerae,* the cause of cholera).
   - **Spirillum** (from Latin *spira* meaning a coil) – a thick, rigid sprial (e.g., *Helicobacter pylori,* the cause of gastritis).
   - **Spirochetes** (from *spira* meaning coil and *chaite* meaining hair) – a thin flexible spiral (e.g., *Treponema pallidum* the cause of syphilis).
4. **Exceptions to the above three basic shapes**

   In addition to three basic shapes, the bacteria are:
   - **Star shaped** (e.g., *Stella*)
   - **Square-shaped** flat cells (e.g., *Haloarcula,* a salt-loving member of *Archaea*).
   - **Triangle-shaped bacteria** (e.g., *Haloarcula gaponica*)
   - ***Y*-shaped bacteria** (e.g., *Pyrodictium abyssi*).

Arrangement (or Group Patterns) of Bacterial Cells

Bacteria reproduce by **asexual binary fission**, that is, each cell splits in half forming new cells. As they increase in number they remain attached to one another forming distinct groups or arrangements. This group pattern which is specific to each bacterium is used an important characteristic in differentiation of bacteria.

Arrangement of Cocci

Division of a coccus takes place in one, two, three or multi planes without breaking, resulting in various arrangements which are termed as:

- **Singly** – Bacteria that appear as single cell, is just called **cocci**.
- **Diplococci (diplococcus)** – These cells are found in pairs and remain attached to each other (e.g., *Streptococcus pneumoniae*).
- **Streptococci** – These cells form chains and remain attached to each other (*Streptococcus pyogenes*).
- **Tetrads** – These cells are found in groups of fours (*Pediococcus*).
- **Sarcinae** – Cocci in packets of 8, 16, 32 or more (*Sarcina ureae*).
- **Staphylococci** – Cocci are arranged irregularly in clusters like grapes (e.g., *Staphylococcus aureus*).

  These group characteristics are frequently helpful in identifying certain cocci.

Arrangement of Bacilli

- **Singly:** Rod-shaped cells that exist in a single cell, called **bacilli** (e.g., *Bacillus cereus*).
- **Diplobacilli:** Two rod-shaped cells attached to each other (e.g., *Coxiella burnetii*).
- **Streptobacilli** – Rod-shaped cells are arranged in long chains (e.g., *Streptobacillus moniliformis*).

KEY POINTS

- The study of size, shape and arrangement of bacterial cells is called **bacterial morphology**.
- Genetically most bacteria are **monomorphic**.
- **Coccus** (spherical), **bacillus** (rod-shaped), and **spiral** (twisted) are the three major basic shapes found in bacteria.
- Bacteria range in size from the smallest rickettsias to the largest spiral forms.

IMPORTANT QUESTIONS

1. Answer in brief:
   (a) What are the three major types of morphology found in bacteria?

(b) Morphological arrangement of cocci with an example of each type.

(c) What is the difference between the terms bacillus and *Bacillus*?

MULTIPLE-CHOICE QUESTIONS

1. One micron (μm) or micrometre, unit of measurement in bacteria, is equal to:

(a) 1×10^{-6} metre
(b) 1×10^{-3} mm
(c) 0.000039 inch
(d) All of the above.

2. Which of the following bacteria is a diplococcus?

(a) *Streptococcus pyogenes*
(b) *Staphyloccus aureus*
(c) *Bacillus cereus*
(d) *Haemophilus influenzae*.

3. A thin flexible spiral-shaped bacterium is called

(a) Vibrio
(b) Spirillum
(c) Spirochete
(d) All of the above.

4. Which of the following terms is used when cocci occur in grape-like clusters?

(a) Sarcinae
(b) Streptococci
(c) Staphylococci
(d) Spirochete.

5. The term used for cocci when occurring in 8 or more in a cluster:

(a) Sarcinae
(b) Streptococci
(c) Staphylococci
(d) None of the above.

ANSWERS TO MCQs

1. (d) 2. (a) 3. (c) 4. (c) 5. (a).

6

Structure and Functions of a Bacterial Cell

STRUCTURE OF A BACTERIAL CELL

Bacteria are prokaryotic unicellular microorganisms. A bacterial cell lacks all membrane-enclosed organelles such as mitochondria, chloroplast, golgi, lysosome, peroxisome, glyoxysome, endoplasmic reticulum and true vauole. Bacteria are also devoid of membrane-bound nucleus and nucleolus.

CELLULAR ORGANIZATION OF BACTERIA

The general cellular organization of a bacterial cell is represented in the form of a flowchart (Fig. 6.1) and diagrammatically (Fig. 6.2).

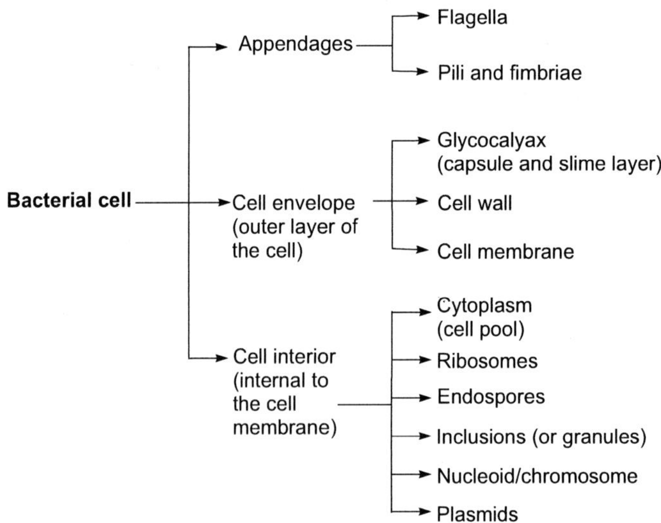

Fig. 6.1 Cellular organization of a bacterial cell.

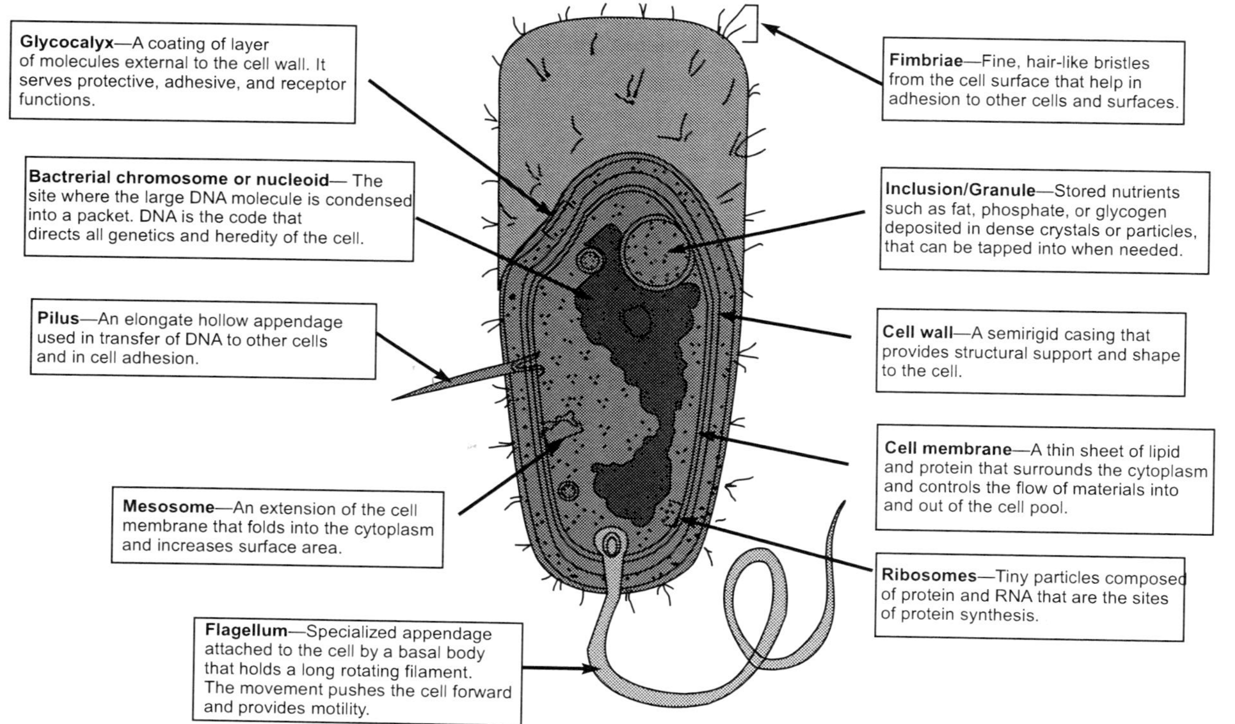

Fig. 6.2 Diagrammatic structure of a generalized bacterial cell. A typical rod-shaped bacterium, showing major external and internal structures with their functions.

GLYCOCALYX

Glycocalyx (sugar coat) is a viscous (sticky) coating or layer external to the cell wall. It is composed of polysaccharide, polypeptide or both. The glycocalyx is called a *capsule* if the coating is firmly attached to the cell wall, and a *slime layer* if it is loosely attached to the cell wall. For capsule visualization, **negative staining** technique is used.

Capsule serves protective function against phagocytosis in several bacterial pathogens (e.g., *Bacillus anthracis, Streptococcus pneumoniae*).

CELL WALL—STRUCTURAL FEATURES

Cell wall is a rigid, murein structure that surrounds the bacterial cell. **Peptidoglycan** (also called *murein*), a polysaccharide, is the major structural component of the cell wall. It is a complex molecule composed of alternating units of two monosaccharides related to glucose: N-acetyl-glucosamine (NAG) and N-acetylmuramic acid (NAM) (from *murus*, meaning wall) cross-linked by short peptides (Fig. 6.3).

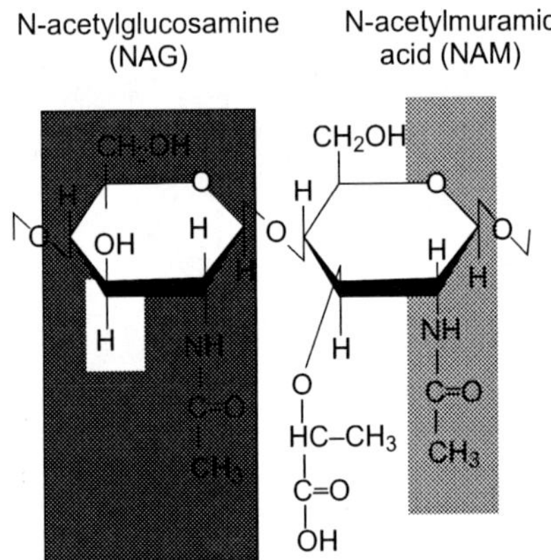

Fig. 6.3 Peptidoglycan molecule. NAG and NAM, the two monosaccharides related to glucose are joined by β-1, 4, linkage.

The major functions of the cell wall are:

- It gives shape, rigidity and support to the cell.
- It prevents the cell against bursting from osmotic pressure (called *lysis*).
- It helps to classify bacteria into two major groups: Gram-positive bacteria and Gram-negative bacteria.

- It offers resistance to harmful effects of environment.
- It contains receptor sites for phages and colicin.

The cell walls of Gram-positive and Gram-negative bacteria (Fig. 6.4) differ in thickness, chemical structure and certain other features as given below:

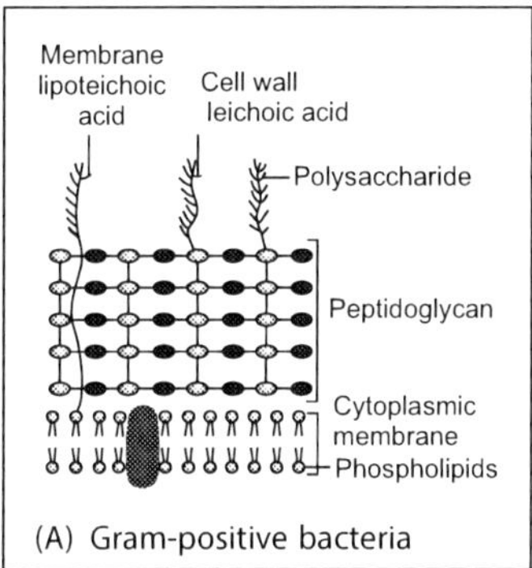

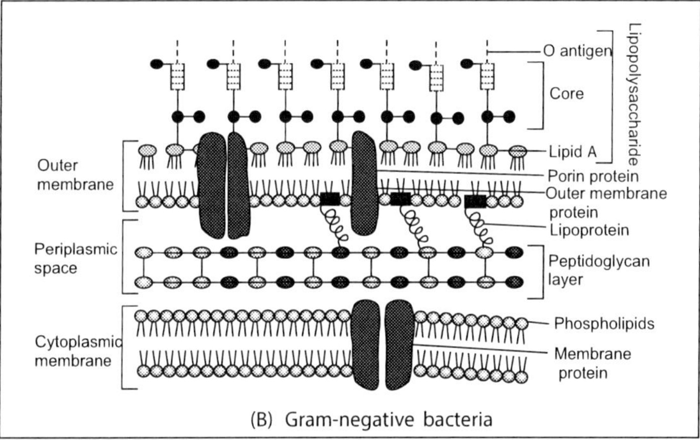

Fig. 6.4 Structure of the cell wall in bacteria both Gram-positive (A) and Gram-negative (B).

1. Gram (+) bacteria have thicker cell walls (20–30 nm), Gram (–) bacteria have thin cell wall (8–10 nm).
2. Gram (+) bacteria have a **thick, multilayered** peptidioglycan layer, Gram (–) bacteria have a **thin, single layer**.
3. Gram (+) have teichoic acids in the cell wall; Gram (–) do not.
4. Gram (+) do not have a periplasmic space; Gram (–) have.
5. Gram (+) do not have porins in their cell walls for nutrient uptake; Gram (–) have porins.
6. Gram (+) have no outer membrane; Gram (–) have this feature.
7. Lipopolysaccharides are high in concentration only in Gram (–) bacteria.

8. Lipid concentration is higher in Gram (–) (15–20%) compared to Gram (+) bacteria (2–4%).
9. Enzyme digestion results in protoplast in Gram (+) and spheroplast in Gram (–) bacteria.
10. Gram (+) stain as **purple** or **blue** (as they retain crystal violet dye), even after rinsing and counter-staining; Gram (–) stain as **pink** or **red** due to the counter-stain (Fig. 6.5).

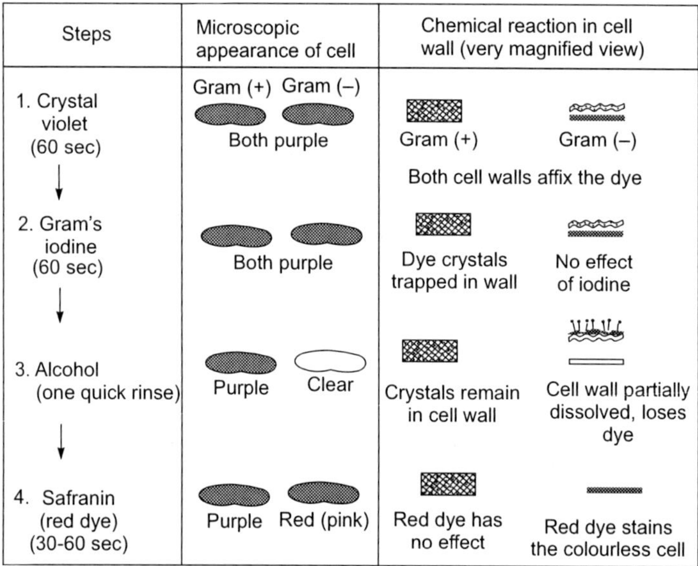

Fig. 6.5 Gram reaction in bacteria as visualized by the gram stain. Gram positive bacteria retain the purple colour of crystal violet and appear purple, whereas Gram-negative lose the colour of the primary stain and take the colour of safranin and appear red or pink.

CYTOPLASMIC MEMBRANE

Cytoplasmic membrane (also called **plasma membrane** and **cell membrane**) (Fig. 6.6) in bacteria is a thin membrane (5–10 nm thick) lying inside the cell wall and enclosing the cytoplasm of the cell. It is made up of 40 % phospholipids and 60 % proteins representing a **fluid-mosaic model** (The model's name is derived from the fact that phospholipids in the membrane are in a fluid state and the proteins are dispersed among the lipid molecules in the membrane, forming a mosaic pattern). Sterols are absent in bacteria except in *Mycoplasma* (the wall-less prokaryotes).

A **phospholipid** molecule contains a polar head, composed of a phosphate group and glycerol that is **hydrophilic** (water-loving) and soluble in water, and nonpolar tails, composed of fatty acids that are **hydrophobic** (water-hating) and insoluble in water (Fig. 6.6).

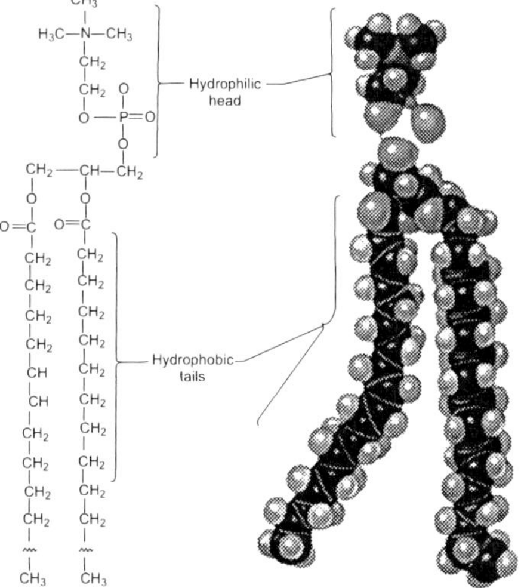

(A) Structure of phospholipid molecule

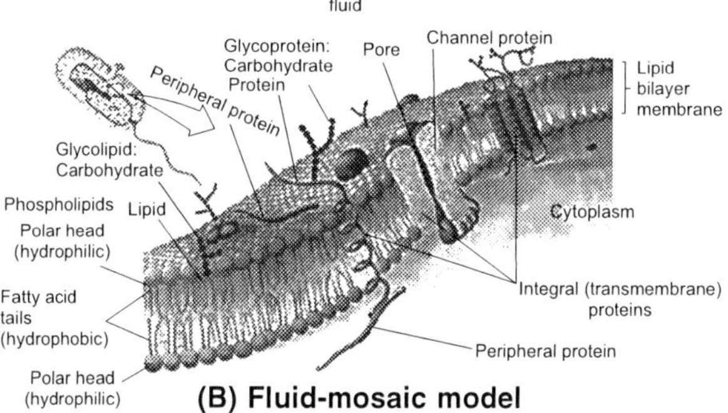

(B) Fluid-mosaic model

Fig. 6.6 Cytoplasmic membrane-structure of a phospholipid molecule and fluid-mosaic model (A). The basic structural component of the membrane the phospholipid molecule. A *phospholipid* has two long fatty acid "tails" of hydrocarbon. The tails are very *hydophobic*–they do not interact with water and form an oily barrier to most water-soluble substances. The "head" of the molecule consists of a charged phosphate group, usually joined to a charged nitrogen-containing group. The head is very hydrophilic – it interacts with water. **(B) The fluid-mosaic model of the cell membrane.** The phospholipids form a bilayer in which the hydrophobic tails form the central core and the hydrophilic heads form the surfaces that face both the interior of the cell and the outside environment. In this fluid bilayer, proteins float like icebergs. Some extend through the bilayer, others are anchored to the inner or outer surface. Proteins and membrane lipids to which carbohydrate chains are attached are called *glycoproteins* and *glycolipids*, repectively. A few bacteria, such as mycoplasmas, have cholesterol molecules in their cell membrane, as do most eukaryotes. *Mycoplasmas lack cell walls*; cholesterol molecules add rigidity to the cell membrane.

Two types of proteins are found in the cell membrane:

- **Peripheral proteins:** They lie at inner or outer surface of the membrane. They function as: enzymes that catalyze chemical reactions; as a scaffold for support; and as mediators of changes in membrane shape during movement.
- **Integral proteins:** They are firmly inserted in the membrane and are involved in transportation.

  Mesosomes: A **mesosome** (or **chondroid**) is a membranous structure formed in a bacterial cell by the invagination of the plasma membrane. They play an important role in:
  - DNA replication and cell division
  - Excretion of exoenzymes.
  - Synthesis of cell wall.

Functions of Cytoplasmic Membrane

- It acts as an osmotic or permeability barrier.
- Location of transport system for specific solutes (nutrients and ions).
- Synthesis of membrane lipids (including lipopolysaccharide in Gram-negative bacteria).
- Synthesis of murein (cell wall peptidoglycan).
- Assembly and synthesis of extra cytoplasmic proteins.
- Coordination of DNA replication and segregation with septum formation and cell division.
- Chemotaxis (both motility per se and cell division).
- Energy generation functions, involving respiratory and photosynthetic electron transport systems, establishment of proton motive force, and transmembranous ATP-synthesizing ATPase.
- Location of specialized enzyme system.

CYTOPLASM

The fluid and all its dissolved or suspended particles is called the **cytoplasm** of the cell. The cytoplasm, or protoplasm, in bacterial cells is a gel-like matrix composed of water (70–80%) which serves as a solvent for the **cell pool**, proteins (enzymes), amino acids, sugars, nucleotides, salts, vitamins, wastes, and gases and contains cell structures such as ribosomes, a circular chromosome (DNA) and plasmids.

All the functions for cell growth, metabolism and replication, the processes necessary for the life of a bacterium, are carried out in the protoplasm.

BACTERIAL CHROMOSOME OR NUCLEOID

The **nucleoid** (Latin: nucis = nut, and *oid* = like) (Fig. 6.2) is the site in the cytoplasm where a single circular strand of DNA designated as the **bacterial chromosome** is condensed into a packet. The DNA comprises a continuous coding sequence of genes and lacking introns which are present in eukaryotes. The DNA carries the genetic information of the cell.

PLASMIDS

Plasmids (Greek: *plasma* = a form + *id* = belonging to) are small, circular, extrachromosomal DNA molecules. They replicate chromosomal DNA independently and are not essential to bacterial growth and metabolism, but confer protective traits such as resisting drugs, and producing toxins and enzymes.

RIBOSOMES

Ribosomes (Greek: *ribose* = a pentose sugar + *soma* = body) are tiny structures composed of protein and RNA that give the cytoplasm a granular appearance. The bacterial ribosomes are 70S (S refers to the Svedberg unit) each composed of a small 30S subunit containing one molecule of rRNA and a larger 50S subunit containing two molecules of rRNA. The eukaryotic ribosomes are 80S ribosomes.

Ribosomes function as the **sites of protein synthesis**.

INCLUSIONS OR GRANULES

Prokaryotic cytoplasm contains several kinds of stored nutrients in an insoluble state such as fat, phosphate or glycogen deposited in dense crystals or particles that can be tapped into when needed. These reserve deposits are called inclusions or granules. Examples include: *metachromatic granules* or *volutin* (they stain red with methylene blue), *polysaccharide granules, lipid inclusions, sulfur granules* and *carboxysomes.*

ENDOSPORES

The bacterial **endospores** (Greek: *endo* = inside + *sporos* = seed) (or simply **spores**) are dormant, non-reproductive, highly dehydrated cells produced by the Gram-positive bacteria, e.g., *Bacillus, Clostridium* and *Sporosarcina*. They are formed internal to the bacterial cell membrane. Their formation is usually triggered by lack of nutrients. Endospore-producing bacteria are termed **sporulating bacteria**.

The primary function of most endospores is to ensure the survival of a bacterium through periods of environmental stress.

Endospore producing bacteria have a two-phase life cycle: a vegetative cell and an endospore (Fig. 6.7). The process of endospore formation within a vegetative cell is known as **sporulation** or **sporogenesis**. An endospore may be located **terminally** (at one end), **subterminally** near one end or **centrally** (inside the vegetative cell) (Fig. 6.8). Return of an endospore to its vegetative state takes place by a process called **germination**. Germination is triggerd by physical or chemical damage to the endospore's coat.

An endospore contains a large amount of an organic acid called **dipicolinic acid** (**DPA**) which is accompanied by a large number of calcium ions and forms a complex within the endospore core. This complex binds free water molecules causing dehydration of the spore. As a result, the heat resistance of macromolecules within the core increases (Fig. 6.8).

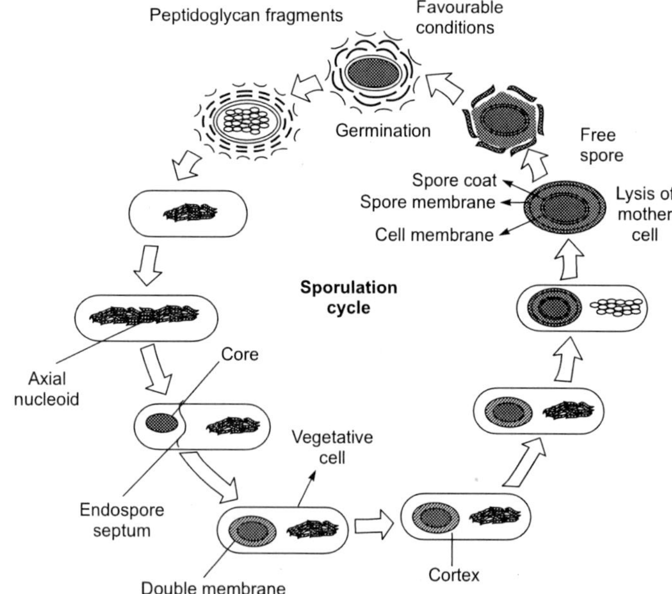

Fig. 6.7 Vegetative and sporulation cycle in bacteria.

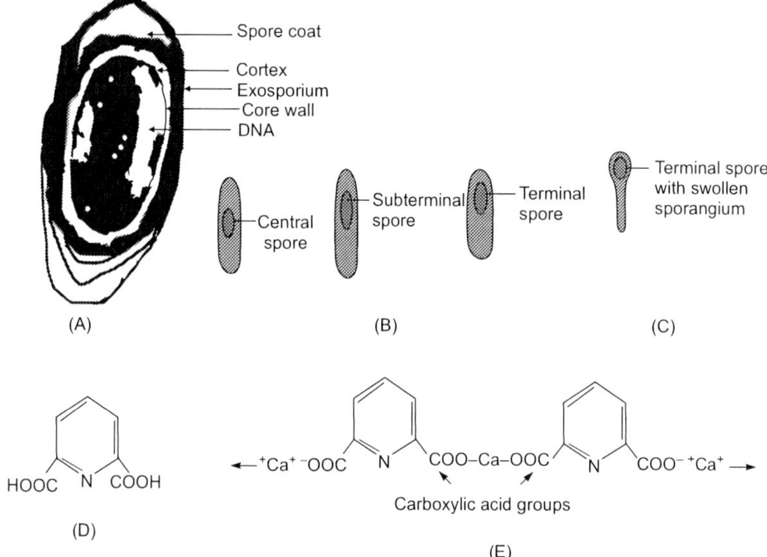

Fig. 6.8 Structure, location and chemical compound in a bacterial endospore. (A) Endospore showing four wall layers. (B) Three different locations of endospore in a cell. (C) Swollen cell due to the large size of the endospore. (D) Structure of dipicolinic acid. (E) Calcium-dipicolinic acid complex.

In bacteria, one vegetative cell forms a single endospore, which, after germination, remains one cell, this sporulation is not a means of reproduction. This process does not increase the number of cells. Bacterial endospores differ from spores formed by prokaryotic actinomycetes and the eukaryotic fungi and algae, which detach from the parent and develop into another organisms, and, therefore represent reproduction.

Endospore walls (Fig. 6.8) are very resistant to penetration of ordinary stains such as simple stains and Gram stains. For endospore staining, a special differential **Schaeffer-Fulton spore stain** method is used that uses two stains: **malachite green** (primary stain) and **safranin** (counter stain) and tap water as a decolorizing agent. Malachite green penetrates the endospores and stains them green and safranin stains the cells red or pink.

Endospores of bacteria can remain dormant for several years. For example, 7500-year old endospores of *Thermoactinomyces vulgaris* from the freezing mud showed germination in a nutrient medium. They are extremely resistant to extreme heat, dry conditions, exposure to radiation and toxic chemicals. Endospores killing requires 121° C for

15 minutes while vegetative cells can be killed by heating at 80°C for 10 minutes (moist heat). Marked resistance is due to several reasons such as:

- the impermeability of their cortex and outer coats;
- their high content of dipicolinic acid and calcium;
- their low water content; and
- their very low metabolic and enzymatic activity.

FLAGELLA

Bacterial **flagella** (sing: **flagellum**, Latin: a whip) (Fig. 6.2) are long, thin (20 nm) whip-like external appendages (external projections) containing the protein **flagellin** that confers **motility** or **self-propulsion,** that is, the capacity of a cell to swim freely through an aqueous habitat.

The flagellar apparatus (Fig. 6.9) consists of the flagellar filament made of polymerized flagellin, the hook-like structure near the cell surface and a system of rings embedded in the cell envelope (the basal body or flagellar motor). The flagellum rotates in a clockwise or counterclockwise direction, in a motion similar to that of a propeller.

Depending upon the presence and absence of flagella, bacteria are of two types: **motile** that can move (e.g., *Vibrio*) and **nonmotile** that cannot move (e.g., *Staphylococcus*). Bacteria that lack flagella are referred to as **atrichous** (i.e., without projections). Motility can be observed microscopically with a hanging drop slide. Different species of bacteria have different numbers and flagellar arrangements (Fig. 6.10). Various types of flagellar arrangement are:

- *Peritrichous* (Gr. *peri* = around + *tricho* = hair): Flagella distributed over the entire surface.
- *Polar:* At one or both ends of the cell.
- *Monotrichous:* (Gr. *mono* = one): A single flagellum at one pole.
- *Lophotrichons:* (Gr. *lopho* = tuft or ridge): A tuft of flagella at one pole.
- *Amphitrichous:* (Gr. *amphi* = on both sides): Flagella at both poles of the cell.

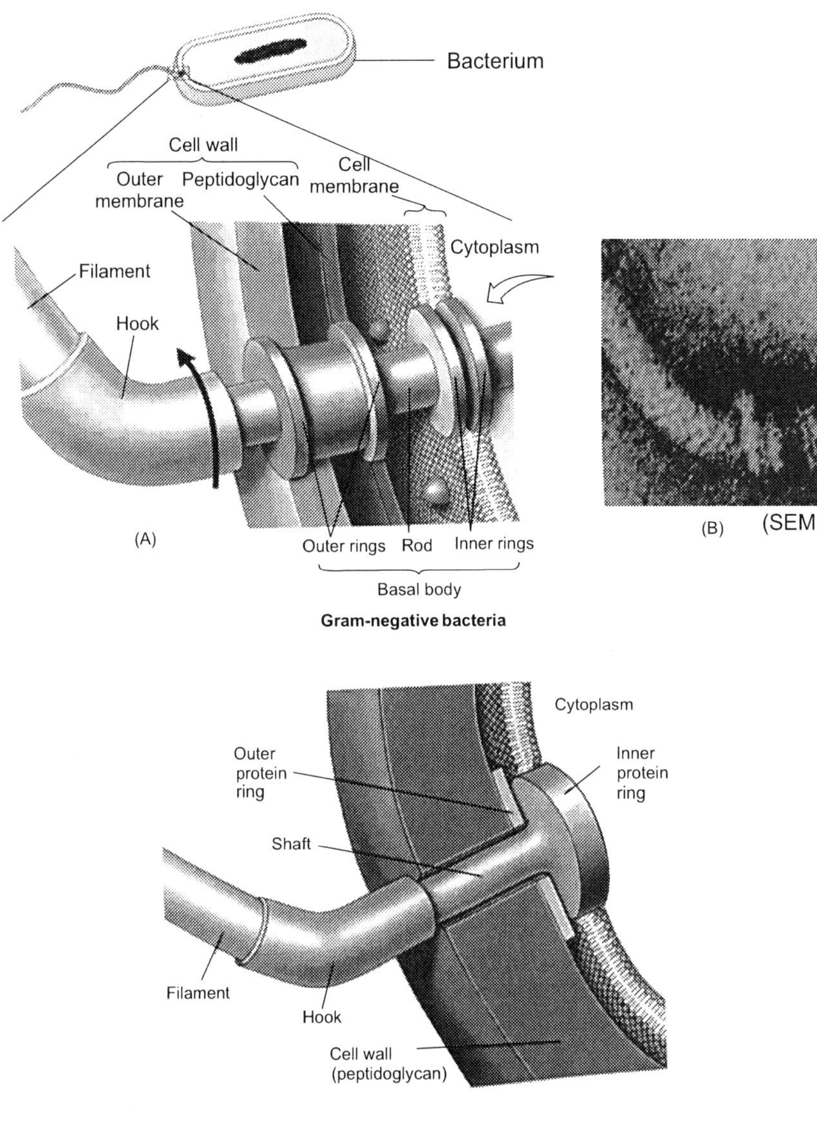

Fig. 6.9 Flagellar apparatus of two different bacterial flagella. (A) Drawing and (B) electron micrograph of the basal region of the flagellum of a Gram-negative bacterium. The flagellum has three main parts: a filament, a hook. and a basal body consisting of a rod surrounded by four rings. (C) Gram-positive bacteria have only two rings, one attached to the peptidoglycan of the cell wall and one to the cell membrane.

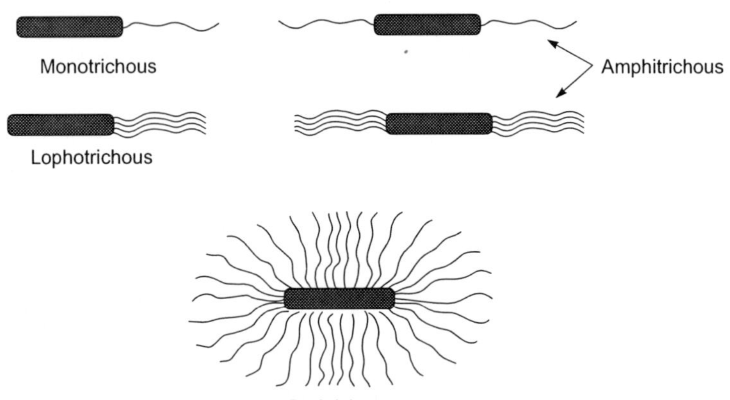

Fig. 6.10 Arrangement of flagella in bacteria. (A) Monotrichous (*Pseudomonas aeruginosa*); **(B) Lophotrichous** (*Pseudomonas fluorescens*); **(C) Amphitrichous** (*Aquaspirillum serpens*); **(D) Peritrichous** (*Salmonella typhi, Escherichia coli*).

Arrangement of flagella in bacteria helps in laboratory identification of pathogens. The flagellar protein called *H antigen* is useful for distinguishing among **serovars** (i.e., variations within a species) of Gram-negative bacteria.

PERIPLASMIC FLAGELLA

A **periplasmic flagellum,** also called **axial filament,** is a type of internal flagellum that is long and coiled and enclosed in the space between the cell wall and cell membrane. These show an unusual wriggly mode of locomotion as shown by cork screw-shaped bacteria, called **spirochetes**.

FIMBRIAE

Fimbriae (sing. **fimbria**, L. a fringe) are proteinaceous tiny bristle-like fibres arising from the surface of bacterial cells. These are shorter and thinner than flagella. They are not involved in locomotion, but have a tendency to attach with each other forming *biofilms* and to surfaces, and help bacteria adhere to eithelial surfaces in the body. For example, in gonorrhea, they help the causative agent *Neisseria gonorrhoae* to colonize mucous membranes.

PILI

Pili (sing. **pilus**, L. hair) are rigid hollow appendages made of a special protein, *pilin*. Pili are longer than fimbriae and there are only a few per bacterial cell. They are found in Gram-negative bacteria while fimbriae are found in both Gram-negative as well as Gram-positive bacteria.

They are involved in a mating process between cells and allowing the transfer of DNA from one cell to another, a process called **conjugation**. Hence, pili are also called **conjugation (sex)** ***pili***.

KEY POINTS

- Bacteria are prokaryotes that lack membrane-enclosed organelles.
- Structures external to bacterial cell wall include **glycocalyx** (capsule slime layer) and appendages (flagella, fimbriae, pili).
- Bacterial cytoplasm (protoplasm) contains **nucleoid** (chromosome without nuclear membrane) ribosomes, mesosomes and inclusions/storage granules.
- Their DNA is a long, circular molecule termed a '**chromosome**'.
- Bacterial chromosome has no introns, instead comprises a continuous coding sequence of genes.
- Bacterial **cell wall** is mainly composed of peptidoglycan (mucopeptide or murein) long chains of N-acetylglucosomine and N-acetylmuramic acid.
- The composition of the bacterial cell wall is used to classify bacteria into two major groups: Gram-positive bacteria and Gram-negative bacteria.
- In Gram staining, Gram-positive bacteria stain purple and Gram-negative bacteria stain red (pink).
- The appendages of bacteria play specific roles: such as flagella (motility), fimbriae (attachment), sex pili (a means of DNA transfer during conjugation).
- Flagellar number and arrangement on the bacterial cell is used in laboratory identification and disease diagnosis.
- Presence and location of **endospore** (terminal, subterminal, central) in a cell helps in bacterial identification.
- **Ribosomes**, the sites of protein synthesis, are 70 S type in bacteria.

IMPORTANT QUESTIONS

1. Draw the structure of a typical bacterial cell with the help of a labelled diagram. Explain the functions of each part.
2. Write short notes on:
   (a) Cell wall in bacteria.
   (b) Cytoplasmic membrane in bacteria.

(c) Glycocalyx.
(d) Endospores.
(e) Differentiate flagella, fimbriae and pili.

MULTIPLE-CHOICE QUESTIONS

1. Which of the following is *not* a part of cell envelope in bacteria?
   (a) Cell membrane (b) Fimbriae
   (c) Cell wall (d) Glycocalyx.
2. The *n*-acetylglucasomine (NAG) and *n*-acetylmuramic acid (NAM) constituents of peptidoglycan present in the bacterial cell wall are what kind of molecules?
   (a) Lipids (b) Proteins
   (c) Carbohydrates (d) None of the above.
3. Peptidoglycan is a major constituent of cell wall of:
   (a) Fungi (b) Algae
   (c) Gram-positive bacteria (d) Gram-negative bacteria.
4. When flagella are distributed all around the cell, the arrangement is called:
   (a) Amphitrichous (b) Monotrichous
   (c) Peritrichous (d) Atrichous.
5. Sedimentation coefficient of bacterial ribosomes is:
   (a) 80 S (b) 70 S
   (c) 60 S (d) 30 S.
6. Which of the following bacterial structures is/are involved in attachment to cell surface?
   (a) Capsule (b) Flagella
   (c) Fimbriae (d) Mesosomes.
7. Which of the following bacteria does not produce endospores?
   (a) *Clostridium* (b) *Bacillus*
   (c) *Escherichia* (d) *Sporosarcina*.
8. Which of the following bacteria has a single polar flagellum?
   (a) *Proteus* (b) *Citrobacter*
   (c) *Salmonella* (d) *Vibrio*.

ANSWERS TO MCQs

1. (b) 2. (c) 3. (c) 4. (c) 5. (b)
6. (c) 7. (c) 8. (d).

7

Bacterial Motility and Locomotion

WHAT IS MOTILITY?

Motility or **self-propulsion** is the ability of a cell or an organism to move or swim freely through an aqueous habitat. Motility confers bacteria an ability to change. Bacterial motility is often associated with flagella and is one characteristic used in the identification of bacteria. Depending upon the presence or absence of flagella, bacteria are of two types:

- **Motile bacteria.** If a bacterium is able to swim in an aqueous habitat it is said to be **motile** (e.g., *Escherichia, Vibrio*). About half of all known bacteria are motile. A motile bacterium propels itself from place to place by rotating its flagella. Almost every bacteria of the family *Enterobacteriaceae* is motile.

- **Nonmotile bacteria.** The bacterial species that lack the ability and structures that would allow them to propel themselves, under their own power, through their enviornment are called **nonmotile bacteria**. These bacteria lack flagella and bacteria without flagella are called **atrichous**. **Cocci** rarely have flagella. *Staphylococcus aureus, Lactobacillus* and diphtheria bacilli are the common examples. The passive type of movement is exhibited by most of these bacteria. It is purely physical. The nonmotile cells oscillate in the same relative space because of bombardment of water molecules, a physical process called the *Brownian movement* (Fig. 7.1).

Motile and nonmotile bacteria can be differentiated by culturing in a stab tube: the nonmotile bacteria will only grow along the stab line while motile bacteria will grow out from the stab line, and the line will appear diffuse and extend into the medium. The words motility, movement and locomotion are used synonymously.

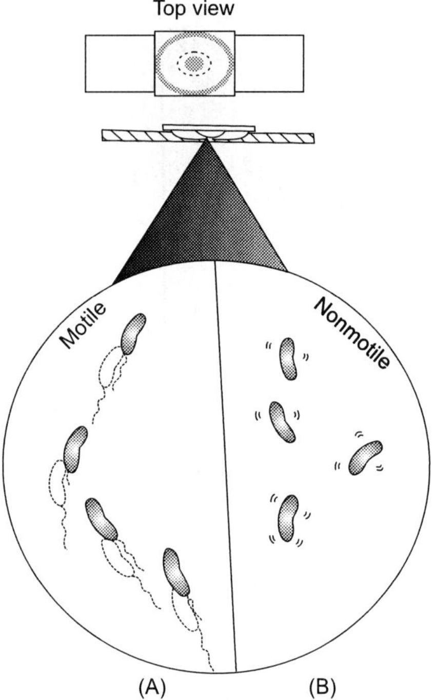

Fig. 7.1 Motility detection and the differentiation between the movement of motile and nonmotile cells by hanging drop slide technique. (A) In true motility, the cell swims and progresses from one point to another. (B) Nonmotile cells oscillate in the same relative space because of bombardment by molecules (i.e., Brownian movement).

TYPES OF MOTILITY OR LOCOMOTION

- Flagellar motility
- Sprochaetel locomotion
- Gliding locomotion

FLAGELLAR MOTILITY

Flagellar motility, also called **true motility**, is caused by rotation of flagella. Bacterial flagella rotate up to 1700 Hz, five times faster than a formula–one racer engine. Flagella can rotate both in clockwise and counterclockwise direction.

A bacterial flagellum has three parts: *filament*, *hook* and *basal body*. The hook, rings and rod function together for rotating the flagellar filament 360° (Fig. 7.2). The integral membrane protein (IMP) initiates and maintains flagellar rotation.

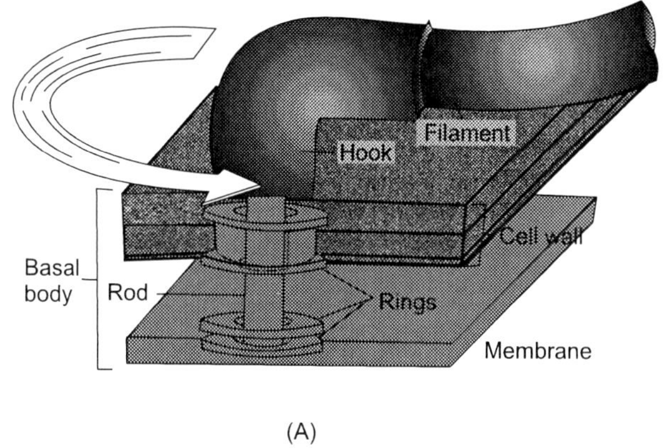

(A)

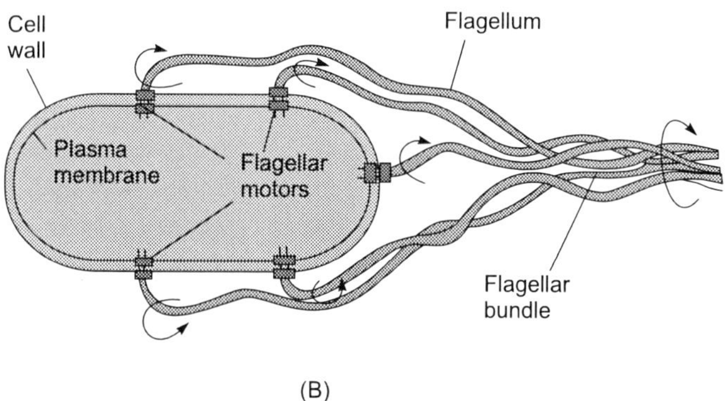

(B)

Fig. 7.2 Flagellum structure and mode of rotation by flagella. (A) Flagellum structure showing the filament, hook and basal body in a gram-negative cell, and mode of rotation. The hook, rings and rod function together as a tiny device that rotates the filament 360°. (B) A bacterial cell showing details of flagellar attachment and their rotation.

Bacteria can move in one direction for a length of time, the movement called a "**run**" (or "**swim**"), or have abrupt changes in direction periodically called **tumbles**.

The number and type of flagellar arrangement has some bearing on the swimming speed of a bacterial taxon. The speediest forms are polar flagellated cells such as *Thiospirillum*, which can zip along at 5.2 mm/minute, and *Pseudomonas aeruginosa*, which can swim at 4.4 mm/minute. Taking into account the small dimensions of these bacteria, such speeds are comparable to "flying speed" for humans. Peritrichous rods, having flagella all over the surface of a cell, such as *Escherichia coli* tend to swim at a relatively slower pace (1 mm/minute).

The rotation of a flagellum is either clockwise or anticlockwise around its long axis. The movement results from rotation of its basal body and is similar to the movement of the shaft of an electric motor. The flagellar motor is powered directly as opposed to indirectly via (ATP) by the protein gradient created across the cytoplasmic membrane by electron transport.

Depending upon the location of flagella, bacteria can swim smoothly, reverse the movement backward or forward or tumble. For example, in peritrichously flagellated bacteria (e.g., *Salmonella, Proteus, Escherichia coli*), when all the flagella present on a cell rotate in a counterclockwise direction, the flagella bundle together and push the bacterium forward in a straight line, the movement called a **run** (Fig. 7.3). On the other hand, when flagella rotate clockwise, the flagellar bundle carries apart, the flagella losing coordination, causing the bacterium to **tumble** randomly. In polar flagellated (one, bi- or multipolar) forms (e.g., *Pseudomonas, Spirillum*), when a polar flagellum rotates in a counterclockwise direction, the cell swims forward and when the flagellum reverses direction and rotates clockwise, the cell stops and tumbles (Fig. 7.3).

Flagellated motile bacteria can detect and move in response to a particular stimulus, known as a **tactic response** or **taxis** (Gr. *taxis* = an ordering). Such stimuli include chemicals (**chemotaxis** pl. chemotaxes), light (**phototaxis**) and magnetic particles (**magnetotaxis**). The movement centre toward (positive taxis) or away (negative taxis) from the stimulus.

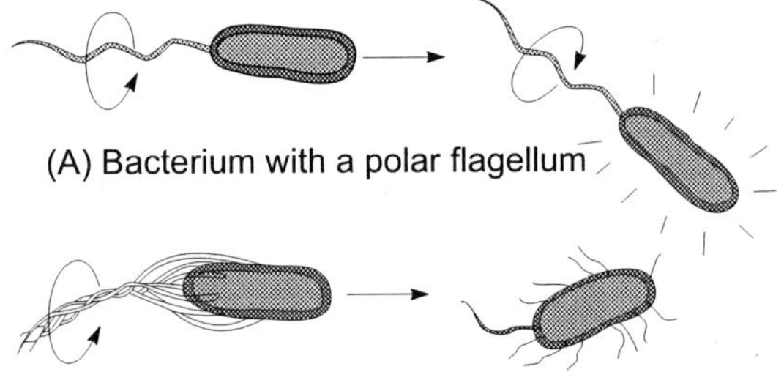

Fig. 7.3 The operation of flagella and the mode of locomotion in bacteria with polar and peritrichous flagella. (A) When a polar flagellum rotates in a counterclockwise direction, the cell swims forward, the movement is called a run. When the flagellum reverses direction and rotates clockwise, the cell stops and tumbles in random directions. (B) In peritrichous forms, all flagella sweep toward one end of the cell and rotate as a single group. During tumbles, the flagella lose coordination.

SPIROCHAETAL MOVEMENT

Spirochaetes, the corkscrew-shaped bacteria, also called helical bacteria (e.g., *Treponema pallidum*, the cause of syphilis; and *Borrelia burgdorferi* the cause of Lyme disease) show **corkscrew motion** (also called **twisting motion**) which allows the bacteria to move about through body fluids. The organelles for motility are **periplasmic flagella** (also called **axial filaments** or **endoflagella**) (Fig. 7.4). These flagella run lengthwise between the bacterial inner membrane and outer membrane in the periplasmic space. These endoflagella are bundled together to form an axial filament. The contraction of the outer filament produces a movement of the outer sheath that propels the spirochetes in a spinning and undulating pattern of locomotion resembling a corkscrew.

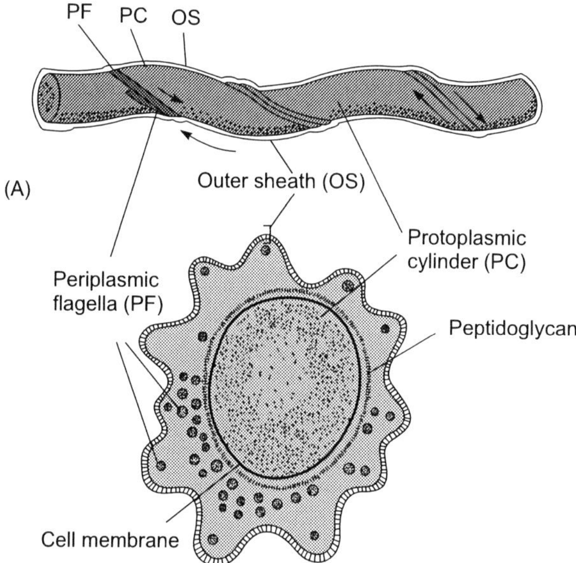

Fig. 7.4 The orientation of periplasmic flagella (axial filament) on the spirachete cell (e.g., *Borrelia burgdorferi*). (A) Longitudinal section. (B) Cross section. Contraction of the filaments imparts a spinning and undulating pattern of locomotion.

GLIDING MOVEMENT

Gliding is defined as the movement of a cell on a surface in the direction of the long axis of the cell. Gliding provides a means for microbes to travel in enviornments with a low water content such as might be found in biofilms, microbial mass and soil. Gliding motility is shown by special bacteria—the Gliding Bacteria Group; such as

Myxococcus, Cystobacter, Cystophaga, cyanobacteria (e.g., *Oscillatoria*). These bacteria do not have flagellar structure and move actively by gliding on the surface by secreting slimy substance like snails during locomotion. The exact mechanism of gliding locomotion is still unknown.

LABORATORY DETECTION OF MOTILITY

Microscopy is the most accurate way to determine bacterial motility for fresh culture of bacteria. Of the two techniques: *Wet mount preparation* and *hanging drop cavity slide,* the latter is a commonly used microscopic technique. Truly motile bacteria will show propelling action forwards definite direction and progressing from one point to another (Fig. 7.1) Nonmotile bacteria will also appear to be motile, however, the movement is zigzag and directionless—oscillating in the same space because of the bombardment of molecules (Fig. 7.3).

IMPORTANCE OF BACTERIAL LOCOMOTION

Chemotactic behaviour and survival

Motility confers bacteria an ability to change direction which is important when bacteria require moving away or towards repellents or attractants, respectively due to their tactic behaviour. It helps in their survival and offers to choose favourable environment having positive stimuli: chemical, light or gravity for bacteria.

Pathogenesis

In most pathogenic motile bacteria such as *Vibrio, Salmonella, Campylobacter,* and saprophytes or opportunists (e.g., *Escherichia*), motility plays an important role in attachment and colonization of intestine and other vital organs.

Root colonization

Colonization of roots is a prerequisite for establishment of a microbe in the rhizosphere. Motile bacteria (e.g., Pseudomonads, *Azospirilla*) are very efficient in attachment and subsequent colonization of their host plants. Motile bacteria can swim towards root exudates or other nutrient gradients earlier as compared to nonmotile bacteria, hence are effective root colonizers.

KEY POINTS

- Transformation of proton energy in the basal body causes rotation of flagella in motile bacteria.

- Bacteria lacking flagella are called **atrichous**.
- Bacteria show three types of locomotion: flagellar, spirochaetal and gliding.
- The movement of a prokaryotic flagellum results from rotation of its basal body.
- Flagellated bacteria show a tactic response (**taxis**): chemotaxis, phototaxis and magentotaxis.
- Periplasmic flagella also called **axial filaments** are involved in spirochaetal movement.
- Wet mount preparation and hanging drop cavity slide are the microscopic techniques used to detect/assay flagellar motility.
- Motility helps bacteria in pathogenesis, root colonization and in their survival.

IMPORTANT QUESTIONS

1. Write brief notes on:
   (a) Describe the three ways bacteria can move.
   (b) Flagellar motility and its application.

MULTIPLE-CHOICE QUESTIONS

1. Which of the following bacteria is nonmotile?
   (a) *Staphylococcus* (b) *Pseudomonas*
   (c) *Salmonella* (d) *Proteus*.
2. Which of the following terms is used for bacteria without flagella?
   (a) Aflagellated bacteria (b) Amphitrichous
   (c) Peritrichous (d) Atrichous.
3. All of the following bacteria have peritrichous flagella EXCEPT:
   (a) *Escherichia* (b) *Salmonella*
   (c) *Pseudomonas* (d) *Proteus*.
4. Which of the following structures is used for bacterial motility?
   (a) Fimbriae (b) Pili
   (c) Flagella (d) All of the above.
5. In *Treponema pallidum*, a spirochete, which of the following is involved in locomotion?
   (a) Axial filaments (b) Flagella
   (c) Pili (d) All of the above.

6. Which of the following bacteria shows gliding movement?
   (a) *Oscillatoria* (b) *Borgel*
   (c) *Treponema* (d) None of the above.
7. Which of the following is used to detect flagellar motility in bacteria?
   (a) Stab inoculation (b) Hanging drop cavity slide
   (c) Gram staining (d) Negative staining.
8. The movement of a flagellated bacterium results from rotation of its basal body. True or false?
9. Bacterial flagella rotate in clockwise and anitclockwise direction by transformation of proton energy powered by basal body. True of false?

ANSWERS TO MCQs

1. (a)	2. (d)	3. (c)	4. (c)	5. (a)
6. (a)	7. (b)	8. True	9. True.	

8

Colonization of Pathogenic Bacteria

Colonization refers to the establisment of a stable population of a microorganism at the appropriate portal of entry without causing clinical evidence of infection. Pathogens usually colonize host tissues that are in contact with the external enviornment such as skin, mouth, airways and urogenital tract.

MECHANISM OF COLONIZATION

The first stage of microbial infection is **colonization**—multiplication and growth of the pathogen called **establishment** at the appropriate portal of entry. Pathogens usually colonize host tissues that are in contact with the external environment. Sites of entry in human hosts include: the digestive tract (mouth), the respiratory tract (airways), the urogenital tract, the conjunctiva, and the skin. Organisms that colonize these regions have the ability to overcome or withstand the constant presence of the host defenses at the surface and have developed tissues adhrence mechanisms.

For many pathogenic bacteria, the initial interaction with host tissues occurs at a mucosal surface. The bacterial colonization normally requires **adherence**—attachment to an eukaryotic cell or tissue surface. Adherence requires the participation of two factors: a **host receptor** (specific carbohydrate or peptide residues on the host's cell surface) and a **bacterial ligand** (called an **adhesin**)—a macromolecular component of the bacterial cell surface. Adhesins and receptors usually interact in a complementary and specific fashion. Adherence allows the establishment of a focus of infection that may remain localized at the site of invasion or may subsequently spread to other tissues through the body (i.e., systemic): Adherence is necessary to avoid innate host defense mechanisms, for example, peristalsis in the gut as the flushing action of mucus, saliva and urine which remove non-adherent bacteria. Successful colonization also requires that bacteria are able to acquire essential nutrients, especially iron for growth.

HOST FACTORS AFFECTING COLONIZATION

Before a bacterial pathogen can colonize and grow in substantial numbers in host tissue, depends on the following:

- To compete successfully with the host's normal microbiota which vary at various sites of entry.
- Appropriate environmental conditions of temperature, pH and redox potential (presence or absence of oxygen).
- Organisms have the ability to use complex nutrients such as glycogen since soluble nutrients (as sugars, amino acids, organic acids) are limited in the vertebrate host.
- Availability of microbial nutrients such as vitamins, growth factors and trace elements, if they are in short supply, can significantly influence establishment of the pathogen.

  For example, the growth of *Brucella abortus*, the cause of abortion of cattle, is very slow, in all the tissues of the cattle except placenta where it grows rapidly due to the high concentration of *erythritol*, a nutrient that enhances the growth of this pathogen.

  Similarly, short supply of trace elements, such as iron greatly influences growth and establishment of a pathogen. Specific proteins called **transferrin** and **lactoferrin**, present in animals bind iron tightly and create iron deficiency for microbes. Some bacteria have the ability to produce **siderophores**—*the iron-chelating compounds*, that help these obtain iron from the environment.
- Colonizers have the ability to overcome the host defense mechanisms and growth conditions of pH, temperature and redox potential. For example, pathogenic bacteria on the skin's surface must withstand environmental conditions and bacteriostatic skin secretions such as lactic acid and fatty acids present in sweat and sebaceous secretions and the lower pH to which they give rise. Of the several antimicrobial peptides, *dermacidin*, made by sweat glands and secreted into sweat, is inhibitory to *Escherichia coli*, *Staphylococcus aureus* and *Candida albicans*, thus protecting the skin against the invading bacteria and fungi.

- The organisms colonizing the respiratory membrane must escape the action of mucus and cilia and those on the lining of portions of digestive tract must withstand peristaltic movements, mucus, digestive enzymes, and acid. *Chlamydia pneumoniae* biofilms that colonize coronary arteries have been implicated in heart disease.

Localization in the Body

A colonizing organism after its initial entry remains localized and multiplies at the site of invasion such as the boil that may arise from *Staphylococcus* skin infections. Alternatively, if the organism enters the lymphatic vessels as well as blood, its spread can result in a systemic infection of the body, with the organism growing in a variety of tissues.

KEY POINTS

- **Bacterial colonization**—the multiplication and growth of bacteria at the site of invasion, is affected by the host defense mechanisms, availability of nutrients especially iron and growth conditions.
- Organisms may grow locally at the site of invasion (**localized**), or may spread throughout the systems of the body (**systemic**).
- The bacterial **adherence** to host mucosal surfaces requires the participation of two factors: a host's **receptor** and a bacterial **ligand** (or **adhesin**).

IMPORTANT QUESTIONS

1. Briefly describe:
   (a) Bacterial colonization of host tissues.
   (b) Host factors that limit or accelerate colonization and growth of a microbe at a local site.

MULTIPLE-CHOICE QUESTIONS

1. The establishment of a stable population of a microbe on or in the host tissue is called colonization. True or false?
2. During bacterial colonization, organisms may grow locally at the site of invasion, or may spread through the body. True or false?

3. In colonization of human tissues, mucosal surface is the invasion site EXCEPT:
   (a) Skin (b) Mouth
   (c) Respiratory tract (d) Urogenital tract.
4. Adhesin (adherence) to the mucosal surface of the invasion site is necessary to avoid innate host defence mechanisms in:
   (a) Invasion (b) Entry of a pathogen
   (c) Colonization (d) Disease development.

ANSWERS TO MCQs

1. True 2. True 3. (a) 4. (c).

9

Reproduction and Mode of Genetic Transfer in Bacteria

Reproduction is the process of producing new organisms: "offsprings" by a sexual or asexual process. All living things reproduce. Reproduction is of two types:

- **Asexual reproduction**—In which offspring are a product of a single organism and are genetically identical. Bacteria normally reproduce by binary fission.
- **Sexual reproduction**—It involves the fussion of two gametes (♂ and ♀) which forms a zygote that potentially develops into an offspring genetically different from the parent organisms. Bacteria do not reproduce sexually.

ASEXUAL REPRODUCTION IN BACTERIA

In asexual reproduction, offspring arise from a single organism, and inherit the genes of that parent only: it does not involve the fusion of gametes, and almost never changes the number of chromosomes. Asexual reproduction is the primary form of reproduction in bacteria.

Four methods for asexual reproduction are:

1. Binary fission
2. Conidial production
3. Budding
4. Fragmentation.

1. BINARY FISSION

In **binary fission** (Fig. 9.1), a the form of asexual reproduction, a single cell divides into two equal, identical cells. During this process, the single *chromosome* (circular double-stranded DNA) undergoes replication, where both the strands and new complementary strands are formed on the original strands resulting in the formation of two identical double stranded DNA molecules. Then, the cell enlarges and divides into two new daughter cells (no spindle formation takes place like mitotic division). The two cells separate by a transverse septum that develops in the middle region of the cell (Fig. 9.1).

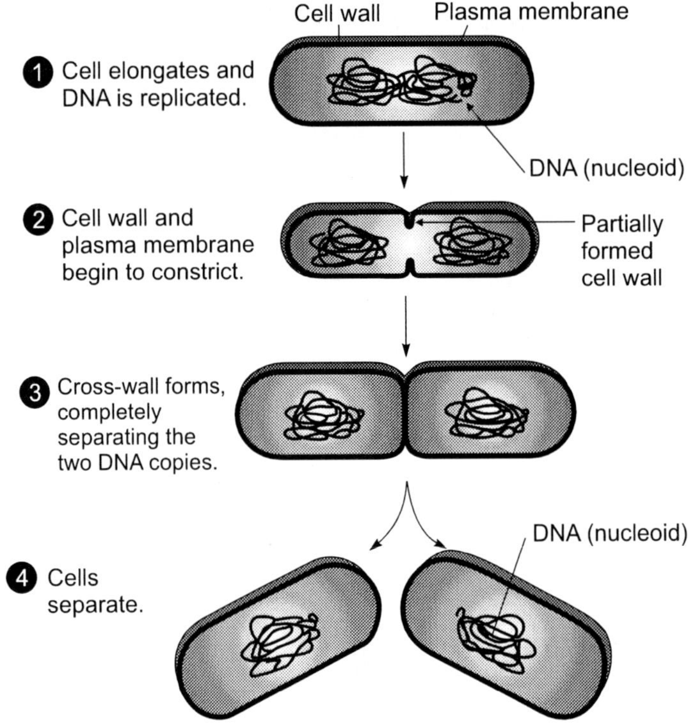

Fig. 9.1 Binary fission in bacteria. Sequence of events in cell division.

The binary fission is a rapid process and cell undergoes division at an interval of 20–30 minutes (*Escherichia coli*). The divison becomes gradually slow after certain time due to the accumulation of toxic substances and exhaustion of nutrients.

2. CONIDIA FORMATION

Some filamentous bacteria such as actinomycetes (e.g., *Streptomyces*) reproduce by producing chains of conidiospores (conidia) externally at the tips of filaments (conidiophores) (Fig. 9.2). After detachment, a conidium germinates and gives rise to new mycelium (filament) as happens in fungi, an eukaryrote.

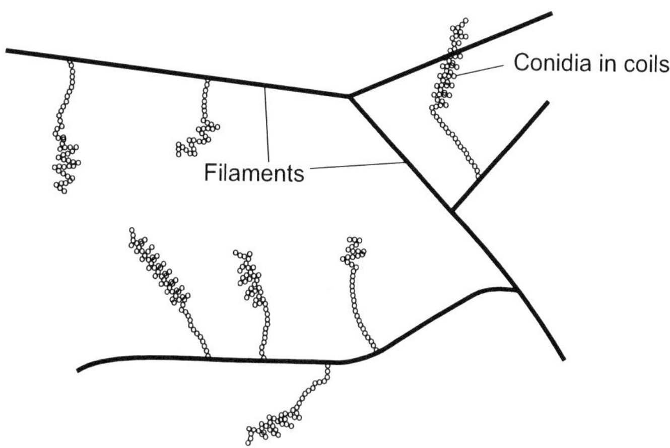

Fig. 9.2 Conidia in coils, asexual reproductive structures, in a filamentous bacterium *Streptomyces*, an actinomycete.

3. BUDDING

Some bacteria (e.g., *Rhodomicrobium, Hyphomicrobium*) reproduce by **budding**. During this process, a bacterial cell develops a small swelling (outgrowth) called a **bud** that enlarges until its size approaches that of the parent cell. Later this bud gets separated from the mother/parent by a partition wall and grows into a cell.

4. FRAGMENTATION

In **fragmentation**, an organism splits into fragments. Each of these fragments develops into matured, fully grown individuals that are identical to their parents. Bacteria that produce extensive filamentous growth, reproduce by fragmentation of the filaments into small bacillary or coccoid cells, each of which gives rise to new cells. Examples include cyanobacteria (e.g., *Oscillatoria*), *Staphylococcus aureus* (single cells separate to form new clusters), and *Neisseria*, a diplococcus, separates into two group of two cells after a round of 2nd cell division.

SEXUAL REPRODUCTION

In bacterial sexual reproduction, there is no meiosis, and no formation of gametes and zygote. Instead it involves transfer of a portion of genetic material (DNA) from a donor cell to a recipient cell. This process is called **horizontal gene transfer** (also called **lateral gene transfer**) or **parasexuality**, a unique process of genetic recombination. Three mechanisms of lateral gene transfer: **transformation, transduction** and **conjugation** (Fig. 9.3) are known and none of which is associated with reproduction. Transfer of genetic material by these mechanisms from one bacterium to another can result in the rapid spread of resistance to antibiotics.

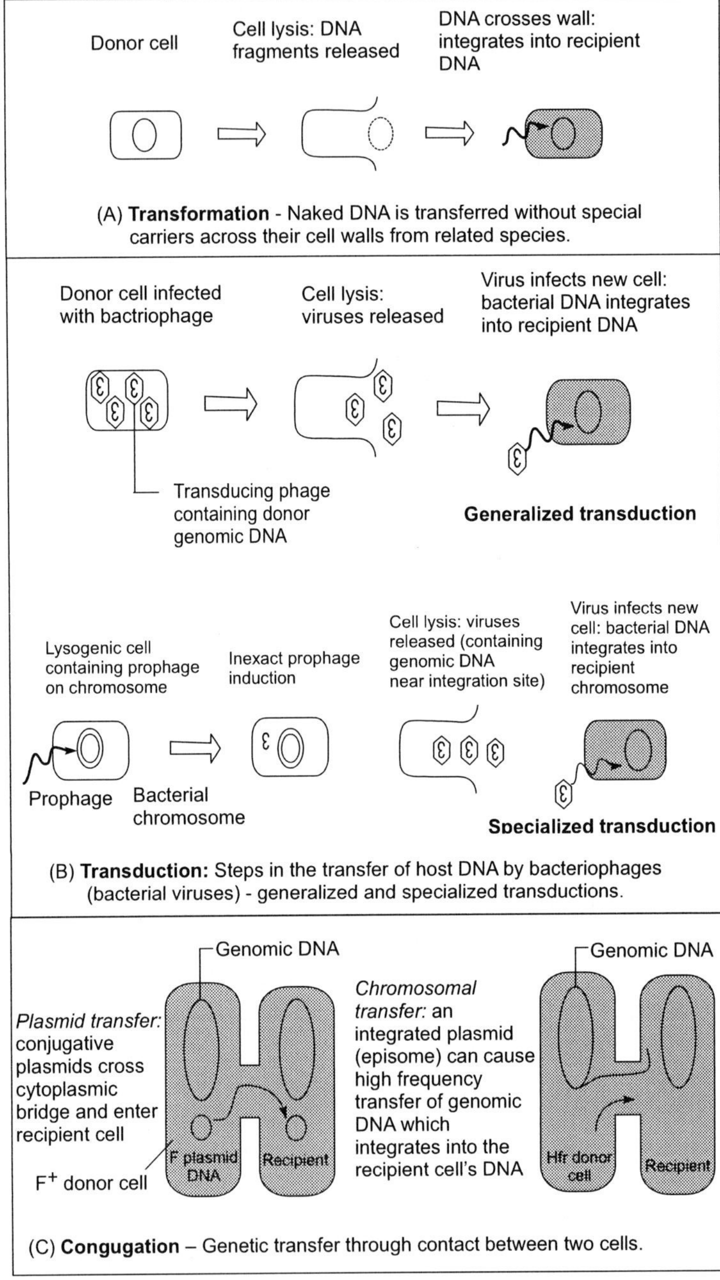

Fig. 9.3 Three different ways: transformation (A), transduction (B) and conjugation (C) in which genes can be transferred between bacteria.

TRANSFORMATION

Transformation (L. *tranc* = across + *formatio* = to form) is defined as the change in an organism's characteristics through the incorporation of naked DNA in its genome from its environment. This phenomenon was discovered in 1928 by **Frederick Griffith**, an English biochemist, working with *Streptococcus pneumoniae* on laboratory mice. He showed that a mixed culture of live, rough and heat-killed smooth pneumococci could produce live, smooth pneunmococci capable of killing mice.

Mechanism of transformation involves the release of naked DNA fragments and their uptake by other cells at a certain stage in their growth cycle through cell wall (Fig. 9.3A) Transformation is used to create recombinant DNA to study gene locations.

TRANSDUCTION

Transduction (L. *transducere* = to lead across) is the transfer of a portion of DNA from one bacterium (donor) to another bacterium (recipient) by bacteriophages (bacterial viruses). This process is known to occur in several bacteria such as *Salmonella*, *Escherichia*, and *Micrococcus*. Transduction is of two types:

- *Generalized transduction*: It involves the transfer of any segment of donor DNA (or gene).
- *Specialized (or restricted) transduction:* It involves the transfer of only a highly specific part of host DNA.

The events in two types of transduction are shown in Figure 9.3 B. Transduction is significant in three ways:

- It transfers genetic meterial and demonstrates a close evolution between prophage and host cell DNA.
- Bacteriophage persistence in a cell suggests a mechanism for viral origins of cancer.
- It provides a possible mechanism for studying gene linkage.

CONJUGATION

Conjugation (L. *conjugates* = yoked together), discovered by **Joshua Lederberg** in 1946 in *Escherichia coli*, is a mode of sexual mating in which a **plasmid** (extrachromosomal DNA molecule) or other genetic material is transferred from one bacterium to another (Fig. 9.3 C). In the two strains of bacteria involved, one acts as a **donor** (or **male**) and the other as a **recipient** (or **female**). The donor cells are known to possess a *sex factor* or *fertility factor* (*F factor*) as a component of its genome, i.e., circular DNA, called the *F^+ strain*.

The recipient cell does not have the factor and hence it is described as *F^- strain*. A conjugation between cells of *F^+* and *F^- strains* always results in the formation of **F^+** bacterial cells in the progeny.

Three mechanisms of conjugation have been observed:

1. In transfer of *F plasmids*, a plasmid is transferred.
2. In *high-frequency recombinations (Hfr)* (Hfr = denotes a cell with an integrated F factor transmits its chromosomal genes at a higher frequency than other cells), parts of F plasmids that have been incorporated into the chromosome (the initiating segment) are transferred along with adjacent bacterial genes.
3. An F plasmid is incorporated into the chromosome and subsequently separated becomes an *F′ plasmid* and transfers chromosomal genes attached to it.

KEY POINTS

- Bacteria reproduce asexually by binary fission, conidial production, budding and fragmentation.
- Bacteria normally reproduce by *binary fission*, a rapid process producing two cells at 20–30 minutes interval.
- Bacteria **lack sexual reproduction**.
- Gene transfer in bacteria occurs by **transformation, transduction** and **conjugation**.

IMPORTANT QUESTIONS

1. In what way binary fission is different from budding and conidia formation in bacteria?

2. Write brief notes on:

(a) Binary fission (b) Transformation

(c) Conjugation (d) Transduction.

MULTIPLE-CHOICE QUESTIONS

1. Transformation, transduction and conjugation are the sexual modes of reproduction in bacteria True or false?

2. Binary fission is the common mode of reproduction in bacteria. True or false?

3. Which of the following bacteria reproduces by conidia?
   (a) *Staphylococcus* (b) *Streptomyces*
   (c) *Hyphomicrobium* (d) *Rhizobium*.
4. Which of the following bacterium reproduces asexually by budding?
   (a) *Hyphomicrobium* (b) *Streptomyces*
   (c) *Staphylococcus* (d) *Lactobacillus*.
5. All of the following pertain to asexual reproduction in bacteria, EXCEPT:
   (a) Binary fission
   (b) Endospores production or sporulation
   (c) Conidia formation
   (d) Budding.
6. Acquisition of naked DNA by a bacterial cell from its environment and incorporation in its genome is called:
   (a) Transformation (b) Transduction
   (c) Conjugation (d) Lysogenic conversion.
7. Transfer of a DNA segment from one bacterium to another bacterium by a bacteriophage is known as:
   (a) Translation (b) Conjugation
   (c) Transduction (d) Transformation.
8. Transfer of genetic material between donor and recipient bacteria through direct contact is known as:
   (a) Sexduction (b) Transformation
   (c) Transduction (d) Conjugation.

ANSWERS TO MCQs

1. False	2. True	3. (b)	4. (a)	5. (b)
6. (a)	7. (c)	8. (d).		

10
Growth and Nutrition of Microorganisms

Growth is an essential characteristic of living organisms. In everyday language, **growth** refers to an increase in size of an organism. We are accustomed of seeing children, other animals and plants growth.

Microbial growth is defined as a process of increase in the number of cells, cell size, cell mass and cell activity.

Bacterial growth refers to increase in cell number (i.e., population). Microbes that are growing and increasing in number, accumulating into **colonies** (groups of cells large enough to be seen with the naked eye) of hundreds of thousands of cells or **populations** of billions of cells.

HOW BACTERIAL GROWTH OCCURS?

Bacterial growth is the **asexual reproduction**, or cell division, of a bacterium into two daughter cells, in a process called **binary fission**.

In binary fission (also called **transverse fission**), one cell's division (i.e., fission cycle) produces 2 cells, two cell's divisions produce 4 cells, and so on. The initial parent stage consists of 1 cell, the **first generation** consists of **2** cells, the 2nd **4**, the 3rd **8** then **16**, **32**, **64** and so on (Fig. 10.1). With the passing of each generation, the population will double, over and over again as long as environmental conditions remain favourable. Growth is thus, by **geometric progression** that can be represented by numbers and the growth rate is **exponential**, i.e., the doubling of the population in a fixed interval of time. Under ideal conditions, one bacterium can multiply to generate 2,097,152 bacteria in just *seven* hours. After *one* more *hour* the number of bacteria will have risen to a colossal 16,777,216 (i.e., within 8 hours).

Bacteria growing on solid media form colonies, and their growth in liquid media (or broth) is diffuse.

Mathematical Expression of Growth. The mathematics of population growth in bacteria can be represented as follows:

Divisions		1st	2nd	3rd	4th	5th	6th
Number of cells	1	2	4	8	16	32	64
Number of generations**		1	2	3	4	5	6**
Exponential value*		2^1 (2×1)	2^2 (2×2)	2^3 $(2 \times 2 \times 2)$	2^4 $(2 \times 2 \times 2 \times 2)$	2^5 $(2 \times 2 \times 2 \times 2 \times 2)$	2^6 $(2 \times 2 \times 2 \times 2 \times 2 \times 2)$

* The exponent increases by *one* in each generation.

** The number of exponent is also the number of the generation.

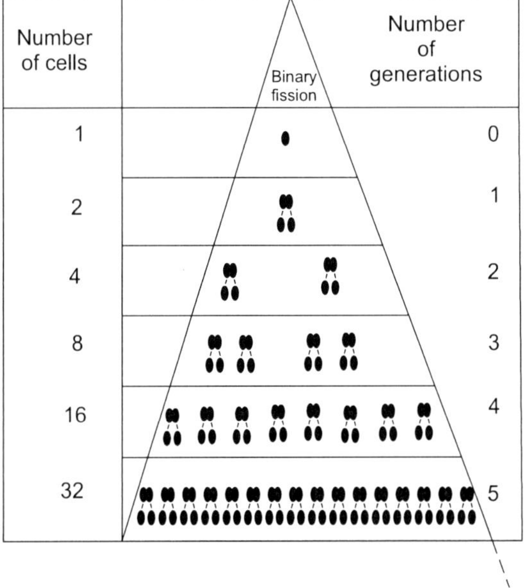

Fig. 10.1 Bacterial replication by binary fission. Starting with a single cell, the population doubles with each new division cycle or generation.

Generation Time or Doubling Time

During the binary fission, the formation of two new daughter cells from a *parent* (or *mother*) cell is known as a **generation** and the time required for a complete fission cycle is called the **generation time** or **doubling time**. The doubling occurs in the log phase of the cycle. The species which have rapid growth rate have the shortest generation time (5–10 minutes) and others which have a very slow growth rate have the longest generation time that ranges from several hours to even days. For example:

• The coli bacilli divide	every 15–20 minutes
• The salmonellae of enteric fever	every 23 minutes
• Pathogenic streptococci	every 30 minutes
• Diptheria bacilli	every 34 minutes
• Tubercle bacilli	every 18 hours
• Leprae bacilli	every 10-30 days.

Growth (or reproduction) in bacteria by binary fission lends certain immortality to a cell because there is never a moment in which first bacterium has died. Bacteria mature, undergo binary fission, and one young organism comes into existence. In other words, *the original bacterium, though millions of years old, is still among us.*

Measurement of Bacterial Growth

In the laboratory, bacterial growth can be seen in the three main forms:

- By the development of **colonies**, the macroscopic product of 20-30 cell divisions of a single cell.
- By the transformation of a clear growth medium (broth) to **turbid suspension** of $10^7 – 10^9$ cells per mL.
- In **biofilm** formation, in which growth is spread thinly (300-400 μm thick) over an inert surface and nutrition obtained from a bathing surface.

Bacterial Counts

Methods commonly used for counting bacteria in a culture medium or clinical specimen are:

- *Direct microscopic counts.* This is done by counting the number of bacteria microscopically in a measured volume of liquid using **counting chambers** (special glass slides) such as **Petroff–Hausser** counting chamber and haemocytometer. This gives the total number of bacteria present in the sample irrespective of whether they are alive or dead.
- *Observing* or *measuring turbidity.*
- *Total cell count* or *viable cell count*: This is done by serial dilutions plate count technique. In this, successive 1:10 dilutions of a liquid bacterial culture are made and transferred onto an **agar plate,** the colonies that arise are counted. Colonies are expressed as *colony-forming units* (*CFUs*), each representing one cell. This method measures only viable (living) bacterial cells.

BACTERIAL GROWTH CURVE (OR PHASES OF BACTERIAL GROWTH)

The characteristic growth curve in bacteria is a **sigmoid curve** which reflects the four phases of growth, in other words, the events in bacterial population, when they are grown in a closed system of microbial culture of fixed volume (i.e., **batch culture**). This curve shows four major phases of growth: the **lag, log, stationary** and **death** phase (Fig. 10.2).

1. **Lag phase:** In this phase, there is **no cell division** and no increase in cell numbers (i.e., population), hence called the **lag phase**. The bacterium adapts to new environment and makes necessary enzymes and intermediates for multiplication to proceed. The time varies from 1 to 4 hours, but the average time of this phase is 2 hours.

2. **Log (logarithmic) or exponential phase:** This phase is characterized by **cell doubling**, bacterial numbers increase **exponentially** or at *logarithmic rate* with a constant generative time, hence *the curve with a constantly increasing slope* (Fig. 10.2). Log phase is used to calculate both the number of generations and the generation time. The average time of this phase is 8 hours. Primary metabolites like amino acids and organic acids major to microbe's function are produced in this phase.

3. **Stationary phase:** The cell division stops due to depletion of nutrients and accumulation of toxic products. Eventually, growth slows down, and the total bacterial population reaches a maxium and stabilizes. The number of new cells produced equals the number of cells dying, thus this phase for a period of time is in a *static condition*, hence called the *stationary phase* of the growth curve, hence it is *horizontal*. The duration of this phase ranges from a few days to a few hours.

   Secondary metabolites like antibiotics and toxins are produced in this phase.

4. **Decline (or death) phage:** This phase is characterized by the *logarithmic decrease in the number of bacterial cells* due to their death. The rate of death exceeds the rate of reproduction, resulting in the decline of viable cells. Autolysis, besides nutrition depletion and build-up of toxic wastes may be the cause of death.

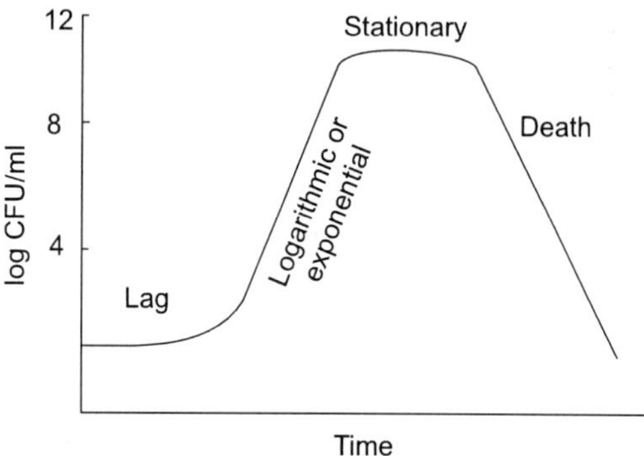

Fig. 10.2 Bacterial growth curve (the graphic representation of the change in bacterial numbers over time) showing the lag, exponential, stationary and death phases of the population.

BACTERIAL NUTRITION

Microbial nutrition (L. *nutrire* = nourishment) is the process of absorbing nutrients from the environment for use in metabolism and growth by a microorganism. Any chemical substance that can be used by a microbe for its growth is called a **nutrient**.

Substances required for survival are called **essential nutrients**. Essential nutrients are of two types:

- **Macronutrients.** Required in large quantities (e.g., proteins, carbohydrates, and other molecules that contain carbon, hydrogen and oxygen).
- **Micronutrients** or **trace elements.** Required in small amounts or traces (e.g., manganese, zinc, copper and nickel).

On the basis of carbon content, the nutrients are classified as: inorganic or organic.

- **Inorganic nutrients.** Atoms or simple molecules that are combination of atoms other than carbon and hydrogen (e.g., ferric nitrate, magnesium sulphate, O_2, CO_2, H_2O).
- **Organic nutrients.** Made up of carbon and hydrogen atoms usually products of living things (e.g., carbohydrates, proteins, lipids, nucleic acids, etc.). Organic nutrients such as amino acids and vitamins that cannot be sythesized and must be provided to promote growth is called a *growth factor*.

Although the basic building blocks required for growth are the same for all cells, bacteria vary widely in their ability to different sources of these molecules. Bacterial growth depends upon an adequate supply of suitable nutrients.

HOW MICROORGANISMS FEED OR NUTRITIONAL CATEGORIES OF MICROORGANISMS

Bacteria are categorized into two basic groups according to how they meet their nutritional needs:

1. **Autotrophy** (Gr. *auto* = self + *troph* = to feed). *"Self-feeding"* is the use of CO_2 as a source of carbon atoms for the synthesis of biomolecules. If the energy needs are met by sunlight, the organism is a *photoautotroph* (e.g., *Chlorobium*), but if it extracts energy from inorganic molecules, it is a *chemoautotroph* (e.g., *Alcaligenes, Nitrosomonas*).
2. **Hetrotrophy** (Gr. *hetero* = other + *troph* = to feed). *"Other feeding"* is the process of intake of nutrition from other sources of organic carbon (i.e., organic compounds) for the synthesis of biomolecules. The heterotrophic organisms cannot produce their own food, hence rely on others for their nutrition. Over 95% of living organisms are heterotrophic. Animals, including humans, are classified as heterotrophs by ingestion, fungi are classified as heterotrophs by absorption. These are mainly of two types:
    - **Saprobe** (or saprophyte). A microbe that feeds upon dead organic matter.
    - **Parasite.** A microbe that feeds from a live host. The disease causing parasites are called *pathogens*.

Classification of microorganisms based on their mode of nutrition, i.e., sources of carbon and energy, are summarized in Table 10.1.

Table 10.1 Nutritional categories of microbes by carbon and energy source

Category	Carbon source	Energy source	Examples
• **Autotrophy**	CO_2	**Nonliving environment**	
Photoautotroph	CO_2	Sunlight	Photosynthetic organisms, such as algae, plants, cyanobacteria
Chemoautotroph	CO_2	Simple inorganic chemicals	Only certain bacteria, such as methanogens, vent bacteria

Contd.

Table 10.1 Contd.

• **Heterotrophy**	**Organic**	**Other organisms or sunlight**	
Photoheterotroph	Organic	Sunlight	Nonsulphur bacteria
Chemoheterotroph	Organic	Metabolic conversion of the nutrients from other organisms	Protozoa, fungi, many bacteria, animals
• Saprobe	Organic	Metabolizing the organic matter of dead organisms	Fungi, bacteria (decomposers)
• Parasite	Organic	Utilizing the tissues, fluids of a live host	Various parasites and pathogens; can be bacteria, fungi, protozoa, animals

FACTORS AFFECTING BACTERIAL GROWTH

Temperature

Temperature is the most important physical factor affecting bacterial growth. An organism exhibits *optimum, minimum,* and *maximum temperatures.* Based on their growth temperature, bacteria can be classified into three categories:

- *Psychrophiles*—which grow at low temperature < 15°C and continue to grow even at 0°C.
- *Mesophiles*—which grow from 10°C to 50°C, best between 20 and 40°C.
- *Thermophiles*—which grow at high temperatures, between 45 and 80°C.

For most of the human pathogenic bacteria, optimum temperature for growth is 37° C (i.e., equal to human's body temperature) with upper and lower temperature limits of 40–50°C and 15–20°C, respectively.

SOLUTE AND WATER AVAILABILITY/OSMOTIC PRESSURE

Actively metabolizing bacteria require some water in their environment. Availability of water (moisture) affects bacterial growth. Water can be drawn into or out of cells according to the relative osmotic pressure created by dissolved substances in the cell and environment. Based on the salt (NaCl) requirement, bacteria can be categorized as:

1. ***Halophiles***—'Salt lovers'- require moderate to large amount of salt for their growth (e.g., *Halobacteria*). Halophiles are of three types:
   - *Mild halophiles*—require 1–6 % salt
   - *Moderate halophiles*—require 6–15 % salt
   - *Extreme halophiles*—require 15–30 % salt.
2. ***Halotolerant***—Grow best in the absence of NaCl, however, can grow at moderate salt concentrations (e.g., cyanobacteria).
3. ***Osmophiles***—Grow in environments of high sugar (e.g., *Enterobacter aerogenes, Micrococcus*).

DRYING/DESICCATION

Microorganisms which thrive in dry environments, i.e., lacking in water are called *xerophiles* (e.g. *Trichosporonoids*). On the other hand, some are not able to grow and survive. For example, *Treponema pallidum*, gonococci and human immunodeficiency virus (HIV) die quickly after drying while tubercle bacilli and staphylococci may survive drying for several weeks.

Bacterial taxa producing endospores (e.g., *Bacillus*) can survive even for thousand years.

Drying in cold and vacuum (*lyophilization*) is used as a method for preservation of bacteria and viruses.

OXYGEN

The quantity of oxygen (O_2) in the environment profoundly affects the growth of bacteria. Based on the O_2 requirement, the bacteria are classified as:

1. **Aerobic bacteria**—Require O_2 for their growth.
   - *Obligate aerobes:* Grow only in the presence of O_2 (e.g., *Vibrio*).
   - *Facultative anaerobes:* An aerobe that prefers a small amount of oxygen but can also grow in the absence of O_2.
   - *Microaerophiles:* Must have only a small amount of oxygen to grow.
2. **Anaerobic bacteria—**Grow in the absence of O_2.
   - *Obligate (strict) anaerobes*—They are killed by free oxygen and can grow only in the absence of oxygen.

- *Aerotolerant anaerobes*—metabolize substances anaerobically but are not harmed by free oxygen.

3. pH
   - Microorganisms are very susceptible to changes in acidity (0-7 pH) and alkalinity (7–14 pH) of the surrounding medium. Optimum pH for most microbes ranges from 6 to 8.

     Acidophiles prefer low pH, and **alkalinophiles** prefer higher pH.

Most of the medically important bacteria can grow at neutral or slightly alkaline pH (7.2–7.6). Some bacteria like lactobacilli and *Vibrio cholerae* grow at acidic and alkaline pH, respectively.

CARBON DIOXIDE

Some bacteria, such as *Brucella abortus* requires extra CO_2 in the air for their growth, and others like pnenmococci and gonococci grow better in the air supplemented with 5–10% CO_2, these organisms are called **capnophiles**.

BAROMETRIC (HYDROSTATIC) PRESSURE

Barometric pressure also affects microbial growth. Some bacteria can withstand extreme **barometric pressures** in deep valleys in the ocean. Such organisms are called **barophiles**.

LIGHT AND OTHER RADIATIONS

Darkness provides a favourable condition for viability and growth, hence incubated under dark conditions during culturing.

Ultraviolet rays from direct sunlight or mercury lamp (254 nm) are *bactericidal*. Ionizing radiations also have a killing affect on bacteria.

NUTRITIONAL FACTORS

Nutritional factors play a very important role in bacterial growth. Bacteria differ in their requirement for essential nutrients or growth factors, their requirements are determined by the kind or number of its enzymes. Hence, microbes have different preferences for different substrates.

KEY POINTS

- Bacteria replicate (or reproduce) by **binary fission**.
- Growth curve graphs represent the state of microbial populations rather than individual microbes.

- Number of cells (CFU per millilitre) counted by the serial dilution plate technique are used to make growth curve.
- **Primary metabolites** (e.g., amino acids, ethanol) and **secondary metabolites** (e.g., antibiotics) are produced during exponental and stationary phases of growth, respectively.
- Bacteria are classified as **obligate aerobes**, **facultative anaerobes**, **obligate anaerobes**, **aeroloterant anaerobes** and **microaerophiles** based on their oxygen requirements.
- Based on temperature requirement, bacteria are classified as **mesophiles**, **thermophiles** and **psychrophiles**.
- Based on salt requirement, they are classified as **halophiles**, **halototerant** and **osmophiles**.
- **Autotrophy** and **heterotrophy** are used by bacteria to meet their nutritional requirements.

IMPORTANT QUESTIONS

1. Answer in brief:
   (a) Generation time or doubling time.
   (b) Colony forming units.
   (c) Secondary metabolites.
2. Write brief notes on:
   (a) Bacterial growth curve.
   (b) Nutritional categories of microorganisms.
   (c) Affect of temperature, oxygen and solute concentration on bacterial growth.

MULTIPLE-CHOICE QUESTIONS

1. Generally, bacterial cells divide by a process called:
   (a) Mitosis (b) Meiosis
   (c) Binary fission (d) Sporulation.
2. Bacterial growth is typically measured by increase in cell size. True or False?
3. In what phase of a typical bacterial growth curve rapid growth of a bacterium is obtained?
   (a) Lag phase (b) log phase
   (c) Stationary phase (d) Decline (death) phase.
4. The growth of a bacterial population follows a geometric progression. True or False?

5. In which of the following phases, antibiotics, a secondary metabolite, are produced during bacterial growth?
   (a) Lag phase (b) Log phase
   (c) Stationary phase (d) Decline phase.
6. Which phase of the bacterial growth curve shows reproduction rate equal to death rate?
   (a) Lag phase (b) log phase
   (c) Stationary phase (d) Decline phase.
7. In which phase of the bacterial growth curve, a logarithmic decrease in number of cells results?
   (a) Lag phase (b) Log phase
   (c) Stationary phase (d) Decline phase.
8. The generation time of *Escherichia coli* is
   (a) 2 minutes (b) 13 minutes
   (c) 20 minutes (d) 50 minutes.
9. Bacteria whose optimum temperature for growth is 37°C are called
   (a) Mesophiles (b) Thermophiles
   (c) Thermotolerant (d) Psychrophiles.
10. An organic nutrient essential to an organism's metabolism that cannot be synthesised by itself is termed a/an
    (a) Trace element (b) Growth factor
    (c) Essential nutrient (d) Micronutrient.
11. An obligate halophile requires high
    (a) pH (b) Temperature
    (c) Salt (d) Pressure.
12. A pathogen would most accurately be described as a:
    (a) Saprobe (b) Parasite
    (c) Symbiont (d) Commensal.

ANSWERS TO MCQs

1. (c) 2. False 3. (b) 4. True 5. (c)
6. (c) 7. (d) 8. (c) 9. (a) 10. (b)
11. (c) 12. (b).

11
Culture Media

Culture medium or **growth medium** (pl. **media**) is a nutrient substrate prepared for the culture or growth of microorganisms in the laboratory. Common culture media are composed of carbon, nitrogen and energy sources with an optimum pH (7.2 – 7.6) for their rapid growth.

A microbe that grows and multiplies in or on a culture medium is called a **culture**.

The original media used by **Louis Pasteur**, a microbiologist, were liquids such as urine or meat broth which were not suitable for getting isolated colonies. **Robert Koch,** the German bacteriologist, devised means of cultivating bacteria on solid media. He initially used **potato slices** followed by **gelatin** (2.5 – 5%) and then **agar** as a solidifying agent which is still in use today. Use of **agar** (also called agar agar), as a solidifying agent for media at the suggestion of **Anglina Hesse**, the American wife of Koch's assistant.

All organisms require six biomolecules: carbon, hydrogen, oxygen, nitrogen, phosphorus and sulphur to grow and reproduce. Nutritional requirements of microbes vary from a few very simple inorganic compounds to a complex list of specific inorganic and organic compounds. At least 500 different types of media are used in culturing and identifying microorganisms.

IMPORTANT INGREDIENTS FOR MEDIA

AGAR

The word agar is derived from **agar-agar**, the Malay name for red algae (*Gracilaria, Gelidium*), the source of its production. Agar is a gelatinous substance, a mixture of two polysaccharides (carbohydrates): Agarose (70%) and agropectin (30%).

It is used as a solidifying agent in culture media since 1882. It has the following features:

- It liquefies on heating at 85°C (180°F).
- It forms a gel (solidify) when cooled to below 45°C (113°F).

- It does not provide any nutrition to bacteria.
- It is not metabolized by any pathogenic bacteria.
- At a concentration of 1 – 2% it yields a suitable gel.

PEPTONE

Peptone is an important ingredient of common culture media. It is derived from meat or milk in which protein is partially digested with the proteolytic enzymes like pepsin, trysin or papain. The major constituents of peptone are: peptides, polypeptides and amino acids. It provides nitrogenous nutrient for the microbes to grow and also acts as a buffer. One per cent peptone can be used for culturing several bacteria.

Other common ingredients of culture media include: casein hydrolysate, yeast extract, meat extract, malt extract, blood and serum.

BACTERIAL GROWTH ON MEDIA

Bacteria grow diffusely in liquid media (broths), and produce discrete visible growth on **agar plates** (Petri plate having solidified agar media). Bacteria have distinct colony morphology and exhibit distinct features such as haemolysis and pigment production which are useful for identifying bacteria.

Solid agar media are used to identify bacteria by studying the colony character, and to purify from the mixed culture of bacteria to get pure, isolated cultures.

TYPES OF CULTURE MEDIA

Culture media have been classified in three ways (Table 11.1).

- Physical form (medium's normal consistency)
- Chemical composition (types of chemicals used)
- Special media (functional type or used for specific purposes)

Table 11.1 Classification of culture media

A. Based on physical form (consistency)
1. Liquid media (or broths)
2. Solid media (agar media)
3. Semisolid media

Contd.

Table 11.1 Contd.

B. Based on chemical composition
1. Simple media (or basal media)
2. Complex media
3. Synthetic or defined media
C. Special media
1. Enriched media
2. Selective media
3. Differential media (or indicator media)
4. Transport media
5. Anaerobic growth media
6. Carbohydrate (sugar) fermentation media
7. Enumeration media
8. Assay media

ROUTINE LABORATORY MEDIA

1. **Basal Media (General-Purpose Media):** Basal media are basically simple media made up of basic nutrients and are used for growth or culture of non-fastidious bacteria that do not need enrichment. These media are generally used as the base for preparing enriched media, hence are called **basal media**. These are generally used for the primary isolation of bacteria.

   Examples: Nutrient broth, nutrient agar and peptone water. *Staphylococus* and members of *Enterobacteriaccae* grow in these media.

2. **Enriched Media:** These media are enriched by adding blood, serum or egg to the constituents of basal media to encourage the growth of a particular microorganism in a mixed culture. Examples of enriched media are:

   - Blood agar—for induction of streptococci.
   - Chocolate agar—for isolation of *Haemophlus*.
   - Bordet-Gengon—for isolation of *Bordetella*.

3. **Selective Media:** These media allow the growth of only the desired microbes by inhibiting the growth of unwanted organisms with salts, dyes or other chemicals. Hence, are used to isolate specific bacteria from specimens where mixed bacterial flora is expected. Examples include:

- Mannitol salt agar—for *Escherichia coli.*
- MacConkey agar—for *Escherichia coli.*
- Lowenstein - Jensen for *Mycobacterium tuberculosis.*
- Blood tellurite agar for *Corynebacterium.*
- Doxychocolate agar (DCA) for *Salmonella* and *Shigella.*

4. **Indicator (Differential) Media:** Differential medium contains an indicator which would produce a visible change in the medium following the growth of a particular bacterium. These media are used for differentiation of bacteria by using different indicators. Examples include.
   - MacConkey agar*:* Neutral red is used as an indicator in the MCA. Used to differentiate lactose fermenters (LF) which produce pink or red colonies and non-lactose fermenters (NLF) due to neutral red indicator: For example, *E. coli* which is a LF, produces red or pink colonies on MCA, *Salmonella, Shigella* and *Vibrio* produce colourless colonies on MCA, hence are NLF.
   - Blood agar: Enriched media like **blood agar** can also act as differential medium on the basis of certain characteristics evident on the medium. Blood acts both as an enrichment material and also as an indicator and used to differentiate bacteria based on whether they are α-, β- or γ-hemolytic (i.e., produce clear zones around the colonies because of the destruction of red blood cells). Blood agar medium is an example of *enriched and differential medium.*
   - EMB (Eosin - methylene blue) agar – is a *selective and differential medium* for enteric Gram-negative rods. On this medium lactose-fermenting colonies are pigmented and non-lactose-fermenting colonies are nonpigmented.
5. **Transport or Holding Media:** A **transport medium** is a holding medium designed to preserve the viability of microorganisms in the specimen without allowing their multiplication. These media are used when clinical specimen cannot be cultured soon after collection and transported from hospital to the laboratory for identification. These media typically contain only buffers and salts and lack carbon, nitrogen and organic factors. Examples include:
   - Ames medium—used for gonococci.
   - Cary-Blair medium—used for faeces that may contain *Salmonella, Shigella, Vibrio* or *Campylobacteria.*
6. **Sugar or Fermenting Media:** These indicator media are used to study "**sugar fermentation**" a parameter used to identify

bacteria based on their fermenting ability to ferment a specific sugar (e.g., lactose, glucose, mannitol) at the rate of 1 per cent). Sugar is added to peptone water containing *Ardrade's indicator*. Durham tube is placed in the medium which is initially colourless, and production of red colour indicates acid production. Gas, if produced, collects in the Durham tube. Production of acid or gas or both is used as a characteristic of identification.

7. **Anaerobic Growth Media: Anaerobic growth media** (also called **reducing media**) contain reducing substances (e.g., thioglycolic acid, cystine) that absorb molecular oxygen (O_2) and permit the growth of strict (obligate) anaerobic bacteria such as clostridia. Examples include:
   - Thioglycolate broth.
   - Cooked meat broth.
8. **Assay Media:** These media are used to test the effectiveness of antimicrobial drugs, as in agar-diffusion assay. Müller-Hinton agar is used for antibiotic susceptibility test.
9. **Enumeration Media:** Culture media used to count the number of organisms in water, milk, food, soil, air and other samples are called **enumeration media**. These are used by food and environmental microbiologists.

KEY POINTS

- Most microorganisms can be cultured on culture media, however, some (e.g., obligate parasites) can be cultured only in living tissue.
- A **culture medium** is a nutrient prepartion used for the growth of microbes in a laboratory.
- Based on the *physical state*, the culture media are classified as liquid (broth), semisolid and solid.
- The cuture media in which exact chemical composition is known are called **synthetic culture media**.
- Enriched, selective, differential, transport, carbohydrate fermentation, reducing, assay and enumeration media are all examples of media designed for special purposes.
- Some media like blood agar can act both as a selective and differential media.

IMPORTANT QUESTIONS

1. Define a culture medium. Classify culture media with an example of each type.

2. Write short notes on:
   (a) Types of culture media.
   (b) Selective, differential and enriched media.

MULTIPLE-CHOICE QUESTIONS

1. Louis Pasteur was the first person to use solid culture media for culturing microbes. True or False?
2. Ames transport medium contains high levels of carbon and nitrogen. True or False?
3. The scientist credited with the first use of solid media for culturing bacteria:
   (a) Louis Pasteur (b) Robert Koch
   (c) Carolus Linnaeus (d) Robert Hooke.
4. Agar was suggested as a solidifying agent for culture media by:
   (a) Walter Hesse (b) Fanne Hesse
   (c) Richard Petri (d) Robert Koch.
5. When a substance is added to a solid medium which inhibits the growth of unwanted bacteria, this medium is called:
   (a) Differential medium (b) Selective medium
   (c) Enriched medium (d) All of the above.
6. MacConkey agar medium is an example of:
   (a) Enriched medium
   (b) Transport medium
   (c) Differential and selective medium
   (d) Selective medium.
7. Reducing media chemically remove CO_2 that might interfere with the growth of anaerobes. True or False?
8. Differential media are used to distinguish different organisms? True or False?
9. Peptone is derived from seaweeds which are partially digested with proteolytic enzymes. True or False?

ANSWERS TO MCQs

1. False	2. False	3. (b)	4. (b)	5. (b)
6. (c)	7. False	8. True	9. False.	

12

Culture Methods

WHAT IS A CULTURE?

In a clinical or microbiology laboratory indications for **culture** are isolation of bacteria in **pure culture**, that is, a population containing only one species. In other words, a population of cells arising from a single cell or spore. A single visible colony represents a pure culture or a single type of bacterium.

FIVE BASIC TECHNIQUES OF CULTURING A MICROBE

In nature, microorganisms including bacteria, never occur alone but usually grow in one of the following forms:

- **Pure culture** – Consists of a single culture of microbe.
- **Mixed culture** – Deliberately contains a mixture of more than one type of microbe.
- **Contaminated culture** – It contains both known and some unwanted, unidentified microorganisms.

But to work with microorganisms, a microbiologist needs a pure culture and thus essential to isolate a pure culture of microorganism.

Microbiologists use five basic techniques, called the **five I's**: inoculation, incubation, isolation, inspection and identification to manipulate, grow, examine and identify microorganisms in the laboratory.

- **Inoculation**—Placing of a sample of culture (i.e., seeding or inoculating) of a microbe into or upon a culture medium.
- **Incubation**—The keeping (incubating) the inoculated sample culture in a temperature controlled environment to encourage growth (i.e., in an incubator).
- **Isolation**—The separation of microbial cells to achieve a pure culture that contains only a single species of microbe.
- **Inspection**—Observing cultures macroscopically for their growth characteristics and microscopically for their morphological features.

Identification—After observing and recording distingushing morphological features of a bacterium, the culture is identified by means of biochemical, genetic and serological methods.

CULTURE METHODS

Different culture methods are required for culturing aerobic and anaerobic bacteria. The methods of aerobic bacterial culture **isolation,** i.e., separating one bacterium from another into a discrete mound called **colony** used in a clinical laboratory include streak plate, spread plate, aerobic pour-plate, lawn culture, stroke culture, stab culture, and shake culture. For the aerobic bacteria, incubation is done in an incubator under normal atmospheric conditions (37°C for most human pathogenic bacteria), 43°C for *Campylobacter*, 30°C for leptospires, 25–28°C for fungi. When prolonged incubation is needed as in tubercle bacilli, screw-capped bottles are used instead of test tubes or plates, to prevent drying of the medium.

CULTURING OF BACTERIA

The normal steps for subculturing a bacterial culture (Fig. 12.1) are: (i) flame the transfer loop until red hot and cooled in air briefly, (ii) uncap the tube, (iii) briefly flame the mouth of the tube, (iv) culture growth is picked up on the sterile loop and transferred to the fresh broth or agar slant, (v) reflame the inoculating loop and recap the culture tube. Microbial cells/conidia can also be transferred to the surface of agar plates. Essentially, the same protocol is followed for inoculating Petri plates except the plate is not flamed.

1. Streak Plate

The **streak plate** or **quadrant streaking method** is one of the most commonly employed methods of streaking a plate for obtaining a pure culture of a bacterium from clinical specimen. In the streak plate, an inoculum is taken with a sterile loop or needle, and a series of streaks are made in one area of the agar plate (Fig. 12.1). The loop is flamed, touched to the first streaked area, and a second series is made in a second area. Similarly, streaks are made in the third and fourth areas, resulting in the spread of different bacteria so that they can develop into discrete/separate colonies on incubation.

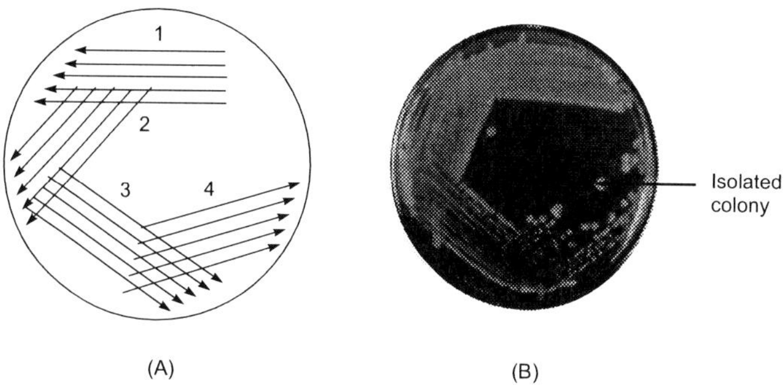

Fig. 12.1 **The streak plate method.** (A) Procedure for streaking an agar plate. Arrows indicate the direction of streaking. Streak series 1 is made from the original bacterial culture. The number of bacterial cells decreases with each series, resulting in well isolated colonies in series 4. (B) A streak plate of *Escherichia coli* on nutrient agar after 24 hours at 37°C.

2. Spread Plate

The **spread plate technique** (Fig. 12.2) is used for the separation of a dilute, mixed population of bacteria so that individual colonies can be isolated. In this method, a small volume (0.1 mL or less) of dilute microbial mixture containing around 30 to 300 cells is transferred to the centre of an agar plate and spread evenly over the surface with a sterile bent glass rod (i.e., glass spreader). The dispersed cells develop into isolated/discrete colonies on isolation.

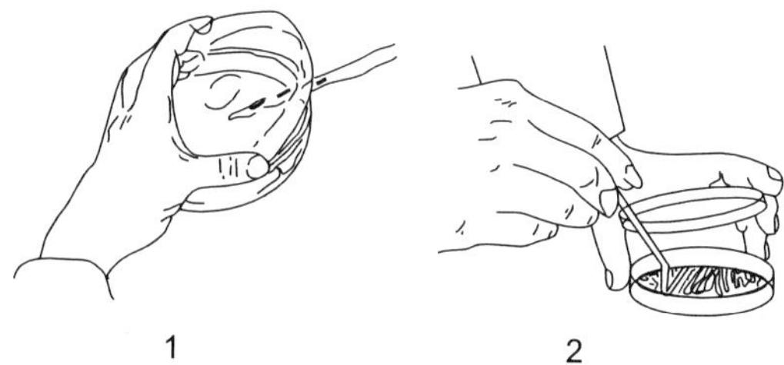

Fig. 12.2 Steps in a spread plate technique.

3. Pour Plate

The **pour plate method** is extensively used for the isolation of bacteria from water, milk and soil. In this method, the original sample is diluted in several tubes of melted agar medium which is to be maintained in a liquid state at a temperature of 45°C to allow thorough distribution of inoculum to reduce the microbial population sufficiently to obtain separate colonies on plating, and small volumes of several diluted samples are added to sterile plates. Liquefied agar, that has been cooled to 45°C, is then poured into the inoculated plates and thoroughly mixed by rotating the plate which is then allowed to solidify. On incubation for 24–48 hours, the bacteria form isolated colonies, where they have been diluted the most.

4. Lawn Culture

Lawn culture, also called **carpet culture**, is prepared by flooding the surface of an agar plate with a bacterial culture or suspension and pipetting off the excess suspension with a swab. Alternatively, the surface of the agar plate may be insulated by applying a swab soaked in the bacterial culture or suspension. On incubation, the bacterial colonies form a uniform growth on the surface and merge to form a field or mat of bacteria, hence termed **bacterial lawn**. This method is useful for antibiotic sensitivity testing and bacteriophage typing.

5. Stroke Culture (Slant Culture)

Stroke culture (also called **slant culture**) is made containing agar slope or slant. Slants are isolated (seeded) by slightly smearing the agar surface with charged loop in a zigzag pattern (not to cut the agar). It is used for providing pure culture of a bacterium for slide agglutination, storage of cultures and other diagnostic tests.

6. Liquid (or Broth) Culture

The desired bacteria are inoculated into a liquid nutrient medium, called **broth**, by touching with a charged loop or by adding the inocula with pipettes or syringes followed by the incubation for 24–48 hours at the desired temperature for the growth of the organism. This is used to grow up large amounts of bacteria for a variety of downstream application.

7. Stab Culture

In **stab culture**, a bacterium is introduced into a test tube containing solidified agar medium (nutrient gelation or glucose agar) via an inoculation needle (charged wire) or a pipette tip being stabbed into the centre of the agar and withdrawing it on the same line to avoid spilling the medium. Bacteria grow on the punctured area. Stab cultures are used for short-term storage, shipment of cultures and demonstration of gelatin liquefaction.

CULTURE OF ANAEROBIC BACTERIA

Exposure to atmospheric levels of *oxygen* is lethal to obligate anaerobes. It is because they lack both the enzyms: **superoxide dismutase** and **catalase** that would convert the lethal superoxide (O^{2-}) formed in their cells due to the presence of oxygen. Death of obligate anaerobes is not by gaseous oxygen but by the toxic superoxide. Hence, they live only in an anaerobic environment (e.g., *Bacteroides* and *Clostridium* species).

Obligate anaerobic bacteria can live and grow only in the absence of oxygen. They are destroyed or killed when exposed to the atmosphere for as briefly as 10 minutes Their culturing in the laboratory is based on to reduce the O^2 content of culture medium and remove any oxygen present inside the system or in the medium by chemical or biological means.

Some of the commonly used techniques to create anaerobic conditions are:

1. **Pyrogallic Acid Technique:** This technique employs pyrogallic acid and sodium hydroxide for the absorption of oxygen thereby producing anaerobic environment in the container in which the microorganisms are incubated.
2. **Shake Culture Technique:** In the **shake culture technique**, the molten and cooled (45°C) nutrient agar is inoculated with loopful of a culture. The tube is shaken, cooled rapidly and incubated. Upon incubation, strict anaerobes will grow in the deeper portions of the culture, facultative anaerobes will be found throughout the preparation, and aerobic bacteria will grow at the surface.
3. **Anaerobic chamber** refers to a plastic anaerobic glove box that contains an atmosphere of hydrogen, carbon dioxide, and nitrogen. Culture media are placed within the chamber by means of an air lock, which can be evacuated and refilled with nitrogen. The media are placed within the main chamber from the air lock. The residual oxygen is removed with reaction to the hydrogen forming water. The water formation is aided by a **palladium** catalyst. The media can be inoculated within the chamber by means of glove ports and incubated within the chamber after rendering it oxygen free.

Pseudomonas aeruginosa, an aerobic bacterium that needs oxygen to grow, inoculated on a nutrient agar plate is kept inside the jar along with the experimental plates, and Methylene blue (MB), a biological indicator that is blue coloured in the oxidized form (i.e., in the presence of air or O_2) and changes to colourless (i.e., reduced leuco compound) in an anaerobic environment. MB is used as a chemical indicator to verify the anaerobic environment in jar.

The **Gas-pak** is now the method of choice for preparing anaerobic jar (Fig. 12.3). Gas Pak is commercially available as a disposable envelope containing chemicals which generate hydrogen and carbon dioxide on the addition of water.

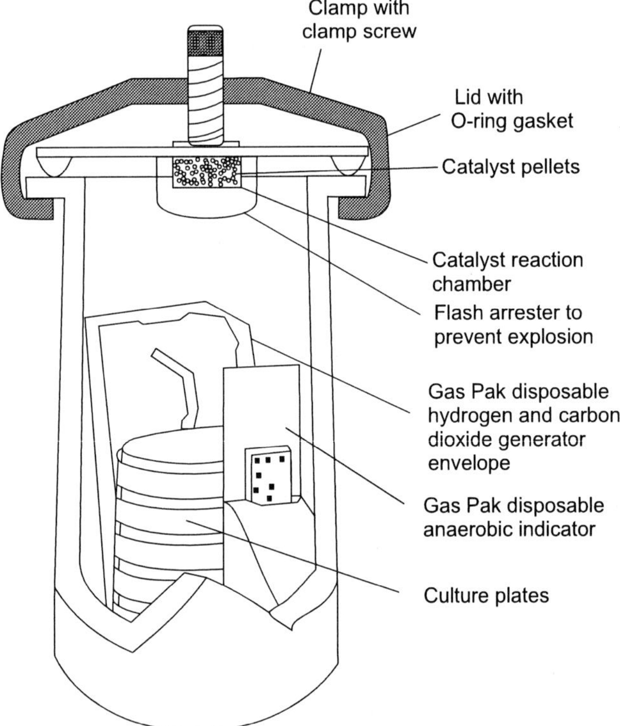

Fig. 12.3 Anaerobic jar with Gas-pak system. The hydrogen released from the generator combines with any oxygen to form water, thereby forming an anaerobic environment. Gas-pak system media are inoculated with anaerobic bacteria and then placed in the jar.

McIntosh Fildes' Anaerobic Jar

This instrument is used to culture anaerobic bacteria which die or fail to grow in presence of oxygen on solid agar media. **Anaerobiosis** (creation of anaerobic environment) by a catalyst (alumina pellets coated with palladium, i.e., **palladimized asbestos or alumina**) which in action uses oxygen forming water with the hydrogen. Hydrogen is pumped into to fill up the jar so that pressure inside equals atmospheric pressure. This is the most reliable and widely used anaerobic jar used in clinical laboratories to culture anaerobic bacteria from clinical specimens. The construction of McIntosh-Fildes' jar is a follows:

- It is a cylindrical tight jar about 20″ × 12.5″
- The body is made up of metal.
- The lid can be placed in an air-tight fashion.
- A screen going through a curved metal strip to secure and holding the lid in place.
- A thermometer to measure the internal temperature.
- A pressure gauge to measure the internal pressure.
- A side tube connected to a gas cylinder or a vacuum for evacuation and introductions of gases.
- A wire cage hanging from the lid to hold the catalyst.

KEY POINTS

- During isolation methods, cells are spread over a large area (**streak** and **spread plate**) or are diluted in a large volume **(pour plate)** so that individual cells are completely separated that grow into colonies.
- Microbial cultures are of three types: **pure**, **mixed** and **contaminated**.
- **Bacterial isolation** means getting of discrete separate colonies on an agar medium.
- Obligate anaerobes are killed not by gaseous oxygen but by a highly reactive and toxic form of oxygen called **superoxide** (O^{2-}).
- *Pseudomonas aeruginosa*, an aerobic bacterium; and methylene blue, an oxygen-sensitive dye; are used as indicators in the anaerobic jars to verify for the anaerobiosis.

IMPORTANT QUESTIONS

1. Answer in brief:
   (a) Meaning of five I's in microbiology.
   (b) Microbial culture.
2. Write short notes on:
   (a) Isolation of pure cultures of microorganisms/bacteria.
   (b) Anaerobic culture methods.

MULTIPLE-CHOICE QUESTIONS

1. Isolation is
   (a) Introduction of inoculum
   (b) Purification of culture
   (c) To grow microorganisms on surfaces
   (d) Separation of a single colony.
2. Diluting the mixed culture is a common step in all the three methods: the streak plate, the spread plate and the pour plate. True or False?
3. In bacterial aerobic culture methods, the agar medium should be maintained in a liquid state at:
   (a) 37°C (b) 45°C
   (c) 67°C (d) 0°C.
4. Obligate anaerobic bacteria usually lack the enzymes: the oxidative enzyme and catalase. True or False?
5. Which is *not* true for obligate anaerobes?
   (a) They are killed by superoxide (O^{2-}), toxic form of oxygen.
   (b) They lack the enzyme catalase that converts hydrogen peroxide (H_2O_2) to water and oxygen.
   (c) They are killed by the toxic effect of superoxide and hydrogen peroxide.
   (d) They are killed by gaseous oxygen.
6. Microaerophiles need a small amount of oxygen for their growth. True or False?
7. Palladinised alumina is used as a catalyst in the McIntos and Fildes' anaerobic jar that coverts water and oxygen to form water. True or False?
8. Which of the following organism is used as an indicator in an anaerobic jar to verify anaerobiosis?
   (a) *Clostridium perfringens*
   (b) *Saccharomyces cerevisiae*
   (c) *Neurospora sitophila*
   (d) *Pseudomonas aeruginosa*.

ANSWERS TO MCQs

1. (d) 2. False 3. (b) 4. False 5. (d)
6. True 7. True 8. (d).

13

Microscope and Microscopy

MICROSCOPY

Microscopy is the science that studies microscope techniques for examining the morphology of cells, their organelles and direct examination of clinical specimens to identify/diagnose a disease. The word microscopy comes from Greek roots: *micros* = small + *skopos* = to look at or view, meaning to view small objects.

Two key characteristics of microscopy are:

- **Magnification**—It is the ability to enlarge small objects. Magnification depends on the objective and ocular lens combination used.
- **Resolving power or resolution**—The ability to distinguish two adjacent lines or points/structures apart. It is a measure of a microscope's capactiy to make clear image of very small objects. Resolution is improved with shorter wavelengths of illumination and with a higher numerical aperture of the lens. The human eye has a resolving power of 0.2 mm.

Both magnification and resolution are important if you want a clear picture of very tiny things.

UNITS OF MEASUREMENT

The standard unit of length is the *metre* (m). Microorganisms are measured in:

- *Micrometre* (μm) = 0.000001 m = 10^{-6} m – to measure microscopic organisms.
- *Nanometre* (nm) = 0.000000001 m = 10^{-9} m – to measure ultramicroscopic organisms.

Bacteria are measured in μm with an **ocular micrometer** (simply a glass disc with etched lines on its surface) that is calibrated with the **stage micrometer** (a special glass slide having in its centre a known distance, one mm). Measurement of microorganisms is called **micrometry**.

MICROSCOPE

A **microscope** is an instrument that magnifies objects otherwise too small to be seen with unaided eye, producing an image in which the object appears larger (or magnified). Most photographs of cells are taken using a microscope, and these are called **microphotographs**.

Based on the lens used, microscopes are of two types:

- **Simple microscope** — It consists of one lens as used by Anton van Leeuwenhoek to see animalcules.
- **Compound microscope** — It consists of multiple lenses.

TYPES OF MICROSCOPE OR MICROSCOPY

Microscopes used in a clinical or diagnostic laboratory are divided into two categories based on the source of illumination:

1. **Optical or light microscopy** - Refers to the use of any kind of microscope that uses visible light to observe specimens. It is of four types:
    - **Bright-field** - Uses visible light as a source of illumination.
    - **Dark-field** - Uses a special disc with an opaque disk that blocks the light from entering the lens directly, the specimen appears light against black background - the dark field.
    - **Phase-contrast** - Uses a special condenser containing an annular ring shaped diaphragm that increases the contrast of an image.
    - **Fluorescent** - Uses an ultraviolet source of illumination that causes fluorescent compounds (green colours) in a specimen to emit light. Fluorescence microscope is very useful to visualize pathogens in clinical specimens – within cells and tissues.
2. **Electron microscopy** - Electron microscopes (EMs) use electron not light waves as an illumination source to provide high magnification 5000× to 1,000,000×) at high resolution (0.5 nm). Instead of glass lenses, electromagnets control focus, illumination and magnification. Electrons have a much lower wavelength than light (1,00,000 times shorter).

    EMs are of two types:

    - **Transmission electron microscope (TEM)** - Analogous to bright-field microscope, is used to see thin sections of organisms to visualize internal details and cell ulltrastructure, magnifies objects 10,000 to 1,000,000× RP is 0.2 nm.
    - **Scanning electron microscope (SEM)** - Corresponds to dark-field microscope is used to see three-dimensional

image of cell and virus surface features. It magnifies objects to 1,00,000 ×, RP is 10 nm.

COMPARISON OF VARIOUS TYPES OF MICROSCOPY

Various types of microscopy, with the applications of each type, are summarized in Table 13.1.

Table 13.1 Comparison of various types of microscopy

Microscope	Maximum practical magnification	Resolution	Important features and uses
Source of illumination: visible light			
Bright-field	2000 ×	0.2 μm (200 nm)	Common multipurpose microscope used for live and preserved stained specimens; specimen is dark, field is white; provides fair cellular detail.
Dark-field	2000 ×	0.2 μm	Best for observing live, unstained specimens; specimen is bright, field is black; provides outline of specimen with reduced internal cellular detail.
Phase-contrast	2000 ×	0.2 μm	Used for live specimens; specimen is contrasted against grey background; excellent for internal cellular detail.
Differential interference	2000 ×	0.2 μm	Provides brightly coloured, highly contrasting, three-dimensional images of live specimens.
Source of illumination: ultraviolet rays			
Fluorescent	2000 ×	0.2 μm	Specimens stained with fluorescent dyes or combined with fluorescent antibodies emit visible light; specificity makes this microscope an excellent diagnostic tool.

Contd.

Table 13.1 Contd.

Source of illumination: electron beams			
Transmission electron microscope (TEM)	10,00,000 ×	0.2 nm	Sections of specimen are viewed under very high magnification; finest detailed structure of cells and virues is shown; used only on preserved material.
Scanning electron microscope (SEM)	1,00,000 ×	10 nm	Scans and magnifies external surface of specimen; produces striking three-dimensional image.

STUDENT LABORATORY MICROSCOPE – LIGHT MICROSCOPE

Most student microscopes are classified as **light microscopes**. In a **light microscope,** visible light passes through the object/specimen (the biological sample you are looking at) and is bent through the lens system, allowing the user to see a magnified image (Fig. 13.1). Students lab microscopes tend to be **bright-field microscopes** meaning that visible light is passed through the sample and used to form an image directly and the field of vision is **brightly illuminated**.

A benefit of light microscopy is that it can often be performed on living cells. These microscopes are used to examine clinical specimens and dividing cells carrying out their normal behaviours such as motility, movement and division to see the morphology, size and shape of cells of stained preparations.

Compound light microscope (Fig. 13.1) is a microscope with one ocular (called **monocular**) or two oculars (called **binocular**), four objective lenses, a mechanical stage, a condenser, an iris diaphragm and a built-in lamp (or provided with a mirror for sunlight). It has a series of lenses and uses visible light as a source of illumination. The principal parts with their functions and the pathway of light with the two stages in magnification of a compound microscope are illustrated in Fig. 13.1.

In this microscope, a series of lenses forms a clearly focussed image that is many times larger than the object itself. As light passes through the condenser, it forms a solid beam that is focussed on the specimen. Light leaving the specimen that enters the objective lens is refracted so

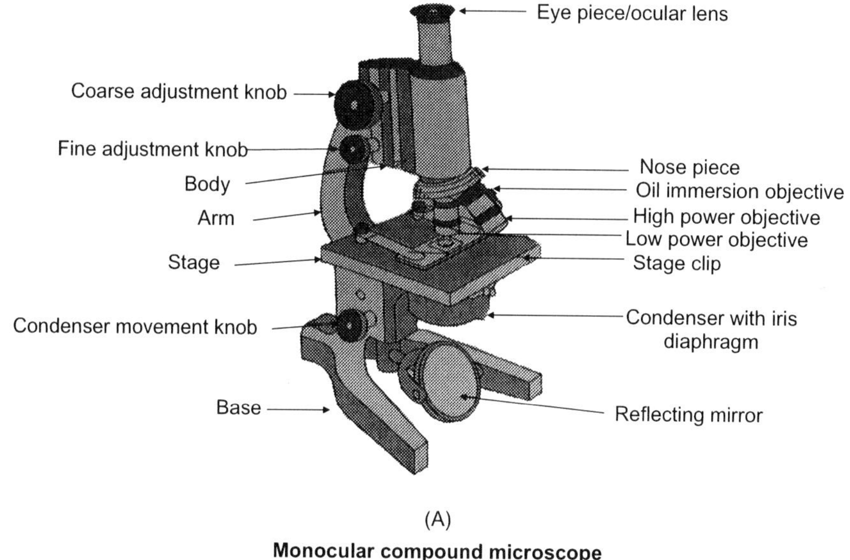

(A)

Monocular compound microscope

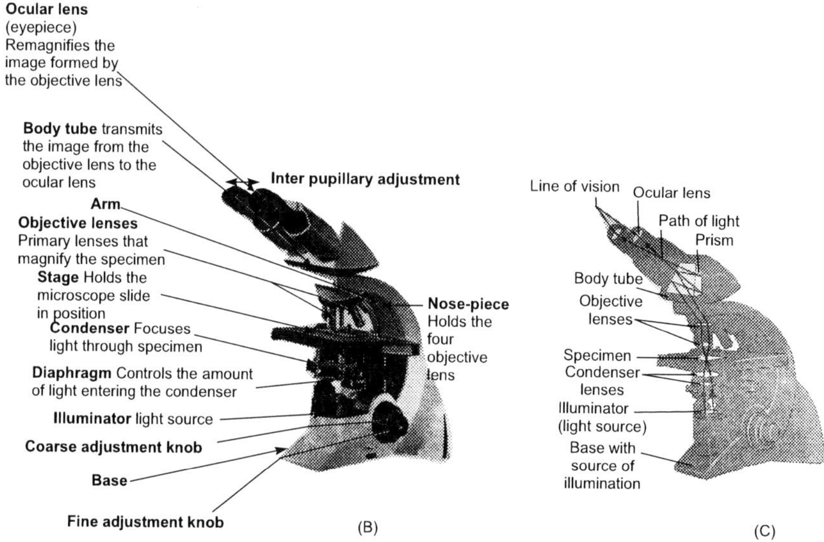

Binocular compound microscope

Fig. 13.1 Compound light microscope. (A and B) principal parts and their functions. (C) the pathway of light (bottom to top) with two stages of magnification enlarged primary image, the **real image** formed by the objective lens and the second image, the **virtual image** formed by the ocular lens.

that an enlarged primary image, the **real image** is formed. One does not see this image. The image is projected through the ocular lens and a second image, the **virtual image** is formed by a similar process. The virtual image is the final magnified image that is received by the retina and perceived by the brain (Fig. 13.1 C).

The total magnification of an object is calculated by multiplying the objective lens magnification (i.e., power) by the ocular lens magnification (power).

Power of objective × Power of ocular = Total magnification
10× (lower power objective) × 10× = 100×
40× (high power objective) × 10× = 400×
100× (oil immersion) × 10× = 1000×

Most of the compound microscopes can magnify an object 1000 times, however, some can achieve a total magnification of 2000× with the oil immersion lens.

Use of immersion oil (e.g., cedar wood oil, a natural oil) is necessary at magnifications greater than 900×. Because the refractive indexes of the glass microscope slide and immersion oil are the same, the light rays do not refract when passing from one to the other when an oil immersion objective lens is used. Use of immersion oil reduces light loss between the slide and the lens for clear visualisation of bacterial cells. Figure 13.2 shows the mode of refraction in the compound microscope using an oil immersion objective lens.

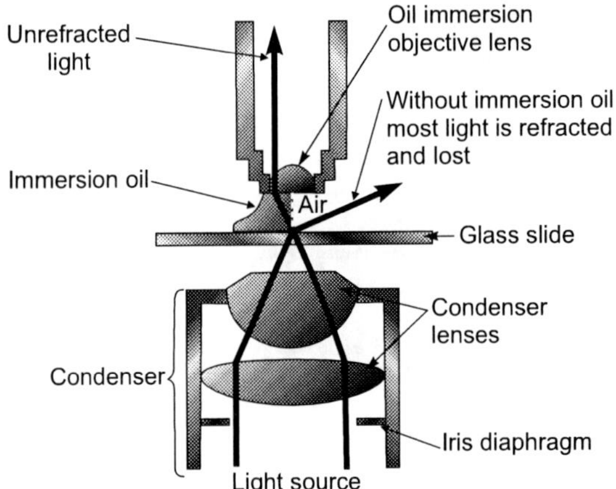

Fig. 13.2 Refraction in the compound microscope using an oil immersion objective lens.

Resolving power (RP) or **resolution,** the ability to distinguish two points, is a measure of a microscope's capacity to make clear images of very small objects. The maximum RP of a bright field compound microscope is 0.2 μm and the maximum magnification is 2000×.

KEY POINTS

- A **simple microscope** consists of a single magnifying lens, whereas a **compound microscope** has two lenses: the ocular (eye piece) lens and the objective lens.
- The most common microscope used in a microbiology or clinical laboratory is the compound light microscope.
- The **compound light microscope** uses visible light, whereas a beam of electrons is used with an **electron microscope**.
- The **total magnification** is the product of the ocular and objective magnifying powers.
- The maximum **resolving power** of a compound light microscope is 0.2 μm and the maximum magnification is 2000×.
- The **real image** and **virtual image** in a compound light microscope, are produced by objective lens and ocular lens, respectively.

IMPORTANT QUESTIONS

1. Write notes on:

(a) Microscopy and its types.

(b) Describe the principal parts and functions of a compound light microscope.

MULTIPLE-CHOICE QUESTIONS

1. In a compound light microscope, real image of an object is produced by:

(a) Ocular lens (b) Eye

(c) Objective lens (d) Condenser.

2. Resolution is the ability to distinguish two objects distinct and separate. True or False?

3. The maximum magnification of a compound light microscope ...... and a transmission electron microscope (TEM) is ......

4. A light microscope that has a total magnification of 1500× with the oil immersion lens has an ocular lens (eyepiece) of what power?

(a) 1.5 × (b) 15 ×

(c) 150 × (d) None of the above.

5. Resolving power of a light microscope is:
   (a) 1 angstron
   (b) 2 micrometre (µm)
   (c) 0.2 micrometre (µm)
   (d) 0.2 mm.
6. Which of the following is *not* a modification of a compound light microscope?
   (a) Fluorescence microscopy
   (b) Electron microscopy
   (c) Bright field microscopy
   (d) Darkfield microscopy.

ANSWERS TO MCQs

1. (c)
2. True
3. (2000 ×, 1,000,000 ×)
4. (b)
5. (c)
6. (b).

14

Staining and Hanging Drop Mount Techniques

WHAT IS STAINING?

Staining means colouring a microorganism with a dye to make structures more visible. **Stain-fixed** mounts are made by drying and heating a thin film of specimen called a **smear** which is used for microscopic examination. A smear is stained with one or more dyes to provide more detailed information on cells such as cell shape, size, arrangement, internal structures and chemical characteristics that are used for bacterial identification.

STAINS OR DYES

A **stain** or **dye** is a molecule that can bind to cellular structure and gives it colour. Most commonly used stains are of two types:

- **Basic (cationic) dyes**—These dyes carry a positive charge and stain bacterial cells because bacteria are negatively charged. This is the basis of positive staining.

  Examples: methylene blue, crystal violet, safranin and malachite green.

- **Acidic (anionic) dyes**—They bear a negative charge, the bacteria repel the dye and stain the background of a bacterial smear.

  Examples: eosin and picric acid.

KINDS OF STAINING TECHNIQUES

In microbiology, three kinds of staining techniques are used:

1. **Simple stain**—It uses just one dye (e.g., methylene blue) and is used to reveal cell morphology (cell shapes and arrangements).
2. **Differential stain**—Requires two or more stains, a primary dye and a contrasting counterstain to differentiate bacteria, useful in diagnosis of pathogenic bacteria.

   Examples: gram stain, acid fast stain and endospore stain.

3. **Special stains**—These are designed to bring out distintive characteristics to reveal the presence of endospores (endospore stain), capsule (negative stain), and flagella (flagella stain). Staining methods classification scheme with the application of each type is presented in Figure 14.1.

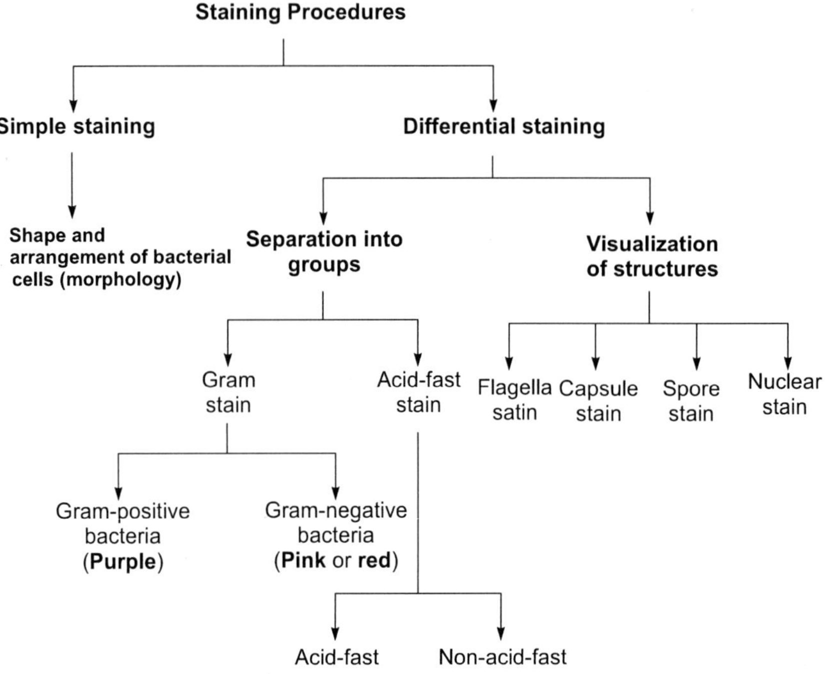

Fig. 14.1 Classification scheme for commonly used staining methods for bacteria.

SMEAR PREPARATION

A thin film of bacteria is called a **bacterial smear**. It is prepared (Figure 14.2) from the organisms growing in liquids (e.g., broths, milk, saliva, urine) and solid media (e.g., nutrient agar, blood agar), in addition to the clinical and food smaples onto a glass slide. A bacterial smear followed by staining is required particularly for the microscopic examination of the specimen or the culture for identifying of bacteria. The purpose of making the smear is to fix the specimen or the bacterial cells onto the glass slide so that it does not get washed during the staining procedure.

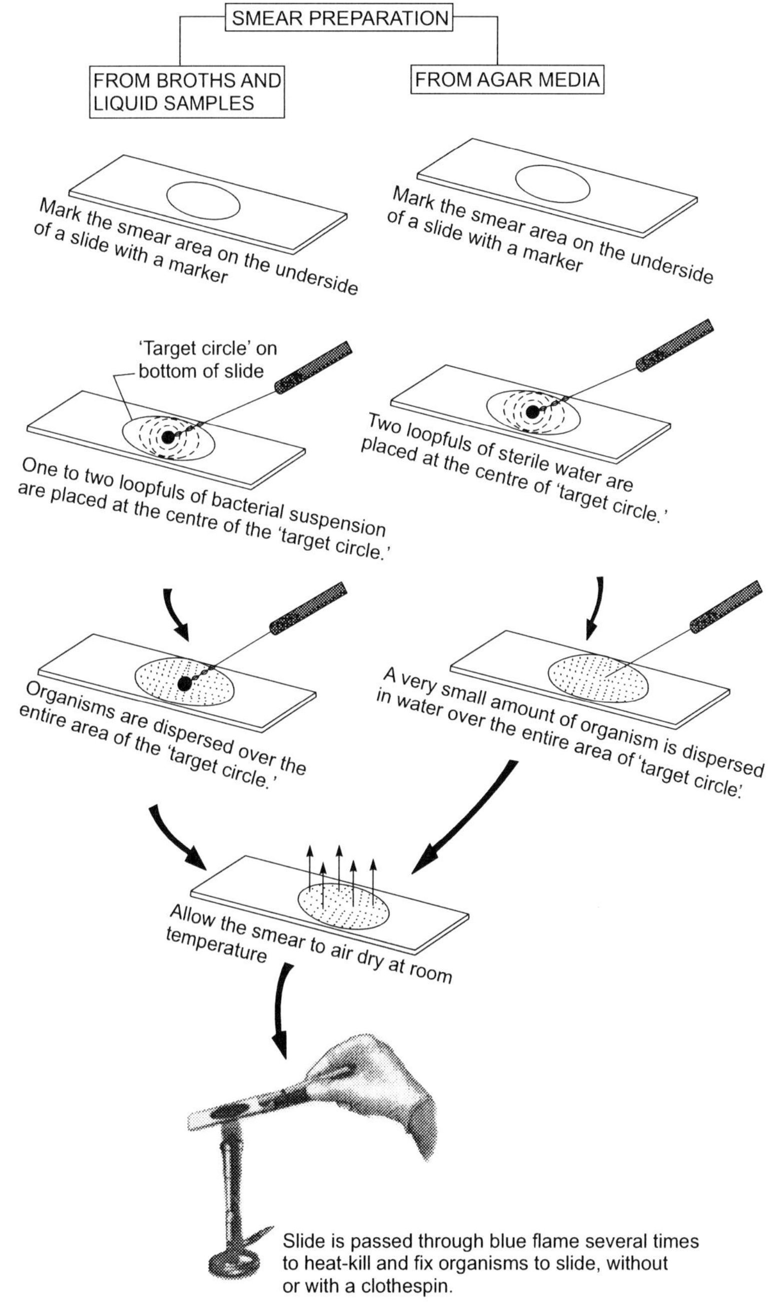

Fig. 14.2 Technique for bacterial smear preparation from solid media, liquid media and specimens.

A bacterial smear is prepared by transferring bacterial cells with a sterile inoculating loop from broth or agar media. If transferred from an agar plate, the cells are mixed thoroughly into a small drop of water on the slide to make a suspension to a glass slide. The bacterial suspension is spread thinly over an area about the size of 10 paise coin with the inoculating loop, followed by air drying at room temperature. This process, called *heat fixation*, accomplishes three things: kills the bacteria, causing them to adhere to the slide, and more.

The scheme of smear preparation is diagrammatically shown in the Figure 14.2.

GRAM STAINING

Gram stain or **Gram staining**, also called **Gram's method** (Figure 14.3), is the most important procedure in microbiology. It was developed by the Danish bacteriologist **Hans Christian Gram** in 1884. This method is used to distinguish and classify bacterial taxa into two large groups: Gram-positive and Gram-negative bacteria by colouring these cells, red or violet. The Gram stain is almost always the first step in the preliminary identification of a bacterial organism and is a valuable diagnostic tool in both clinical and research settings. Nearly all clinically important bacteria can be detected/visualized using Gram staining method, the only exception being: *Chlamydia, Mycoplasma* and spirochetes.

The Gram stain procedure uses a purple stain (crystal violet), iodine as a **mordant**, an alcohol **decolorizer**, and a red counterstain (safranin). Gram-positive bacteria retain the **purple** stain after the decolorization step; Gram-negative bacteria do not and thus appear **pink** from the counterstain. This difference is based on the composition of their cell wall: Gram-positive bacteria (e.g., *Staphylococcus, Bacillus, Clostridium*) have a thick layer of peptidoglycan 90% of the cell wall. Gram-negative bacteria (e.g., *Pseudomonas, Escherichia, Salmomella, Vibrio*) have a thin layer of peptidoglycan 10% of cell wall and high lipid content.

Difference in colour reaction in Gram-positive and Gram-negative: The higher amount of lipid present in Gram-negative bacteria is readily dissolved by C_2H_5OH resulting in the formation of large pores in the cell wall facilitating the leakage of **Crystal - violet - iodine (CV-I)** complex resulting in decolorization of the bacterium which later takes the counterstain and appears **pink** (or **red**).

In contrast, the Gram-positive cell walls, when treated with C_2H_5OH, results in dehydration and closure of cell wall pores, thereby not allowing the loss of CV-I complex and cells remain purple (Figure 14.3).

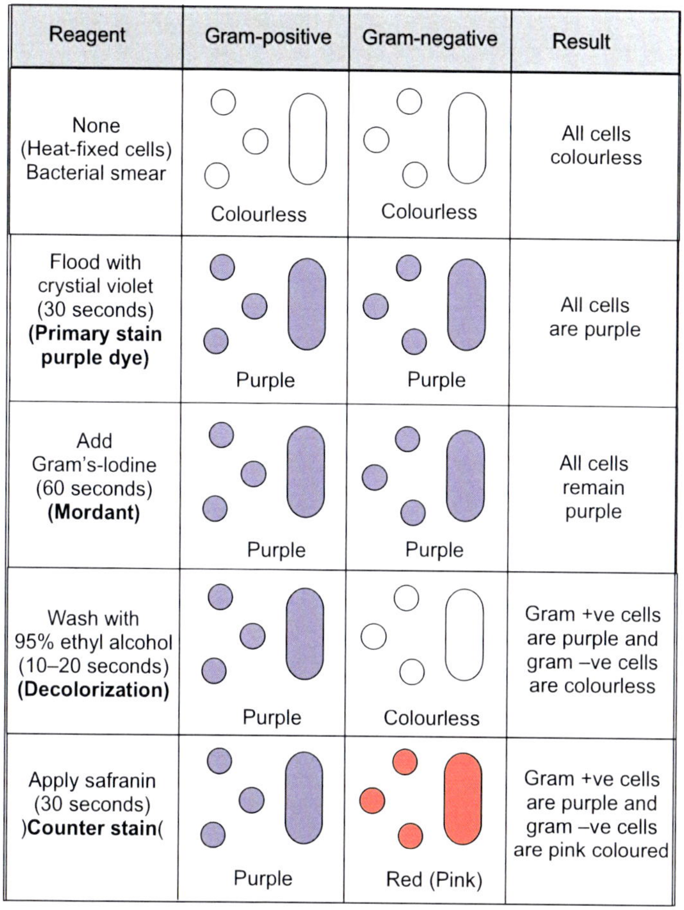

Reagent	Gram-positive	Gram-negative	Result
None (Heat-fixed cells) Bacterial smear	Colourless	Colourless	All cells colourless
Flood with crystial violet (30 seconds) **(Primary stain purple dye)**	Purple	Purple	All cells are purple
Add Gram's-Iodine (60 seconds) **(Mordant)**	Purple	Purple	All cells remain purple
Wash with 95% ethyl alcohol (10–20 seconds) **(Decolorization)**	Purple	Colourless	Gram +ve cells are purple and gram –ve cells are colourless
Apply safranin (30 seconds) **)Counter stain(**	Purple	Red (Pink)	Gram +ve cells are purple and gram –ve cells are pink coloured

Fig. 14.3 Procedure of Gram staining.

ACID - FAST STAINING

Acid-fast stain was initially developed in 1882 by **Paul Ehrlich**, a German physician. **Franz Jiehl** and **Friedrich Neelsen** independently modified the original method, hence it is called **Ziehl Neelsen acid-fast** staining method.

Acid-fast stain is an important diagnostic tool used to diagnose tuberculosis (TB) and leprosy caused by mycobacteria and infections cauused by *Nocardia* in a sample of blood, sputum, urine, stool, bone marrow and skin tissue.

Carbolfuchsin, an acid-fast stain, binds strongly to bacteria that have a waxy material called **mycolic acids** present in their cell wall and appear red or pink after acid-alcohol decolorization, hence are said to be acid-fast organisms (e.g., *Mycobacterium* and *Nocardia*). **Non-acid-fasts** lose this stain and take up the methylene blue counterstain and appear blue.

In acid-fast staining, bacterial smear is treated with the staining dye, carbol fuchsin, over boiling water for 5 minutes, followed by heat fixing and washing with acid alcohol (15-20 minutes) and finally counterstaining with methylene blue (30 seconds). Acid-fast bacteria show red cells and non-acid-fast reveal blue cells.

WET MOUNTS AND HANGING DROP MOUNTS

Live samples of microorganisms are placed in wet mounts or hanging drop mounts (Fig. 14.4), so that they can be observed as near to their natural state as possible. The cells are suspended in a suitable fluid (sterile water, broth or saline) that temporarily maintains viability and provides space and a medium for locomotion. These mount permits examination of the characteristics of live cells such as motility, shape and arrangement, as heating required for staining methods can alter these characteristics.

WET MOUNT

Wet mount is a microscopic technique in which a drop of fluid/ medium containing the living organisms is placed on a microscopic glass slide and covered with a cover glass. It allows the examination of live cells which is useful for evaluating their natural size, and shape in addition to their motility.

Wet mounts are also useful to observe fungi as they allow the observation of live cells, unstained cells especially spores (conidia), sporulating structures (sporangiophores, conidiophores) and hyphae (septate, aseptate), criteria used in their identification.

HANGING-DROP MOUNT

The hanging-drop technique is a special type of wet mount often used to observe flagella and motility in bacteria, a significant method in bacterial identification.

The hanging-drop technique (Fig. 14.4) is performed by placing a loopful of bacterial suspension on a coverslip, ringed with petroleum jelly, followed by inverting and placing over the well in a cavity (or depression) slide and observing it under the microscope, often with dark-field illumination. The bacteria are observed as a drop that is suspended under a cover glass in a concave depression slide.

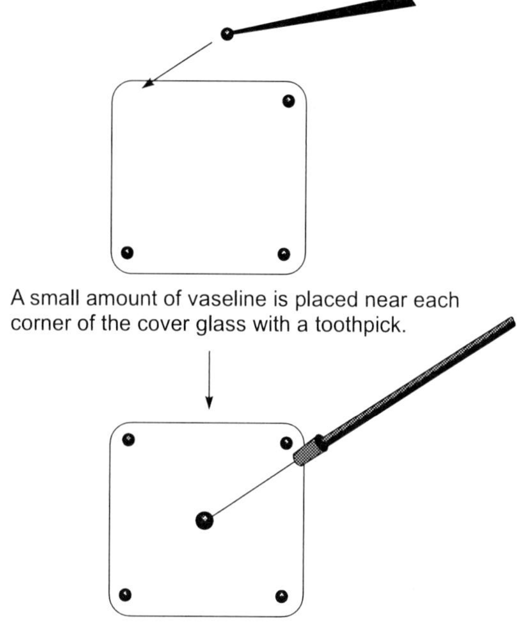

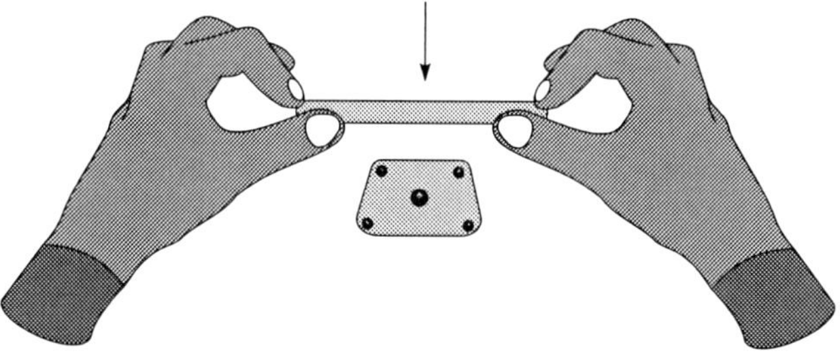

Depression slide is pressed against vaseline on cover glass and quickly inverted.

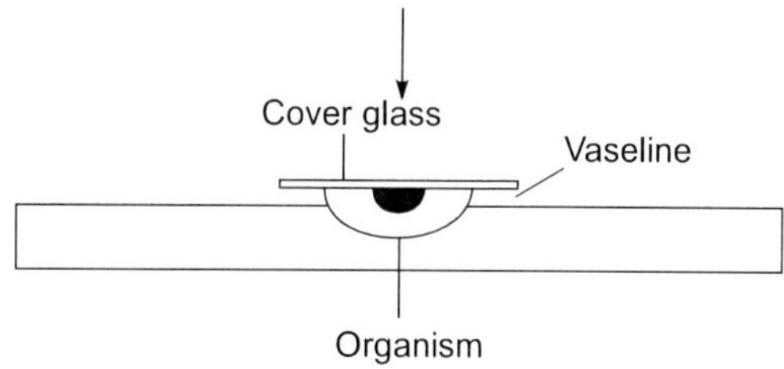

The completed preparation is examined under oil immersion.

Fig. 14.4 Procedure for the preparation of hanging drop mount.

KEY POINTS

- **Staining** means colouring a microorganism with a dye (stain) to make cell structures more visible.
- A **smear** is a thin film of material used for microscopic examination.
- **Fixing** uses heat or alcohol to kill and attach microorganisms to a slide.
- Bacteria are negatively charged, and coloured positive ion of a basic dye stain bacteria cells.
- Gram-positive bacteria retain the colour of the primary stain, hence appear **purple** and Gram-negative bacteria do not hence appear **pink** (or **red**) from the counterstain.
- **Acid-fast bacteria** (e.g., *Mycobacterium* and *Nocardia*) retain the carbol fuchsin and appear red, and non-acid fasts take up the colour of counterstain and appear blue.
- **Wet mounts** or **hanging drop mounts** permit examination of the characteristics of live cells.

IMPORTANT QUESTIONS

1. Write notes on:
   (a) Gram staining
   (b) Acid-fast staining
   (c) Hanging-drop mounts.

MULTIPLE-CHOICE QUESTIONS

1. Bacteria tend to stain more readily with cationic (positively charged) dyes because:
   (a) Bacterial surfaces are negatively charged
   (b) Bacterial surfaces are positively charged
   (c) Are neutral
   (d) Have thick walls.
2. Live samples of microbes are observed by:
   (a) Smear technique (b) Hanging-drop mounts
   (c) Gram stain (d) All of the above.
3. Acid-fast staining technique was initially developed in 1882 by:
   (a) Hans Christian Gram (b) Niehl-Neelsen
   (c) Paul Ehrlich (d) Robert Koch.

4. The stain used to classify bacteria based on their cell wall contents belong to:

(a) Negative stain (b) Gram stain

(c) Endospore stain (d) Simple stain.

5. The stain used frequently to identify mycobacteria whose cell walls contain high amount of lipid is:

(a) Malachite green (b) Capsular stain

(c) Acid-fast stain (d) Negative stain.

6. The function of heat fixation in a bacterial smear is:

(a) Causes bacteria to adhere to the slide

(b) Causes bacteria to shrink and adhere to the slide

(c) Causes bacteria to adhere to the slide, kills them and makes them to accept the stain more readily

(d) More quickly dries the specimen.

7. In Gram stain, Gram-positive bacteria appear pink and Gram - negative bacteria appear violet. True or False?

ANSWERS TO MCQs

1. (a) 2. (b) 3. (c) 4. (b) 5. (c)
6. (c) 7. False.

15

Bacterial Classification/Taxonomy

WHAT IS TAXONOMY?

The science of classification, especially the classification of living forms, is called **taxonomy** (*taxis* from the Greek for orderly arrangement). It provides an orderly basis for the naming of organisms and for placing organisms into a category, rank or level. Each category is called a **taxon** (pl: **taxa**).

Microbial taxonomy is concerned with:

- to establish the criteria for identifying microorganisms;
- to arrange related organisms into groups based on their mutual similarity (genetic or phenotypic); and
- to provide important information on how organisms evolved (called **phylogeny** or **systematics**).

Thus, taxonomy deals with three basic concepts:

- Classification
- Nomenclature
- Identification.

The Swedish botanist, **Carolus Linnaeus** in 1735 laid down the basic rules for taxonomic categories or taxa, and gave the **binomial nomenclature** – a two name—**genus** and **species** identification system for each living organism, and classified all organisms into two kingdoms: *Plantae* and *Animalia*. He is known as the **father of taxonomy**.

BACTERIAL TAXONOMY

The science devoted to identifying, naming and classifying bacteria is called **bacterial taxonomy**.

Identification. The process of assigning a pre-existing taxon name to an individual organism is called **identification**. In clinical practice, microbiologists are generally concerned with the correct naming of isolates according to agreed systems of classification.

Identification is performed by the use of keys that allow the organization of bacterial traits based on growth, morphology, nutritional requirements, staining (especially Gram stain), biochemistry and molecular analysis. Some tests are definitive of a genus or species.

Scientific (or binomial) nomenclature: A two-name identification system for each living organism: these names are the genus name and the species name, both names are underlined or italicized. The first letter of the genus name is always capitalized and is always a noun. The species name is in lowercase (small letter) and is usually an adjective (e.g., *Escherichia coli*).

Nomenclature requires agreement so that the same name is used unambiguously by everyone. Rules for assigning names to bacteria are established by the International Code of Botanical Nomenclature.

Classification is defined as the arrangement of bacteria into taxonomic groups called **taxa** on the basis of similarities and differences. Its purpose is to show relationship among bacteria which have been identified and named as per the scientific (binomial) nomenclature.

Taxonomic Hierarchy (or Taxonomic Ranks)

All organisms are grouped into series of subdivisions according to their relatedness that make up the taxonomic hierarchy. The taxonomic hierarchy shows evolutionary or phylogenetic relationships among organisms.

Species is the basic taxonomic group (called taxa) in taxonomy. Species that are closely related are grouped into a genus, related genera make up a family, families orders, classes phyla, phyla kingdoms and kingdoms a domain.

The taxonomic ranks used in the classification of bacteria 'based on the latest phylogenetic tree' are as follows:

Rank or level	Example
• Domain	*Bacteria*
• Kingdom	Not assigned for bacteria
• Phylum (Division)	*Proteobacteria*
• Class	*Gammaproteobacteria*
• Order	*Enterobacteriales*
• Family	*Enterobacteriaceae*
• Genus	*Escherichia*
• Species	*E. coli.*

It was an American scientist **Carl Woese** who gave a new taxonomic category, the domain, above the level of kingdom.

Closely related **strains** constitute a **bacterial species**. A group of bacteria derived from a single cell is called a **strain**.

TYPES OF CLASSIFICATION

Bacterial classification is the orderly arrangement of bacteria into groups (taxa) preferably in a format that shows evolutionary relationships.

It is categorized into three types:

1. **Classical classification (or taxonomy).** In this several phenotypic characteristics are assessed, and the data is used to group bacteria up the taxonomic ladder from species to domain. Characteristics considered are morphology, nutrition, physiology and habitat.
2. **Molecular taxonomy (or chemotaxonomy).** It uses base composition of DNA, 16 S rRNA sequencing, DNA: DNA hybridization, ribotyping (molecular fingerprinting), multilocus sequence typing, protein profiling and fatty acid profiling.
3. **Numerical taxonomy.** Organisms are compared on the basis of a large number of characteristics and grouped according to the percentage of shared characteristics, resulting in a probable evolutionary tree.

CLASSIFICATION SYSTEMS IN BACTERIA

Following the binomial system of nomenclature used throughout biology, prokaryotes (bacteria) are given genus name and species name. It is regulated by the rules of the **International Code of Nomenclature of Prokaryotes (ICNP)** formerly **the International Code of Nomenclature of Bacteria (ICNB)** or the **Bacteriological Code (BC)**. The code covers the rules for naming all species, genera, families, and orders of prokaryotes (*Bacteria* and *Archaea*).

Classification is different from identification which refers to the determination of correct place of an organism in a previously establishd plan of classification.

Of the various classification systems, the accepted reference on the classification and identification of bacteria is the **Bergey's Manual**. It has served the community of microbiologists since 1923 and is a compendium of information on all recognized species of prokaryotes. Ninth edition of *Bergey's Manual of Systematic Bacteriology* published in 1994 is widely used for bacterial classification. Cell wall composition, morphology, differential staining, oxygen requirements and biochemical tests have been used as the criteria for classifying bacteria in this manual.

As per this manual, the kingdom *Prokaryotae* is divided into four major divisions (based on the nature of the cell wall alone) and a total of 7 classes (Table 15.1).

- **Gracilicutes** (L. *gracilus* = thin + *cutin* = skin): have Gram-negative cell walls, and thus are thin-skinned.
- **Firmicutes** (L. *firmus* = strong): have Gram-positive cell walls that are thick and strong.
- **Tenericutes** (L. *tener* = soft): lack a cell wall and thus are soft.
- **Mendosicutes** (L. *mendosus* : to be false): primitive prokaryotes (archaea) with unusual cell walls and nutritional habits.

Table 15.1 Scheme of prokaryotic classification as per 9th edition of Bergey's Manual of Systematic Bacteriology — major taxonomic groups

Division I Gracilicutes: Gram-negative bacteria	
Class I	**Scotobacteria:** Gram-negative non-photosynthetic bacteria
Class II	**Anoxyphotobacteria:** Gram-negative photosynthetic bacteria that do not produce oxygen (purple and green bacteria)
Class III	**Oxyphotobacteria:** Gram-negative photosyntheic bacteria that evolve oxygen (cyanobacteria)
Division II Firmicutes: Gram-positive bacteria	
Class I	**Firmibacteria:** Gram-positive rods or cocci
Class II	**Thallobacteria:** Gram-positive branching cells (the actinomycetes)
Division III Tenericutes	
Class I	**Mollicutes:** Bacteria lacking a cell wall (the mycoplasmas)
Division IV Mendosicutes	
Class I	**Archaebacteria:** Bacteria with atypical compounds in the cell wall and membranes

A practical system that uses a few morphological and biochemical features to categorize the major, medically important families has been given in the next chapter.

The latest classification scheme for bacteria has been devised in the Second Edition of the *Bergey's Manual of Systematic Bacteriology* (published in 5 volumes between 2001 and 2012). In this manual, prokaryotes are divided into two domains: *Bacteria* and *Archaea*. Each domain is divided into phyla. The classification is based on similarities in nucleotide sequences in RNA. Classes are divided into orders, orders into families, families into genera; and genera into species. A

prokaryotic species is defined simply as a population of cells with similar characteristics.

BACTERIAL PHYLOGENY

Based on the sequencing of ribosomal RNA genes, phylogenetic tree of bacteria for the 18 known phyla (lineages) has been proposed. In the tree, the most phylogentically ancient phylum contains the genus *Aquifex* and relatives, all of which are hyperthermophiles, hydrogen oxidizing chemolithotrophs. Proteobacteria is the largest and final phylum on the tree. It consists of five clusters (alpha, beta, gamma, delta and epsilon) each containing several genera.

CRITERIA USED FOR CLASSIFYING BACTERIA

Bacteria were classified earlier on the basis of their morphology, staining reactions, oxygen requirement and mode of reproduction. With the advancement in the technology, other properties nowadays used include features related to growth, nutritional requirements, physiology, biochemistry, genetics and molecular analysis (such as properties of DNA, rRNA sequencing and protein profiling). These criteria have been summarized in Table 15.2.

Table 15.2 Criteria used for classifying bacteria

S. No.	Criteria	Examples	Uses in classification
1.	**Morphology**	Size and shape of cells; arrangement in pairs, clusters, or filaments; presence of flagella, pili, endospores, capsules	Primary distinction of genera and sometimes species
2.	**Staining**	Gram-positive, Gram-negative, acid-fast	Separates bacteria into divisions
3.	**Growth**	Characteristics in liquid and solid cultures, colony morphology, development of pigment	Distinguish species and genera
4.	**Nutrition**	Autotrophic, heterotrophic, fermentative with different products; energy sources, carbon sources, nitrogen sources, needs for special nutrients	Distinguish species, genera and higher groups

Contd.

Table 15.2 Contd.

5.	**Physiology**	Temperature (optimum and range); pH (optimum and range), oxygen requirements, salt requirements, osmotic tolerance, antibiotic sensitivities and resistances	Distinguish species, genera and higher groups
6.	**Biochemistry**	Nature of cellular components such as cell wall, RNA molecules, ribosomes, storage inclusions, pigments, antigens; biochemical tests	Distinguish species, genera, and higher groups
7.	**Genetics**	Percentage of DNA bases (G + C ratio); DNA hybridization	Determine relatedness within genera and families
8.	**Serology**	Slide agglutination, fluorescent-labelled antibodies	Distinguish strains and some species
9.	**Phage typing**	Susceptibility to a group of bacteriophages	Identification and distinguishing of strains
10.	**Sequence of bases in rRNA**	rRNA sequencing	Determine relatedness among all living things, phylogenetic relatedness
11.	**Protein profiles**	Separate proteins by two-dimensional PAGE (electrophoresis)	Distinguish strains

KEY POINTS

- The science devoted to identifying, naming and classifying organisms is called **taxonomy**.
- **Gram stain** is the major staining technique used to classify bacteria into two groups: Gram-positive (violet) and Gram-negative (red).
- Bacteria are formally classified by phylogenetic relationships and phenotypic characteristics.

IMPORTANT QUESTIONS

1. Answer in brief:
   (a) Binomial nomenclature
   (b) Bergey's Manual.
2. Write brief notes on
   (a) Bacterial taxonomy
   (b) Bacterial classification systems
   (c) Criteria used for classifying bacteria.

MULTIPLE-CHOICE QUESTIONS

1. Which one of the following terms is used for the classification of organisms?
   (a) Nomenclature (b) Taxonomy
   (c) Microbiology (d) Classificology.
2. Using binomial nomenclature, the first name designates the genus while the second name designates the
   (a) Specific epithet (b) Taxon
   (c) Strain (d) Isolate.
3. Which of the following scientists gave binomial system of nomenclature for living organisms?
   (a) Linnaeus (b) Cohn
   (c) Hooke (d) Leeuwenhoek.
4. If typed, the genus and species names should be italicized, if written they should be ———.
   (a) Highlighted
   (b) Underlined separately
   (c) Underlined with a common line
   (d) Written in bold ink.
5. Which scientist suggested that a new taxonomic category, the domain, be created above the level of kingdom?
   (a) G.E. Fox
   (b) Carl Woese
   (c) T. Cavalier Smith
   (d) Norman R. Pace.
6. Which one of the following characteristics is considered with respect to cell shape, cell size, motility and pigmentation?

(a) Physiological (b) Phylogenetic
(c) Morphological (d) None of these.

7. Which of the following tools is used to classify a bacterium?
(a) *Black's Manual of Taxonomy*
(b) The Internet
(c) *Bergey's Manual of Determinative Bacteriology*
(d) *Pasteur's Dictionary of Bacteriology*.

8. In the bacterium *Escherichia coli*, what is the species name?
(a) *Escherichia* (b) *coli*
(c) *E. coli* (d) None of the above.

ANSWERS TO MCQs

1. (b)	2. (a)	3. (a)	4. (b)	5. (b)
6. (c)	7. (c)	8. (c).		

16

Laboratory Methods for Identification of Bacteria

WHAT IS BACTERIAL IDENTIFICATION?

Identification deals with the determination of correct place of an organism in a previously established plan of classification. Identification is the first step performed by a microbiologist in **taxonomy** that includes: classification, nomenclature and identification. Most importantly correct and rapid identification of the bacteria in clinical samples is important in patient management and antimicrobial therapy. Most specimens for bacteriological examination whether from humans, animals or the environment contian mixtures of bacteria (mixed culture), and is essential to obtain **pure cultures** (that is, isolation from all other forms of life) of individual isolates before embarking on identification. Isolation and laboratory growth are also necessary for discovery and verification of new species.

LAB PROCEDURES USED TO IDENTIFY BACTERIA

MICROSCOPY

Morphological characteristics and staining reactions of individual organisms generally serve as preliminary criteria to place an unknown species to an appropriate biological group.

Gram stain smear suffices to show the Gram reaction (+ve or –ve) size, shape and grouping of the bacteria, in addition to the arrangement of any endosposes. This is one of the first steps in identifying bacteria. Most bacteria are either Gram-positive or Gram-negative.

Acid-fast stain although useful for a limited group of bacteria is useful in identifying mycobacteria and other acid-fast bacteria.

An unstained **wet film** with dark-ground illumination in the microscope is used to observe the morphology of delicate spirochetes.

Hanging-drop preparation examined under bright-field microscope is used to observe motility in bacteria, a diagnostic feature to differentiate motile and non-motile bacteria.

Presumptive identification of certain bacteria in pathological specimens is made simply by direct microscopic observation (e.g., tubercle bacilli in sputum; *T. pallidum* in exudate from a chancre).

CULTURAL CHARACTERISTICS OR MACROSCOPIC MORPHOLOGY

Macroscopic morphology, i.e., the characteristics of colony on a nutrient agar medium such as texture, size, shape, pigment, colour, elevation, and its translucency (clear, translucent or opaque), speed of growth and patterns of growth in broth and gelatin media are unique for a bacterium.

Changes brought about in a medium (e.g., haemolysis in a blood agar medium) is a diagostic test for some bacteria.

The ability of bacteria to grow in the presence of oxygen (aerobe) or absence of oxygen (anaerobe), in the presence of CO_2, or on media containing selective inhibitory factors (salts), low or high pH, are also of diagnostic significance.

BIOCHEMICAL OR PHYSIOLOGICAL TESTS

Biochemical activities are widely used to differentiate bacteria. Even closely related bacteria can usually be separated into distinct species by subjecting them to biochemical tests. Examples include test for fermentation of sugar; capacity to digest or metabolize complex polymers such as proteins and polysaccharides; production of gas; and presence of enzymes such as catalase, oxidases and decarboxylases. All members of the family *Enterobacteriaceae* which cause diarrhoeal illness are oxidase-negative. Enteric bacteria can be diagnosed on the basis of their ability to ferment lactose into acid and gas (e.g., *Escherichia, Enterobacter, Citrobacter* and many more) from the non-lactose fermenters (e.g., *Salmonella* and *Shigella*).

IDENTIFICATION

Data from a cross section of such tests can produce a unique profile for each bacterium. Final differentiation of any unknown bacterial isolate is accomplished by its profile with the characteristics of known bacteria in tables, charts and dichotomous keys.

Many of the identification systems are automated and clinically computerized to process data and provide a **'best fit'** identification.

RAPID IDENTIFICATION METHODS

Rapid identification methods are designed for groups of clinically significant bacteria such as enterics. Such tools are designed to perform several biochemical tests simultaneously and can identify bacteria within hours. This is somehow called **numerical identification** because the results of each test are assigned a number.

Test kits are now available for a number of different groups of organisms. DNA microassay based approach is currently used for quick detection and identification of bacteria using species-specific *obligonucleotide probes* designed for specific regions of various targetted genes. The technique is important for patient management and anti-microbial therapy.

MEDICALLY IMPORTANT GENERA

Same of the medically important bacterial genera with their features, the diseases they cause, their classification (families), an informal working classification system is given in Table 16.1.

Table 16.1 A simple classification scheme of medically important families and genera of bacteria with the major diseases caused, based on microscopy, staining and biochemical technique.

I. Bacteria with Gram-positive cell wall structure
• *Cocci in clusters or packets that are aerobic or facultative* Family Micrococcaceae: *Staphylococcus* (members cause boils, skin infections)
• *Cocci in pairs and chains that are facultative* Family Streptococcaceae: *Streptococcus* (species cause strep throat, dental caries)
• *Anaerobic cocci in pairs, tetrads, irregular clusters* Family Peptococcaceae: *Peptococcus, Peptostreptococcus* (involved in wound infections)
• *Spore-forming rods* Family Bacillaceae: *Bacillus* (anthrax), *Clostridium* (tetanus, botulsim, gas gangrene)
• *Non-spore forming rods*
Family Lactobacillaceae: *Lactobacillus, Listeria* (milk-borne disease)
Family Propionibacteriaceae: *Propionibacterium* (involved in acne)

Contd.

Table 16.1 Contd.

Family Corynebacteriaceae: *Corynebacterium* (diptheria)
Family Mycobacteriaceae: *Mycobacterium* (tuberculosis, leprosy)
Family Nocardiaceae: *Nocardia* (lung abscesses)
Family Actinomycetaceae: *Actinomyces* (lumpy jaw), *Bifidobacterium* (gastrointestinal tract microbiota)
Family Streptomycetaceae: *Streptomyces* (important source of antibiotics)
II. Bacteria with Gram-negative cell wall structure
Family Neisseriaceae
• *Aerobic cocci* *Neisseria* (gonorrhoea, meningitis), *Branhamella*
• *Aerobic coccobacilli* *Moraxella, Acinetobacter*
• *Anaerobic cocci* Family Veillonellaceae *Veillonella* (dental disease)
• *Miscellaneous rods* *Brucella* (undulant fever), *Bordetella* (whooping cough), *Francisella* (tularaemia)
• *Aerobic rods* Family Pseudomonadaceae: *Pseudomonas* (pneumonia, burn infections) Miscellaneous: *Legionella* (Legionnaires' disease)
• *Facultative or anaerobic rods and vibrios* Family Enterobacteriaceae: *Escherichia, Edwardsiella, Citrobacter, Salmonella* (typhoid fever), *Shigella* (dysentery), *Klebsiella, Enterobacter, Serratia, Proteus, Yersinia* (one species causes plague)
Family Vibronaceae: *Vibrio* (cholera, food infection), *Campylobacter, Aeromonas*
• Miscellaneous genera: *Chromobacterium, Flavobacterium, Haemophilus* (meningitis), *Pasteurella, Cardiobacterium, Streptobacillus*
• *Anaerobic rods* Family Bacteroidaceae: *Bacteroides, Fusobacterium* (anaerobic wound and dental infections)

Contd.

Table 16.1 Contd.

• *Helical and curviform bacteria* Family Spirochaetaceae: *Treponema* (syphilis), *Borrelia* (Lyme disease), *Leptospira* (kidney infection)
• *Obligate intracellular bacteria* Family Rickettsiaceae: *Rickettsia* (Rocky Mountain spotted fever), *Coxiella* (Q fever) Family Bartonellaceae: *Bartonella* (trench fever, cat scratch disease) Family Chlamydiaceae: *Chlamydia* (sexually transmitted infection)
III. Bacteria with no cell walls
Family Mycoplasmataceae: *Mycoplasma* (pneumonia), *Ureoplasma* (urinary infection)

KEY POINTS

- A bacterial species can be properly identified only if it is grown in pure culture.
- Medical identification of a bacterial pathogen uses a more informal system of classification based on Gram stain, morphology, biochemical reactions, and metabolic requirements.
- Microscopy, cultural characterisitcs and biochemical reactions are the laboratory methods for identifying a bacterium in a clinical diagnostic laboratory.

IMPORTANT QUESTIONS

1. Beriefy describe the laboratory methods used for identification of a pathogenic bacterium.

MULTIPLE-CHOICE QUESTIONS

1. A bacterial species can be properly identified only if it is available as.
   (a) Pure culture
   (b) Mixed culture
   (c) Growing in broth
   (d) Growing on an agar medium.

2. All of the following are laboratory methods used to identify a bacterium EXCEPT:

(a) Gram stain

(b) Wet mount

(c) Gene probe

(d) Oxidase test.

ANSWERS TO MCQs

1. (a) 2. (c).

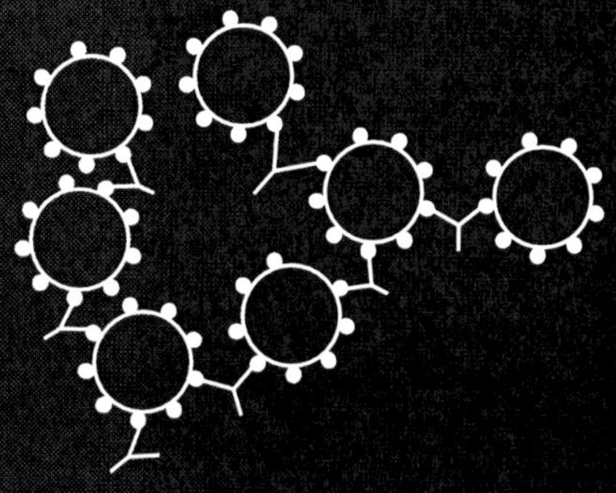

Unit III

INFECTION CONTROL

(Methods of Infection Control and Role of Nurse in Hospital Infection Control Programme)

- Asepsis, Infection and Disease
- Sterilization and Disinfection
- Antimicrobial Chemotherapy and Antibiotics
- Standard/Universal/Safety Precautions in Healthcare
- Handwashing and Hand Hygiene
- Biomedical (Hospital) Waste Treatment
- Hospital Acquired Infections and Hospital Infection Control Programme
- Role of Nurse in Hospital Infection Control Programme
- Protocols for Collection and Transport of Specimens/ Samples for Microbiological Investigations and Responsibilities of Nurses

17

Asepsis, Infection and Disease

WHAT IS ASEPSIS?

Asepsis (from the Greek *a* = no or none + *sepsis* = decay or putrid) refers to any practice that prevents or reduces the risk of microbial contamination in an operative field of surgery or medicine to prevent infection.

The goal of asepsis is *not* to achieve **sterility** (i.e., free from all kinds of pathogenic and non-pathogenic microorganisms) but to prevent contamination. Asepsis can be achieved by the use of sterile devices, materials and instruments and by creating an environment that is too low in microbes number.

HISTORY OF ASEPSIS

The modern concept of asepsis evolved in the 19th century. **Inaz Semmelweis** showed that washing hands prior to delivery reduced puerperal fever. After the suggestion of Louis Pasteur, **Joseph Lister** in 1865 introduced the use of **carbolic acid** as an antiseptic to reduce surgical infections. Lister being the first to use **aseptic techniques** in surgical infections is considered the **father of antiseptic surgery**. Aseptic techniques are important in surgery to minimize contamination from the instruments, operating personnel and the patient.

TYPES OF ASEPSIS

Asepsis is of two types: medical asepsis and surgical asepsis.

Medical Asepsis

Medical asepsis is also known as a **clean technique**. All practices that reduce the number, growth, transfer and spread of pathogenic microorganisms come under the umbrella of medical asepsis. These practices include: hand washing, bathing, gloving, gowning, mask wearing, covering hair and shoes, cleaning indoor environment, disinfecting articles, changing patient's bed linen and waste disposal.

Following these practices, growth and spread of pathogenic microorganisms is inhibited thus preventing **cross infection**, i.e., spread of disease from one person to another in hospital environment.

Principle of medical asepsis is also followed in kitchen (washing hands prior to food preparation to prevent food-borne contamination); and after using toilet to prevent faecal-borne contaminants (infections).

SURGICAL ASEPSIS

Surgical asepsis is also known as a **sterile technique**. The practices in surgical asepsis keep an area or objects free from all microorganisms both non-pathogenic and pathogenic including endospores and viruses. It prevents infectious agents from reaching a wound.

The practices (steps) in surgical asepsis carried out by the nursing staff earlier than a patient enters the operating room include: removal of hair, cleaning and disinfecting skin with an antiseptic that removes skin oils and microorganisms from the area of the skin to be opened. Betadine, Iodine, Loprep and Surgidine are the often used antiseptics.

WHAT IS INFECTION?

Infection is defined as the invasion and growth of pathogens within or on the host's body. Examples of pathogens include: bacteria, fungi, viruses, protozoa, prions and helminths.

WHAT IS DISEASE?

Disease is defined as an abnormal state in which part or all of the body is incapable of carrying out normal functions.

The terms *infection* and *disease* are sometimes used interchangeably.

TYPES OF INFECTIONS

- **Primary infection.** It is an acute infection that causes the initial illness.
- **Reinfection.** Subsequent infection by the same pathogen in the same host is called reinfection.
- **Secondary infection.** The infection caused by another (second) pathogen after the host is weakened from a primary infection is called the secondary infection.
- **Local infection.** It affects a smaller area of the body.
- **Systemic infection.** It spreads throughout the body via the circulatory system.

- **Focal infection.** It is a condition where due to infection at localized sites, like appendix and tonsil, general effects are produced.
- **Mixed infection.** One type of infection caused by several pathogens simultaneously.
- **Acute infection.** Relatively severe infection that appears suddenly and has a short course.
- **Chronic infection.** It persists over a long period of time.
- **Subclinical (or inapparent) infection.** Clinical effects (i.e., symptoms) are not apparent in the host.
- **Nosocomial infection.** Cross infection ocurring in a hospital.
- **Latent infection.** The infection remains in a latent or hidden form for sometimes and clinical symptoms appear after the resistance is lowered.

SOURCES OF INFECTION

A **source of infection** refers to the immediate origin of an infectious agent. The place from where a pathogen originates (i.e., its habitat) is called the **reservoir**.

Sources are categorized into two types:

- **Endogenous infection.** Caused due to the organisms from the host's normal flora.
- **Exogenous infection.** Caused by the organisms which are derived from a source outside the body.

ENDOGENOUS INFECTIONS

These are also called **autoinfections**. The normal flora will only invade if circumstances permit such as:

1. *Escherichia coli* and *Enterococcus faecalis*, normal resident of intestine cause **urinary tract infection**.
2. **Inhalation of stomach contents** may cause pneumonia followed by a lung abscess.
3. Enterobacteriaceae and *Bacteroides fragilis* invade the peritoneal cavity following bowel perforation causing peritonitis and septicaemia.
4. **Infective endocarditis** is caused by viridans streptococci, the normal resident of the mouth, following the tooth extraction and rheumatic heart disease.

EXOGENOUS INFECTIONS

Sources of exogenous infections: Other humans, animals, insects, environment, faecal-oral, and sexual transmission.

1. **Humans:** The most important source of human infection is man himself who may be a patient or carrier. For example, AIDS, syphilis, whooping cough, hepatitis B and measles are acquired from sick persons.
2. **Animals:** Animal pathogens may be spread to humans by direct contact or in food. Such infections are called zoonoses and the animals are called the **reservoir hosts**. Examples include: bovine tuberculosis, *E. coli* 0157, *Salmonella* food poisoning, variant creutzfeldt jakob disease (vCJD), rabies, *Microsporum canis, Trichophyton uerrucosum.*
3. **Insects:** Insects that feed on blood (e.g., mosquitoes, ticks, mites, flies, lice) act as a source of a wide range of human infections. Insect transmitting pathogens are called ***vectors*** and the infections are called **vector-borne** (e.g., malarial infection).
4. **Environment:** Soil, food and water that contain pathogens act as a source of wide range of infections. The examples of infections transmitted by these sources are:
   - **Soil:** Endospores of tetanus or gas gangrene bacilli, fungi causing mycetoma, sporotrichosis and histoplasmosis.
   - **Water:** *Shigella, Salmonella, Vibrio cholerae,* polio virus, hepatitis A and E virus.
   - **Food:** Gastroenteritis, diarrhoea, and dysentery.
   - **Air:** Influenza.

PORTALS OF ENTRY

A ***portal of entry*** is the site through which microorganisms enter the body and cause an infection/disease. Common portals of entry for infectious agents include the skin and the mucous membranes of the digestive, respiratory and urogenital systems. Openings to the outside of the body include: the ears, nose, mouth, eyes, anus, urethera and vagina.

Examples include:

- **Upper respiratory tract:** through inhalation (e.g., influenza)
- **Gastrointestinal tract:** ingestion of food (e.g., gastroenteritis)

- **Urogenital tract:** sexual contact (e.g., *Chlamydia*)
- **Skin and mucous membranes:** open wounds or punctures, burns (*Pseudomonas aeruginosa*)
- **Blood:** Needlestick injury (e.g., hepatitis B).

PORTALS OF EXIT

A **portal of exit** is the site from where microoraganisms leave the body. Pathogens have definite portals of exit, which are generally the same sites where they entered initially (Figure 17.1). The various portals of exit are:

- **Respiratory tract** via
  - coughing
  - sneezing
- **Gastrointestinal tract** via
  - saliva from the oral cavity
  - faeces/diarrhoea from the bowel
  - vomitus
- **Urogenital tract** via
  - semen from the penis
  - vaginal secretion from the vagina
  - infected urine
- **Blood**
  - infected blood
- **Skin and mucous membranes**
  - discharges from the infected skin lesions and infected wounds.

Of the above portals of exit, respiratory and gastrointestinal tracts are the most common portals.

Examples of the pathogens that cause tuberculosis, whooping cough, influenza, mums, measles, chickenpox, pneumonia are discharged through the respiratory route. Cholera, typhoid fever, amoebic dysentry, salmonella, shigellosis pathogens through faeces; rabies, mumps through saliva; typhoid fever and brucellosis through urine; and ringworms, herpes through skin.

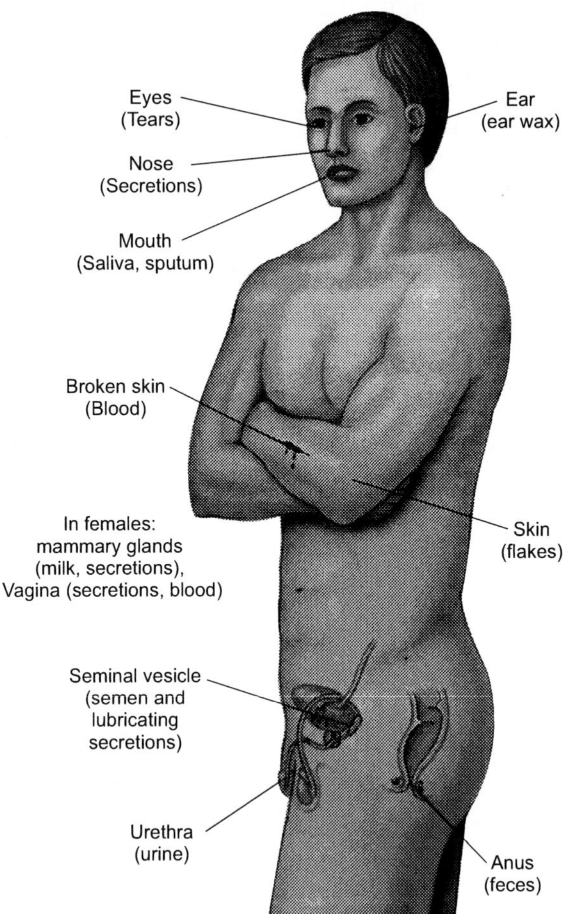

Fig. 17.1 Portals of exit for human pathogens. Besides those portals common to males and females, additional portals in males include the seminal vesicles, and in females the mammary glands and vagina.

MODES OF SPREAD (OR TRANSMISSION) OF INFECTION

Modes of spread of pathogens from infected person to the healthy have been grouped into three categories: **contact, vehicle** and **vector**.

1. **Contact transmission:** It is of three types:
    - **Direct contact:** Person-to-person: syphilis, gonorrhoea, herpes, staphylococcal infections.
    - **Indirect infection:** By fomites (inanimate objects): tetanus, ringworms, common cold.
    - **Droplets:** via saliva or mucus in coughing or sneezing: influenza, common cold, whooping cough, pneumonia, and fever.

2. **Vehicle transmission:** By a medium (vehicle) such as water food, air and hands:
   - **Waterborne:** cholera, shigellosis.
   - **Airborne** (including dust particles): TB, chickenpox, influenza, histoplasmosis, coccidiodomycosis.
   - **Foodborne:** salmonellosis typhoid fever, tapeworms, hepatitis A.
   - **Handborne:** dysentery.
3. **Vector transmission:** By arthropod vectors
   - Mechanical (on insect bodies): *E. coli,* diarrhoea, salmonellosis, trachoma.
   - Biological: Plague, malaria, yellow fever, Rockey mountain spotted fever.

KEY POINTS

- **Asepsis** refers to the absence of microbial contamination and it prevents the spread of infection.
- **Medical asepsis** is a clean technique and **surgical asepsis** is a sterile technique.
- **Aseptic techniques** are important in surgery to minimize contamination.
- **Infection** refers to the invasion and growth of parasites/ pathogens within or on the host's body.
- Source of infection can be **endogenous** (from the body itself) and **exogenous** (outside the body).
- **Portal of entry** refers to the specific route (e.g., skin or mucous membranes) by which a pathogen gains access to the body.
- **Infection spread** occurs via contact, vehicle and vectors.

IMPORTANT QUESTIONS

1. What is asepsis? Differentiate between medical asepsis and surgical asepsis.

2. Write brief notes on:

   (a) Sources of infection.

   (b) Modes of spread of infection.

   (c) Portal of entry or exit of human pathogens.

MULTIPLE-CHOICE QUESTIONS

1. Asepsis refers to sterility. True or False?
2. Medical asepsis refers to a sterile technique and surgical asepsis refers to a clean technique. True or False?
3. Which of the following scientists is known for preventing the spread of infection?
   (a) Louis Pasteur (b) Robert Koch
   (c) Joseph Lister (d) Philipp Semmelweis.
4. The use of aseptic techniques in surgical operations was first introduced by
   (a) Joseph Lister (b) Philipp Semmelweis
   (c) Robert Koch (d) None of the above.
5. Which of the following is often associated with prevention of cross infection?
   (a) Surgical asepsis (b) Medical asepsis
   (c) Asepsis (d) Sterilization.
6. Infections that are transmitted from animals to humans are called
   (a) Vectors (b) Zoonoses
   (c) Carriers (d) Reservoirs of infection.
7. Which of the following is *not* a portal of entry for pathogens?
   (a) Blood (b) Digestive tract
   (c) Respiratory tract (d) Urogenital tract.
8. Nonliving objects that can harbour and aid in spread of infections are called
   (a) Vectors (b) Fingers
   (c) Fomites (d) Reservoirs of infection.
9. Which of the following infection is not spread by the respiratory route?
   (a) Mumps (b) Measles
   (c) Common cold (d) Hepatitis B.

ANSWERS TO MCQs

1. False	2. False	3. (c)	4. (a)	5. (b)
6. (b)	7. (a)	8. (c)	9. (d).	

18

Sterilization and Disinfection

STERILIZATION

Sterilization is the process of killing or removing all microorganisms in a material or on an object. Any material or object that is free from all microbial life (both pathogenic and non-pathogenic) is said to be **sterile**.

DISINFECTION

Disinfection is the process of reducing the number of pathogenic organisms on objects or in materials to a desired concentration so that they pose no threat of disease.

APPLICATIONS OF STERILIZATION AND DISINFECTION

Both these processes have applications in:

- **Practical microbiology** – Need of sterile culture media, glassware, equipment and other tools to work with microbial cultures.
- **Practice of medicine** – Prevention of hospital infection requires the use of sterile instruments, dressings and parenteral drops.
- **Surgery** – Use of antimicrobial agents to disinfect surgical areas, inanimate objects, operating room environment and tools used in surgery to prevent transmission of infectious microorganisms.
- **Food and pharmaceutical industries** – To prevent spoilage and preservation of foods, creation of microbes-free environment in pharmaceutical industries.
- **At home** – Disinfection of toilets and kitchen to prevent infections.
- **In agriculture** – Disinfection of sewer water before its disposal into the agriculture fields.

TERMS RELATED TO STERILIZATION AND DISINFECTION

The terms often used in relation to sterilization and disinfection are defined below:

1. **Sterile.** Any object or material free from all kinds of pathogenic and non-pathogenic microbes.
2. **Sterility.** It is a microbiologically germs-free state of all surgical materials and items.
3. **Antiseptic.** A chemical agent used externally on the living tissue (skin or mucosa) to inhibit or reduce the number of viable microorganisms.
4. **Antisepsis.** Destruction or prevention of microorganisms in living tissues.
5. **Disinfectant.** A chemical agent used on inanimate objects to destroy microorganisms. Most disinfectants do not kill spores.
6. **Sanitizer.** A chemical agent typically used on food-handling equipment and eating utensils to reduce the level of contaminants so as to meet public health standards. **Sanitization** simply refers to thorough washing with only soap or detergent.
7. **Germicide.** An agent capable of killing microbes rapidly.
    - *Bactericide* – An agent that kills bacteria. Most such agents do not kill spores.
    - *Viricide* – An agent that inactivates viruses.

      Fungicide – An agent that kills fungi.

      Sporicide – An agent that kills bacterial endospores or fungal spores.
8. **Bacteriostatic agent.** An agent that inhibits the growth of bacteria.
9. **Fungistatic agent.** An agent that inhibits the growth of fungi.

METHODS/AGENTS FOR STERILIZATION AND DISINFECTION

Sterilization and disinfection can be achieved by various physical and chemical methods, as summarized below.

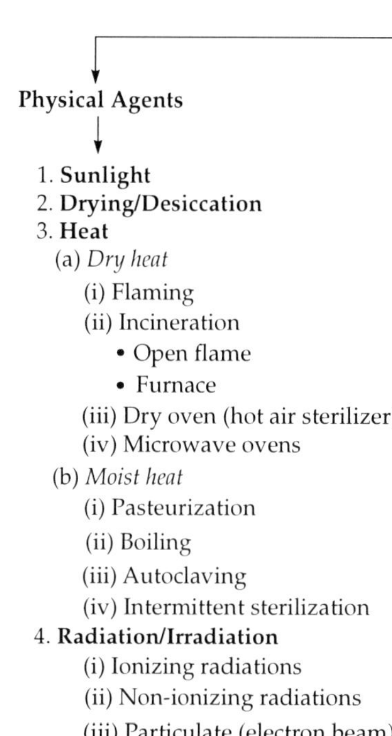

Chemical Agents

1. Detergents and soaps
2. Alcohols
3. Halogens
4. Phenolics
5. Hydrogen peroxide
6. Heavy metals
7. Aldehydes
8. Gases and aerosols

PHYSICAL AGENTS

1. Sunlight

Sunlight possesses germicidal activity due to the presence of ultraviolet rays. This acts as one of the natural methods of water sterilization in tanks, rivers and lakes due to UV and heat rays.

2. Drying/desiccation

Metabolic inhibition of air-borne microbes due to gradual withdrawal of water from cells by exposure to room air, especially during the summer months. This method is useful in preservation of foods, but is not effective for controlling infections.

3. Dry heat sterilization

Heat is considered to be the most reliable method of sterilization of objects that can withstand heat. Heat as **dry** and **moist heat** are the most common sterilizing agents.

In dry heat treatment, hot air is used to sterilize metal objects and glassware.

Killing by dry heat is due to:

- Coagulation of proteins
- Oxidative damage
- Melting lipids.

(A) FLAMING

Mouths of culture tubes, conical flasks, needles, scalpel blades, glass slides and cover slips are passed over flame without allowing them to become red hot. Only non-endospore producing bacteria are destroyed by flaming.

(B) INCINERATION IN OPEN FLAME

Inoculating wires and bacterial loops, forceps, spatulas are sterilized by holding them for a few seconds in *open flame* of Bunsen burner (800°C to 1800°C) until red hot.

(C) INCINERATION IN FURNACE

Incinerator chamber equipped with flame (600° – 1200°C) that burns materials to ashes. It is an efficient method for decontamination and safely destroying contaminated materials such as soiled dressing, animal carcasses, bedding and, clinical and industrial wastes.

(D) HOT AIR OVEN

Hot-air oven (or sterilizer) (Fig. 18.1) is a closed chamber which uses dry heat and temperature for sterilization. Dry heat affects killing of DNA due to oxidation of cells and denaturation of proteins and DNA. Hot air oven was originally developed by **Louis Pasteur**.

The oven is electrically heated double walled insulated closed chamber fitted with a thermostat that maintains the chosen temperature from 50° to 300°C. There is an air circulating fan that keeps the hot air moving around at a constant temperature throughout the body. It is fitted with a adjustable wire mesh, plated trays or aluminium trays for keeping the articles as well as indicators and control for temperature and holding time. Holding time for sterilization in hot air oven is 20 minutes at 180°C, 60 minutes at 170°C, 120 minutes at 160°C, 180 minutes at 140°C and 600 minutes at 120°C. It is timed as beginning when the thermometer first shows 180°C or 120°C, respectively.

Sterilization controls: The efficiency of the oven during use can be tested by:

- **Biological Indicators:** Filter paper strip impregnated with endospores of *Bacillus subtilis* subsp. *niger* contained in an envelope is placed within the load. No growth of the bacterium in tryptone soy broth at 37°C for 5 days indicates proper sterilization.

- **Chemical Indicator:** A Browne's tube containing red solution is kept along with the load and a colour change from red to green shows proper sterilization.

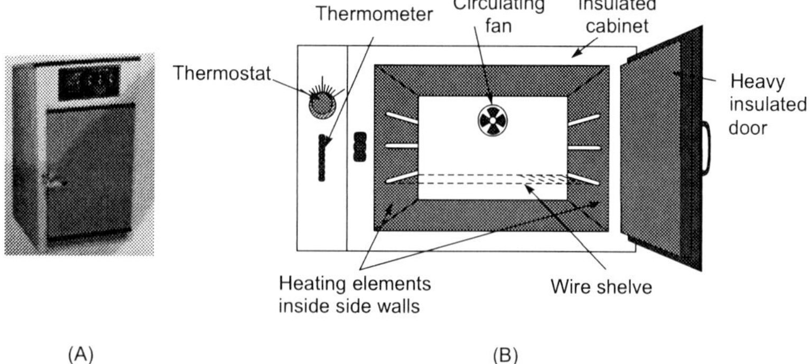

Fig. 18.1 Hot air oven for dry heat sterilization. (A) External and (B) internal view.

(E) MOIST HEAT STERILIZATION AND DISINFECTION

Moist heat in the form of steam or hot water is used to kill microorganisms including bacterial endospores (**sterilization**) or to destroy vegetative microbial cells (**disinfection**) by denaturing enzymes (proteins).

The process in which saturated steam under pressure is used to sterilize an object is called **moist heat sterilization**.

Application of moist heat to control microorganisms is brought about by four ways:

1. Saturated steam under pressure (15 psi/121°C 10-40 minutes)—Autoclave.
2. Intermittent sterilization—Free floating steam 100°C – Arnold sterilizer.
3. Boiling water (100°C)—Water bath
4. Pasteurization (< 100°C)—HTST pasteurizer

AUTOCLAVE

An **autoclave** (also called **steam sterilizer**) (Fig. 18.2) is a sealed heating device which uses moist heat (steam) under pressure to sterilize an object. The material is exposed to 121°C (15 psi) for 15–20 minutes. This process, called **autoclaving**, is the most effective method of moist heat sterilization.

The name autoclave is derived from Greek *auto*—meaning self, and Latin *clavis* meaning key, i.e., a self-locking device. It was developed in 1884 by **Charles Chamberland**, one of the Pasteur's associates. A very basic autoclave is similar to a pressure cooker used in kitchens, both use the power of steam to kill microbes, endospores and germs resistant to boiling water and powerful detergents.

Autoclaving is used to sterilize various medical and laboratory products like culture media, instruments, dressings, line, intravenous equipment, applicators, aqueous solutions, syringes, etc. However, autoclaving is not recommeded for oils, waxes and powders that repel moisture.

Principle: Autoclave is based on the principle that moist heat (saturated steam) under pressure at elevated temperature (> 100°C) effects sterilization. The higher the pressure in the autoclave, the higher the temperature, the relationship between the two is shown in Table 18.1. Steam at pressure of 15 pounds per square inch (= 100 kPa), i.e., 121°C (= 250°F) will kill *all* organisms and their endospores in 15 minutes (but not prions). Saturated steam heats an object > 2500 times more efficiently than does the hot air (dry) at the same temperature. Lethal action of steam is due to coagulation of proteins/enzymes which is caused by breakage of hydrogen bonds. For effective sterilization the steam must directly contact the material to be sterilized. In addition all the air must be expelled from the autoclave so that the articles are exposed to pure steam due to three reasons.

- The admixture of air with steam results in lower temperature being achieved.
- Air hinders penetration of steam into interstices of porous materials, surgical dressings and syringes.
- The air being denser to steam forms a separate and cooler layer in the lower part of the autoclave thereby preventing proper sterilization of the articles.

Table 18.1 The relationship between the temperature of steam and pressure at sea level

Pressure (psi)	Temperature (°C)
0	100
5	110
10	116
15	121
20	126
30	135

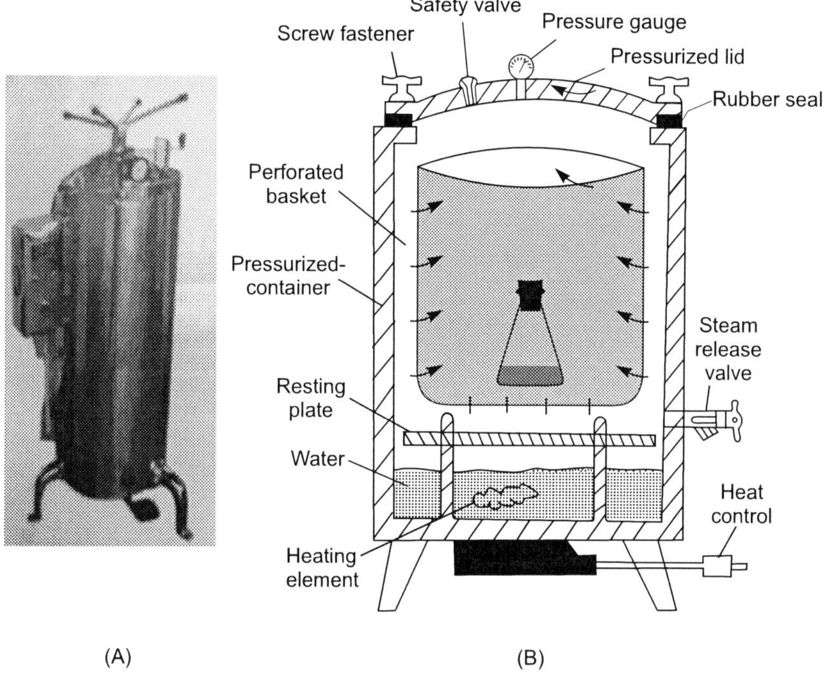

Fig. 18.2 Vertical autoclave. (A) external and (B) internal view.

Construction

A simple autoclave (Fig. 18.2) is a double-walled vertical or horizental cylinder of gunmetal or stainless steel, one end of which is open to receive the articles to be sterilized. The lid is tightened by screw clamps and rendered air-tight by asbestos gasket. It is provided with the pressure gauge, steam cock (exhaust value), and safety valve. Basket, provided with holes all around for free circulation of the steam, is used for keeping the articles. Perforated metallic separators are used, if more materials are to be sterilized.

Operation/Working

- Sufficient water is added in the vessel so that the heating element submerges in it.
- The articles are placed in the basket/chamber.
- The lid is closed by tightening the fastener diagonally with the discharge tap open and the safey valve adjusted to the desired pressure (15 psi).
- Swith on the power supply.

- As heating continues, the steam and air mixture expels.
- When the temperature reaches 100°C, it indicates all the air from inside the autoclave has been removed, the steam release valve is now closed.
- Steam valve opens when the pressure reaches 15 psi (i.e., 121°C), from this point the **holding time** (15 minutes) is counted for sterilization to take place.
- Heating is stopped by switching off the electric supply when the holiding time is over.
- The autoclave is allowed to cool till the pressure falls to zero mark which indicates that inside pressure has reached to atmospheric level.
- The discharge tap is now opened allowing the entery of atomspheric air in the autoclave.
- Now unlock and open the autoclave lid/door and remove the sterilized articles and put these on the asbestos.

Precautions

- Heating element must always be submerged in water.
- Articles should be loosely placed in the basket so that steam can easily penetrate them.
- Air (initial) should be evacuated (expelled) so that steam fills the chamber.
- Dry paper (not aluminium foil) should be used for wrapping the dry objects (e.g., bandages, glassware) for penetration of steam.
- Never open the lid when the pressure inside the lid is high otherwise the liquid media will boil violently and may explode.
- The articles are not allowed to remain in the autoclave after the normal atmospheric pressure has reached inside the chamber resulting in water evaporation that will be lost from the media.
- For liquids, a container is usually not filled past 75% of its capacity.

Controls for efficacy of the instrument or sterility

1. **Bacterial endospores** (biological indicator). A commercially available spore test ampule having *Bacillus stearothermophilus* (heat-resistant endospore produing bacterium) or filter paper

strip impregnated with the spores of this bacterium, is placed with the load in the coolest and least accessible part of the autoclave. No growth of the autoclaved endospores after 5 days at 56°C in the inoculated tryptone soy broth from the ampoule/strip means spores have been killed indicating proper sterilization of the articles.

2. **Chemical indicator.** A Brown's tube containing red solution of a dye (used as indicatior) is placed within the load. A change of colour from red to green when exposed to 121°C for 15 minutes in an autoclave, indicates proper sterilization of the articles.

INTERMITTENT STERILIZATION

Intermittent sterilization (also called **tyndallization**) uses free flowing unpressurized steam (at 100°C) applied for 20 minutes on three successive days. This is a fractional method of sterilization.

First exposure to steam kills all vegetative bacteria, and any spores present being in a favourable nutrient medium will germinate, and are killed during the subsequent heating.

This method is useful for substances that cannot be autoclaved especially the media containing sugars, egg serum and certain canned foods which may be damged at higher temperature of the autoclave.

The instrument commonly used is **Koch's** or **Arnold's steamer** that employs moist heat at 100°C. It is simply a vertical metal cylinder with a removable lid having a small outlet for the steam escape and at its bottom it contains water which is heated up. Above the water level, there is a perforated shelf for keeping the articles to be sterilized.

PASTEURIZATION

Pasteurization named after **Louis Pasteur** who discovered that spoilage organisms could be inactivated in wine by applying heat at temperature below its boiling point. It is the process of application of heat (< 100°C) to a liquid or a food product in order to kill disease producing microorganisms, to inactivate spoilage causing enzymes, and to reduce or destrory spoilage microorganisms. Pasteurization does not kill all the microorganisms in an article hence it is a process of **disinfection** and therefore not synonmous with sterilization.

Pasteurization is of three types:

- **Low temperature long time pasteurization (LTLT)** (*Vat pasteurization*)—62.8°C (145°F) for 30 minutes.

- **High temperature short time pasteurization–(HTST)**—71.7°C for 15 seconds.
- **Ultra-high temperature pasteurization (UHT)**—140°C for 4 seconds.

Pasteurization is used for packaged and non-packaged foods, beverages and other food processing industries to achieve food preservation and food safety. Common pasteurized products are milk, butter, cheese, cream, vinegar, nuts, yogurt, commerical sauerkraut, beer, wines, eggs, juices, water and canned foods.

BOILING AT 100°C

Immersion in **boiling water at 100°C** for 10–30 minutes is a moist heat method that destroys pathogenic microorganisms. Boiling kills many regetative cells and viruses within 10 minutes. Endospore producing bacteria require prolonged periods of 2 or more hours. Boiling is a method of disinfection rather than sterilization. Therefore, it is not recommended for sterilization of instruments for surgical procedures.

Boiling is used in clinics and homes to disinfect dishes, clothing, utensils, baby's articles and beddings.

FILTRATION

Filtration is the passage of a liquid or air through a filter with pores (openings) small enough to retain microorganisms. During filtration microbes including viruses are trapped, the process called *filter sterilization*.

This is used to sterilize heat-sensitive liquids, e.g., vaccines sera, antibiotics, media, water in the laboratories and removal of microorganisms from air in hospital rooms, isolation units, laminar flow cabinet, and clean rooms. **Surgical masks** and **cotton plugs** used on culture vessels (flasks and tubes) work on the principle of filtration.

Types of Filters

- **Membrane filters** (also known as *millipore filters*) composed of biologically inert cellulose esters, nitrocellulose, polycarbonate with porosities from 0.015-12 µm. Used to filter out bacteria, viruses, and even large proteins.
- **Air filters**—*high-efficiency particulate air (HEPA) filters* with porosities 0.3 µm. Used in ventilation system to supply microbes

free air in operating rooms, burn units, intensive-care units and laminar flow transfer hoods in laboratories.

- Earthenware filters, asbestos (seitz) filters, sintered glass filters and syringe filters are the others filters used in filtration.

RADIATION STERILIZATION

Radiation sterilization is a method of **cold sterilization** that uses energy in the form of waves (**electromagnetic**) and particles (e.g., electrons, protons and neutrons) to kill microbes. Two types of radiation are used for sterilization: ionizing radiation and non-ionizing radiation.

Ionizing Radiation (IR)

IR is the use of short wavelength, high-intensity radiation to kill microorganisms by causing direct damage to DNA by the formation of breaks and mutations. IR can dislodge electrons from atoms creating ions, hence named. Types of IR include: gamma rays, X-rays, cathode rays (high-speed electron beams); of these gamma rays being most effective have a high degree of penetration and exert their effect by ionizing water by forming highly reactive hydroxyl radicals.

Applications of gamma radiation emitted by cobalt 60 are:

- To sterilize heat-sensitive, medical materials in packages (e.g., plastic sringes, cathaters, gloves and intravenous sets).
- To sterilize, prevent spoilage and increase storage time of various foods (e.g., sea foods, meats, poultry and fruits).

However, their application is more expensive and dangerous than other methods.

Non-ionizing Radiation

Infrared and ultraviolet (UV) radiation are the two forms of non-ionizing radiation. These excite, but do not ionize atoms, hence named non-ionizing radiations.

UV radiations in the range of 240 nm to 280 nm wavelength are lethal, of these 260 being highly germicidal. In everyday practice, the source of UV radiation is the germicidal lamp which generates radiation of 254 nm. Sunlight contains UV rays, consequently it has definite germicidal effects.

These cause cell damage by acting on DNA molecule by making thymine dimers that interfere with the replication of DNA. Most vegetative bacteria, fungi and protozoa are susceptible to UV radiations. Endospores are highly resistant and susceptibility of viruses is variable. These can penetrate only a few mm in liquids and not at all into solids. Therefore, their use is best restricted to disinfection rather than sterilization.

UV light has been used for many years to sanitize just about everything from water to surfaces in the healthcare and medical industries, as well as labs.

Major applications of UV light are:

- to disinfect air in hospital rooms, operating rooms, food preparation areas, schools and dental offices to reduce the chances of air borne infections and food spoilages;
- to sterilize the interiors (indoors) of biological saftey cabinets;
- to treat drinking water, water in pools and spas and to purify other liquids (milk and fruits juices);
- to treat sera, vaccines and drugs;
- to disinfect surfaces of solid, non-porous materials such as walls and floors, as well as meat, nuts, tissues for grafting and drugs;
- to disinfect effluent (sewage) water; and
- hanging laundry outdoors on bright sunny days is used to kill microbes on clothing by UV light present in the sunlight.

Disadvantages of UV radiation

- UV rays can cause skin burns and damage eyes, hence direct exposure must be avoided.
- Presence of DNA repair mechanism in some bacteria can overcome the damage caused by UV rays.
- Due to the lower penetration power, UV radiation does not penentrate glass, paper, aluminium and plastic.

CHEMICAL AGENTS

Since the first use of chloride water to treat wounds and washing of hands before surgery by **Ignaz Semmelweis** in 1800s and use of carbolic acid (phenol) during surgical operation by **Joseph Lister** in 1860s, several chemical agents have been used to disinfect (*disinfectants*) and antisepticize (*antiseptics*): sterilize (*sterilants*) and sanitize (*sanitizers*) materials as a means of preventing infection; and agents to prevent microbial spoilage of foods (*preservatives*) and other harmful microbial activities.

Classes of Chemical Agents

Nine major classes of antimicrobial chemical agents are:

1. *Phenol and phenol derivatives*—phenol, cresol, hexachlorophene, chlorohexidine
2. *Alcohols*—ethanol, isopropanol
3. *Halogens*—chlorine, iodine and its derivatives
4. *Heavy metals*—mercurials, silver salts
5. *Aldehydes*—formaldehyde, gluataraldehyde
6. *Gaseous agents*—ethylene oxide
7. *Dyes*—aniline, acridine
8. *Detergents*
9. *Quaternary ammonium compounds*

The antimicrobial chemical agents damage microorganisms by damaging the cell membrane, denaturing proteins (enzymes) and modifying functional groups of proteins and nucleic acids.

1. Phenol and Phenol Derivatives

Phenol is obtained by distillation of coal tar. It is credited to be the first disinfectant used in the form of **carbolic acid** by **Joseph Lister** in 1867. Phenol and its derivatives are used as disinfectants in laboratories and hospitals.

Phenol is very effective as 5% aqueous solution. It has the distinction of being the standard against which other disinfectants of a similar chemical structure are compared to determine their antimicrobial efficacy (*phenol-coefficient method*).

Phenolics are powerful **microbicidal** (*bactericidal, fungicidal* and *virucidal*) but not sporicidal. They act on the microbes by distrupting cell membranes (the cell contents leak out and the microbes die) and precipitating proteins.

Applications

- *Phenol* at a concentration of 0.5% is used to preserve sera and vaccines.
- *Lysol* (a mixture of 1–3% orthophenylphenol in soap) is used as a cleaner and disinfectant in housekeeping, excreta, floors and sterilization of infected glass wares.
- It is used in air sprays and hospital disinfectants.
- *Savlon* (chlorohexidine and cetrimide)—widely used in wounds, preoperative disinfection of skin and as bladder irrigant.

- *Dettol* (chloroxyenol)—used as an antiseptic for medical (cuts, scratches) and is a household disinfectant on home surfaces and in laundry.
- *Hexylresorcinol* is used as mouth wash, throat lozenges and topical antiseptic.
- *Cresote* (a mixture of 3 cresols)—used commercially as a wood preservative for fence posts and telephone poles.

2. Alcohols

The two most popular alcohols used in sterilization are: *ethanol* (ethyl alcohol) and *isopropanol* (isopropyl alcohol). *Methanol* (methyl alcohol) is also germicidal but is not generally used due to its highly poisonous nature. Its fume may cause permanent damage to the eyes.

Ethanol is affective in concentrations between 50 and 90 %, the ideal concentration is 70% which kills all the vegetative bacteria, fungi, lipid containing viruses, but not endospores (i.e., the alcohols are not sporicidal).

Alcohols, used as an antiseptic and disinfectant, act as surfactant and exert their action by denaturing proteins and dissolving membrane lipids. They are also dehydrating agents.

Applications

- Seventy percent ethyl alcohol is frequenthy used as a skin disinfectant to treat skin before a venipuncture or injection (alcohol-based hand rubs)
- C_2H_5OH is used to preserve cosmetics, homoepathic medicines and syrups.
- It is used to disinfect thermometers and delicate instruments (70% C_2H_5OH for 10 minutes). Isopropyl alcohol is preferred over ethyl alcohol for clinical thermometers as it is a better fat solvent, more bactericidal and less volatile.

3. Halogens

The word **halogens** means **salt-former** is derived from the Greek (*halos* meaning salt or sea and *gen* meaning to produce). Chlorine (Cl_2) and iodine (I_2) are the two halogens commonly used (alone or as their compounds) as disinfectants.

Chlorine

Chlorine is widely used to kill pathogens in water in 3 forms: Elemental chlorine (Cl_2), hypochlorites and chloramines. These act on the microbes by denaturation of protein by disrupting disulphide bonds and by oxidizing cellular components. Chloride is sporicidal in nature, kills all kinds of microbes including endospore producing bacteria. Formation of *hypochlorous acid* when Cl_2 is added to water is responsible for the germicidal action of Cl_2.

Iodine (I_2) – Iodine is an effective antimicrobial agent in three different forms:

Povidone-iodine (PVP-I), also called **iodopovidone** (trade names Betadine, Pyodine), is an antiseptic used for skin disinfection before and after surgery. Also used to disinfect the skin of the patient and hands of the healthcare providers as well as a mouth wash.

Tincture of iodine (2-7 % elemental iodine and potassium iodide dissolved in a mixture of ethanol and water) was one of the first skin antiseptics to come into use since 1908.

Iodine solution (25 ppm idophor) is used to sanitize the surface of fruit and vegetables against bacteria and viruses (not safe for protozoan parasites).

4. Heavy Metals and their Compounds

Metals with relatively high densities, atomic weight or atomic numbers are called **heavy metals**. The ions of heavy metals (e.g., mercury, sliver, arsenic, zinc and copper), act as biocidal even in low concentrations, this activity is referred to as **oligodynamic action** (*oligo* means a few).

They are **bacteriostatic antiseptics** and act by precipitation of proteins and oxidation of sulfhydryl groups. Examples:

- **Sliver nitrate** (10% solution) is widely used to guard against an infection of the eyes called gonorrhoeal neonatal opthalmia caused by *Neisseria gonorrhoeae*.
- **Sliver sulphadiazine**, a combination of silver and sulfadiazine, is used as an antiseptic topical component for extensive burns.
- **Organic mercury compounds** have been used as topical disinfectants (thimerosal, nitromersol and merbromin) and preservatives in medical preparations (thimerosal) and grain products (both methyl and ethyl mercurials). **Mercury was used for syphilis treatment in old days**.
- **Arsenic**—For many decades, arsenic had been used medicinally to treat syphilis.
- **Selenium sulphide** kills fungi, including spores. Selenium preparations are commonly used to treat fungal skin infections. Shampoos that contain selenium are effective in treating dandruff caused by fungi.

- **Zinc iodide** and **zinc sulphate** are used as topical antiseptics. **Zinc chloride** is a common ingredient in mouthwashes and deodorants, and **zinc pyrithione** as an ingredient in anti-dandruff shampoos.

5. Surface-Active Agents (Surfactants)

The term **surfactant** (or **surface-active agent**) is used to describe organic chemicals which can decrease surface among molecules of a liquid in which it is dissolved. These compounds are **amphiphilic** with two opposing portions, one part is **hydrophilic** (water-attracting) and the other is **hydrophobic** (water-repelling). Such agents include soaps and detergents.

Surfactants are classified into: cationic, anionic, non-ionic and amphoteric in nature.

- **Cationic detergents**—These are known as **quaternary ammonium compounds** (or **Quats**). They are strongly bactericidal to Gram-positive bacteria and fungi but not sporicidal. By distrupting plasma membrane, quats allow cytoplasmic constituents to leak out of the cell resulting in death of the organism.

  Examples: **Benzalkonium** and **cetylpyridinium chlorides** are quats used in environmental disinfection as cleansers in clinics and the food industry, and as preservatives.
- **Anionic detergents (soaps):** They are water-soluble sodium or potassium salts of fatty acids and are anionic surfactants (i.e., having negative charge). They have weak antimicrobial properties but assist in removing microorganisms in addition to removal of grease and soil on skin, utensils, and environmental surfaces.

6. Aldehydes

An **aldehyde** is an organic compound containing a terminal carbonyl group (RCHO). **Formaldehyde** (or **formalin**) and **glutaraldehyde** are the two aldehydes which are among the most effective chemical disinfectants. They are microbicidal in action. They kill cells by alkylation of amino and nucleic acids (in other words, inactivation of proteins and nucleic acids).

Formaldehyde (FAH)—It is used in both the liquid and vapour states.

- As a gas, it is used in hosptials as a disinfectant for clothing, woollen blankets, mattresses, respirators, heat-senstive instruments and for sterilization of rooms and furniture.

- FAH in liquid form is used as a water and methanol solution called **formalin** for preserving biological and anatomical specimens.

  It is to be stored and used in a fume-hood or well-ventilated area because **it is a well-known human carcinogen**.

  Glutaraldehyde it is a saturated dialdehyde ($C_5 H_8 O_2$) and is a transparent oily liquid with a pungent odour. It is sold under several brand names, e.g., Cidax, Glutarol, Aldensen, Wavicide. Glutaraldehyde and has gained wide acceptance as a high-level disinfectant and cold chemical sterilant effective against a range of microorganisms including bacterial spores.

  Major applications include: Two per cent buffered solution is used to disinfect and clean heat-sensitive medical, surgical and dental equipment such as cystoscopes, bronchoscopes, endoscopes, thermometers, face masks, plastic and polythene tubings.
- It is used for industrial water treatment and as a chemical preservative.
- It is used to treat warts on the bottom of feet.

7. Dyes

Two groups of dyes: *aniline* dyes (triphenyl methane) and *acridine* dyes that possess antimicrobial properties are often used by microbiologists for staining.

Aniline dyes (e.g., crystal violet, malachite green, brilliant green) are used extensively as skin and wound antispectics.

Crystal violet (**gentian violet**) has antibacterial, antifungal and antihelminthic proerties. It acts by interferring with cell wall synthesis and/or cellular oxidation processes. It is a primary stain used in Gram stain and can be used to treat infections caused by *Candida albicans* (a yeast) and *Trichomonas* (a protozoan).

Acridine dyes (e.g., acriflavine, euflavine, proflavine, aminacrine) exhibit selective activity against bacteria especially staphylococci and gonococci. They interfere with the synthesis of nucleic acids and proteins. They are used to treat burns and wounds and for opthalmic application and bladder irrigation.

8. Gaseous Agents

Ethylene oxide and beta propiolactone are effective sterilizing gaseous agents for heat-sensitive objects.

Ethylene oxide (ETO) (C_2H_4O) exists as liquid at temperature below 10.8°C (51.4°F) and vaporizes rapidly when the temperature moves up. This gas is most frequently used for sterilization. It penetrates most materials and kills all microorganisms (including spores) by protein denaturation.

ETO is the only approved gaseous sterilant. It is used to sterilize disposable plastic Petri dishes and syringes, heart lung machnie components, catheters, blankets, pharmaceutical products (crude drugs and powders), spices, contaminated plastic equipment and the plastic wraps; space programme by both the USA and Russia for decontaminating spacecraft.

Beta-propiolactone (BPL) is a condensation product of ketone and formaldehyde $\left(\begin{matrix} CH_2 - CH_2 \\ | \quad\quad | \\ O - C = O \end{matrix}\right)$. The gas becomes liquid at 20°C.

BPL is a broad spectrum microbicide that kills bacteria, fungi and viruses. It destroys microbes more readily than ethylene oxide, but lacks penetrating power of ethylene oxide and is also a carcinogen, hence its use is restricted. It is used to sterilize vaccines and sera (in liquid form) and to disinfect rooms and biological materials.

9. Hydrogen Peroxide

Hydrogen peroxide (H_2O_2), a versatile microbicide, is a pale blue, clear liquid, slightly more viscous than water. It acts on microbes by producing highly active hydroxyl-free radicals and damage proteins and DNA molecules. It also decomposes to water and O_2 gas which are toxic to anaerobes, strong solutions are sporicidal. Its uses include:

- 3% H_2O_2 acts as a mild antiseptic and is used for skin and wound antisepsis and a mouth rinse to help remove mucus and to relieve minor mouth irritation (due to canker/cold sores, gingivitis) and to disinfect utensils.
- Strong H_2O_2 (6–25%) can be used to sterilize equipment.

KEY POINTS

- **Sterilization**—The process of killing or removing of all microorganisms from an object.
- **Sterile**—The material free from all microbial life.
- **Disinfection**—Reducing the number of pathogenic organisms on objects or in materials so that they pose no threat of disease.
- **Antiseptic**—A chemical substance applied to living tissue/skin for preventing the growth of disease causing microorganisms.

- **Disinfectant**—A chemical agent applied on non-living (inanimate) objects to destroy microorganisms.
- **Physical agents to reduce/inhibit, kill microorganisms** include sunlight, drying, heat (dry and moist heat), radiation, filtration and ultrasonic and sonic vibrations, heat being the major agent in medicine.
- **Antimicrobial chemical agents** include phenol and phenol derivatives, alcohols, halogens, heavy metals, surface-active agents, aldehydes, dyes, gaseous agents and hydrogen peroxide.
- Moist heat (steam) under pressure (15 psi) (121°C temperature) used to sterilize an object in an **autoclave** is called **autoclaving** or **steam sterilization**.
- Dry heat is used to sterilize an object in an **oven** (also called **sterilizer**).
- **Sanitizer** is a compound (e.g. soap or detergent) used to reduce the level of contaminants and the process is called **sanitization**.

IMPORTANT QUESTIONS

1. Define sterilization, disinfection, antiseptic and disinfectant. Describe in brief the applications of sterilization and disinfection.
2. Describe the role of moist and dry heat in sterilization.
3. Name various types of disinfectants. Discuss the uses and mode of action of alcohols, halogens and moist heat.
4. Write short notes on:
   (a) Autoclave
   (b) Hot-air oven
   (c) Pasteurization
   (d) Role of UV radiations in sterilization
   (e) Halogens or aldehydes as antimicrobial agents.

MULTIPLE-CHOICE QUESTIONS

1. All of the following processes kill endospores EXCEPT:
   (a) Incineration
   (b) Hot-air sterilization
   (c) Autoclaving
   (d) Pasteurization.
2. Incineration is an efficient method for:
   (a) Sterilizing points of forceps
   (b) Destroying contaminated materials

(c) Sterilizing scalpel blades and needles
(d) Sterilizing all glass syringes.

3. Exposure of material to moist heat at 100°C for 20 minutes on three consecutive days is known as:
   (a) Pasteurization (b) Autoclaving
   (c) Tyndallization (d) Inspissation.
4. The temperature pressure combination for an autoclave is
   (a) 100°C and 4 psi
   (b) 115°C and 9 psi
   (c) 121°C and 15 psi
   (d) 131°C and 16 psi.
5. Nonionizing radiation acts on microbes by:
   (a) Producing superoxide ions
   (b) Making pyrimidine dimers
   (c) Breaking disulphide bonds
   (d) Denaturing proteins.
6. Phenol is bactericidal at a concentration of:
   (a) 0.1% (b) 0.2%
   (c) 0.5% (d) 1.0%.
7. Which of the following is most suitable to sterilize heat-sensitive materials (rubber and plastic) and bulk materials (e.g., mattresses)?
   (a) UV radiation (b) Dry heat
   (c) Autoclaving (d) Ethylene oxide.
8. Dry heat damages microbes by
   (a) Denaturing nucleic acid
   (b) Denaturing proteins
   (c) Destructive oxidation of essential cell constituents
   (d) None of the above.
9. Which of the following methods can be used to sterilize a liquid without damaging heat-labile proteins in the solution?
   (a) Autoclaving
   (b) Boiling
   (c) Filtering through 0.5 μm filter
   (d) Filtering through 0.22 μm filter.
10. Silver nitrate is used:
   (a) To disinfect water
   (b) In antiseptic of burns

(c) To treat genital gonorrhoea

(d) As a mouth wash.

11. Which of the following is an approved sterilant?

(a) Betadine (b) Ethyl alcohol

(c) Chlorhexidine (d) Ethylene oxide.

ANSWERS TO MCQs

1. (d)	2. (b)	3. (c)	4. (c)	5. (b)
6. (d)	7. (d)	8. (c)	9. (d)	10. (c)
11. (d).				

19
Antimicrobial Chemotherapy and Antibiotics

CHEMOTHERAPY

The term chemotherapy is derived from Greek words: *Chemieia* = chemistry and *theraapeia* = service to the sick. In simple words, treatment of diseases by chemical compounds is called **chemotherapy**. The chemical agents used in medical practice are called **chemotherapeutic agents** or **drugs**. But to most people, the word chemotherapy means drugs used for cancer treatment. It's often shortened to **"chemo"**.

The term chemotherapy was coined in early 1900s by the German physician **Paul Ehrlich** to treat microbial diseases by the use of chemical substances without harming the host.

ANTIMICROBIAL CHEMOTHERAPY

Antimicrobial chemotherapy is defined as the treatment of microbial (infectious) diseases by the use of chemical agents. A chemical agent used to treat a disease caused by a microbe (or parasite) is called an **antimicrobial agent**. And the prevention of infections by use of antimicrobial drugs is called **antimicrobial prophylaxis**.

Paul Ehrlich was the first to treat African sleeping sickness, the disease caused by a trypanosome, by the dye **trypan red** in 1904. This dye with antimicrobial activity was referred to as a **"magic bullet"**. It was followed by the use of **salvarsan** (arsenobenzol) to treat syphilis (caused by *Treponema pallidum*) by **Ehrlich** and **Sakahiro Hata** in 1910. Use of salvarsan marked the beginning of the era of chemotherapy, the foundation laid by Ehrlich. Hence, **Paul Ehrlich** is known as the **father of modern chemotherapy**.

TYPES OF ANTIMICROBIAL THERAPY

Based on the effectivity of an antimicrobial drug against a kind of microbe is of five types:

(i) *Antibacterial chemotherapy*—treats bacterial infections (e.g., penicillin, sulfoniamides).

(ii) *Antifungal chemotherapy*—treats mycoses (fungal infections) (e.g., amphotericin B, griseofulvin).

(iii) *Antiviral chemotherapy*—treats viral infections (e.g., ribavirin, idoxuridine).

(iv) *Antiprotozoan chemotherapy*—treats protozoan infections (e.g., chloroquine, metronidazole).

(v) *Antihelminthic chemotherapy*—treats helminth (or worm) infections (e.g., mebendazole, niclosamide).

ANTIBIOTICS

Antibiotic literally means "against life", is derived from Greek words: *anti* = against + *bios* = life. An **antibiotic** is defined as a chemical substance produced by microorganisms which has the ability to kill or inhibit the growth of pathogenic microorganisms in low concentration.

Antibiotics are low-molecular weight, non-proteinaceous molecules produced as **secondary metabolites** mainly by soil-inhabiting microorganisms. Commercially used antibiotics have been derived from five taxa: *Streptomyces* (streptomycin, tetracyclines), *Bacillus* (polymyxin, bactericin); *Penicillium* (penicillin, griseofulvin), *Cephalosporium* (cephalosporin) and *Micromonospora* (gentamycin).

In contrast to antibiotics, antimicrobial compounds made by chemical synthesis are called **synthetic drugs** (sulfonamids, trimethoprim); and the antimicrobial agents made partly by microorganisms and partly by laboratory synthesis are known as **semisynthetic drugs** or **semisynthetic antibiotics** (amoxicillin, ketoconazole).

The current trend is to use the term **antimicrobic** for all antimicrobial drugs, regardless of their origin; and **antibioic** for all antimicrobials which destroy pathogens within the body.

PROPERTIES OF ANTIBIOTICS

- Antibiotics are low molecular weight, non-proteinaceous molecules.
- They are produced as secondary metabolites by microorganisms.
- They either inhibit microbial growth (*microbistatic*) or kill bacteria (*bactericidal*) or other microogansims (*microbicidal*).
- They are derived from microorganisms that normally reside in soil.

- They exhibit selective toxicity.
- They are either **broad spectrum** (effective against a variety of species), **narrow-spectrum** (effective against Gram-positive or Gram-negative bacteria), and **limited spectrum** (effective against a single organism or disease).
- They are selective in their effect on different microorganisms.
- Antibiotics are potentially capable of eliciting various types of hypersensitivity.
- They vary in their toxicity for animals and human beings.
- They taget certain essential functions of the microbe resulting in growth inhibition or death.
- Sensitivity of an antibiotic gradually changes after contact with an organism for varying periods resulting in resistance.
- Medically used antibiotics do not interfere with essential functions of the microbe's host.

MODE OF ACTION OF ANTIMICROBIAL DRUGS

Antimicrobial drugs/antibiotics target certain essential functions of the pathogen resulting in killing (microbicidal) or inhibiting growth (microbistatic) thereby controlling infection and treating the patient.

Mechanisms of action of antimicrobial agents are categorized into five types:

1. **Inhibitors of cell wall synthesis**
    - Natural and semisynthetic penicillins
    - Cephalosprins (cephalothin, cefixime, cefactor)
    - Polypeptide antibiotics (bacitracin, vancomycin)
    - Isoniazid
    - Capsofungin
    - Cycloserine
2. **Inhibitors of plasma membrane functions**
    - Polymyxin B
    - Amphotericin B
    - Azoles
3. **Inhibitors of protein synthesis**
    - Chloramphenicol
    - Aminioglycosides (streptomycin, neomycin, gentamicin)
    - Tetracyclines (plain tetracycline, chlorotetracycline, doxycycline).

- Macrolides (erythromycin, azithromycin, clarithomycin)
- Clindamycin
- Fusidic acid

4. **Inhibitors of nucleic acid replication and transcription (i.e., nucleic acid synthesis)**
    - Rifamycins (rifamycin)
    - Quinolones (nalidixic acid, ciprofloxacin, gatifloxacin)
5. **Inhibitors of the synthesis of essential metabolites**
    - Sulfonamides (trimethoprim)
    - Isoniazid

SOME COMMONLY USED ANTIMICROBIAL DRUGS

PENICILLIN

Penicillin (PCN or Pen) refers to a group of antibiotics which include *penicillin G, penicillin V* and *benzathine penicillin*. These are characterized by a common chemical nucleus (6 – aminopenicillanic acid) which contains a β-*lactam ring*. This ring is responsible for its antibacterial activity, i.e., **inhibition of cell wall synthesis** of Gram-positive bacteria.

Penicillin G (or **benzlpenicillin**) was isolated from the mold *Penicillium notatum* in 1928 by Scottish scientist **Sir Alexander Fleming**. It was the first antibiotic discovered and became the first clinically effective antibacterial antibiotic against many bacterial infections caused by staphylococci and streptococci.

Pencillins act by preventing the cross-linking of the peptidoglycans, which interferes with the final stages of the construction of the cell walls, thus inhibiting the cell wall synthesis, primarily of Gram-positive bacteria. They have a narrow-spectrum of activity and are **bactericidal** in rapidly multiplying bacteria.

Penicillin G is the drug of choice in treating infections caused by Gram-positive bacteria, including streptococci, clostridia, pneumococci and several spirochetes. It is adminstered **parenterally** (a route of drug administration other than the gastrointestinal tract), that is, **intramuscularly** or **intravenously**, but never through the gut (orally) since most of it is broken down by stomach acids.

Two major disadvantages of penicillin are:

- Allergy to penicillin among adults (1-10%), serious allergy only in 0.03%.
- Development of resistance in bacteria that produce the enzyme-penicillinases (β-lactamases), most notably species of *Staphyloccocus*.

CEPHALOSPORINS

Cephalosporins are bactericidal **β-lactam antibiotics** similar to **penicillin**. The first cephalosporin was isolated from the fungus *Cephalosporium acremonium* (now named *Acremonium*) by an Italian scientist **Gluseppe Brotizu** in 1945. Cephalosporins are bactericidal (kill bacteria) and act in a similar way to penicillin. They bind to and block the activity of enzymes responsible for making peptidoglycan, an important compound of the bacterial cell wall, thus **inhibiting cell wall synthesis**.

Structures of cephalosporins have been modified to make them more effictive against a wide range of bacteria. Currently, five generations of cepalosphorins exist. These have been referred to as the first, second, third, fourth, and fifth generation cephalosporins.

Examples include:

• *First generation*	Cephalothin-cephalexin	Effective aganist Gram-negative bacteria.
• *Second generation*	Cefacbor (oral) cefamdole (IV)	More active against Gram-negative bacteria.
• *Third generation*	Ceftazidime Cefixime Cefdinir	Most active against Gram-negative bacteria, including pseudomonads.
• *Fourth generation*	Cefepime	Most extended spectrum of activity.
• *Fifth generation*	Ceftaroline	Active against MRSA (methicillin resistant *Staphylococcus aureus*), Gram-positive and Gram-negative bacteria.

Cephalosporins are used as alternatives to penicillin where resistance is found and in cases where penicillin allergies exist. They are used to treat respiratory tract infections, urinary tract infections and skin infections caused by bacteria.

TETRACYCLINES

Tetracyclines are **broad-spectrum** (inculding chlamdias and rickettsias) antibiotics, produced by *Streptomyces* species. These are characterized by **four-ring nucleus** with attached side chains. They act by inhibiting the protein synthesis by binding to 30S portion of the 70S ribosome thereby interfering with the binding of tRNA to mRNA.

The first tetracycline discovered was aureomycin (=choloro-tetracycline) from a soil bacterium (*Streptomyces aureofaciens*) in 1948 by an American botanist, **Benjamin Minge Duggar**. It was patented in 1953 and came into commercial use in 1978. Currently, it is on the World Health Organization's List of Essential Medicines, the most effective and safe medicine in a health system.

Of the eight kinds of tetracyclines, *oxytetracycline* (terramycin), *chlorotetracycline* (aureomycin) and *tetracycline* itself are more commonly used. Being broad-spectrum in nature, they are used to treat many urinary tract infections, chlamydial and rickettsial infections, mycoplasmal pneumonia, syphilis and gonorrhea.

Their use is to be avoided in children as they cause brownish discoloration of the teeth and in pregnant women they damage the liver. Tetracyclines may also cause superinfections of the gastrointestinal tract by *Candida albicans* due to the suppression of useful normal microbiota.

CHLORAMPHENICOL

Chloramphenicol, an antibacterial, first broad-spectrum antibiotic was isolated in 1947 from *Streptomyces venezuelae* by **David Gottlieb**. Due to the presence of chlorine in the molecule it was named chloramphenicol. It is the first antibiotic to be artificially synthesized in 1949, instead of extraction from a microorganism.

It inhibits protein synthesis by binding to the 70S ribosomes of prokaryotic cells.

Chloramphenicol (brand named: Chloromycetin) is an effective drug used for treatment of serious infections caused by bacteria (e.g., typhoid, cholera, plague and meningitis) when other medicines are ineffective. It is often used as an eye ointment or eye drops to treat conjunctivites.

BACTERIAL RESISTANCE TO ANTIBIOTICS

Resistance to an antibiotic means that a bacterium formerly susceptible/sensitive to the action of an antibiotic/drug is no longer affected by it. The spread of drug-resistant pathogens is one of the most serious threats to the successful treatment of infectious diseases. Bacterial resistance to antibiotics leads to longer hospital stay, higher medical costs and increased mortality. Morever, it is one of the biggest threats to global health, food security and development. A growing number of infections such as pneumonia, tuberculosis, gonorrhoea and salmonellosis are becoming harder to treat due to the development of drug resistance.

Bacteria that are resistant to large number of antibiotics are designated as **superbugs.** Overuse and misuse of antibiotics has resulted in an explosion of microorganisms resistant to all common drugs. Notable examples include: methicillin-resistant *Staplylococus aureus* (MRSA), penicillin-resistant *Enterococcus faecium*, and multidrug-resistant *Mycobacterium tuberculosis* (MDR-TB) which is resistant to two TB drugs (isoniazid and rifampicin), vancomycin-resistant *Enterococcus* (VRE), and carbapenem-resistant Enterobacteriaceae gut bacteria.

Mechanisms of Antibiotic Resistance

Antibiotic resistance occurs when bacteria develop the ability to defeat the drugs designed to kill them. When bacteria become resistant, antibiotics cannot fight them, and the surviving bacteria continue to multiply causing more harm to the host. In some cases, antibiotic resistance infections can lead to serious disability or even death.

Major mechanisms (Fig. 19.1) by which bacteria become resistant to antibiotics include:

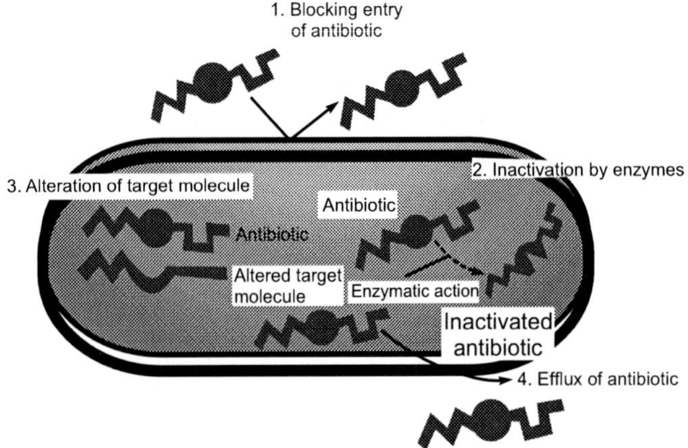

Fig. 19.1 A few mechanisms of bacterial resistance to antibiotics.

- blocking entry of the antibiotic into the bacterial cell;
- synthesis of enzymes that inactivate the antibiotic;
- change in the number or affinity of the drug's receptor sites;
- modification of the essential metabolic pathways of the host formerly attacked by the drug;
- efflux of the drug from the cell;
- when an organism survives exposure to an antibiotic;

- due to mutations on the chromosomal DNA-drug resistant mutants arise spontaneously once in 10^7 to 10^{10} cell divisions; and
- **R-factors** (resistance R plasmids) act as very important mode of transferable drug resistance in bacteria.

Knowledge of drug resistance mechanisms in microorganisms is critical for understanding the limitations of antibiotics' use.

ANTIBIOTIC SENSITIVITY TESTING

Antibiotic sensitivity (or **antibiotic susceptibility**) is defined as the susceptibility of bacteria to antibiotics. Antibiotic susceptibily test (AST) is performed in a clinical laboratory as to which antibiotic will be most effective in treating a bacterial infection *in vivo* which forms the basis of an ideal antibiotic therapy.

Sensitivity of bacteria to antibiotics is determined by exposing them to the agents in laboratory cultures. Several methods—disk diffusion, dilution, serum-killing power and automated methods are available to do this. Of these, disk diffusion method is often used.

DISK-DIFFUSION METHOD

Disk-diffusion method (Fig. 19.2), an agar diffusion technique, was developed in the early 1960s by **William M. Kirby** and **A.W. Bauer** hence also termed **Kirby–Bauer** method. It is the most commonly used method for testing antibiotic (drug) sensitivity.

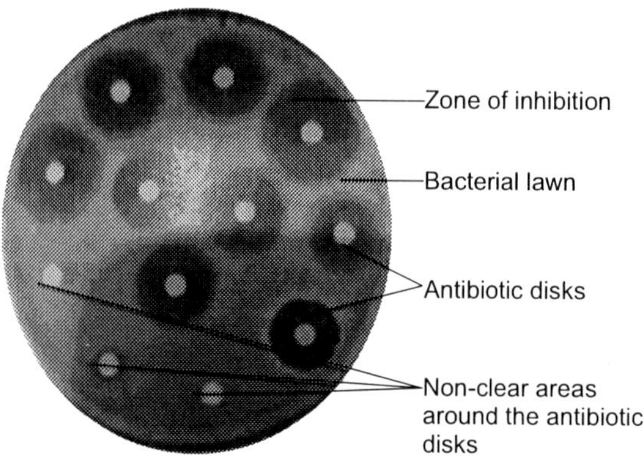

Fig. 19.2 The Kirby-Bauer (disk-diffusion) antimicrobial susceptibility test. Of the 12 antibiotics tested against a bacterium, nine inhibited growth around disks, indicating their effectiveness and three disks did not inhibit the growth (no clear areas around disks) indicating resistance of these antibiotics.

It this test, paper disks, each containing a measured amount of a particular antibiotic, are placed into a **Müeller–Hinton agar** plate preswabbed with a test bacterium. A clear ring, or zone 24-48 hours post-incubation, around a disk represents inhibition of test bacterium by the antibiotic (i.e., sensitive to the antibiotic). The antibiotic diffuses in the area surrounding each disk resulting in bacterial lysis (clear zone). Non-clear areas indicate resistance to that antibiotic.

The diameters of zones of inhibition are measured after 24–48 hours incubation and compared to a standard table for that drug and concentration to know whether the tested organism is sensitive, moderately sensitive, or resistant to the drug.

KEY POINTS

- **Chemotherapy** is the treatment of infections by chemical compounds.
- **Chemotherapeutic agents** or **drugs** are chemical agents in medical practice.
- Paul Ehrlich, the discoverer and first user of trypan red and salvarsan to treat infections is the **father of modern chemotherapy**.
- **Antibiotic** is a microbially produced chemical substance that kills or inhibits the growth of pathogenic microorganism in low concentration.
- **Antibiotic (drug) resistance** means that a bacterium does not respond to the therapeutic dose of the drug clinically designed for it.
- Mode of action of an antimicrobial drug (antibiotic) on microorganisms is either by inhibiting cell wall synthesis, protein synthesis, DNA synthesis, essential metabolite or functions of the plasma membrane.
- **Disk-diffusion** (or **Kirby-Bauer**) method, based on the agar diffusion technique, is the method of choice for antibiotic sensitivity testing.

IMPORTANT QUESTIONS

1. Describe briefly:
   (a) Antibacterial antibiotics
   (b) Chemotherapy
   (c) Mode of action of antibacterial antibiotics
   (d) Antibiotic resistance mechanisms
   (e) Antibiotic sensitivity testing.

MULTIPLE-CHOICE QUESTIONS

1. Which of the following scientists is known as the father of modern chemotherapy?
   (a) Alexander Fleming (b) Joseph Lister
   (c) Paul Ehrlich (d) Robert Koch.
2. Quinine (chloroquinine) used to treat malaria is obtained from -
   (a) Plants (b) Animals
   (c) Bacteria (d) Molds.
3. Which of the following antibiotics acts by causing injury to the plasma membrane?
   (a) Polymyxin B (b) Penicillin
   (c) Tetracycline (d) All of the above.
4. Penicillins and cephalosporins act on microorganisms by interfering with:
   (a) Protein synthesis
   (b) DNA synthesis
   (c) Cell wall synthesis
   (d) Cell membrane functions.
5. Protozoan infections are treated with:
   (a) Primethamine (b) Metronidazole
   (c) Mabendazole (d) Griseofulvin.
6. Cephalosporins resemble which antibiotic in their structure and mode of action:
   (a) Penicillin (b) Tetracycline
   (c) Erythromycin (d) Chloramphenicol.
7. An antibiotic that contains β-lactam ring in its molecule is:
   (a) Tetracycline (b) Bacitracin
   (c) Penicillin (d) Polymyxin B.
8. Which of the following drug is used to treat fungal infections?
   (a) Amphotericin B (b) Penicillin
   (c) Mabendazole (d) Ribavirin.
9. Which term is used when a bacterium does not respond to the therapeutic dose of the drug clinically designed for it?

ANSWERS TO MCQs

1. (c) 2. (a) 3. (a) 4. (c)
5. (b) 6. (a) 7. (c) 8. (a)
9. Antibiotic or drug resistance.

20

Standard/Universal/Safety Precautions in Healthcare

UNIVERSAL PRECAUTIONS

Universal blood and body fluid precautions or **universal precautions (UPs)** is a "set of guidelines designed by the CDC to protect the health-care workers from exposure to infections such as HIV, Hepatitis B virus and other pathogens which are transmitted by blood and other body fluids of the patient in healthcare settings". Examples of bodily fluids (also called body fluids and biofluid) to which UPs apply include blood, semen, vaginal tissue, cerebrospinal, synovial (joint cavity), pleural, peritoneal, pericardial, and amniotic fluids. As per CDC, UPs do not apply to urine, faeces, sputum vomitus, sweat, tears, and nasal secretions, as long as these do not contain visible blood.

Universal precautions apply to *all* patients, not just those infected with the viruses that cause AIDS or hepatitis B, hence the term *universal*.

The universal precautions for preventing illness includes:

- Wear gloves and gown if soiling of hands, exposed skin, or clothing with blood or body fluids is *likely*.
- Wear both masks and protective eyewear or chin length plastic faceshields whenever splattering or splashing of blood or body fluids is *likely*.
- Wash hands before and after patient contact, and after removal of gloves. Change gloves with *each* patient.
- Use disposable mouth piece/airway for cardiopulmonary resuscitation (i.e., the process of reviving a person from unconsciousness or apparent death).
- Immediately discard contaminated needles and other sharp items into a *nearby* puncture-proof container.
- Needles must *not* be bent, clipped or recapped
- Clean spills of blood or contaminated fluids by:
  1. Putting on gloves and any other barriers needed.
  2. Wiping up with disposable towels.

3. Washing with soap and water.
4. Disinfecting with a 1:10 solution of household bleach and water for minimum 10 minutes.

STANDARD PRECAUTIONS

Standard precautions in healthcare are defined as "the minimum level of infection control precautions (or measures) used when providing care to the patients". They have been designed to prevent the transmission of infectious organisms from patient to healthcare worker, healthcare worker to patient, patient to patient, hospital environment to patient, and hospital waste to community. They are the cornerstones of nosocomial infection prevention and are to be used by every nurse for every patient every time in all healthcare settings (medical and dental).

Standard precautions recommedations are the result of merger of two practices (universal precautions and body substance isolation) by CDC in 1996.

Healthcare Facility Recommendations for Standard Precautions (WHO, 2007) are given below.

1. **Hand hygiene:** It refers to both washing hands with soap and water, and alcohol gel. Hand washing is a major component of standard precautions and one of the most effective methods to prevent transmission of pathogens associated will healthcare.

   Hands should be washed immediately and thoroughly if contaminated with blood or other body fluids, after gloves are removed before and after any direct patient contact and between patients before handling an invasive device, and after contact with inanimate objects in the immediate vicinity of the patient.
2. **Gloves:** These should be worn when touching blood and body fluids, mucous membranes, and nonintact skin and when handling items or surfaces soiled with body fluids. These should be changed after contact with each patient and even between tasks and procedures on the same patient. Follow the **glove pyramid** – to aid decision making on when to wear (and not wear) gloves.
3. **Facial protection (eyes, nose and mouth):** Masks and protective eyewear or face shields should be worn during activities that are likely to generate splashes of blood or other body fluids.
4. **Gown:** Gown or aprons should be worn to protect the skin and prevent soiling of clothing during procedures that are likely to generate splashy or sprays of blood or other body fluids.

5. **Prevention of needlestick injuries:** Extensive care should be taken while handling needles, scalpels, other sharp instruments, or cleaning used instruments. Used needles or sharp instruments should be placed in puncture-resistant containers for disposal.
6. **Respiratory hygiene and cough etiquette:** Persons with respiratory symptoms should cover their nose and mouth when coughing/sneezing with tissue or mask, dispose of used tissue masks properly. Perform hand hygiene after contact with respiratory secretions, and spatial separation of persons with acute febrile respiratory symptoms.
7. **Environmental cleaning:** Adeqate procedures should be used for routine cleaning and disinfection of environmental and other frequently touched surfaces.
8. **Linens:** Used linens should be handled, transported and processed in a manner to avoid transfer of pathognes to other patients and/or the environment.
9. **Waste disposal:** Ensure safe management of clinical waste in accordance with local regulations.
10. **Patient care equipment:** Clean, disnifect and reprocess resuable patient care equipment appropriately before use with another patient, and handle equipment contaminated with blood and body fluids.
11. **Personal protective equipment (PPE):** Use of PPE (gloves, gown, mask, protective eyewear) should be guided by risk assessment and extent of contact anticipated with blood and body fluids, or pathogens. In addition, provision of adequate staff and supplies, together with leadership and equation of health workers, patients, and visitors, is critical for an enhanced safety climate in healthcare settings.

KEY POINTS

- **Universal precautions** also called **unversal blood and body fluid precautions** are a set of CDC guidelines designed to protect the healthcare workers from exposure to infection transmitted by blood and body fluids.
- **Standard precautions** are the result of merger of universal precautions and body substance isolation by CDC and designed to prevent infection from health workes to patient and vice versa, nosocomial infections and from hospital waste to community.

IMPORTANT QUESTIONS

1. Write briefly on:
   (a) The Universal Precautions for preventing illness/disease
   (b) Recommendations for standard precautions in healthcare.

MULTIPLE-CHOICE QUESTIONS

1. Standard precautions don't include:
   (a) Washing hands before and after patient contact
   (b) Use of aseptic techniques
   (c) Use of gloves and gowns at all times in health care
   (d) Appropriate handling of contaminated clinical waste.
2. Universal safety precautions are a set of guidelines designed to protect the:
   (a) patient's samples (b) patient's relatives
   (c) healthcare workers (d) patients.
3. Standard precautions include:
   (a) Appropriate use of personal protective equipment
   (b) Appropriate handling of sharp equipment
   (c) Hand hygiene
   (d) All of the above.
4. Personal protective equipment (PPE) doesn't include:
   (a) Mask (b) Gloves
   (c) Protective eye wear (d) Linens.
5. Universal precautions apply to all of the following bodily fluids EXCEPT:
   (a) Semen (b) Tears
   (c) Blood (d) Amniotic fluid.

ANSWERS TO MCQs

1. (c) 2. (c) 3. (d) 4. (d) 5. (b).

21

Handwashing and Hand Hygiene

Thousands of people die every day around the world from infectious diseases acquired while receiving healthcare. Hands are the main routes of germ transmission during healthcare.

Hands contaminated with toilet are the cause of transmitting diarrhoeal pathogens from person to food contact surfaces after using the toilet that include:

- *Salmonella, Shigella, Escherichia, Campylobacter* (bacterial pathogens).
- Hepatitis A, norovirus, rotavirus (viral pathogens).
- *Taenia* (helminths).
- *Giardia, Cryptosporidium* (protozoa).

Eye infections (trachoma), skin (impetigo), and respiratory infections (influenza H_1N_1 or common cold, SARS coronavirus) are also transmitted by hands.

Staphylococus aureus, streptococci, Gram-negative bacilli (*Escherichia coli, Pseudomonas*) and viruses, resident hand microbiota which is difficult to remove by simple hand washing also cause human diseases.

ROLE OF HANDS IN DISEASE TRANSMISSION: HISTORICAL

Ignaz Semmelweis, a Hungarian physician, the **father of hand hygiene**, was the first person to report in 1847—the agent causing childbed fever, is transmitted through hands to the doctor and medical students attending on woman in labour in Vienna hospital. In the same year, he also observed that handwashing by healthcare workers reduced the incidence of infections in patients. **Lord Joseph Lister,** a famous British surgeon, the **father of antiseptic surgery**, in 1867 used carbolic acid (later called phenol) to wash hands before and attending the patients to prevent transmission of infections.

HAND HYGIENE

Hand hygiene refers to cleaning of hands for the purpose of removing soil, dirt, and pathogenic microorganisms. It includes washing hands with plain or antibacterial soap and water, and rubbing of hands with alcohol gel.

Since most of the nosocomial and diarrhoeal pathogens are transmitted by contaminated hands, hand hygiene is, therefore, the most important measure to avoid the transmission of harmful germs and prevent infections throughout the entire community from your home and work place to childcare facilities and hospitals. Hand hygiene is the most important component of standard precautions in healthcare.

May 5th is celebrated every year the **"World Hygiene Day"** globally highlighting the importance of hand hygiene in healthcare to prevent infections including sepsis.

Each year **Global Handwashing Day (GHD)** is celebrated on October 15th since 2008 as a global campaign to raise awareness, to motivate and mobilize people around the world to emphasize the significance of cleaning hands with soap as it is a **"do - it - yourself vaccine"** that prevents infection and saves lives.

HOW TO PERFORM HAND HYGIENE?

- **Handwashing**—Washing of hands with soap and water when hands are visibly dirty or visibly soiled with blood or other body fluids or after using toilet.

  If exposure to potential spore forming bacterial pathogens is strongly suspected or proven including outbreak of *Clostridium difficile*—(the cause of watery diarrhoea and colitis) handwashing with soap and water is the preferred choice.
- **Handrubbing**—Cleaning of hands by rubbing them with an alcohol-based formulation that contains 60% alcohol. It is the preferred means for routine hygienic hand antisepsis if **hands are not visibly soiled**. Handrubbing is faster, more effective and better tolerated by your hands than washing with soap and water (i.e. handwashing).

WHEN HANDWASHING IS A MUST FOR HEALTHCARE WORKERS

- Before and after touching a patient.
- Immediately touching blood and body fluids.
- Before handling an invasive device.

- When moving from a contaminated to clean site of the patient.
- After touching patient surroundings – any object or furniture, changing bed linen.
- After coughing or sneezing into a tissue.

KEY TIMES FOR HANDWASHING BY EVERY HUMAN BEING

- Before, during and after preparing food.
- Before eating food.
- After using the toilet.
- After touching garbage.
- After cleaning kitchen's shelf.
- After changing diapers or cleaning up a child who has used the toilet.
- After blowing your nose, coughing or sneezing.
- After touching an animal, animal feed or animal waste.

HANDWASHING WITH SOAP AND WATER

Steps:

- Wet your hands with clean, running water (normal or warm).
- Apply enough soap to cover all hand surfaces.
- Rub hands together to make enough lather and lather the backs of your hands, between yours fingers, and under your nails.
- Scrub your hands for at least 15 seconds (using a timer) or hum the "Happy Birthday" song from beginning to end twice.
- Rinse your hands well under clean, running water.
- Dry your hands using a clean paper towel or air dryer.
- Entire procedure of handwashing takes 40-60 seconds.

HANDRUBBING WITH ALCOHOL BASED SANITIZER

Steps:

- Apply a palmful of the alcohol based hand rub or gel in a cupped hand (often left) with right hand.
- Rub hands together thoroughly.
- Spread the gel over all surfaces of your hands (palm and back) and fingers.

- Continue rubbing until the hands are dry.
- Entire procedure takes 20–30 seconds.

KEY POINTS

- **Hand hygiene** refers to the cleaning of hands for the purpose of removing soil, dirt and pathogenic microorganisms to prevent healthcare associated and community infections.
- Wash hands (handwashing) with soap and water visibly soiled.
- Rub hands (handrubbing) with alcohol gel for hand hygiene.

IMPORTANT QUESTIONS

1. Write notes on
   (a) Hand hygiene
   (b) Differentiate between handwashing and handrubbing.

MULTIPLE-CHOICE QUESTIONS

1. Alcohol based handrub may be used instead of soap and water when hands are not visibly soiled. True or False?
2. Hand hygiene is the most important way to prevent the spread of germs. True or False?
3. There is no need to perform hand hygiene after using a tissue for coughing or sneezing. True or False?
4. What is the best way to prevent the spread of germs?
   (a) Eat healthy
   (b) Cover your mouth with your hands when you sneeze
   (c) Wash your hands often
   (d) Wear gloves at work.
5. Which of the following statement is true about the use of alcohol based hand rubs?
   (a) Apply a large amount of gel into wet palms.
   (b) Hand rub should be used when hands are visibly soiled.
   (c) Rub hands until dry before performing another task.
   (d) Rinse product off with warm water after 15 seconds.
6. During handwashing which of the following is important to remember?
   (a) Lather and rub hands together for 15 seconds
   (b) Wash hands with hottest water possible

(c) Turn faucet off after disposing of your paper towel
(d) The focus of good handwashing is the palms.

7. Which of the following scientists is called the father of hygiene?
(a) Joseph Lister (b) Ignaz Semmelweis
(c) Paul Ehrlich (d) Edward Jenner.

8. Since 2008, every year Handwashing Day is celebrated on:
(a) 5th May (b) 15th June
(c) 15th October (d) 1st December.

ANSWERS TO MCQs

1. True 2. True 3. False 4. (c) 5. (c)
6. (a) 7. (b) 8. (c).

22

Biomedical (Hospital) Waste Treatment

WHAT IS BIOMEDICAL WASTE TREATMENT?

Biomedical waste treatment deals with the segregation, transportation, storage, treatment and disposal of medical waste. Proper management of hospital waste is part of hospital infection prevention measures. Being a mandatory legal requirement, it is a duty of every healthcare facility to strictly follow the *Biomedical Waste Management (Management and Handling) Rules*, 1998, revised in 2011, 2016 promulgated by the Government of India.

WHAT IS BIOMEDICAL WASTE?

Biomedical waste (BMW) or **medical waste** refers to any waste generated from biological or medical sources during testing, diagnosis, immunization or treatment of either humans or animals. In simple words, BMW refers to "**by-products of the healthcare industry**".

Common examples of BMW is used microbial culture dishes, glassware, bandages, gloves, discarded sharps like needles and scalpels, swabs, and human and animal wastes.

BMW is produced by hospitals, health clinics, nursing homes, dental clinics, home healthcare, emergency medical services, medical research facilities, clinical laboratories, veterinary clinics, offices of physicians, dentists, veterinarians, and funeral homes.

Different names for medical waste include:

- Medical waste
- Biomedical waste (BMW)
- Clinical waste
- Biohazardous waste
- Healthcare waste
- Infectious medical waste
- Regulated medical waste (RMW)

HEALTH HAZARDS OF BMW

Medical waste can pose several health hazards to healthcare employees, waste workers and the general public. These include:

- **Hazards from sharps and infectious waste:** Pathogens in infectious waste may enter the human body through a puncture, cut or abrasion in skin resulting in infection. Infections of concern are HIV (AIDS) and hepatitis viruses B and C.
- **Hazards from pharmaceutical and chemical wastes:** Many of the chemical disinfectants and pharmaceuticals used as medicine are toxic, genotoxic, flammable, reactive and explosive. They may cause burns, injuries or intoxication.
- **Hazards from radioactive waste:** Radioactive exposure may lead to headache, dizziness, vomiting and sometimes serious complications.
- **Pollution from infectious waste:** Improperly treated waste may cause soil, water and environmental pollution.

TYPES OF MEDICAL WASTE

In our country, the amount of waste generated in healthcare settings has been estimated as 0.5-2 kg/bed/day. On an average 1/5 (i.e., 20%) is medical waste and the rest 80% is general waste.

The BMW is composed of infectious waste (15%), chemical and pharmaceuticals (3%), sharps (1%), radioactive, genotoxic and heavy metals (1%).

Based on their harmful effects on humans, BMW is mainly of two types:

- **Biohazardous medical waste** includes sharps, human tissue fluids and contaminated supplies.
- **General medical waste** includes non-contaminated equipment and animal tissues.

  WHO has categorized BMW into 8 types: sharps, infectious, radioactive, pathological, pharmaceutical, chemical, genotoxic and general non-regulated medical waste.
- **Sharps waste** includes all things that can pierce the skin such as needles, scalpels, lancet, razor, ampules, staples, wires, trocars and broken glass.
- **Infectious (or biohazardous) waste** includes all infectious or potentially infectious things such as swabs, tissue, excreta, lab cultures and equipment. These are the source of pathogenic

microbes that can infect healthcare workers, patients and the general public.

- **Radioactive waste** includes unused radiotherapy liquid, lab research liquid, in addition to any glassware or other supplies contaminated with this liquid.
- **Pathological waste** includes human fluids, tissue, body parts, blood, bodily fluids, and contaminated animal carcasses.
- **Pharmacological waste** includes all unused time expired vaccines and drugs (e.g., antibiotics, injectables and pills).
- **Chemical waste** includes disinfectants, solvents used in lab, batteries and heavy metals from medical equipment (e.g., mercury from broken thermometers).
- **Genotoxic waste** includes cytotoxic drugs (i.e., carcinogenic, tetragonic or mutagenic) which are used to treat cancer patients.
- **Non-hazardous waste** also called **general non-regulated medical waste**, includes all those who don't pose any particular chemical, biological, physical or radioactive damage. Examples are paper, cardboard, cartons, flowers and ordinary office or kitchen waste akin to domestic waste.

WASTE SEGREGATION

Waste segregation refers to the basic separation of different categories of waste generated at source. Segregation is the most crucial step in BMW management reducing the risks and cost of handling and disposal.

Disposal occurs **off-site**, at a location that is different from the site of generation. Off-site treatment involves having of a BMW disposal service (also called a truck service) whose employees collect and haul away the waste in special containers, usually cardboard boxes, or reusable plastic bins, based on the colour-coded segregation system as per the Government of India, *Biomedical Waste Management Rules* 2016.

The latest guidelines for segregation of BMW recommend the following five colour coding: red, yellow, blue, white and black.

- **Red bag** is used for syringes (without needles), soiled gloves, catheters, IV tubes. These are later incinerated.
- **Yellow bag** is used for all dressings, bandages and cotton swabs with body fluids, blood bags, human anatomical waste, body parts, soiled bed sheets, and microbiology laboratory waste.
- **Card board box with blue marking/sticker** is used for glass vials, ampules and other glassware.

- **White translucent puncture-proof container (PPC)** is used for needles, sharps and blades.
- **Black bag** is used for non-biological waste, e.g., stationary, leftovers, packaging including that from medicines, disposable caps, masks, shoe-covers, and tea cups, cartons, sweeping dust, vegetable peels and kitchen waste.

TREATMENT OF BMW

Different methods used for treating BMW are:

1. **Incineration (burning to ashes):** This is a high temperature (1050–1100°C) thermal process employing combustion of waste to ash (inert material). Three types of incinerators (multiple health type, rotary kiln and controlled air types) are used for hospital waste.

   This technology is recommended for pathological human anatomical waste, animal waste, cytotoxic drugs, discarded medicines and soiled non-plastic waste.
2. **Autoclaving (steam sterilization under pressure):** It is an effective method for disinfecting and treating biohazardous (infectious) waste to non-hazardous waste and disposal to solid waste landfills. Two types of autoclaves (gravity flow autoclave, vacuum autoclave) are used.

   In gravity flow autoclave, autoclaving is performed
   - 121°C (15 psi) for 60 minutes
   - 135°C (31 psi) for 45 minutes
   - 149°C (52 psi) for 30 minutes

   Autoclave treatment has been recommeded for microbiology and biotechnology waste, sharps waste, soiled and solid wastes.
3. **Microwaving:** It is a process which disinfects the waste by moist thermal disinfection technology in which microwave heats the targetted material from inside out, providing a high level of disinfection. The moisture content within the waste is rapidly heated by microwaves and the infectious components are destroyed by heat conduction. It is recommeded for biohazardous waste.
4. **Chemical disinfection:** Several chemical disinfectants are used to treat sharps, solid and liquid wastes as well as chemical wastes. It is also an important preliminary process before final treatment for sputum or pus to be disinfected before buried or autoclaved.

The most effective and economical disinfectant is 1% hypochlorite (sodium or calcium) that is allowed to act for 30 minutes.

5. **Biological processes:** Biological enzymes are used for treating BMW. Biological reactions does not decontaminate the waste but also cause the destruction of all the organic constituents so that only plastics, glass and other inert will remain in the residue.

WASTE DISPOSAL

Disposal of BMW occurs **off-site**-at a location that is different from the site of generation (**on-site**). *Land filling, deep burial, sharp pits* and *sewage* are used for disposal of BMW.

Secured landfill: Ash from incinerators, cytotoxic drugs, and expiry drugs are disposed of in secured landfills. These have contaminant measures such as liners and a leach collection system to prevent migration of materials into the surrounding soil and water.

Deep burial: Deep burial is used for disposing of the treated human and animal infectious waste. A pit or trench should be dug about 2 m deep. It should be half filled with waste, followed by covering with lime within 50 cm of the surface, before filling the rest of the pit with soil. The pits should always be distant from habitation, and sited so as to ensure that no contamination occurs in surface or groundwater, and the location should not be prone to flooding or erosion.

Sharp pits: Circular or rectangular pits are used to dispose of sharps such as blades and needles after disinfection. Such pits are lined with brick covered with a heavy concrete slab, pretreated by a steel pipe with internal diameter of 20 mm projecting 1.5 m above the slab for depositing the sharps. This is the safest method for sharps disposal.

Sewage: Liquid waste from BMW should undergo primary, secondary, and tertiary treatment in effluent treatment plants (ETF) followed by disinfection and sludge treatment and finally into the drainage system.

KEY POINTS

- Bioproduct of the healthcare industry is called the **biomedical (or hospital) waste**.
- BMW is to be segregated at the point of generation (i.e., source) as 80% of the waste is non-hazardous.
- BMW is segregated based on color coding for its safe management.

IMPORTANT QUESTIONS

1. Describe briefly:
   (a) Segregation of waste in hospital/clinic.
   (b) Treatment of biomedical waste.
   (c) Classification of biomedical (hospital) waste.

MULTIPLE-CHOICE QUESTIONS

1. In which container cytotoxic waste should be placed?
   (a) Yellow (b) Red
   (c) Black (d) Blue.
2. Black bag is used for non-biological waste. True or False?
3. Hospital waste should be segregated at the point of treatment. True or False?
4. Disposal of hospital waste often occurs **off-site**. True or False?
5. For which hospital waste incineration is recommended?
   (a) Pathological human waste
   (b) Microbiology and biotechnology waste
   (c) Sputum
   (d) None of the above.
6. What is the colour coding of the bag used in hospitals to dispose of human anatomical wastes such as body parts?
   (a) Black (b) Red
   (c) Yellow (d) Blue.
7. Which is the most suitable temperature-time combination for autoclaving BMW?
   (a) 121°C – 15 minutes (b) 121°C – 30 minutes
   (c) 121°C – 60 minutes (d) 121°C – 45 minutes.
8. Which of the following methods is used for decontamination/treatment of infectious waste before final disposal?
   (a) Shredding (b) Autoclaving
   (c) Incineration (d) Chemical disinfection.
9. All are non-infectious hazardous wastes EXCEPT:
   (a) Chemical waste (b) Radioactive waste
   (c) Pathological waste (d) Pharmacological waste.

ANSWERS TO MCQs

1. (a)	2. True	3. False	4. True	5. (a)
6. (c)	7. (c)	8. (b)	9. (c).	

23

Hospital Acquired Infections and Hospital Infection Control Programme

WHAT IS A HOSPITAL-ACQUIRED INFECTION?

Hospital-acquired infection (**HAI**) (also called **hospital infection**, **healthcare associated infection**, and **nosocomial infection**) is defined as an infection acquired in hospital by a patient who was admitted for a reason other than that infection. This infection was not present or incubating at the time of hospitalisation and becomes obvious in the patient within 48 hours of stay in the hospital.

The term **nosocomial** is derived from Greek words: *nosos* = meaning disease and *komeo* = meaning to take care of, refers to hospital, i.e., any infection acquired while in hospital. The causative agent that causes the HAI is called a **nosocomial pathogen**. *Escherichia coli* and *Staphylococcus aureus* cause the vast majority of HAI. Of these, urinary tract infection is the most common.

Nosocomial infection is a result of the interaction of three factors: microorganisms in the hospital environment, compromised (or weakened) status of the host (patient) and chain of transmission in the hospital.

PUBLIC HEALTH IMPORTANCE AND CONSEQUENCES

HAI is one of the leading causes of death. At any time 1.4 million people suffer from HAIs and their complications. The prevalence of HAIs is 5–10% in developed countries and up to 10–30% in developing countries, i.e., 2-20 times higher than the developed countries. HAIs affect both the patient and the community.

Major consequences of HAI:

- Results in serious illness or death.
- Economic burden due to extra cost for hospitalisation, cost of medicine, and haematological, biochemical, microbiological and radiological tests.

- Additional morbidity and mortality rates.
- Chance of development of multiresistant organisms which may be endemic in the hospital and epidemic in community due to spread causing a serious issue.
- Physical and physiological sufferings to the patient.

MICROBIAL AGENTS OF HAI

HAI can be caused by any bacterium, virus, fungus and parasite. The frequencies of various bacterial and fungal pathogens involved are diagrammatically shown in Fig. 23.1.

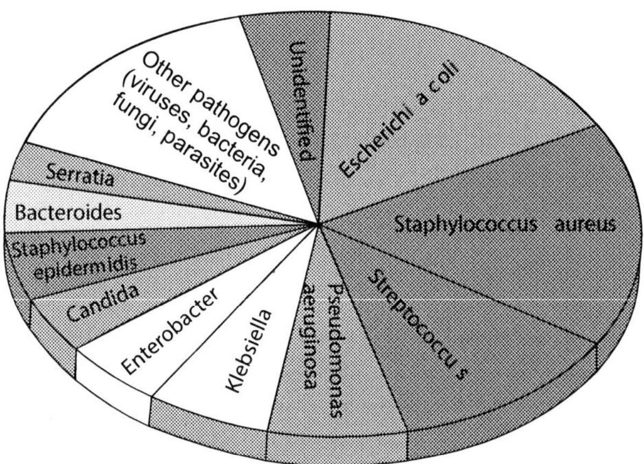

Fig. 23.1 Diagram showing frequencies of causative agents of hospital-acquired infections. *Staphylococcus* (especially MRSA) and *Escherichia coli* are the most common causes of HAI.

Bacterial taxa causing HAI are Gram - positive cocci: staphylococci (*Staphylococcus aureus* and coagulase-negative), streptococci (*Streptococcus pneumoniae, S. pyogenes*), and Gram-negative rods: *Escherichia coli* and *Pseudomonas aeruginosa*. However, commonly occurring and problematic strains of these are resistant to antibiotics such as vancomycin and methicillin *S. aureus*: MASA and carbapenem resistant *P. aeruginosa*.

Among fungi, *Candida* especially *C. albicans*, the cause of UTI and systemic bloodstream infection, is the most serious nosocomial fungal pathogen. Mucormycosis or "**black fungus infection**" caused by species of *Mucor* has been found to be a fast emerging fungal infection in India, especially among the COVID-19 patients.

Viruses are currently recognized as important causes of several HAIs, affecting both the patients and healthcare workers. Major viral pathogens are: HIV, hepatitis B and C viruses (acquired by contact with blood and blood contaminated products), influenza and respiratory syncytial virus (RSV) (acquired by respiratory route), viral diarrhoea, chicken pox and measles.

COMMON SITES AND TYPES OF HAI

Commonly occurring major HAIs based on the body site includes: urinary tract infection, surgical wound infection, lower respiratory tract infection and bloodstream infection. Gasteroenteritis, skin and eye infections are the other nosocomial infections.

Common procedures causing HAI are catheter related bloodstream infection, venilator associated pneumonia, and catheter related UTI.

Urinary Tract Infections

UTI, the most prevalent type of nosocomial infection, accounts for 35% to 40% of total nosocomial infections. These infections occur after catheterization and instrumentation of urethera, bladder and kidneys.

Initial infection of urinary tract is caused by the bacteria – *Escherichia coli, Staphylococcus epidermidis* and *Enterococcus* followed by invasion of *Klebisiella, Proteus, Serratia, Pseudomonas aeruginosa,* and the yeast *Candida albicans.*

Surgical Incision – Site Infections

These infections account for 20% of nosocomial infections. These are caused by *Staphylococcus aureus, Pseudomonas aeruginosa* (important cause of infection in burns of diabetic patients), *Streptococcus pyogenes* and other Gram-negative bacilli.

Respiratory Tract Infections

Respiratory infections account for 15% of nosocomial infections. *Ventillator associated pneumonia:* VAP (also called nosocomial pneumonia) is the major cause of illness and death in critically ill patients that are in an intensive care unit receiving mechanical ventillation. It is mainly caused by *Pseudomones aeruginosa, Klebsiella pneumoniae* and *Staphylococcus aureus.*

Blood Stream Infections (BSIs)

BSIs (bacteremia or septicaemia or sepsis) which account for 14% of nosocomial infections, are a leading cause of death especially in the United States of America. These may occur as a consequence of infections at any site, but are commonly caused by infected intravenous cannula.

The most common pathogens causing BSIs are coagulase-negative staphylococci, *Staphylococcus aureus* (MRSA), *Enterococcus faecalis*, *Escherichia coli* and *Candida* spp.

Gasteroenteritis Infections

Nosocomial gasteroenteritis (food poisoning) accounts for 12% of HAIs which can be potentially fatal for a hospitalized patient. Nosocomial diarrhoea is the most common infection in children, who are typically affected by rotavirus. In adults, gasteroenteritis is often caused by *Clostridium difficile* which is particularly dangerous for the patients since the bacterial strain has become resistant to many antibiotics. Food and contaminated hands act as the mode of spread of these pathogens.

Skin Infections

Skin infections account for 8% of nosocomial infections. *Staphylococcus aureus* and *Streptococcus pyogenes* are the two common bacteria involved in these infections which are *endogenous* in origin. The bacteria originate from the patient's own skin microflora, become opportunistic after surgery or other procedures that compromise the protective skin carrier.

Eye Infections

Bacterial conjunctivitis, a highly contagious inflammation of the conjunctiva in young children, is a common bacterial eye infection in intensive care units. *Pseudomonas aeruginosa* is often involved and infects during surgery.

SOURCES OF HOSPITAL INFECTIONS

Source refers to the origin of an infecting organism. Hospital infections may be acquired from an endogenous source or exogenous source.

Endogenous infection: Self-infection from another site in the body where the infecting organisms originate from the patients own microbiota. It occurs during surgical operation, instrumental manipulation or nursing procedures.

Exogenous infections: Cross-infection from another human, or environmental source.

- **Human sources** include other patients, hospital staff and occasionally visitors who are incubating an infection or are healthy carriers of virulent strains of *Staphylococcus aureus* and *Streptococcus pyogenes*.
- **Environmental sources:** Contaminated objects (fomites), food, water or air.
- Skin cells, hair, clothing and bedding.
- Medical equipment: endoscopes, catheters, cytoscopes, needles, spatula, washbowls, ventilators, respiratory equipment, toilet thrash can.
- Disinfectants (quaternary ammonium compounds).
- Floor and surfaces contaminated by patient's secretions and body fluids.
- Dust-borne microorganisms that can withstand drying.
- Contaminated food.
- Contaminated distilled water used to prepare a variety of pharmaceuticals.

SPREAD OF HOSPITAL INFECTIONS

Nosocomial infections are spread or transmitted by the same routes as infections spread in the community. Three main routes of spread are contact, air and vehicles.

1. **Contact spread:** It is the principal mode of transmission. It takes place by two routes:
    - *Direct contact*: It is called **cross-infection**. Person-to-person spread between an infected patient, staff member, or visitor (staphylococcal and streptococcal species); varicella-zoster virus (VZV).
    - *Indirect contact*: Contact of contaminated objects results to infection in patients (enteric Gram-negatives, e.g., *Salmonella, Pseudomonas*).
2. **Airborne spread:** Spread occurs via:
    - *Droplets* (Examples: influenza, respiration syncytial virus (RSV), *Streptococcus pyogenes*-pharyngitis).
    - *Dust from bedding and floors: Mycobacterium tuberculosis, Streptococcus pyogenes*, aspergilli, Varicella-zoster virus (VZV) causing chickenpox.

- *Aerosols:* Produced by nebulizers, humidifiers and air conditioning apparatus. *Legionella pneumophila,* a Gram-negative, aerobic bacillus, is ubiquitous in aquatic environments including potable water supplies, infects the respiratory tract causing legionnaire's disease, a form of labour pneumonia.

3. *Vehicle-borne spread:* Common vehicles which transmit various pathogens:
   - Blood and blood products (HIV, Hepatitis B virus).
   - IV fluids (Gram-negative rods).
   - Contaminated antiseptic solution (*Pseudomonas aeruginosa*).
   - Foodborne: *Salmonella* and *Campylobacter.*

PREVENTION OF HOSPITAL ACQUIRED INFECTIONS

CDC estimates that 36% of all infections acquired in hospitals can be prevented. HAIs are often caused by breaches of infection control practices and procedures, unclean and nonsterile environmental surfaces, and/or, ill hospital staff.

Hospital infections can be prevented by three main strategies:

- Excluding the source of infection from the hospital environment.
- Interrupting the transmission of infection from source and origin to susceptible host (i.e., breaking the chain of infection).
- Enhancing the host's ability to resist infection (i.e., boosting immunity and reducing risk factors).

Control measures aimed at nosocomial infections by implementing *Standard Precautions* (also known earlier as *Universal Precautions*), the guidelines designed by CDC, while caring for patients (discussed earlier in Chapter 20). These have been designed to reduce the risk of transmission of drug-resistant microorganisms and blood-borne pathogens between patients and from healthcare workers to patients (cross-infection). These include:

1. Apply hand hygiene: Thorough handwashing before and after any procedure involving nursing care or close contact with the patient or inanimate objects. It is the most important method to control the spread of infection within a hospital.
2. Use of sterile instruments, dressings, surgical gloves, face-masks, theatre clothing and fluids.
3. Mandatory use of gloves, gown, mask and protective eyewear by healthcare workers.

4. Use of disposable mouthpiece/airway for cardiovascular resuscitation.
5. Proper preoperative disinfection of patient's skin.
6. Use of sterile antiseptics for irrigation of wound site at operation, or for mucosal surfaces such as bladder after urological surgery and peritoneum during dialysis.
7. Appropriate use of prophylactic antibiotics.
8. Use of isolation rooms and wards.
9. Proper investigation of nosocomial infection and treatment of the patient and carrier.
10. Discarding contaminated needles and other sharp items *immediately* into a *nearby*, special puncture-proof container.

HOSPITAL INFECTION CONTROL PROGRAMME

"The first requirement of a hospital is that it should do the sick no harm" was **Florence Nightingale's** dictum. Each healthcare facility needs to develop an infection control programme to ensure the well-being of both patients and staff.

The **Infection Prevention and Control Program (IPC Program)** though initially implemented in hospitals in the United States in the 1960s was considered to be a critical component of a hospital in 1985 after the publication – **Study on the Efficacy of Nosocomial Infection Control (SENIC Project)** in reducing HAIs by 32%.

What is IPC Programme?

IPC programme at the hospital is a planned, systematic approach to monitor and evaluate the quality and appropriateness of infection control procedures and practices (Fig. 23.2). The programme to be developed by each heathcare facility is a plan of action which is designed to identify infections that occur in patients and staff that have the potential for disease transmission. Various steps involved in it are:

- Identify opportunities for the reduction of risk for disease transmission.
- Recommend risk reduction practices by integrating principles of sound infection control management into patient care, education and training of employees.
- Sterilization and disinfection practices at the hospital.
- Manage surveillance through internal audits and various reporting tools.

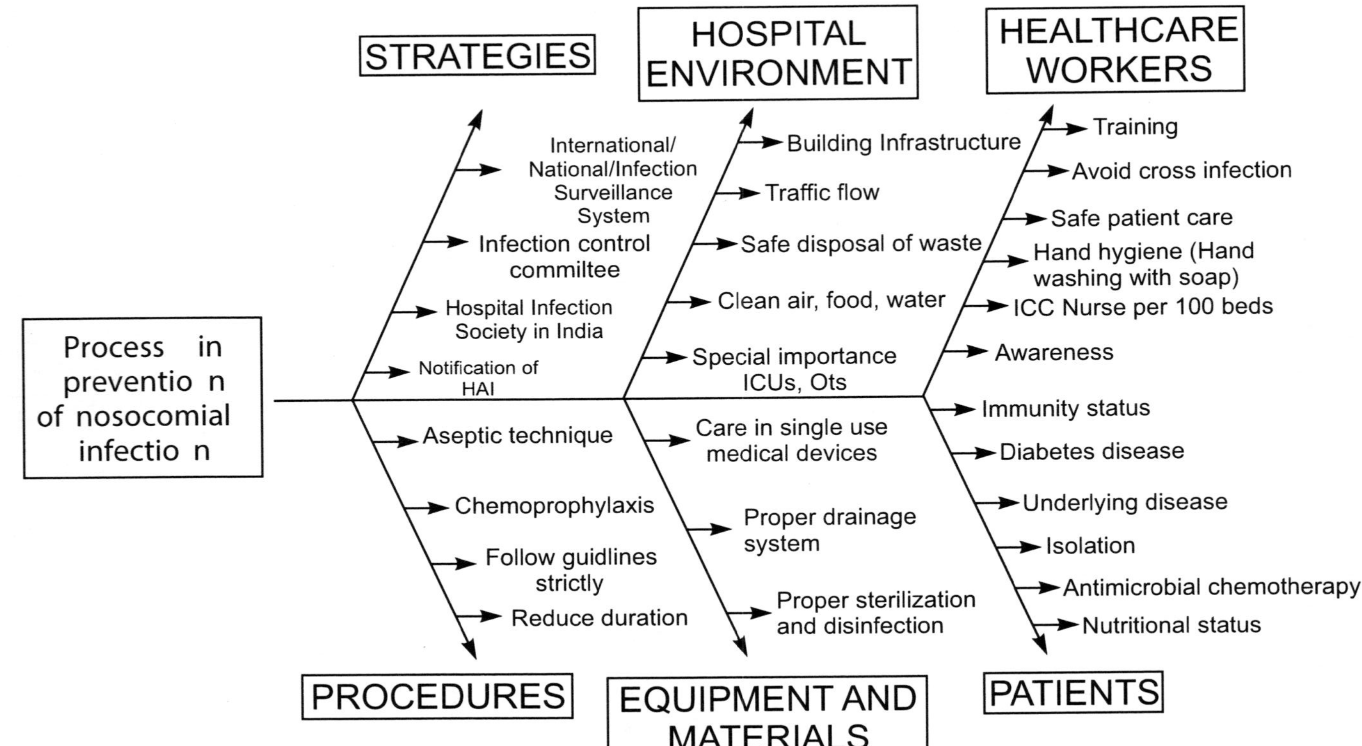

Fig. 23.2 Fish model showing prevention and control of hospital acquired infection.

An effective hospital infection control programme involves: to educate staff, create a multidisciplinary team, collection and analysis of data, data reporting, implementation of policies and action plans, constant vigilance, and stay up-to-date on policies and news.

Aim of IPC Programme

The main aim of the infection control programme is to lower the risk of infection during the period of hospitalization. Hospital infection control programme can prevent 33–36% of nosocomial infections.

Objectives of the Infection Control Programme

1. **Monitoring of hospital associated infections** by developing survillance system. **Survillance** implies that the observed data are regularly analyzed and reported to those who are in position to take appropriate action. Survillance is the one essential component of an IPC programme necessary to reduce rates of HAIs.
2. **Training of staff in prevention and control of HAI.**
3. **Investigation of outbreaks** that often provide critical information about the epidemically important pathogens.
4. **Controlling the outbreak by rectification of technical lapses**, if any.
5. **Monitoring of staff health** to prevent staff-to-patient and patient-to-staff spread of infection.
6. **Advice on isolation procedures and infection control measures**.
7. **Infection control audit** including inspection of waste disposal, laundry and kitchen.
8. **Monitoring and advice on the safe use of antibiotics.**

INFECTION CONTROL ORGANIZATIONS IN A HOSPITAL

Infection control organizations are essential features of an infection prevention control programme in a hospital. These organizations include:

1. Infection Control Committe (ICC)
2. Infection Control Team (ICT)
3. Infection Control Officer (ICO), usually a medical microbiologist
4. Infection Control Nurse (ICN)
5. Infection Control Manual (ICM).

KEY POINTS

- **Hospital acquired infection (HAI)** or **nosocomial infection** is defined as any infection acquired by a patient while in hospital.
- HAI can be acquired from an *exogenous source* or an *endogenous source*.
- Staphylococci (especially MRSA) and *Escherichia coli* are the most common causes of infection in hospitals.
- One-third (33–36%) of all infections acquired in hospital are preventable, if standard precautions are strictly implemented.
- Urinary tract infections, 35–40% of total, are the most common nosocomial infections.
- Hospital infections are spread by the same routes as infections spread in the community (i.e., air, contact and vehicle).
- Hospital infections can be prevented by excluding sources of infection, interrupting transmission and enhancing patient's resistance by following the standard precautions.
- The major objective of hospital infection control programme is to ensure the well-being of both, patients and staff.

IMPORTANT QUESTIONS

1. Define hospital acquired (or nosocomial) infection. What are the major nosocomial pathogens.
2. Write short notes on the following:
   (a) Sources of hospital infection
   (b) Major types of hospital acquired infections
   (c) Prevention of hospital acquired infections
   (d) Hospital infection control programme.

MULTIPLE-CHOICE QUESTIONS

1. All of the following names are used for hospital acquired infections EXCEPT:
   (a) Nosocomial infection
   (b) Latrogenic infection
   (c) Healthcare associated infection
   (d) Hospital infection.
2. Hospital acquired infection occurs by:
   (a) Airbone spread
   (b) Contact spread

(c) Vehicle-borne spread
(d) All of the above.

3. Which of the following pathogens is transmitted via disinfectants?
(a) *Pseudomones aeruginosa*
(b) *Staphycococcus aureus*
(c) *Salmonella typhimurium*
(d) *Streptococcus pyogenes.*

4. Which of the following pathogens can be transmitted by water in hospitals?
(a) HIV (b) Hepatitis B virus
(c) *Legionella* (d) *Staphylococus aureus.*

5. Which of the following is the most prevalent hospital-acquired infection worldwide?
(a) Bloodstream infection
(b) Urinary tract infection
(c) Respiratory pneumonia
(d) Gastroenteritis infection.

6. All of the following can help to prevent nosocomial infections EXCEPT:
(a) Hand hygiene
(b) Use of gloves
(c) Patient remaining in bed
(d) Judicious use of antibiotics.

7. Hospital infections are spread by the same routes as infections spread in the community. True or False?

8. What percentage of nosocomial infections can be prevented through hospital infection control programme?
(a) 100% (b) 63–66%
(c) 33–36% (d) 13–23%.

ANSWERS TO MCQs

1. (b) 2. (d) 3. (a) 4. (c) 5. (b)
6. (c) 7. True 8. (c).

24

Role of Nurse in Hospital Infection Control Programme

WHAT IS HOSPITAL INFECTION CONTROL PROGRAMME?

Hospital infection control programme refers to the prevention or to minimize the potential for nosocomial infections in patients as well as in staff by breaking the chain of transmission of nosocomial pathogens.

HIC programme involves sterilization, isolation, knowledge related to safety measure, vaccination, waste management, staff education and action plan to reduce the exogenous hospital acquired infections.

To fulfill the objective of hospital infection control programme, every hospital has an **infection control committee (ICC)** to formulate and update policies for the whole hospital with the following roles:

- The surveillance of hospital infection.
- The investigation of outbreaks, i.e., tracking the source and modes of transmission.
- Procedures designed to prevent/manage outbreaks.

The ICC is composed of infection control officer (a physician or microbiologist) and an infection control nurse.

Nurses play a crucial role in implementing the HIC programme in a hospital.

ROLE OF NURSE IN HOSPITAL INFECTION COTROL PROGRAMME

Nurses in all roles and settings can demonstrate leadership in prevention and control by using their knowledge of microbiology, skill and judgement to initiate appropriate and immediate infection control procedures. Implementation of the patient care practices for infection control in a hospital is the role of nursing staff. Nurse's roles in control programme can be categorized as:

- Senior nursing administrator
- Nurse incharge of a ward
- Nurse incharge of infection control

Nurse's roles and responsibilities include.

1. Responsibilities of Senior Nursing Administrator (or Nurse Administrator)

- Acting both as a leader and team builder in a hospital.
- Participitating in the infection control committee.
- Responsible for large-scale policy planning, and staff management.
- Promoting the development and improvement of nursing techniques as per the Standard (Universal) Precautions.
- Developing training programme for members of the nursing staff for updating their knowledge.
- Monitoring of adherence of nursing staff to policies of ICC.
- Cordinating and supervising the delivery of best possible care to their patients.

2. Responsibilities of Nurse Incharge (Incharge Nurse) of a Ward

Incharge nurse is responsible for immediate function of a ward (or unit) and plays the following roles.

- Making sure that all the patients receive adequate care.
- Maintaining hygiene by monitoring aseptic techniques, proper handwashing and use of isolation.
- Reporting of any new infection appearing in patients under the nurse care.
- Initiating the process of collection of specimen.
- Ordering the specimen culture to diagnose the infectious microbe.
- Initiating patient isolation.
- Proper segregation of waste for its safe disposal.
- Limiting patient exposure to exogenous infections from other patients, hospital staff, visitor's or equipment used for diagnosis or treatment.
- Proper maintenance of safe and adequate supply of vaccines, drugs, patient-care supplies and ward equipment.

3. Responsibilities of Infection Control Nurse (Nurse Incharge of Infection Control)

The infection control nurse (ICN) is a key member of the infection control committee (ICC).

- Surveillance of hospital infections.
- Investigation of outbreaks, tracking the source and routes of spread/transmission.
- Investigation to determine if inadequate procedures may have contributed, in conjunction with technical officer.
- Prepare strategies and action plans for preventing infections.
- Ensure compliance with local and national regulations.
- Liaison with appropriate personnel concerned with notifying hospital infections.
- Provide expert consultative advice to staff and other hospital programmes related to spread of infections.

KEY POINTS

- Every hospital has an **infection control committee (ICC)** and **infection control team (ICT)** of workers to formulate and update the information on infection control and to manage outbreaks of nosocomial infection.
- There are three **types of nurses**: The senior nursing administrator, nurse incharge of a ward, and infection control nurse, involved in the hospital infection control programme.
- The **infection control nurse (ICN)** is a key member of the infection control team.

IMPORTANT QUESTIONS

1. Briefly describe:
   (a) Hospital infection control programme.
   (b) Role of a nurse in hospital infection control programme.

MULTIPLE-CHOICE QUESTIONS

1. Which of the following is a key member of the infection control committee?
   (a) Infection control officer
   (b) Infection control nurse
   (c) Senior nursing administrator
   (d) Nurse incharge of a ward.

2. The infection control nurse is a key member of the infection control programme. True or False?
3. Hospital infection control programme refers to the prevention or to minimize the potential for nosocomial infections both in the patients and staff. True or False?

ANSWERS TO MCQs

1. (b) 2. True 3. True.

25

Protocols for Collection and Transport of Specimens/Samples for Microbiological Investigations and Responsibilities of Nurses

WHAT IS A SPECIMEN?

A **specimen** is a sample collected from the patient's tissue, body fluids or other materials for examination or study in the laboratory to assist medical diagnosis and treatment. It is derived from a Latin word *specere*—meaning "to look".

There is not much difference between the two words: **sample** and **specimen**, but both refer to the material, not the equipment. A **sample** is limited quantity of a material. Common examples include throat swabs, sputum, urine, stool, blood and tissue biopsies.

ROLE OF A NURSE IN SPECIMEN COLLECTION

Nurses need to be aware of how to properly gather specimens, both for self-protection, and to prevent the spread of diseases. Specimen collection, preparation and handling are important tasks performed by nurses.

The core responsibilities and role of nurses in specimen collection are:

- Ensuring right amount of sample, right specimen in a right container from the right patient.
- Proper labelling of specimens for analysis.
- Making sure all selected supplies are suitable for collection.
- Ensuring timely transfer of specimen to the diagnostic/microbe's culture laboratory.
- Patient interaction.

RESPONSIBILITIES OF A NURSE IN A HOSPITAL

A. Placement of an Order in the Hospital Information System (HIS)

It should include the following information:

- Patient name
- Patient age and sex
- Patient room number
- Physician name
- Date and time of specimen collection
- Specific anatomic culture site
- Antimicrobials, if any, patient is receiving
- When appropriate, include clinical diagnosis, special culture request, and relevant patient history
- Test or procedure requested.

A separate order is needed for each test, including anaerobic bacterial cultures.

Special requests for culture of unusual bacterial pathogens (e.g., *Corynebacterium diphtheriae, Leptospira, Actinomyces, Nocardia, Brucella, Hemophilus ducreyi, Bordetella pertussis,* etc.,) require prior notification to the laboratory, in addition to ordering the tests.

B. Labelling of Specimen Container

It should include the following information:

- Patient name
- Date and time of collection
- Hospital number or DOB
- Culture site
- Initials of collector.

SAFETY CONSIDERATIONS FOR NURSES DURING SPECIMEN COLLECTION

- Follow Universal Precautions Guidelines—treat all specimens as potentially hazardous.
- They should use appropriate protection such as gloves and gown.

- Minimize direct handling of specimens in transit from the patient to the lab.
- Do not contaminate the external surface of collection container and /or its accompanying paper work.
- Use plastic sealable bags with a separate pouch for the laboratory requisition or transport carrier (such as small buckets with rigid handles).

PROTOCOLS/BASIC GUIDELINES FOR COLLECTION AND TRANSPORTATION OF SPECIMENS

- Collect specimens for microbiological investigations before the initiation of antimicrobial therapy.
- Use strict aseptic technique.
- Collect an adequate amount of sample to allow for all tests.
- Avoid contamination with indigenous microbiota.
- Collect the specimen at the acute phase of infection.
- Use sturdy, sterile, screw-cap, leak-proof containers that do not create aerosols when opened.
- Transport microbiological specimens promptly within 2 hours, to the lab for examination/analysis.
- Use appropriate temperature (i.e., 37°C or 4°C) for storage of samples between collection and transportation.
- Use sterile tools/devices for collecting samples.
- Expiry dates need to be checked before using any collection device.
- Fill the test request form completely and label the specimen properly mentioning the patient's name, identification number/ or date of birth.
- Mention an appropriate time between collection of the specimen and delivery to the lab.
- Identify the specimen source and/or specific site so that proper culture media can be used for processing a sample.
- Provide proper instructions to the patient when they themselves have to collect the sample (e.g., sputum, faeces or urine).

SPECIFIC PROCEDURES FOR COLLECTION AND TRANSPORTATION OF COMMON SPECIMENS

Throat Swab

- Wash your hands thoroughly.
- Put on gloves, surgical mask and protective eye-wear.
- Have the patient facing a strong light to ensure the back area of the throat to be swabbed is visible.
- Aseptically remove two swabs (one for smear and other for culture) from the package.
- Have the patient tilt their head backwards, open their mouth and check for inflamed area using a sterile wooden tongue depressor.
- Now ask him/her to say 'AHHH' and firmly rub the sterile swabs at the inflamed area of throat, tonsils and pharyngeal mucosa.
- Place the inoculated swab into sterile transport system vial (or sterile tube) immediately.
- Take care not to contaminate the swab with saliva.
- Replace cap and tighten to secure.
- Label the vial/culture tube with appropriate patient's information.
- Complete the request form.
- Transport the labelled throat specimen to the microbiology laboratory promptly.
- It can be maintained at room temperature (37°C) for 24 hours.

Sputum

- Nurse will explain the procedure to the patient and give a special sterile wide-mouthed plastic container (cup) for collecing the sputum sample.
- As soon as the patient wakes up in the morning (before eating or drinking any thing), brush the teeth and rinse mouth with plain water (do not use mouthwash or toothpaste).
- Ask the patient to take deep breath and hold the air for 5 seconds, slowly breath out, take another deep breath and cough hard until some sputum comes up into the mouth.
- Spit the sputum into the sterile container.

- Repeat the above step until the sputum reaches 5 mL (about 1 teaspoon).
- Close the container immediately after collecting the sputum.
- Ask the patient to wipe his mouth with tissues.
- Write the date and time of collection on the container.
- Put the container into the box or bag given by the nurse.
- Give the sputum container to the nurse or your clinic.
- Record the characteristics of sputum: quantity, colour, consistency as well as the time and date in the nursing notes (sputum from the lungs is usually thick and sticky).
- Deliver the specimen to the lab as soon as possible (stroage can be done in the refrigerator, never in freezer or room temperature) for diagnosis of TB).

Stool/Faeces

Stool (faeces) sample is collected to determine the presence of blood, ova, pathogens, parasites, bile, fat or substances such as ingested drugs. Gastroenteritis, inflammatory bowel disease (e.g., Crohn's disease, ulcerative colitis) are diagnosed by testing stool.

- Since stool sample is collected by the patients themselves, nurse should explain the procedure to the patient.
- Take a clean sterile, dry, leak-proof, screw-cap container for specimen collection.
- Label the container with the date, name and date of birth of the patient.
- Place something in the toilet to catch the stool, e.g., a potty, or an empty plastic food container, or an empty match box, or spread clean newspaper or plastic wrap over the rim of the toilet.
- Make sure the sample doesn't touch the inside of the toilet.
- Using sterile spoon or spatula, transfer the sample to the container and screw the lid shut. If the stool is semisolid, a small quantity is sufficient; if liquid, as in the case of cholera, it should fill a third of the container.
- Put anything you used to catch the stool in a plastic bag, tie it up and put it in the bin.
- Wash your hands thoroughly with soap and warm running water.
- Stool samples should be handed to the nurse as soon as possible.
- Place the stool sample container in a sealed plastic bag and submit to the laboratory.

- The fresh stool specimen must be processed for culturing within 1 and 2 hours of passage.
- If delay is unavoidable, then store it in a fridge (2–8°C), but for no longer than 24 hours.

Urine

- Nurse to explain the procedure and precautions to be taken by the patient while collecting a urine sample.
- Provide the patient, a labelled sterile screw-cap container with the name, DOB and date.
- Collect the sample when urine has been in your bladder for 2-3 hours.
- Wash and dry your hands thoroughly.

Boys and Men

- Urinate a small amount into the toilet bowl and then stop the flow of urine.
- Collect a sample of urine "mid-stream" into the labelled sterile container/cup, until it is half full.
- Remove the container from the urine stream.
- Finish urinating into the toilet bowl.

Girls and Women

- Sit on the toilet with your legs apart.
- Use your two fingers to spread open your labia and clean the genital areas including urethera (opening where urine comes out) with towellelte prior to urinating.
- Keeping your labia spread open, pass an amount of urine into the toilet and then stop the flow of urine.
- Hold the container a few inches (or a few centimetres) from the urethera and urinate until the container is half full.
- Finish urinating into the toilet bowl.
- Put the lid back on the specimen container.
- Wash your hands thoroughly.
- Return the specimen to the nurse.
- Transport urine specimen to the microbiology laboratory promptly (or refrigerate 4°C) within 30 minutes not more than 1-2 hours.

(Urine specimens must be **refrigerated** if there is delay in delivery to the laboratory.)

Cerebrospinal Fluid (CSF)

A **lumber puncture** or **"spinal tap"** is used to collect CSF for culture.

- The patient is asked to lie on side with knees pulled up toward the chest, and chin tucked downward.
- After the back is cleaned, the nurse will inject a local numbing medicine (anaesthesia) into the lower spine.
- A sterile wide-bore needle is inserted between 4th and 5th lumber vertebrae.
- The CSF is allowed to drop into a sterile dry container.
- A sample of 3–5 mL of CSF is collected.
- The needle is removed, the area is cleaned, and a bandage is placed over the needle site.
- The patient is asked to remain lying down for a short time after the test.
- Immediately deliver the sample with a request form to the laboratory.

  (If transporting is delayed, then store the CSF sample at 37°C. *Do not refrigerate.*)

Wound, Abscess or other Discharges

- Perform hand hygeine and put on clean gloves.
- Thoroughly rinse the wound/affected area of the skin with sterile saline solution.
- Remove the gloves, perform hand hygiene, and put on clean gloves.
- Swab the wound by gently rotating and use enough pressure to express fluid from within the wound tissue. Place the swab in a sterile container (better to collect 2 swabs—one for direct microscopic examination and the 2nd for culture).
- In case of discharge, 1-2 mL of sample is collected in a sterile container.
- Label the container properly and send it to the lab as soon as possible.

BLOOD (VENIPUNCTURE TECHNIQUE)

- Assist the patient to a comfortable position in a chair, or sitting or lying in a bed.
- Disinfect your hands.
- Using a pressure cuff, locate a suitable vein in the arm.
- Select site for venipuncture.
- Put on gloves and clean the drawing site with 70% isopropyl alcohol (or ethanol) by swabbing in a circular motion for 30 seconds.
- Allow the area to air dry for 30 seconds.
- Remove dust caps from both the culture bottles – blue cap (for aerobic) and burgundy cap (for anerobic bacteria).
- Wipe the culture bottle's top using an ethanol-ether swab.
- Put the needle in the syringe.
- Using a syringe and needle, draw 10 cc of blood from the patient.

Remove the syringe and needle from the arm while applying pressure to the venipuncture site with cotton ball or gauze pad. Ask the patient apply pressure to the site. Place a band-aid over the patient's venipuncture site.

- Replace needle on the syringe with another sterile needle.
- Inject 5 cc of blood into the aerobic culture bottle, while retaining the needle in the bottle, disconnect it from the syringe for allowing the entry of air into the culture bottle.
- Replace the needle on the syringe with another sterile needle and inject 5 cc of blood into anaerobic culture bottle; do not allow air to enter the bottle without delay, gently mix the blood with the broth, not allowing the blood to clot in the culture medium because the bacteria will become trapped in the clot.
- Using a fresh ethanol-ether swab, wipe the top of culture bottles and replace the tape or protective cover.
- Label both bottles with the patient's details.
- Complete the laboratory request form.
- As soon as possible transport the specimen to the laboratory for incubating the inoculated culture bottles. If not possible, keep in incubator (37°C) or at room temperature. *Never refrigerate.*

KEY POINTS

- **Sample** and **specimen** both refer to the material, and a sample is a limited quantity of a material.
- A sample collected from the patient for examination or study in the laboratory is called a **specimen**.
- All microbiological specimens must be transported promptly within two hours of collection for proper diagnosis.
- **Never refrigerate** CSF samples and blood culture bottles after inoculation.
- Urine specimens must be refrigerated (4°C) if there is a delay in delivery to the microbiology laboratory.
- In suspected urinary infections, mid-stream clean-catch urine sample needs to be collected.
- Stool samples should be transported to the microbiology laboratory immediately after collection, if delayed, they should be stored in a fridge (4°C), but for no longer than 24 hours.

IMPORTANT QUESTIONS

1. Discuss methods of collection and transportation of common specimens for culturing/diagnosis.
2. Write short notes on:
   (a) Guidelines for collection of specimens
   (b) Collection of urine for culture
   (c) Collection of throat swab specimen
   (d) Collection of blood specimen for aerobic and anaerobic cultures.

MULTIPLE-CHOICE QUESTIONS

1. Blood culture bottles are to be refrigerated in case of delay in the transport or processing of specimen. True or False?
2. Throat swab specimens are to be stored at room temperature if not transported immediately. True or False?
3. All the specimens can be refrigerated, in case of delay in transport to the lab EXCEPT:
   (a) CSF (b) Urine
   (c) Stool (d) Sputum.

4. Ideally, the specimens for microbiological investigations should be collected:
   (a) After completion of antimicrobial therapy
   (b) Before the start of antimicrobial therapy
   (c) After finishing half of antimicrobial therapy
   (d) It is irrelevant.

5. All are *true* for collection of specimens for microbiological investigations EXCEPT:
   (a) Use strict aseptic technique
   (b) Use appropriate containers for collection and transport of specimens
   (c) All microbiological specimens, if not transported promptly within two hours of collection, should be stroed in the refrigerator (4°C)
   (d) Provide proper instructions to the patient when they themselves have to collect the sample (e.g., sputum, urine, faeces).

6. All the unusual bacterial pathogens that require prior notification to the laboratory and special requests for culture by a nurse EXCEPT:
   (a) *Hemophilus ducreyi*
   (b) *Bordetella pertussis*
   (c) *Escherichia coli*
   (d) *Corynebacterium diphtheriae*.

ANSWERS TO MCQs

1. False 2. True 3. (a) 4. (b) 5. (c)
6. (c).

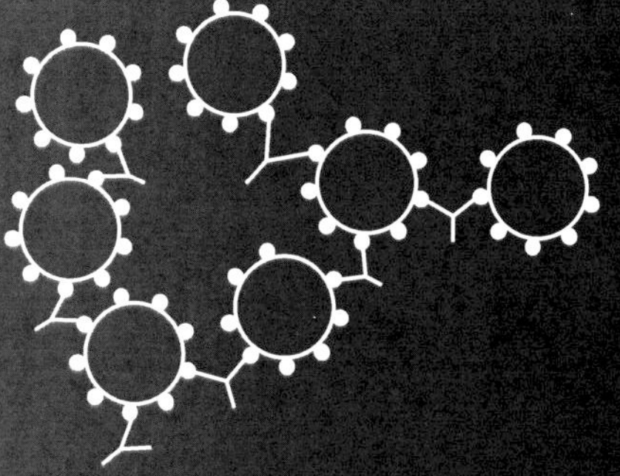

Unit IV A

BACTERIA-MEDICAL BACTERIOLOGY

- *Staphylococcus*: A Gram-positive Coccus Forming Grape-like Clusters
- *Streptococcus*: A Gram-positive Aerobic Coccus Forming Chains
- *Pneumococcus*: A Gram-positive Diplococcus (*Streptococcus pneumoniae*)
- *Enterococcus*: A Gram-positive Gastrointestinal Diplococcus (Fecal streptococci)
- *Neisseria*: A Gram-negative Coffee-bean Shaped Diplococcus
- *Bacillus*: An Aerobic Endospore-forming Gram-positive Bacillus
- *Clostridium*: A Gram-positive Strictly Anaerobic Endosporic Bacillus
- Gram-negative Bacilli of Medical Importance and *Enterobacteriaceae*
- *Escherichia*: A Gram-negative Non-endosporic Bacillus
- *Klebsiella, Enterobacter, Serratia* and *Citrobacter*: Coliforms other than *Escherichia*
- *Proteus, Morganella* and *Providencia*: Noncoliform Enteric Bacilli
- *Salmonella*: A Gram-negative Motile, Nonsporing Enteric Bacillus
- *Shigella*: A Gram-negative Bacillus
- *Pseudomonas*: A Gram-negative, Aerobic Motile Bacillus
- *Brucella*: A Gram-negative Aerobic Coccobacillius
- *Bordetella*: An Aerobic Encapsulated Gram-negative Coccobacillus
- *Legionella*: An Aerobic Motile Gram-negative Bacillus
- *Yersinia*: A Gram-negative Pleomorphic Coccobacillus
- *Haemophilus*: A Gram-negative Pleomorphic Bacillius
- *Gardnerella*: A Pleomorphic Gram-variable Bacillus or Coccobacillus
- *Mycobacterium*: An Acid-fast Aerobic Bacillus
- Spirochaetes: *Treponema, Borrelia, Leptospira*
- Mycoplasmas: *Mycoplasma, Ureaplasma*
- *Rickettsia* and *Coxiella*
- Chlamydiae: *Chlamydia*
- *Vibrio*: Curved Gram-negative Motile Rods
- *Campylobacter* and *Helicobacter*: Gram-negative Curved Flagellated Rods

26

Staphylococcus: A Gram-positive Coccus Forming Grape-like Clusters

Skin infections; Toxic shock syndrome; Food poisoning; Endocarditis

WHAT IS A COCCUS?

A **coccus** (pl. **cocci**) is a spherical, ovoid or round bacterium. Based on the Gram-stain reaction, cocci are of two types: Gram-positive (purple/blue) cocci and Gram-negative (red) cocci. Cocci are among the most significant infectious agents of humans. They are often called **pyogenic cocci** because of their ability to stimulate pus formation.

COCCI OF MEDICAL IMPORTANCE

Gram-positive cocci: *Staphylococcus, Streptococcus, Enterococcus* and *Micrococcus.* Of these, two former genera are most important human pathogens.

Gram-negative cocci: *Neisseria, Haemophilus, Moraxella, Acinetobacter* and *Kingella.* Of these, *Neisseria* has the greatest clinical significance.

STAPHYLOCOCCUS: A GRAM-POSITIVE COCCUS

Staphylococcus (Fig. 26.1) is a Gram-positive, spherical (coccus) bacteium that forms grape-like clusters. This bacterium is a catalase-positive, facultative anaerobe, capable of growth both aerobically and anaerobically.

Staphylococcus was discovered in 1871 by **von Reckiinhausen** from human pyogenic lesion. **Sir Alexander Ogston**, a Scottish surgeon, in 1880 named it *Staphylococcus* (from the Greek words: *staphyle* = bunch of grapes + *kokkos* = + berry or grain) due to the typical occurrence of cocci in grape-like clusters both in pus and culture.

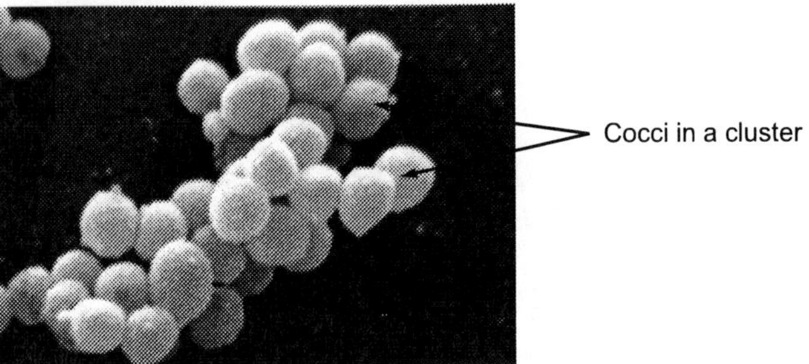

Fig. 26.1 ***Staphylococcus aureus*** **(SEM).** Yellow-pigmented, Gram-positive cocci in grape-like clusters, diagnostic feature of this bacterium.

The genus *Staphylococcus* includes 40 species. Of these, 9 have two subspecies each, and one has three subspecies and one has four subspecies. It has been found to be a nectar inhabiting microbe. Most of the species are harmless and reside normally on the skin and mucous membranes of humans and other organisms. *S. aureus* is the most serious human pathogen.

Systematic Position

Domain	:	Bacteria
Phylum	:	Firmicutes
Class	:	Bacilli
Order	:	Bacillales
Family	:	Staphylococcaceae
Genus	:	*Staphylococcus*

Based on their ability to clot blood plasma, species are classified into two groups:

- *Coagulase-positive staphylococci* (*Staphylococcus aureus*).
- *Coagulase-negative staphylococci* (*S. epidermidis, S. saprophyticus* and *S. haemolyticus*).

STAPHYLOCOCCUS AUREUS

The species *Staphylococcus aureus* was named for its tendeney to produce a golden-yellow pigment (Fig. 26.2) from the Latin word *aurum* meaning gold by **Friedrich Julius Rosenbach**, a German physician and microbiologist, in 1889. This coagulase-positive and Gram-positive bacterium is the most resistant of all spore forming pathogenic bacteria and considered the most dangerous pathogen of humans responsible for causing a wide range of infections in man and animals (Table 26.1). It is characterized by its ability to clot blood plasma by the action of the enzyme **coagulase**. All other known species of *Staphylococcus* lack this enzyme.

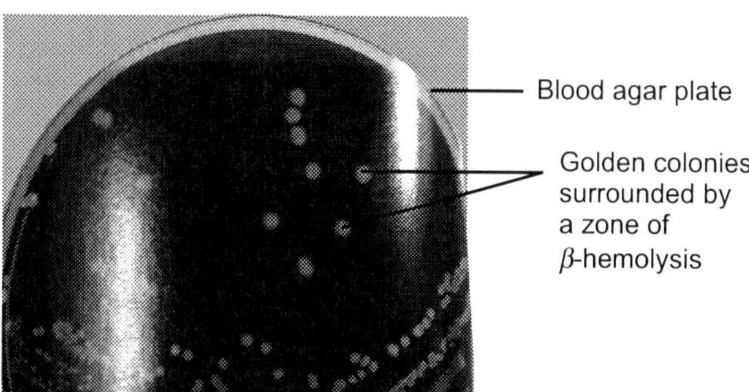

Fig. 26.2 ***Staphylococcus aureus* on blood agar.** At 35°C, after 24-40 hours, the colonies (6-8 mm, cream coloured, opaque, β-hemolytic) produce the golden pigment that led to its species name.

Table 26.1 Infections caused by *Staphylococcus aureus*

Skin infections	Life-threating diseases
• Pimples, impetigo, boils, cellulitis, folliculitis, carbuncles, abscesses.	• Pneumonia, meningitis, osteomyelitis, endocarditis, staphylococcal toxic shock syndrome, bacteremia, sepsis.
• Scalded skin syndrome	• Food intoxication (poisoning)
• Wound infections following surgery in hospitals	

MORPHOLOGY

This bacterium is a Gram-positive, spherical, non-motile, non-sporing coccus, 1 μm in diameter, arranged characteristically as grape-like clusters (Fig. 26.1). However, in pathological specimens, cocci may occur as single cells or pair of cells.

CULTURE CHARACTERISTICS

S. aureus can be grown on a variety of media (e.g., nutrient agar, blood agar, MacConkey agar) between 10 and 40°C (37°C being the optimum) under aerobic conditions (i.e., in air). On nutrient agar (at 37°C after 24 hours), the colonies are circular, 2-3 mm in diameter with a smooth shiny surface producing golden-yellow pigment that led to its species name (Fig. 26.2).

Mannitol salt agar, a selective and differential medium, which contains a high concentration of salt (7–10% NaCl), is used for isolating and presumptive identification of this bacterium from food, faeces and clinical materials (e.g., nasal swabs).

DISTINCTIVE BIOCHEMICAL TESTS FOR *S. AUREUS*

1. Beta-haemolysis on blood agar
2. Golden yellow pigment production
3. Positive coagulase test (ability to clot plasma)
4. Deoxyribionuclease (DNase) production
5. Thermostable endonuclease production
6. Mannitol fermentation
7. Gelatin liquefaction
8. Phosphatase production
9. Clumping factor production
10. Tellurite reduction.

PATHOGENESIS AND VIRULENCE

Staphylococcus aureus causes infection most commonly at sites of lowered host resistance, e.g., damaged skin or mucous membranes. It produces disease by one of the two mechanisms:

- *Toxin mediated disease:* Disease results due to the production of toxin by the bacterium either in the infected host or preformed *in vitro*. Toxins act as the virulent factors.
- *Direct invasion of tissue:* The bacteria gain access to damaged skin, mucosal or tissue sites, colonize by adhering to cells, evade host defense mechanisms, multiply and cause destruction of tissues.

S. aureus infections range from superficial skin infections (e.g., folliculitis, boil, abscesses, impetigo), to systemic infections, (e.g., pneumonia, endocarditis, scalded-skin syndrome).

VIRULENCE FACTORS

S. aureus produces an array of virulence factors that enable the bacteria to resist phagocytosis, destroy host tissue and invade the blood. Enzymes and toxins act as the main virulence factors. Overall pathogenicity is due to a combination of virulence factors which enable the bacterium to cause both local and systemic infections. Other factors involved in virulence are:

- Cell surface polymers – peptidoglycan and teichoic acid.
- Cell surface proteins – Protein A, clumping factor and fibronectin binding protein.
- Exoproteins – α-lysin, β-lysin, γ-lysin, δ-lysin and panton-valentine leucocidin.

ENZYMES AS VIRULENCE FACTORS

Various enzymes produced by *S. aureus* with their functions are as follows.

- **Coagulase**—It is an extracellular enzyme produced by the bacterium that reacts with **coagulase-reacting factor (CRF)** present in plasma, causing the plasma to clot by the conversion of fibrinogen → fibrin in blood.

  Coagulase test, which measures the ability to clot plasma, a confirmatory characteristic, is used to distinguish *S. aureus* from other bacteria that appear similar. This test is performed by two methods: slide coagulase test and tube coagulase test.
- **Hyalouronidase** – Also called the **"spreading factor"**, hydrolyses the intracellular glue (hyaluronic acid) that binds connective tissue in host tissues, thus facilitating the spread of the bacterium to adjacent tissues.
- **Staphylokinase (fibrinolysin)** – Digests blood (fibrin) clots allowing spread of infection to contiguous tissues.
- **Deoxyribonuclease (DNase)** – Degrades DNA. This characteristic is used to aid in the differentiation of *S. aureus* from coagulase-negative staphylococci (CNS).
- **Lipase** – Degrades lipid that helps bacteria to colonize oily skin surfaces.
- **Penicillinase** – Enzyme inactivates penicillin and other antimicrobial drugs, giving them multiple drug resistance and resulting in development of several resistant strains which cause serious problems in hospitals.

TOXINS AS VIRULENCE FACTORS INVOLVED IN PATHOGENESIS

S. aureus produces a wide variety of toxins which act as important virulence factors involved in pathogenesis. These include:

1. Haemolysins

Four antigenically distinct types of haemolysin – alpha, beta, gamma and delta are produced. All these are **exotoxins** (toxins released into the surrounding medium). Of these, alpha-haemolysin is most important in pathogenicity. It is cytotoxic, leucocidal and dermonectric. It also damages the muscle tissues and circulatory system.

2. Enterotoxins

S. aureus produces at least *eight* distinct **enterotoxins** (toxin acting on the gastrointestinal tract): A, B, C, D, E, G, H, I. Of these, **enterotoxin A**, a peptide encoded by a chromosomal gene, is responsible for the food poisoning (= food intoxication). It can withstand boiling at 100°C for a few minutes, is a superantigen, acts directly on ANS and produces **gastroenteritis**. The disease is characterized by nauesea, vomiting, diarrhoea, headache which most commonly occurs within 2-6 hours of consuming contaminated food containing preformed toxin. Meat, fish, milk, milk products, poultry, egg, salads are involved.

3. Toxic shock syndrome toxin (TSST-1)

Some strains of *S. aureus* cause the *toxic shock syndrome* (TSS) characterized by sudden fever (102°F or more), vomiting, diarrhoea, dizziness, fainting when standing up, or a rash that looks like a sunburn. Highest incidence is recorded in women under 30 years of age. This multisystem disease is caused by staphylococcal TSST-1, or enterotoxin or both. The absence of circulating antibodies to TSST-1 is a factor in the pathogenesis of this syndrome.

4. Epidermolytic toxins

S. aureus produces two types of epidermolytic (Gr. *epi* = over or upon + *derma* = skin + *lysis* = loosening) toxins. Both the toxins cause separation of the skin layers called **exfoliation**. Toxin A, which remains localized, causes **bullous impetigo** and toxin B which circulates to distant sites, causes **scalded skin syndrome (SSS)** in which skin is peeled off in sheets. Outbreaks of bullous impetigo is a frequent problem in hospital nurseries, where the condition is called **pemphigus neonatorum** (or **impetigo of the newborn**).

DISEASES CAUSED BY *S. AUREUS*

Diseases caused by *S. aureus* are classfied into six types, as described below.

Category	Examples
1. *Cutaneous infections*	Boils, carbuncles, pustules, impetigo, wound and burn infections
2. *Deep and systemic infections*	Osteomycelitis, tonsillitis, pharyngitis, pneumonitis, sinusitis, bacteremia and septicaemia
3. *Food poisoning*	Staphylococcal food poisoning (or intoxication)
4. *Hospital acquired infections*	Urinary tract infections and respiratory tract infections
5. *Exfoliate diseases*	Staphylococcal scalded skin syndrome (SSSS), bullous impetigo
6. *Toxic shock syndrome*	Multisystem illness

LABORATORY DIAGNOSIS

S. aureus is diagnosed from one or more of the following specimens: pus, tissue exudates, sputum, faeces or vomit, urine or blood.

- **Gram staining**—Gram-positive cocci (violet coloured) in clusters is the characteristic feature of this bacterium. The cocci may appear singly or in pairs or in short chains in specimens.
- **Culture**—On blood agar within 18 to 24 hours at 35–37°C, yellow or golden yellow colonies with or without β-hemolysis are observed.
- **Mannitol fermentation**—On mannitol salt agar (MSA), plates within 24 to 48 hours at 35–37°C, show yellow or gold colonies.
- **Coagulase test**—Rabbit plasma (collected with EDTA) tube inoculated with *S. aureus* culture at 35-37°C after 4 hours, results in **clot formation** (i.e., coagulase-positive), a confirmatory test for its identification.

ANTIMICROBIAL RESISTANCE

S. aureus developed resistance after penicillin was introduced due to two reasons: **production of beta - lactamase (*penicillinase*)** which inactivates penicillin by splitting the β-lactam ring, and changes in bacterial surface receptors which reduce bonding of antibiotics to cells.

An increasing problem with *S. aureus* is its resistance to methicillin, and vancomycin resulting in methicillin resistant *S. aureus* (MRSA) and vancomycin resistant *S. aureus* (VRSA) strains, respectively, one of the most common causes of nosocomial infections.

TREATMENT

Staph infections treatment should be based on antibiotic susceptibility test since drug resistance is common among staphylococci.

- Benzyl penicillin is the most effective antibiotic if the disease causing strain is sensitive because this antibiotic is narrow-spectrum and bactericidal.
- If the patient is hypersensitive to penicillin, cefazolin, an alternative drug, is used.
- Cloxacillins are effective against penicillinase producing strains.
- Clindamycin and teicoplanin in case of cefoxitin resistance are used.
- Vancomycin is used in case of MRSA strains.

COAGULASE-NEGATIVE STAPHYLOCOCCI

Staph bacteria that lack the enzyme coagulase are called the **coagulase-negative staphylococci (CNS)**. These slime-producing bacteria are the most common causative agents of infection by indwelling devices. Once they have adhered to the surface, they began to divide and finally the entire surface is coated with a biofilm contaninig these organisms. CNS have relatively low virulence but frequently associated with nosocomial and opportunisitic infections in immunocompromised patients. Of the over 30 CNS, *S. epidermidis* and *S. saprophyticus* are serious human pathogens.

STAPHYLOCOCCUS EPIDERMIDIS

S. epidermidis is the cause of **endocarditis** (infection of the heart valves and parts of the inside lining of the heart muscle), intravascular devices (prosthetic heart valves, shunts) and in prosthetic joints, catheters, large wounds and septicaemia. Septicaemia is especially prevalent resulting from neonatal infections particularly in very low birth weights. High incidence of *S. epidermidis* in the hospital settings is due to the contamination of patient care equipment and evironmental surfaces by it. Presence of a polysaccharide outer layer (glycocalyx), allowing adherence and subsquent formation of a multilayered biofilm which binds strongly to plastic. Glycocalyx acts as an important virulence factor and is essential for pathogenesis of device related infection in *S. epidermidis*.

DIAGNOSIS

The diagnosis of *S. epidermidis* is made by:

- Coagulase-negative reaction
- White colonies with little or no pigment on blood agar at 35–37°C (Fig. 26.3)
- Susceptibility to novobiocin.

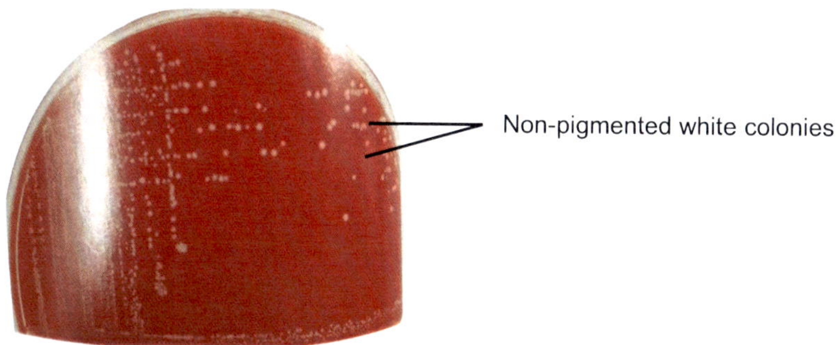

Fig. 26.3 ***Staphylococcus epidermidis*** **on blood agar (at 35°C for 24 hours).** *S. epidermidis*, in contrast to both *S. aureus* and other CNS, produces a white colony with little to no pigment.

TREATMENT

Because it is a multidrug resistant bacterium, vancomycin or rifampin is used to treat the infection caused by this pathogen.

STAPHYLOCOCCUS SAPROPHYTICUS

S. saprophyticus, a member of the normal genitourinary tract microbiota, is a leading cause of cystits, a urinary tract infection, particularly in young sexually active females.

DIAGNOSIS

- **Colonial characteristic.** On 5% sheep blood agar, colonies are large (5–8 mm in diameter), glossy, smooth, white, cream, yellow or orange.
- **Novobiocin susceptibility** on Mueller-Hinton agar exhibits resistance to the antibiotic novobiocin (no zone of inhibition), a distinguishing feature of this species.
- **Coagulase test** - Coagulase-negative.

TREATMENT

Treated with trimethoprim-sulfamethoxazole, or norfloxacin. Susceptibility to ampicillin and ceftriaxone has also been found.

KEY POINTS

- **Gram-positive cocci** (*Staphylococcus, Streptococcus, Enterococcus, Micrococcus*) and **Gram-negative cocci** (*Haemophilus, Neisseria, Acinetobacter*) are among the most clinically significant cocci of humans.
- Members of the genus *Staphylococcus*, called **staphylococci**, cause 13% of the total nosocomial infections annually.
- *Staphylococcus aureus*, the most serious pathogen among cocci, is identified by the production of coagulase, haemolysis, golden yellow colonies and several types of virulence factors.
- Based on the coagulase test, staphylococci are classified as **catalase-positive staphylococci** (*Staphylococcus aureus*) and **catalase-negative staphylococci** (*S. epidermidis, S. saprophyticus, S. haemophilus*).
- Enterotoxins produced by *S. aureus* cause serious food poisioning **(food intoxication)** due to consumtion of contaminated food (e.g., custards, sauces, cream pasteries, meats, ham, etc).

IMPORTANT QUESTIONS

1. Describe briefly:
   (a) Toxins of *Staphylococcus aureus*
   (b) *Staphylococcus aureus* enzymes as virulence factors
   (c) Laboratory diagnosis of *Staphylococcus aureus*
   (d) Coagulase-negative staphylococci of medical signficance.

MULTIPLE-CHOICE QUESTIONS

1. All are Gram-negative cocci EXCEPT:
   (a) *Haemophilus* (b) *Acinetobactor*
   (c) *Staphylococcus* (d) *Neisseria.*
2. All are coagulase-negative staphylococci EXCEPT:
   (a) *Staphylococcus epidermidis*
   (b) *Staphylococcus aureus*
   (c) *Staphylococcus saprophyticus*
   (d) *Staphylococcus haemolyticus.*

3. Which of the following bacteria is/are novobiocin resistant?

(a) *Staphylococcus saprophyticus*

(b) *Staphylococcus aureus*

(c) *Staphylococcus epidermidis*

(d) All of the above.

4. Which of the following staphylococci has a polysacharide outer layer which bonds strongly to plastics and forms biofilm that helps in pathogenesis?

(a) *Staphylococcus aureus*

(b) *Staphylococcus saprophyticus*

(c) *Staphylococcus epidermidis*

(d) *Staphylococcus haemolyticus.*

5. All are true for *Staphylococcus aureus* EXCEPT:

(a) A golden yellow pigment

(b) Coagulase positive

(c) Ferment mannitol

(d) Resistant to the antibiotic novobiocin.

6. Which of the following is the drug of choice for methicillin-resistant *Staphylococcus aureus* (MRSA)?

(a) Metronidazole (b) Vancomycin

(c) Azithromycin (d) None of the above.

ANSWERS TO MCQs

1. (c) 2. (b) 3. (a) 4. (c) 5. (d)
6. (b).

27

Streptococcus: A Gram-positive Aerobic Coccus Forming Chains

Strep throat; Rheumatic fever; Acute glomerulonephritis; Pneumonia; Meningitis

The genus *Streptococcus* comprises Gram-positive, catalase-negative, aerobic cocci that typically grow as pairs or chains, may appear bent or twisted (from the Greek words: *strepto* = twisted + *kokkos* = berry, spherical, meaning berries in chain) (Fig. 27.1). Viennese surgeon **Albert Theodor Billroth** in 1877 coined the term *Streptococcus*. It belongs to the **Lactic acid bacteria** group. Its members commonly colonize mucosal membranes and are a predominant component of the respiratory, gastrointestinal and genital tracts.

SYSTEMATIC POSITION

Streptococci are facultative anaerobes, catalase and oxidase negative that metabolize carbohydrate by fermentation producing mainly lactic acid. Currently, the genus comprises 50 species classified as:

SYSTEMATIC POSITION

Domain	:	Bacteria
Phylum	:	Firmicutes
Class	:	Bacilli
Order	:	Lactobacillales
Family	:	Streptococcaceae
Genus	:	*Streptococcus*

CLASSIFICATION

Streptococci (for the genera *Streptococcus* and *Enterococcus*) have been grouped by the phenotypic characteristics of the **haemolysis**:

- **α-haemolysis**—distinctive green colour around the colonies;
- **β-haemolysis**—colonies surrounded by a clear zone of serveral centimetres;
- **γ-haemolysis**—colonies showing no haemolysis on blood agar.

Other features used for grouping are: Lancefield antigen composition, biochemical (physiological) and pathological potential.

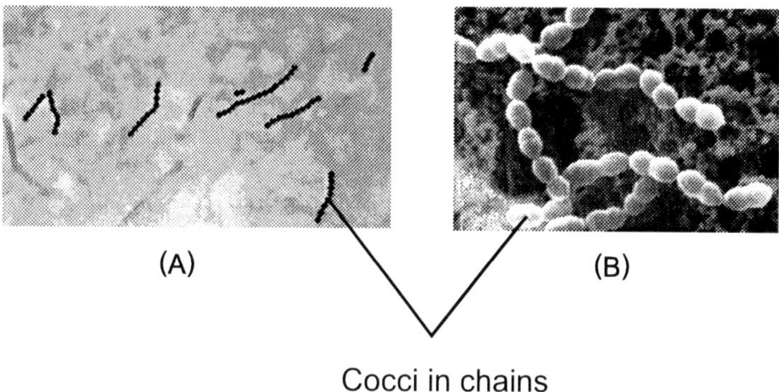

Fig. 27.1 ***Streptococcus pyogenes.*** (A) Gram-positive cocci (spherical to oval) present in chains, characterisitc feature of the genus. (B) Enlarged view showing dividing (oval) cells (SEM).

The **Lancefield grouping or classification system** was developed by **Rebecca Lancefield**, an American bacteriologist at Rockefeller University, for distinguishing β-haemolytic (pyogenic) streptococci. It is a serotype classification that describes specific polysaccharide (carbohydrate) present on the bacterial cell wall (referred to as **Lancefield antigen**). The 20 described serotypes are named Lancefield groups A to V (excluding I and J). Most members of the Lancefield groups are beta-haemolytic belonging to groups A and B (also known as "**group A strep**" and "**group B strep**").

PATHOGENESIS

Clinically significant streptococci with their classification are listed in Table 27.1

TABLE 27.1 *Streptococcus* species of clinical importance

Species	Type of haemolysis	Lancefield group	Major diseases
S. pyogenes	β	A	Pharyngitis, pyoderma, rheumatic fever, glomerulonephritis
S. agalactiae	β	B	Neonatal meningitis and sepsis
S. pneumoniae	α	O	Pneumonia
S. bovis	α or none	D	Endocarditis, UTI
S. mitis	α	O	Endocarditis
S. sanguinis (= *S. sanguis*)	α	H	Endocarditis, dental caries
S. mutans	None	Not designated	Dental caries

STREPTOCOCCUS PYOGENES—GROUP A BETA-HEMOLYTIC *STREPTOCOCCUS*

Streptococcus pyogenes (Fig. 27.1) is a beta-haemolytic, Gram-positive and catalase-negative bacterium. It is commonly called **group A beta-haemolytic *Streptococcus* (GABHS)**.

The species name is derived from Greek words: *streptos* meaning a chain and *coccus* (Latinized for *kokkos*) meaning berries, *pyo* (pus) and *genes* (forming) because streptococcal cells tend to link in chains of round cells and a number of infections caused by the bacteria produce pus.

MORPHOLOGY

The cells are round (cocci), 0.5 µm – 1 µm (diameter), arranged in long chains (Fig. 27.1) due to the division of cells in one plane only and the daughter cells remaining attached to each other. The cells appear violet with Gram stain (Gram +ve bacterium).

CULTURE/GROWTH

S. pyogenes readily grows on enriched media containing blood serum or sugars (e.g., blood agar medium). This is an aerobic and facultative

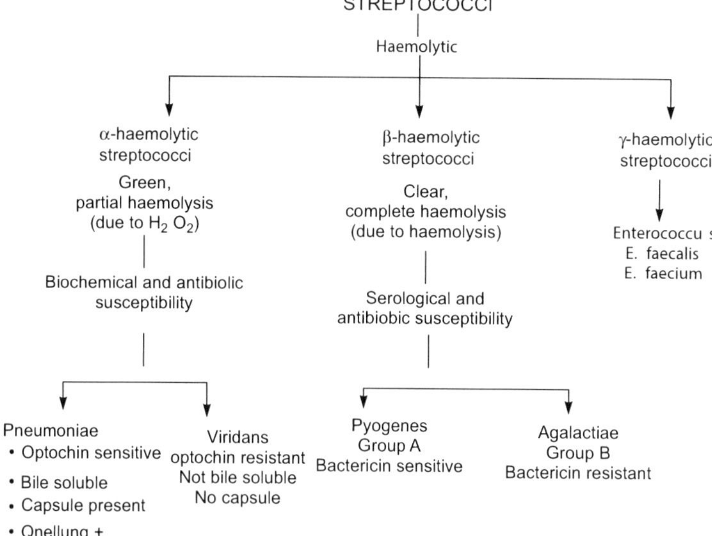

Fig. 27.2 **Classification of streptococci** (*Streptococcus and Enterococcus*) primarily based on the type of haemolysis produced on blood agar, a key characteristic used in identifying *Streptococcus* spp.

bacterium, i.e., can tolerate high levels of oxygen too. Growth and haemolysis are promoted by 5–10% CO_2. Best growth occurs at 37°C (range 22–42°C) between 7.4 and 7.6 pH producing light golden yellow colonies surrounded by large *clear zone of* β*-hemolysis*, several times greater than the colony size (Fig. 27.3).

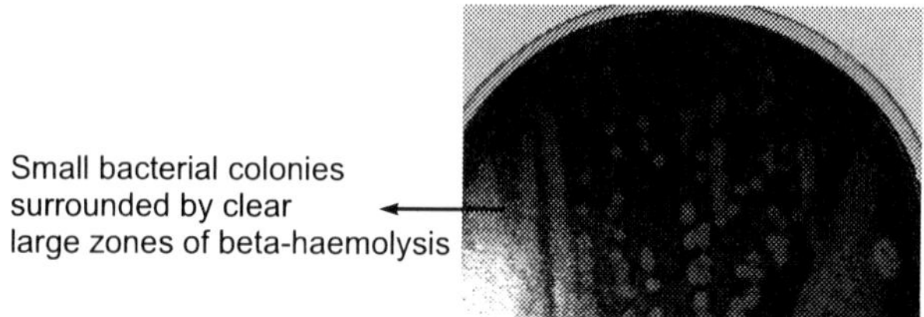

Fig. 27.3 ***Streptococcus pyogenes*** **on blood agar.** This bacterium produces a large zone of beta-haemolysis around a relatively small colony.

BIOCHEMICAL REACTIONS

- Catalase-negative
- PYR-positive (to detect enzyme pyrrolidonyl arylamidase)
- Fements a number of sugars (fructose, glucose, galactose, lactose, maltose) producing acid but no gas
- Insoluble in 10% bile (unlike *Streptococcus pneumoniae*).

CELL SURFACE ANTIGENS

Antigenic components involved in virulence, especially colonization, evasion of phagocytosis and host immune responses include:

- *Capsular polysaccharide* (hyaluronic acid)
- Cell wall peptidoglycan and lipoteichoic acid (LTA)
- Surface proteins—M proteins, fimbrial proteins, fibronectin-binding proteins (e.g., protein F)
- Cell-bound streptokinase
- The antigen, group A polysaccharide, is an integral part of the cell wall.

TOXINS AND ENZYMES AS VIRULENCE FACTORS

Strep pyogenes elaborates many exotoxins (streptolysin, eryothrogenic toxin) and enzymes (hyaluronidase, streptokinase and streptodornase).

STREPTOLYSIN EXOTOXINS

Streptolysin, an exotoxin, is a type of *haemolysin* (i.e., red blood cells destroyer) produced by *S. pyogenes*. Streptolysin is of two types: *streptolysin* O (SLO) (O stands for oxygen because it is inactivated by atmospheric oxygen) (i.e., oxygen-labile) and *streptolysin S* (SLS) (S stands for oxygen stable and serum soluble). Both streptolysins cause lysis of RBCs, white blood cells (whose function is to kill the streptococci) and platelets by forming pores in their cell membrane.

Streptolysin O is a potent cell poison responsible for the lysis of WBCs and RBCs, and is also cardiotoxic because streptolysin O is immunogenic and serves as an antigenic compound and helps in diagnosis of this bacterium **(antistreptolysin O titre)**.

SLS toxin is responsible for the haemolytic zone around GAS colonies grown under routine aerobic conditions on blood agar plates. It can also induce the release of lysosomal contents with subsequent cell death after engulfment by phagocytes. In contrast to SLO it is not immunogenic.

PYROGENIC EXOTOXINS

Pyrogenic exotoxins, because of their ability to induce fever (also called **erythrogenic toxins** from the Greek: *erythro* = red + *gennan* = producing), are produced by *S. pyogenes*. These are superantigens that damage the plasma membranes of blood capillaries under the skin and produce a typical bright red rash (typical symptom of scarlet fever) and it also induces fever by acting upon the temperature regulatory centre. Only lysogenic strains of *S. pyogenes* that contain genes from a temperate bacteriophage can synthesize this toxin.

Pyrogenic toxins are of three types: A, B and C (SPEA, SPEB and SPEC). SPEA is most toxic and is lethal followed by SPEB that causes mycocardial necrosis.

HYALURONIDASE

Hyaluronidase (hyaluronate lyase or **spreading factor)** is an extracellular enzyme that breaks down hyaluronic acid, a glue-like material, that binds the cells of connective tissue. It causes disintegration of tissues (necrotizing fasciitis) and promoting rapid invasion of *S. pyogenes* at the rate of one inch per hour.

STREPTOKINASE

Streptokinase (**fibrinolysin**) dissolves blood clots through the activation of a pathway leading to the digestion of human fibrin clots. Pathogens trapped in blood clots free themselves to spread to other tissues thus playing a role in invasion.

Since streptokinase has the ability to disslove human blood clots, it is used as an antithrombic agent in the management of blood clots affecting the blood vessels of the heart, lungs, etc. It is given intravenously for the treatment of early myocardial infarction (heart attack) due to blockage of blood flow to the heart muscle, pulmonary embolism and arterial thromboembolism.

STREPTODORNASE

Streptodornase (***Streptococcus* DNase**), an enzyme released by streptococci, digests DNA released from dead cells, reduces the viscosity of pus allowing the bacterium greater motility.

It is used medicinally (often in combination with streptokinase) to dissolve clotted blood, and fibrinous and purulent accumulations of exudate.

DISEASES

Streptococcus pyogenes causes infections of three types:

- **Suppurative** (pus producing)—Infections of upper respiratory tract and of skin and soft tissue (e.g., pharyngitis, cellulitis, erysipelas, lymphadenitis).

- **Non-suppurative (non-pyogenic)**—Post-infections, not associated with local bacterial multiplication and pus formation (e.g., acute glomerulonephritis and rehumatic fever following both skin and throat infections).
- **Toxic manifestations**—Scarlet fever.

STREP THROAT (PHARYNGITIS OR TONSILLITIS)

Strep throat is a common bacterial infection in children, more common in late winter and early spring. Potential complications include rheumatic fever and peritonsillar abscess.

Symptoms: **Sore throat**—throat feels raw, and it hurts to swallow, fever of 101°F or higher, red, swollen tonsils with exudates (pus), white patches on the throat, nausea, vomiting and enlarged lymph nodes in the neck. Symptoms typically begin one to three days after exposure and last 7 to 10 days.

Transmission: *S. pyogenes* lives in the nose and throat. The pathogen spreads through airborne droplets when someone with the infection coughs or sneezes, or through shared foods or drinks or by touching something that has droplets on it and then touching the eyes, mouth or nose.

Diagnosis: Diagnosis is made based on the results of **a rapid antigen detection test** or **throat culture** in those who have symptoms.

Teatment: Paracetamol (acetaminophen) and nonsteroidal anti-inflammatory drugs (NSAIDS) such as ibuprofen are used to relieve pain. **Penicillin** (benzathine penicillin G in India and penicillin V in the United States) **is the drug of choice**. Erythromycin or clindamycin is an alternative medicine for severe penicillin-allergic patients.

Prevention: To avoid getting strep throat, follow:

- Washing hands immediately after having contact with an infected person.
- Do not share toothbrushes and eating and drinking utensils.

RHEUMATIC FEVER AND RHEUMATIC HEART DISEASE

Rheumatic disorder refers to an inflammatory disease causing chronic pain of joints (arthritis) and or connective tissue.

Rheumatic fever (RF) (or **acute rheumatic fever, ARF**) is a post-streptococcal sequela that can involve the joints, heart, skin and brain. The disease typically develops 2–4 weeks after *Streptococcus* *pyogenes* throat infection. RF is most common in the developing world and among indigenous peoples in the developed world. Currently, 3,25,000 children between the ages of 5 and 14 have RF.

Symptoms—Fever (100.8–102.0°F), multiple painful joints, involuntary muscle movements and occasionally a characteristic nonitchy rash, called **erythema marginatum**.

Rheumatic heart disease (RHD)—Damage to heart valves is called **RHD**. RHD usually results in heart failure, atrial fibrillation, and infection of the valves. The disease usually occurs after repeated attacks of RF.

Diagnosis—Diagnosis is based on infection history, clinical symptoms (e.g., inflammation of joints, rash or skin nodules, heart abnormalities, ECG or EKG, echocardiogram) and presence of strep bacteria (throat culture and blood).

Treatment—**Aspirin is the drug of choice for relieving pain and inflammation**. However, gastritis and salicylate poisoning are the major side effects in addition to the **Reye's syndrome,** a serious and potentially deadly condition. Ibuprofen is alternative to aspirin.

Patients having RF and RHD, prolonged treatment of penicillin at monthly intervals for 5 year and 40 years, respectively is sometimes recommended.

In severe RHD, valve replacement surgery or valve repair is required since the damaged valves may result in heart failure.

ACUTE GLOMERULONEPHRITIS

Glomerulonephritis (GN) refers to an inflammation of the tiny filters of the kidney, the glomeruli, hence the name. The causes of GN include: infections (bacterial, viral or parasitic pathogens), drugs, systemic disorders (SLE, vasculitis) or diabetes.

Acute glomerulonephritis (AGN) is a sudden inflammation of glomeruli, that occurs after a week or two after streptococcal pharyngitis (strep throat), for which it is also known as **post-infection** or **post-streptococcus glomerulonephritis (PSGN)**. Annually, 1.5 million people are infected with over 20,000 deaths worldwide due to AGN.

SYMPTOMS

- Pink or cola-coloured urine from RBCs in the urine (*haematuria*).

- Fluid retention (*oedema*) with swelling evident on the face, feet, hands and abdomen.
- High blood pressure (hypertension).
- Fever (headache, malaise, anorexia, nausea).

DIAGNOSIS

- Diagnosed clinically, based on history and examination of the patient.
- Urine examination.
- Blood chemistry studies.
- Serologically, specifically the **streptozyme test** to measure streptococcal antibodies.
- Kidney biopsy.
- Complement profile.

TREATMENT

- Treatment of AGN requires the management of high blood pressure with low-sodium diet.
- Thiazide or loop diuretics can be used to simultaneously reduce oedema and control hypertension; however, electrolytes such as potassium must be monitored.
- It is a self limited episode that resolves without any permanent damage, hence does not require the use of penicillin.

STREPTOCOCCUS AGALACTIAE (GROUP B STREPTOCOCCUS)

Streptococcus agalactiae (also known as **group B streptococcus**) is a harmless commensal member of human microbiota that resides in vagina, pharynx and large intestine. Nevertheless, it can cause severe invasive infections in the newborn.

CHARACTERISTICS

- Gram-positive cocci, 2.0 μm, occurring in pairs and short chains.
- Facultatively anaerobic.
- Beta-haemolysis on blood agar-narrow zone of haemolysis relative to the colony size.
- Catalase negative.
- Hippurate positive.
- CAMP (Christie Atkins Munch-Peterson) test positive.

DISEASES

Diseases of the newborn in humans and cow mastitis (inflammation of the mammary gland).

Neonatal diseases include: Septicaemia (90%), pulmonary involvenent (40%) and meningitis (30%).

PATHOGENESIS

Adult infections include pneumonia, UTI peritonitis, meningitis, endocarditis; and osteomyelitis.

Early onset of disease acquired in the uterus from the colonized bacterium in mother or during passage through the birth canal and can have a case fatality rate of 50%, late onset of disease with onset from 1 week to 3 months after birth have a case fatality rate of 20% and probably acquired by contact spread between babies in nursery after birth. Survivors of meningitis cases can be left with hearing loss, blindness, cerebral palsy, mental retardation and/or epilepsy.

EPIDEMIOLOGY

Worldwide, *S. agalactiae* mainly causes diseases in infants months of age with low birth weight, and in the elderly predispositions include diabetes, HIV and cancer.

TREATMENT

Administration of penicillin or ampicillin at the oneset and throughout labour to women who are colonized with group B bacterium and who are at high risk of delivering an infected infant (premature).

Combination of penicillin and gentamicin is used to treat serious infection.

GROUP D STREPTOCOCCI

Group D streptococci were earlier classified into two groups:

- **Enterococcus group** (enterococci or faecal enterococci)—Because they are the normal colonists of the human intestine)—currently, these bacteria are classified in the genus *Enterococcus*.
- **Nonenterococcal group**—Because they colonize other animals and rarely humans (e.g. *Streptococcus bovis* and *S. equinus*).

VIRIDANSSTREPTOCOCCI (ALPHA-HAEMOLYTIC STREPTOCOCCI)

Viridans streptococci are Gram-positive bacteria that are alpha-haemolytic and nonhaemolytic producing a green colouration on blood agar plates (hence, the name viridans from Latin, *viridis* meaning green). They are the commensal members of the oral cavity (gingiva, cheeks, tongue, saliva) and are also found in the nasopharynx, genital tract and skin.

VGS group includes: *Streptococcus mitis, S. mutans, S. milleri, S. salivarius, S. sanguis* and *S. intermedius*.

CHARACTERISTICS

VGS streptococci are catalase-negative and Gram-positive cocci, present in chains, leucine aminopeptidase positive, pyrrolidonyl arylamidase negative, and do not grow in 6.5% NaCl and on bile esculine agar.

DISEASES

Several viridans species are associated with:

- Dental caries and subacute bacterial endocarditis, particularly in patients with damaged heart valve (*S. mutans* and *S. sanguinis*). These bacteria have the unique ability to synthesize dextrans from gulcose which allows them to adhere to fibrin-platelet aggregates at damaged heart valves.
- Deep abscesses, partically in the brain and liver (*S. intermedius*). Dental extraction or injury to the mucosa can lead to their introduction into the blood stream which is followed by endocarditis.

TREATMENT

Antibiotics found effective to treat viridans streptococci are:

- Oral – roxithromycin, amoxicillin and rifampin.
- Intravenous – penicillin, cephalothin and vancomycin.

KEY POINTS

- **Streptococci** are catalase-negative Gram-positive cocci arranged in chains and pairs.
- Streptococci are classified immunologically by their cell wall antigens **(Lancefield groups)**
- *Streptococcus pyogenes*, group A β-haemolytic pathogen, is extremely pathogenic due to the presence of many virulence factors.

- *Streptococcus agalactiae*, group B β-haemolytic pathogen, is a common opportunistic agent of wound, skin and neonatal infections.
- *Streptococcus faecalis* found in the intestine, is currently considered a *Enterococcus*.
- Viridans group streptococci (VGS), alpha-hemolytic, Gram-positive cocci occur in pairs and short chains, cause dental caries as well as subacute bacterial endocarditis following dental extraction or injury to the oral mucosa.
- Penicillin G is the drug of choice to treat most streptococcal infections.

IMPORTANT QUESTIONS

1. Describe the morphology, classification and treatment of streptococci.
2. Write short notes on:
   (a) *Streptococcus pyogenes*
   (b) Virulence factros of *Streptococcus pyogenes*
   (c) Viridans streptococci
   (d) Streptococcal sore throat
   (e) Acute rheumatic fever and rheumatic heart disease.

MULTIPLE-CHOICE QUESTIONS

1. All of the following streptococci show β-hemolysis on blood agar, EXCEPT:
   (a) *Streptococcus pyogenes*
   (b) *Streptococcus agalactiae*
   (c) *Streptococcus mitis*
   (d) None of the above.
2. All are *true* for *Streptococcus pyogenes* EXCEPT:
   (a) Catalase-positive
   (b) PYR positive
   (c) Insoluble in 10% bile
   (d) Ferments a number of sugars producing acid but no gas.
3. *Streptococcus pyogenes* can be differentiated from other haemolytic streptococci on the basis of:
   (a) Penicillin sensitivity
   (b) Erythromycin sensitivity
   (c) Bacitracin sensitivity
   (d) Vancomycin sensitivty.

4. The bacterial sore throat is caused by
   (a) *Haemophilus* spp.
   (b) *Staphylococcus aureus*
   (c) *Streptococcus pyogenes*
   (d) *Streptococcus mitis.*
5. The bacteria involved in the production of dental caries is/are
   (a) *Streptococcus agalactiae*
   (b) *Streptococcus mutans*
   (c) *Streptococcus pyogenes*
   (d) *Streptococcus anginosus.*
6. Which of the following enzymes/virulence factors is involved in dissolving blood clots?
   (a) Hyaluronidase (b) Streptokinase
   (c) Streptodornase (d) None of the above.
7. Rheumatic fever damages the———, and acute glomerulonephritis damages the ———.
   (a) Skin, heart
   (b) Heart valves, kidney
   (c) Joints, bone marrow
   (d) Brain, kidney.

ANSWERS TO MCQs

1. (c) 2. (a) 3. (c) 4. (c) 5. (b)
6. (b) 7. (b).

28

Pneumococcus: A Gram-positive Diplococcus (*Streptococcus pneumoniae*)

Pneumonia; Otitis media

Pneumococcus (named for its role as a cause of pneumonia in 1886) was termed *Diplococcus pneumoniae* because of its characteristic appearance (lancet-shaped diplococci) in Gram-stained sputum in 1920. In 1974, this bacterium was renamed *Streptococcus pneumoniae* because it shared characteristics with streptococci. *Pneumococcus* is a normal inhabitant of the human upper respiratory tract.

The beginning of the *era of molecular genetics*—the genetic material consists of DNA—is based on the transformation experiments carried out on pneumococcus by **Frederick Griffith** in 1928 and **Oswald Avery**, **Colin MacLeod** and **Maclyn McCarty** in 1944.

DISEASES

S. pneumoniae (or pneumococcus) is the most leading cause of community acquired pneumonia (CAP) and otitis media (middle ear infection). In addition, it can cause bacterial meningitis, bacteraemia, sinusitis, septic arthritis, osteomycelitis, peritonitis and endocarditis.

Pneumonia is a serious infection of the lungs which can be fatal, especially in the elderly and infants. Of the various infections, each year over 2 million children under the age of 2 die due to pneumococcal infections.

MORPHOLOGY

Its cells are Gram-positive, lancelolate or flame-shaped (one end broad and other pointed), non-motile, capsulated, 1 μm cocci, appearing in pairs (diplococci), hence the genus was initially named as *Diplococcus* (Fig. 28.1).

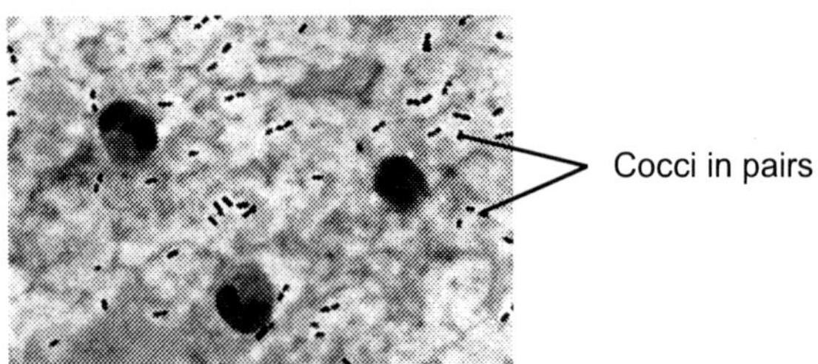

Fig. 28.1 ***Streptococcus pneumoniae.*** Gram stain of direct smear of sputum specimen showing lancet-shaped, Gram-positive cocci in pairs (diplococci).

CULTURAL CHARACTERISTICS

It grows only on enriched media requiring blood or serum for growth (e.g., blood agar), under aerobic and anaerobic conditions, optimally at 35–37°C. Growth is enhanced in CO_2 (5–10%).

On blood agar, colonies are alpha-haemolytic (green) and mucoid due to capsule, as the colonies age, they tend to be described as concave and can appear to have a "punched-out" centre due to autolysis of organisms in the centre of the growing colony (Fig. 28.2). Green discolouration around the colonies resembles to that of viridan streptococci. On blood agar, at 37°C, the bacterium has a doubling time of 20–30 minutes.

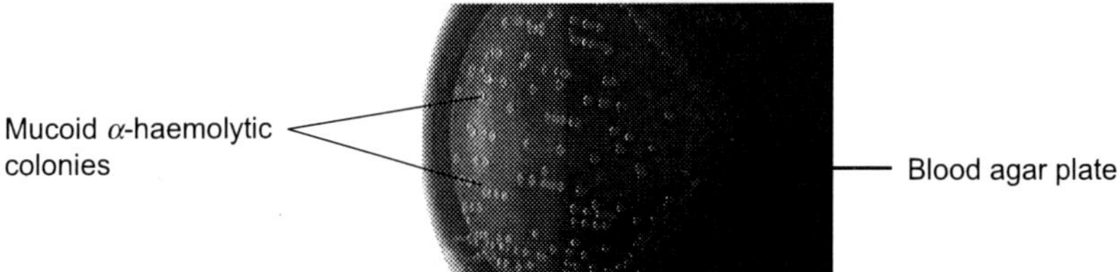

Fig. 28.2 ***Streptococcus pneumoniae*** **on blood agar.** Mucoid colonies produce a zone of alpha-haemolysis and centre of each colony appears to be 'punched out' due to autolysis of bacteria in the centre of the growing colony.

BIOCHEMICAL CHARACTERISTICS

- Catalase-negative
- Oxidase-negative
- Soluble in 10% bile (differentiates *S. pneumoniae* from *S. pyogenes*)
- Fermentation of inulin (differentiates it from other streptococcus)
- Sensitive to optochin antibiotic

- Ferments various sugars producing acid without gas (similar to other streptococcus).

DIAGNOSTIC FEATURES

Bile solubility and optochin susceptibility tests are most widely used to identify *S. pneumoniae*.

Strains of *S. pneumoniae* have been defined by their capsular antigens, and currently over 90 serotypes have been defined which differ in virulence, prevalence and extent of drug resistance.

Swelling of the capsule in the presence of specific antiserum/type specific antibodies is referred to as a **quellung reaction**. Alternatively, strains can be typed using commercially available agglutination.

VIRULENCE FACTORS

S. pneumoniae produces a range of colonization and virulence factors: polysaccharide capsule, surface proteins, enzymes, and the toxin pneumolysin (PLY), contributing to pathogenesis and the disease development.

- **Polysaccharide capsule**—It inhibits phagocytosis by polymorphonuclear leukocytes in blood, leading to invasion of bloodstream and cerebrospinal fluid.
- **Pneumolysin** (PLY)—It is a toxin produced by the bacterium which inhibits antibody synthesis and lymphocyte proliferation.
- **Autolysin**—It is an enzyme that releases cell wall products.

MODE OF SPREAD

Humans are the only reserviors of pneumococcus and the pneumococcal infection is spread when an infected person talks, coughs or sneezes small droplets containing infectious agents into the air, by the *droplet mechanism* from up to 6 feet away. Infection can also spread by contact with hands, tissues and other articles soiled by infected nose and throat discharges. Disease results when the host resistance is lowered.

Pneumococcal infections are more common during the winter and may be triggered by viral infections.

SIGNS AND SYMPTOMS

Infections usually involve lungs, middle ear, sinuses, bloodstream, and meninges.

Major symptoms of pneumococcal pneumonia

- Fever
- Chills and shaking
- Chest pain when breathing in or out
- Shortness of breath
- Cough
- Blood stained or 'rusty' sputum (phlegm)
- Elderly people reveal confusion or drowsiness (excessive sleepiness).

Major symptoms of pneumococcal meningitis

- High fever
- Headache
- Stiff neck
- Nausea and vomiting
- Photophobia (discomfort when looking at light)
- Symptoms in infants: Child may only appear to be inactive, irritable, feeding poorly and may be vomiting.

Major symptoms of acute otitis media, AOM (or inflammation of the middle ear):

- Affects children before the age of three
- Ear pain
- Presence of pus in the middle ear
- Eardrum inflamed (i.e., bulging)
- Fever
- Most common bacterial pathogens of AOM are *Streptococcus pneumoniae* (40%), *Haemophilus influenzae* (30%) and *Moraxella catarrhalis* (15%).

INCUBATION PERIOD

Symptoms usually appear 3 to 4 days (sometimes 1 to 10 days) after infection of an individual.

DIAGNOSIS

By microscopic examination and culture of bacteria from sputum, blood (pneumonia); fluid aspirated from middle ear, Gram stained films of CSF (meningitis).

PREVENTION/VACCINES

Two vaccines are available for pneumococcal infections for specific groups.

Prevenar-13: For children 6 weeks of age, 4 and 12 months of age; and for the persons with chronic medical conditions and associated with an increased risk of pneumococcal infection.

Pneumovax-23: For persons 65 years of age and over, children four years of age who have a chronic medical condition and considered at high risk of increased complications from pneumococcal infection.

Pneumovax-23 must not be given to children less than two years of age.

TREATMENT

Penicillin is the antibiotic of choice to treat pneumococcal infections provided the infecting strain is sensitive to penicillin; and ceftriaxone for the strains that have reduced susceptibility to penicillin. For empiric treatment (i.e., therapy based on the experience) of meningitis, use of ceftriaxone in conjunction with vancomycin or rifampin is recommended.

Amoxicillin is the drug of choice for the treatment of acute otitis media.

KEY POINTS

- The causative agent of pneumonia has been variously named *Pneumococcus, Diplococcus pneumoniae* and *Streptococcus pneumoniae.*
- *Streptococcus pneumoniae* is a Gram-positive, capsulated, producer of lanceolate cocci arranged in pairs (diplococci). Colonies α-hemolytic, mucoid on blood agar and sensitive to optochin antibiotic.
- Pneumonia, meningitis and otitis media are the major pheumococcal diseases.
- Vaccines (prevanar -13 and pneumovax-23) are available for both at high risk and healthy children.
- Ceftriaxone antibiotic is an alternative to the first drug penicillin to treat pneumococcal infections.
- Amoxicillin, a broad-spectrum semi-synthetic penicillin, is usually the first choice to treat otitis media in children.

IMPORTANT QUESTIONS

1. Describe briefly pneumonia.

MULTIPLE-CHOICE QUESTIONS

1. These names have been used for the causative agent of pneumonia EXCEPT:
   (a) *Pneumococcus*
   (b) *Streptococcus pneumoniae*
   (c) *Streptococcus agalactiae*
   (d) *Diplococcus pneumoniae.*
2. Which of the following is true for *Streptococcus pneumoniae*?
   (a) Optochin sensitive
   (b) Bile insoluble
   (c) Produces streptolysin
   (d) Has CAMP factor.
3. An effective vaccine exists to prevent infections from
   (a) *Streptococcus pyogenes*
   (b) *Streptococcus pneumoniae*
   (c) *Staphylococcus aureus*
   (d) *Neisseria gonorrhoeae.*
4. Most common bacterium causing otitis media (middle ear infection)is
   (a) *Streptococcus pyogenes*
   (b) *Moraxella catarrhalis*
   (c) *Streptococcus pneumoniae*
   (d) *Staphylococcus aureus.*

ANSWERS TO MCQs

1. (c) 2. (a) 3. (b) 4. (c).

29

Enterococcus: A Gram-positive Gastrointestinal Diplococcus (Fecal streptococci)

Opportunistic Urinary, Wound and Surgical nosocomial infections

Members of the genus *Enterococcus* (from Greek *entero* – intestine and kokkoc, *coccus* – granule) were earlier classified as group *D Steptococcus* until 1984, when genomic DNA analysis indicated a separate genus, *Enterococcus* by **Schleifer** and **Kilppër-Bälz** under the Family Enterococcaceae (Lactobacillales).

SYSTEMATIC POSITION

Domain	:	Bacteria
Division	:	Firmicutes
Class	:	Bacilli
Order	:	Lactobacillales
Family	:	Enterococcaceae
Genus	:	*Enterococcus*

There are over 20 species in this genus. The members are facultative anaerobic, alpha or non-haemolytic, Gram-positive cocci that often occur in pairs (diplococci) or short chains (Fig. 29.1) and are tolerant to a wide range of environmental conditions: extreme temperature (10–45°C), pH (4.5–10.0) and high sodium chlroide concentrations.

Enterococci, part of normal intestinal microbiota, are found in soil and water. Clinically important species belong to *E. faecalis* (90–95%) and *E. faecium* (5–10%).

Enterococci are most emerging as serious nosocomial opportunists due to the rising incidence of multi-drug-resistant strains and the ease with which they are transferred from person to person. Enterococcal isolates with reduced susceptibility to the antibiotic vancomycin can be categorized as *van A*, *van B* and *van C*, the first two are more resistant. Major diseases caused by them are urinary tract infections, endocarditis, and severe septicaemia after surgery and in the immunocompromised patients.

ENTEROCOCCUS FAECALIS

Enterococcus faecalis (formerly called *Streptococcus faecalis*) is a Gram-positive, commensal bacterium inhabiting the gastrointestinal tract of healthy humans and other mammals. However, it can cause life-threating nosocomial infections. It has been frequently found in reinfected, root-canal treated teeth. Resistance to vancomycin in *E. faecalis* is becoming more common.

CHARACTERISTICS

Gram-positive cocci often in pairs and short chains, more ovate appearance than the streptococci (Fig. 29.1).

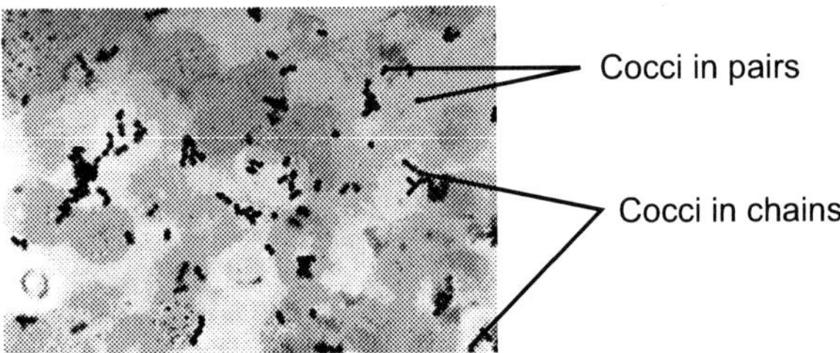

Fig. 29.1 ***Enterococcus faecalis.*** Gram-positive cocci in pairs and short chains from blood culture.

On blood agar after 24 hours of incubation at 35°C, colonies are nonhaemolytic, flat, grey, smooth with translucent edge, 1–2 mm in diameter (Fig. 29.2). Characteristically, they are able to grow in 6.5% NaCl (i.e., salt tolerant), at 45°C (heat tolerant), bile esculin positive, catalase-negative, capable of aerobic and anaerobic respiration.

DISEASES

Major diseases caused are urinary tract infections, endocarditis, septicaemia, meningitis, peridontitis and wound infection. A plasmid-encoded haemolysin, called the cytolysin plays an important role in pathogenesis. Role of toxins and other virulence factors have not been demonstrated.

Fig. 29.2 ***Enterococcus faecalis.*** Colonies on blood agar are nonhaemolytic, flat, grey each with a smooth, translucent edge.

SYMPTOMS

Symptoms depend on the type of infection and include: fever, chills, fatigue, headache, abdominal pain, pain or burning during urination, nausea, vomiting, diarrhoea, fast breathing or shortness of breath, stiff neck and swollen, red tender and bleeding gums.

TRANSMISSION

Most infections are thought to be endogenously acquired, but cross-infection may occur in hospitalized patients, especially through faecal contaminated hands (transferred to food or onto surfaces, e.g., doorknobs, telephones, computer keyboards, taps) and other equipment.

TREATMENT

Ampicillin is the preferred antibiotic used to treat *E. faecalis* infections.

For vancomycin resistant (VRE) strains, linezolid or daptomycin are treatment options.

Combination of antibiotics—ampicillin or vancomycin plus gentamicin or streptomycin are used to treat severe infections, such as endocarditis or meningitis.

PREVENTION

The preventing measures include: thorough handwashing with soap and water after using washroom, before preparing or eating food; avoid sharing personal items with patients; wiping TV remotes, doorknobs, telephones with antibacterial disinfectant; disinfection of medical devices (thermometers, blood pressure cuffs, catheters, DVs). Use of prophylactic antibiotics to prevent endocarditis, before dentistry or surgery on the gut or urinary tract.

KEY POINTS

- Enterococci are Gram-positive, catalase-negative, alpha or no haemolytic cocci often occur in pairs and small chains.
- *Enterococcus faecalis* (*Streptococcus faecalis*), normal commensal of intestine, causes opportunistic urinary, wound and surgical infections
- Hand hygiene plays an important role to prevent *E. faecalis* infections.

IMPORTANT QUESTION

1. Write briefly about enterococci or faecal streptococci.

MULTIPLE-CHOICE QUESTIONS

1. Gram-positive, salt tolerant cocci that occur in pairs or short chains and produce alpha or no haemolytic colonies on blood agar are most likely:
   (a) *Streptococcus algalactiae*
   (b) *Streptococcus pyogenes*
   (c) *Enterococcus faecalis*
   (d) *Streptococcus pneumoniae.*
2. Which of the following taxa was formerly classified in the genus *Streptococcus*?
   (a) *Escherichia* (b) *Staphylococcus*
   (c) *Neisseria* (d) *Enterococcus.*
3. Which of the following belongs to faecal streptococci?
   (a) *Escherichia* (b) *Enterococcus*
   (c) *Streptococcus* (d) *Staphylococcus.*

ANSWERS TO MCQs

1. (c) 2. (d) 3. (b).

30

Neisseria: A Gram-negative Coffee-bean Shaped Diplococcus

Meningitis; Gonorrhoea; Conjunctivitis

The genus *Neisseria* (Fig. 30.1) named after its discoverer **Albert Neisser**, a German bacteriologist, is a Gram-negative bacterium that produces characteristic kidney bean-shaped diplococci formed inside polymorphonuclear leukocytes.

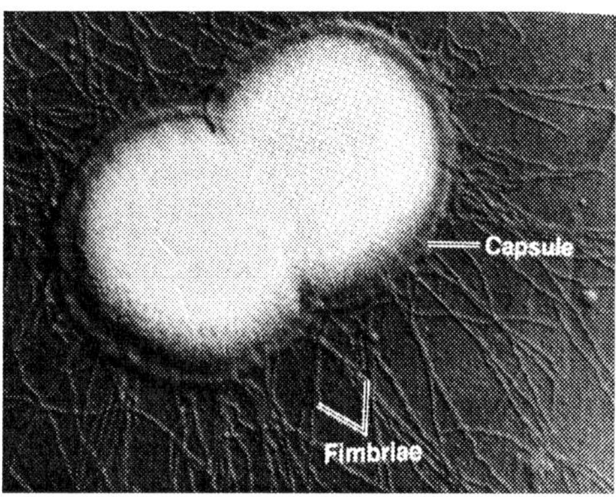

Fig. 30.1 ***Neisseria.*** Gram-negative capsulated cocci in paired arrangement (called diplococci) with fimbriae (SEM).

Neisseria contains 25 species classified in the family Neisseriaceae among the Proteobacteria, a large group of Gram-negative bacteria. These normally colonize the mucous membranes of mammals. Of the 11 species that colonize humans, only two are pathogens:

- *Neisseria meningitidis* (meningitis, septicaemia).
- *N. gonorrhoeae* (gonorrhoea, conjunctivitis in the newborn and vulvovaginitis in young girls).

SYSTEMATIC POSITION

Domain	:	Bacteria
Phylum	:	Proteobacteria
Class	:	Betaproteobacteria
Order	:	Neisseriales
Family	:	Neisseriaceae
Genus	:	*Neisseria*

NEISSERIA MENINGITIDIS

Neisseria meningitidis, often called **meningococcus**, is an aerobic, Gram-negative, kidney or coffee-bean shaped diplococcus with a polysaccharide capsule that is important to its virulence.

The bacterium was first of all observed in the cerebrospinal fluid (CSF) in 1884 followed by its isolation in 1887 from the CSF and named as *Diplococcus intracellularis meningitidis* by **Anton Weichselbaum.**

MORPHOLOGY

Meningococci are Gram-negative, oval or spherical (0.6–1.0 μm), arranged in pairs (hence diplococci), typically kidney bean-shaped owing to the flattened side where the two cocci appear to touch (Fig. 30.2).

Cocci are capsulated as demonstrated by Quellung reaction.

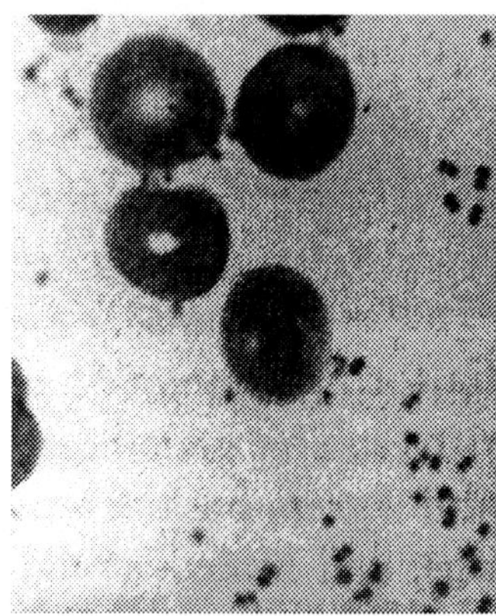

Fig. 30.2 ***Neisseria menigitidis.*** Kidney bean-shaped, Gram-negative diplococci from blood culture.

CULTURAL CHARACTERISTICS

It is a fastidious aerobic bacterium which grows best at 35–37°C with 5% CO_2 (or in candle jar) between pH 7.0 and 7.4. Blood agar, chocolate agar, Mueller-Hinton starch casein hydrolysate agar (without the addition of blood or serum) are used for its culturing.

On blood agar, the colonies are grey and unpigmented, round, smooth, moist, glistening and convex with a clearly defined edge at 35–37°C after 18–24 hours. It is a very delicate organism that dies within a few days at room temperature. Death results within 5 minutes at 55°C.

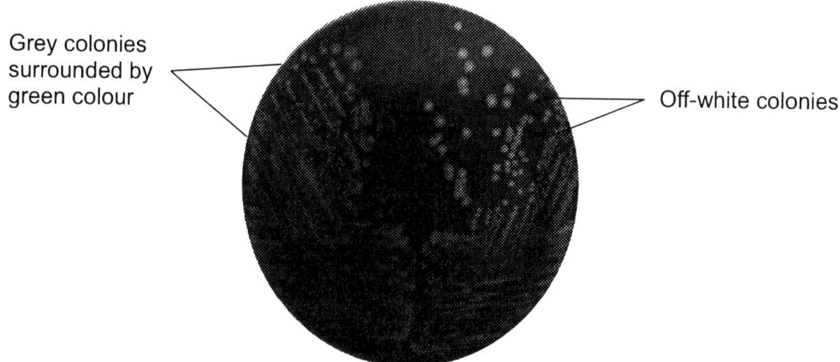

Fig. 30.3 Colonies of *Neisseria meningitidis and N. gonorrhoeae.* On chocolate agar, *N. meningitidis* grows as a grey colony surrounded by green colour (left) while *N. gonorrhoeae* produces an off-white colony with no discolouration of the agar (right).

BIOCHEMICAL REACTIONS

- Oxidase and catalase-positive
- Ferments carbohydrates–maltose, sucrose and glucose with the production of acid.

ANTIGENIC CLASSIFICATION

Based on the antigenic structure of the polysaccharide capsule, 13 subtypes in *N. meningitidis* have been identified. Of these, six—A, B, C, W135, *X* and *Y* serotypes are responsible for most meningococcal infections worldwide. Serotype A is most prevalent in Asia and Africa.

DISEASES

Meningococcus causes **meningococcal meningitis**, a common disease in children and teens; **meningococcal septicaemia**, a life threatning sepsis; and **urethritis** in men.

Meningococcal meningitis is a global problem. WHO estimates that annually about 1.2 million cases and 1,35,000 deaths occur worldwide.

VIRULENCE FACTORS

- **Lipooligosaccharide (LOS),** a component of the outer membrane of the bacterium, acts as an endotoxin and is responsible for septic shock and haemorrhage due to the destruction of red blood cells.
- **Polysaccharide capsule** which prevents host phagocytosis and aids in invasion of the host immune response.
- **Fimbriae**, mediate attachment of the bacterium to the epithelial cells of the nasopharynx.
- IgA protease, an enzyme, that allows the bacteria to evade the humoral immune system.

TRANSMISSION

Meningococcus is frequently present in the nose and throat (nasopharynx) of carriers without showing symptoms which act as reservior of infection. It is spread through saliva and other respiratory secretions during coughing, sneezing, kissing and chewing of toys. Inhalation of respiratory droplets from a carrier or close contact with a carrier can transmit the bacteria.

In susceptible individuals, the pathogen invades the blood stream causing systemic infection, sepsis, disseminated intravascular coagulation, breakdown of circulation and septic shock.

The incubation period is short, from 2 to 10 days.

SYMPTOMS

The symptoms of meningococcal meningitis are mostly caused by an endotoxin that is produced very rapidly and is capable of death within just a few hours.

The most distinguishing feature is a rash that does not fade when pressed.

DEVELOPMENT OF THE DISEASE

Meningococcal meningitis reveals three steps:

It typically begins with a **throat infection**, leading to **meningococcal bacteremia** (also called **meningococcaemia**, bloodstream invasion) and eventually **meningitis**.

It usually occurs in children under 2 years. Significant number of these children have residual damage, such as **deafness**.

Death can occur within a few hours after the onset of fever, without chemotherapy, mortality rates approach 80%.

LABORATORY DIAGNOSIS

Meningococcal infections are diagnosed:

- Presence of Gram-negative diplococci in centrifuged sample of CSF and sometimes inside the white blood cells, on microscopic examination.
- Colonial characteristic by growing on chocolate agar plate and Thayer-Martin agar from sterile body fluid (CSF or blood).
- Oxidase and catalase positive test.
- Positive sugar (maltose and sucrose) utilization test.
- Serogrouping (to determine subgroups) by slide agglutination with hyperimmune sera.
- PCR tests to identify on molecular basis.

TREATMENT

- **Penicillin is the drug of choice**, a single dose of intramuscular antibiotic is to be given immediately after diagnosis confirmation.
- Cephalosporin (e.g., cefotaxime, ceftriaxone) is used for patients allergic to penicillin.

PROPHYLAXIS (PREVENTIVE MEASURES)

Chemoprophylaxis: The agent of choice is usually oral rifampicin for a few days for adolescents and for those who had direct exposure to the patient through kissing, sharing utensils or mouth-to-mouth resuscitation.

Immunoprophylaxis

- A meningococcal polysaccharide vaccine (MPSV4) is used for people above 55 years.
- Two meningococcal conjugate vaccines (MCV4) are the preferred vaccines for people 2 through 55 years of age.
- A combination vaccine, **menhibrix**, approved in 2012, to prevent disease caused by *N. meningitidis* subgroups C and Y and *Haemophilus influenzae* type b (Hib) for infants (6 weeks to 18 months old).
- **Trumenba**, first vaccine against serogroup B, for use in 10 to 25 years old persons, has been approved for use in Oct, 2014.

NEISSERIA GONORRHOEAE

Neisseria gonorrhoeae (syn. *Gonococcus neisseri*), commonly known as **gonococcus,** is an aerobic, Gram-negative diplococcus that causes gonorrhoea, a sexually transmitted infection (STI).

N. gonorrhoeae is named for **Albert Neisser,** who isolated it in 1878 as the causative agent of the disease gonorrhoea (from the Greek words *gonos* means seed + *rhoia* means flow, i.e., flow of seed, referring to the condition in which white discharge flows from the penis without erection.

Gonorrhoea, a very common STI, with more than 10 million cases recorded per year in India alone, may lead to infertility in males, if untreated.

MORPHOLOGY

The cocci are Gram-negative, spherical (0.6–1 μm), noncapsulated, coffee-bean shaped diplococci, found predominantly in polymorphonuclear leukocytes in pus cells (Fig. 30.4).

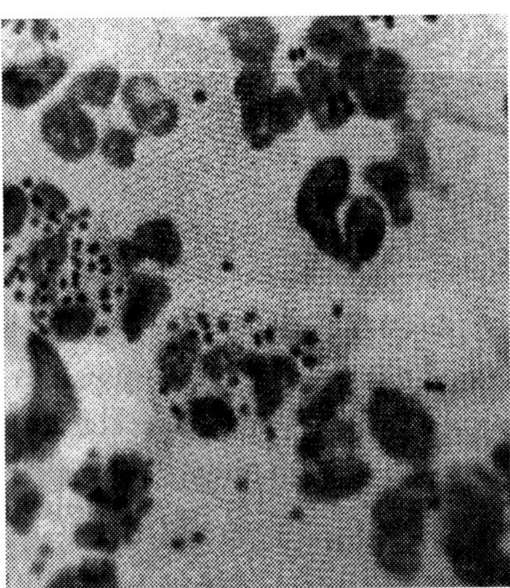

Fig. 30.4 ***Neisseria gonorrhoeae.*** Urethral smear showing intracellular Gram-negative, kidney bean-shaped diplococci.

CULTURE CHARACTERISTICS

N. gonorrhoeae requires enriched media such as chocolate agar. Best growth occurs at 37°C and pH 7.4. It produces an off-white colony with no discolouration of the agar (in contrast to *N. meningitidis* grows as a grey colony and imparts a green colour to the agar immediately surrounding the colony) (Fig. 30.3).

BIOCHEMICAL CHARACTERISTICS

- Oxidase-positive
- Ferments only glucose sugar (and not maltose)
- Positive superoxal test—used to differentiate from other *Neisseria* spp. This test is similar to the catalase test except that it is performed with 30% H_2O_2 rather than the standard 3%.

DISEASES

- Gonorrhoea (especially gonococcal urethritis)
- Disseminated gonococcal diseases (e.g., gonorrhoeal meningitis)
- Gonococcal opthalmia neonatorum.

GONORRHOEA

Gonorrhoea, also known as **"the clap"**, is a sexually transmitted disease (STD) that usually spreads by having vaginal, oral, or anal sex. Globally, there are an estimated 78 million new cases of gonorrhoea diagnosed each year.

SYMPTOMS

N. gonorrhoeae attaches the mucosal cells of the oral-pharyngeal area, genitals, eye and rectum by means of fimbriae. The bacteria start multiplication in warm-moist areas of the body. Symptoms appear within 1 to 14 days of infection. Infection can come from any type of sex with an infected partner. In addition, infection can come through contact with the mouth, throat, eyes, urethera, vagina, penis, or anus.

In males, the infection extends along the urethera to the prostate, seminal vesicles and epidymis. The primary symptom of genitourinary infection is **urethritis**-burning with painful urination **(*dysuria*)**, increased urge to urinate, pus containing discharge, and **epididymitis** (an inflammation of the epididymis (coiled tube) at the back of the testicle that stores and carries sperms).

Infection may spread to prostate resulting in **prostatitis** sometimes leading to prostate cancer.

In women, the primary symptoms of genitourinary are increased greenish yellow or whitish discharge from the vagina, burning when urinating, pain and spotting after intercourse and swelling of the vulva **(vulvitis)**. Untreated infection leads to **pelvic inflammatory disease** (PID) in 10–20% of females, if the infection spreads into the pelvic peritoneum.

Infected throat reveals swollen glands and burning in the throat (**pharyngitis**) (oral sex) and infection of the anus/rectum **(proctitis)** (anal sex).

Specific arthritis of joints (gonorrhoeal arthritis) can be caused in both sexes if the infection is not treated well in time.

LABORATORY DIAGNOSIS

Gonorrhoea is diagnosed by **Gram-staining** of smear prepared from the discharge (urethera, cervix), **culturing** of the pathogen on chocolate agar at 35–37°C under 5–10% CO_2, by **ELISA** or nucleic acid amplification.

PREVENTION

Latex barriers such as condoms or dental dams should be used during intercourse and during oral and anal sex, as well.

TREATMENT

The current treatment recommended by CDC is a dual antibiotic therapy that includes: an injected single dose of ceftriaxoze along with oral administration of azithromycin because of the development of penicillin-resistant gonococcus strains, hence penicillin is no longer the antibiotic of choice.

GONOCOCCAL OPHTHALMIA NEONATORUM

Ophthalmia neonatorum (or **neonatal conjunctivitis**), a nonveneral infection of the eye caused by gonococcus, is acquired by infants during the passage through the birth canal of an infected mother. Conjunctivitis occurs within 2–5 days after birth which is severe. The eye infection can lead to corneal scarring or perforation, ultimately resulting in blindness.

In the newborn, it can be prevented by the application of erythromycin gel to the eyes at birth as a public health measure.

KEY POINTS

- *Neisseria,* named after Albert Neisser, is an aerobic, Gram-negative bacterium that produces characteristic coffee-bean shaped diplococci that normally colonize mucous membranes of many mammals.

- *Neisseria meningitidis* (commonly called meningococcus) is the cause of meningococcal meningitis, a serious disease in children and teens.
- *Neisseria gonorrhoeae* (gonococcus) causes gonorrhoea a STD and ophthalmia neonatorum, an eye infection.

IMPORTANT QUESTIONS

1. Write brief notes on:
   (a) Laboratory diagnosis and prevention of meningococcal infections.
   (b) Gonorrhoea.
   (c) Meningococcal meningitis.

MULTIPLE-CHOICE QUESTIONS

1. All are true for *Neisseria* EXCEPT:
   (a) Normally colonizes the mucous membranes of mammals
   (b) Was discovered as a causative agent of gonorrhoea
   (c) Gram-positive coccus
   (d) Diplococci resembling coffee beans.
2. *Neisseria meningitidis* is a serious cause of bacterial infection which
   (a) Can result in septicaemia
   (b) Can cause pneumonia
   (c) Is due to excessive activation of T lymphocytes
   (d) Is treated with anti-TNF monoclonal antibodies.
3. Untreated gonorrhoea leads to the diseases, _______in men and ______ in women.
   (a) AIDS/Herpes
   (b) Testicular cancer/Vaginal cancer
   (c) Epididymitis/Pelvic inflammatory disease (PID)
   (d) PID/Chlamydia.
4. Gonorrhoea, a sexually transmitted disease, is caused by
   (a) Kissing many different people
   (b) Dirty toilet seat
   (c) Drinking after too many people
   (d) None of the above.

5. The gonorrhoea is treated with:
  (a) Antibiotics
  (b) Alcoholic beverages
  (c) Surgery
  (d) Hands on cleaning by a doctor.

6. *Neisseria gonorrhoeae* can be differentiated from other species of *Neisseria* by:
  (a) Oxidase test
  (b) Catalase test
  (c) Superoxal test
  (d) None of the above.

ANSWERS TO MCQS

1. (c) 2. (a) 3. (c) 4. (d) 5. (a)
6. (c).

31

Bacillus: An Aerobic Endospore-forming Gram-positive Bacillus

Anthrax; Food poisoning

GRAM-POSITIVE BACILLI OF MEDICAL IMPORTANCE

Bacilli (sing. **bacillus**) (from Latin *bacillus* = rod) refers to bacteria that are rod-shaped. Gram-positive bacilli accounts for a number of significant infectious diseases such as bubonic plague, typhoid fever, tetanus and leprosy.

Gram-positive bacilli can be divided into four general groups:

- **Endospore-forming bacilli**
    - Aerobic : *Bacillus*
    - Anaerobic : *Clostridium*
- **Non-endospore forming bacilli**
    - Regular in morphology: *Listeria, Erysipelothrix*
    - Irregular in morphology:
        - Aerobic : *Corynebacterium*
        - Anaerobic : *Propionibacterium*
- **Acid-fast bacilli**
    - *Mycobacterium*
    - *Nocardia*
- **Non-acid-fast branching filamentous bacilli**
    - Actinomycetes

BACILLUS

The genus *Bacillus* is a Gram-positive aerobic, spore-forming bacillus, present in chains that can grow both aerobically and anaerobically. **Christian Gottfried Ehrenberg** in 1835 named this genus and currently contains 216 ubiquitous species which are harmless saprobes widely distributed in soil, dust and water, and classified as follows:

SYSTEMATIC POSITION

Domain	:	Bacteria
Phylum	:	Firmicutes
Class	:	Bacilli
Order	:	Bacillales
Family	:	Bacillaceae
Genus	:	*Bacillus*

Two clinically signficant species are:

B. anthracis – the cause of anthrax

B. cereus – the cause of food poisoning

Bacillus species are also an important source of antibiotics.

BACILLUS ANTHRACIS

Bacillus anthracis is an aerobic, non-motile, Gram-positive, endospore forming, rod-shaped bacterium that causes anthrax in humans and animals. The endospores survive for 50 years in soil. The name is derived from the Greek word for coal, *B. anthrakis,* because of its ability to cause black, coal-like cutaneous eschars. It was the first bacterium to be used to prove that bacteria caused diseases, when **Robert Koch** in 1877 produced anthrax spores and infected them into animals.

MORPHOLOGICAL CHARACTERISTICS

The bacilli are large (4 – 10 µm × 1 – 1.5 µm), Gram-positive, spore-forming, encapsulated occurring in long chains. The endospores are oval, central in position, without causing significant swelling (bulging) of the cells.

In tissues, the cells are found singly, in pairs or in short chains lacking endospores, the entire chain surrounded by a polypeptide capsule. Spores are formed only after the organism is shed from the body (Fig. 31.1).

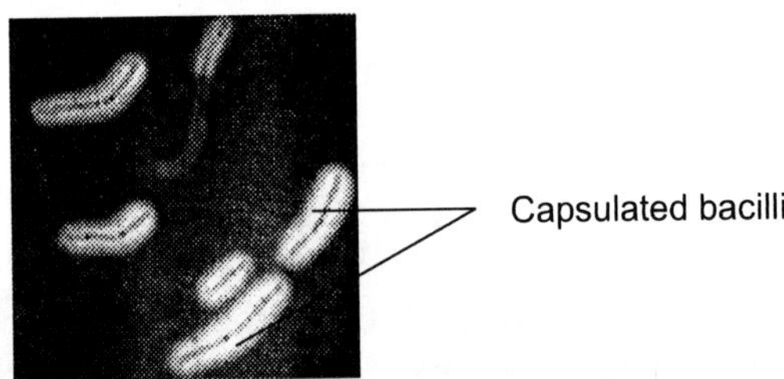

Fig. 31.1 Negative stain (India ink stain) of *Bacillus anthracis.* Polypeptide encapsulated bacilli as seen in clinical specimens.

GROWTH CHARACTERISTICS

B. anthracis is a strong aerobic bacterium that can be grown on an ordinary nutrient medium at 35°C (12–45°C) under aerobic conditions.

After overnight incubation at 35°C on nutrient agar, colonies are 2-3 mm in diameter, with a wavy margin and small projections resembling locks of matted hair, so called **medusa head appearance** (Fig. 31.2).

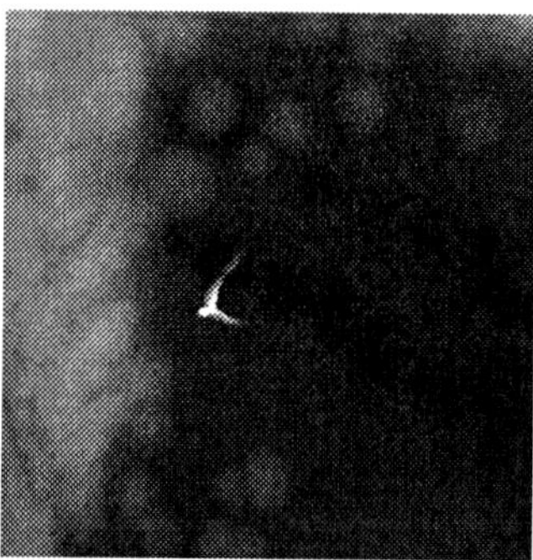

Fig. 31.2 Bacillus anthracis on blood agar. After overnight incubation at 35°C, colonies measure 2 to 5 mm in diameter and appear with curled hair projections resembling a *medusa head.* These are tenacious and behave like beaten egg with white when lifted with an inoculating loop.

ENDOSPORES AND RESISTANCE

The endospores are higly resistant, surviving extemes of temperature (resist dry heat at 140°C for 1 to 3 hours, boiling or steam at 100°C for 5–10 minutes), low-nutrient environments, drying and harsh chemical disinfectants (including 95% ethanol). Because of these attributes, the endospores are extraordinarily well-suited to use (both in powder and aerosol form) as **biological weapons**.

An endospore is actually a dehydrated cell with thick walls and additional layers (e.g., a **thin outer endospore coat**, a **thick spore cortex**, and an **inner spore membrane**) surrounding the endospore core which contains **dipicolinic acid (DPA)**.

Endospores are never found in tissues, but appear when the bacterium is shed or grown on culture media; they stain only with special spore staining technique (flooding a heat-fixed smear with 10% aqueous malachite green for up to 45 minutes, followed by washing with water and counter-staining with aqueous safranin for 30 seconds (spores staining green and vegetative cells pinkish red).

VIRULENCE FACTORS

Two principal virulence factors involved in lethality of anthrax are:

- **Anthrax toxin** (tripartite protein toxin): it is a mixture of three protein components:
  - (i) Protective antigen (PA)
  - (ii) Edema factor (EF)
  - (iii) Lethal factor (LF)

This toxin complex increases vascular permeability which leads to shock.

- **Antiphagocytic capsule** (Fig. 31.1)—which is unusual in being a polypeptide of D-glutamic acid (i.e., polyglutamic acid).

ANTHRAX

Anthrax caused by *Bacillus anthracis*, a serious illness, is an extremely rare disease (fewer than 5 thousand cases per year in India). The name ***anthrax*** is derived from the Greek word for coal. It usually affects farm animals like cows and sheep. People at risk are those who handle animals, hides, wool, and other animal products, travellers, postal workers and military personnel. Symptoms begin between one and two months after the infection is contracted. It spreads by contact with the bacterium's endospores which often appear in infectious animal products. Contact is by breathing, eating or through an area of broken skin. It does not thoroughly spread directly between people. It affects humans in four forms:

- Cutaneous anthrax
- Gastrointestinal anthrax
- Inhalational (lung) anthrax
- Injection.

CUTANEOUS ANTHRAX

The swelling and formation of a black scab that forms around the point of infection is a characteristic of anthrax skin lesion (Fig. 31.3). It results from contact with material containing endospores. Skin infections represent more than 95% of the anthrax. If the bacteria enter the bloodstream, mortality without antibiotic treatmant can reach 24%.

GASTROINTESTINAL ANTHRAX

It is caused by ingestion of undercooked food containing endospores. Symptoms include: nausea, vomiting, bloody diarrhoea, abdominal pain, ulcerative lesions in intestine, in addition to mouth and throat. The risk of death is from 25–75%.

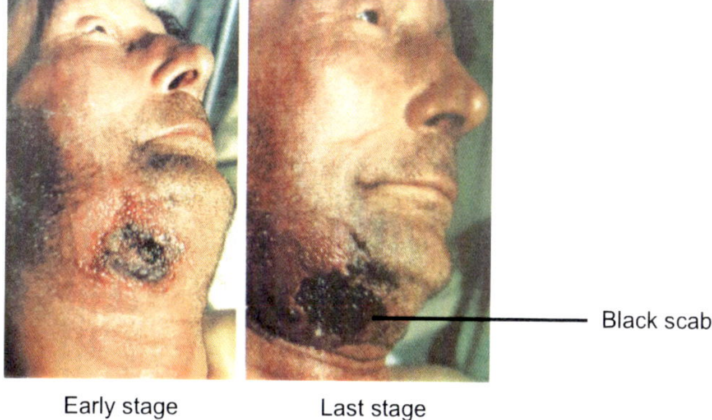

Fig. 31.3 **Cutaneous anthrax** by ***Bacillus anthracis.*** The swelling and formation of a black scab (eschar) that forms around the point of skin infection is a characteristic of cutaneous anthrax (basis for the derivation of the name *anthrax* for coal).

PULMONARY (INHALATIONAL) ANTHRAX

It occurs due to inhalation of dust containing endospores from infected wool and is common in wool factory workers. The disease is commonly called **wool-sorters** disease. As the bacteria enter the bloodstream and proliferate, the illness progresses in 2 or 3 days into septic shock leading to death of the patient within 24 to 36 hours. The mortality rate is high (50–80%), even with treatment.

DIAGNOSIS

- *Gram-strain*—Gram-positive bacilli in long chains.
- *Endospore stain*—A green, centrally located endospore in pinkish red cells.
- *Characterisitic colonies*—Medusa head appearance.
- *Non-haemolytic on horse blood agar.*
- *Encapsulated bacilli* in clinical specimens.
- *Direct fluorescent antibody test (DFA).*
- Rapid diagnostic technique—*polymerase chain reaction* (PCR).

TREATMENT

Ciprofloxacin is the antibiotic of choice. Other antibiotics that can be used are: Doxycycline, penicillin, erythromycin and chloramphenical.

PREVENTION

- Formalin disinfection of hides.
- Decontamination of contaminated articles by boiling in water for 30 minutes.
- Burning clothing is an effective method to destroy spores.
- Immunization of veterinarnarians and laboraory workers at risk.

BACILLUS CEREUS AND FOOD-BORNE ILLNESS

Bacillus cereus (Fig. 31.4) is a Gram-positive, motile, spore-producing, non-encapsulated, rod-shaped, beta-hemolytic, aerobic-to-facultatively anaerobic bacterium, commonly found in soil and food. Some strains can cause two different forms of food-associated illness: Emetic and diarrhoeal, while other strains can be beneficial as probiotics for animals. It grows on a simple agar medium (e.g., nutrient agar) producing very large, β-haemolytic, ground-glass colonies at 37°C (Fig. 31.5).

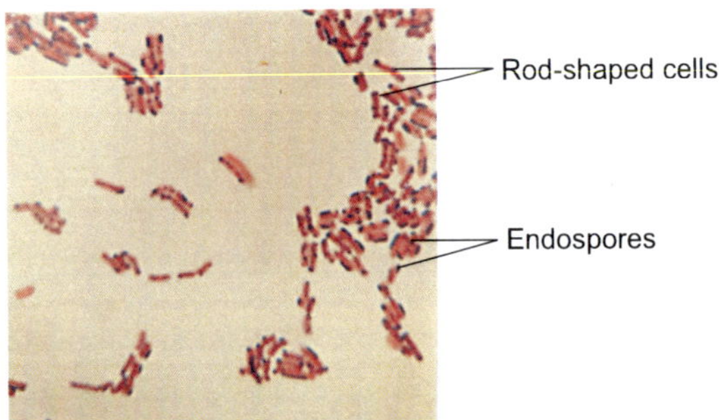

Fig. 31.4 Gram stain of *Bacillus cereus*. Gram-positive (violet coloured) rod-shaped cells appear in a palisade manner (rathan than in long chains as in *B. anthracis*).

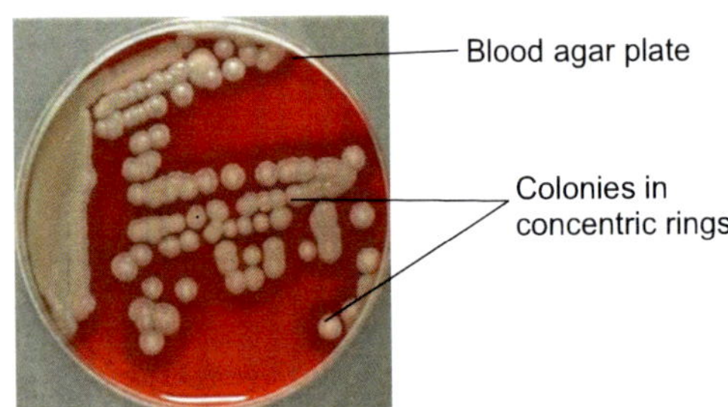

Fig. 31.5 *Bacillus cereus* on blood agar. The colonies are large (approximately 7 mm in diameter), beta-haemolytic, circular, greenish, and with a ground-glass appearance.

EMETIC (VOMITING) SYNDROME

This syndrome is commonly caused by fried rice cooked for a time and temperature insufficient to kill endospores present and later imporperly referigerted. The surviving endospores germinate at room temperature (between 10°C and 50°C) and produce heat-stable enterotoxin, ***cereulide*** that can withstands temperature of 121°C (= 250°F) for 90 minutes, hence is not destroyed by heating later (e.g., fried rice). Consumption of emetic toxin containing fried rice leads to nausea and vomiting within 1 to 5 hours (hence it is a type of food-borne intoxication). The toxin is resistant to heat, proteolysis and acid conditions.

DIARRHOEAL SYNDROME

It is also called the long-incubation form of ***B. cereus*** **food poisoning** since the onset of symptoms occurs after 8-16 hour of consumption of foods like cereal dishes that contain corn and cornstarch, mashed potatoes, minced meat, sauces, soups or other foods that have been set out for long at room temperature. Bacteria are ingested with the food, heat-labile enterotoxin (that can be inactivated after heating at 56°C for 5 minutes) is produced in the gut resulting in watery diarrhoea and cramp-like gastrointestinal pain. The enterotoxin involved is composed of three toxins: **haemolysin BL, nonhaemolytic enterotoxin** and **cytotoxin K**.

TREATMENT AND PREVENTION

- Both the emetic and diarrhoeal syndroms are shortlived and self-limiting, hence antibiotic treatment is not required.
- Get rest and drink plenty of fluids to prevent dehydration.
- Hygienic preparation and proper storage of food.
- Storing cooked food in a wide shallow container and its refrigeration as soon as possible.
- Referigerated foods should be reheated thorough before serving.
- For cooked foods to be stored longer than two hours at room temperature, keep hot foods hot above 50°C (122°F) and cold foods cold below 10°C (50°F).

KEY POINTS

- *Bacillus anthracis* is an endospore-forming aerobic, non-motile, Gram-positive, encapsulated, chain forming, rod-shaped bacterium.

- Anthrax caused by *Bacillus arthracis* is a zoonosis.
- Based on the mode of infection, anthrax in humans is of three types: cutaneous (skin), intestinal and pulmonary, all the three treated with ciprofloxacin.
- *Bacillus cereus* is an endospore-forming, motile, non-capsulated Gram-positive, rod-shaped bacterium.
- *Bacillus cereus* causes two different forms of food associated illness: emetic (food intoxication) and diarrhoeal (food-borne infection) syndrome.
- Hygienic preparation and proper storage of food can prevent the *Bacillus cereus* food-borne illness.

IMPORTANT QUESTIONS

1. Write short notes on:
   (a) Anthrax
   (b) *Bacillus cereus* food associated illness.

MULTIPLE-CHOICE QUESTIONS

1. All are *true* for *Bacillus anthracis* EXCEPT:
   (a) Causes food poisioning
   (b) Medusa head appearance
   (c) Non-motile
   (d) Produces Edema and lethal factors.
2. Anthrax caused by *Bacillus anthracis* directly spreads from person to person. True or False?
3. The capsule in *B. anthracis* is unusual because it is a polypeptide of D-glutamic acid. True or False?
4. Which of the following is a non-endospore-forming bacillus?
   (a) *Bacillus cereus* (b) *Bacillus anthracis*
   (c) *Clostridium* (d) *Lactobacillus*.

ANSWERS TO MCQs

1. (a) 2. False 3. True 4. (d).

- *Coliforms:* Enteric bacteria that ferment lactose rapidly i.e., within 48 hours – *Escherichia, Klebsiella, Enterobacter, Hafnia, Serratia* and *Citrobacter.*
- *Noncoliforms:* Normal gut flora that lack the ability to ferment lactose – *Proteus, Morganella, Providencia* and *Edwardsiella.*

Based on their biochemical characteristics, *Enterobacteriaceae* are divided into three tribes:

I. ***Escherichiae:***

Examples: *Escherichia*
Edwardsiella
Citrobacter
Salmonella
Shigella

II. ***Klebsiellae:***

Examples: *Klebsiella*
Enterobacter
Hafnia
Serratia

III. ***Proteae:***

Examples: *Proteus*
Morganella
Providencia

KEY POINTS

- Gram-negative bacilli are pink stained, non-sporing, rod-shaped bacteria with a thin peptidoglycan cell wall.
- Family *Enterobacteriaceae* contains the most important Gram-negative bacilli of medical significance.

IMPORTANT QUESTIONS

1. Write brief notes on:
   (a) Gram-negative bacilli
   (b) Enterobacteriaceae.

MULTIPLE-CHOICE QUESTIONS

1. All are *true* for Gram-negative bacilli EXCEPT:
   (a) They are rod-shaped
   (b) Composed of thin cell wall of lipopolysaccharide

(c) They contain endospores.

(d) Pink coloured when Gram-stained.

2. All are facultative anaerobic Gram-negative bacilli of medical importance EXCEPT:

(a) *Pseudomonas* (b) *Escherichia*

(c) *Salmonella* (d) *Shigella.*

3. Which of the following is not an aerobic Gram-negative bacillus of medical significance?

(a) *Pseudomonas* (b) *Brucella*

(c) *Klebsiella* (d) *Bordetella.*

4. All are coliforms EXCEPT:

(a) *Escherichia* (b) *Proteus*

(c) *Klebsiella* (d) *Enterobacter.*

ANSWERS TO MCQs

1. (c) 2. (a) 3. (c) 4. (b).

34

Escherichia: A Gram-negative Non-endosporic Bacillus

UTI; Diarrhoea

Escherichia is a Gram-negative, non-spore-forming, facultatively anaerobic, rod-shaped, motile bacterium belonging to the family *Enterobacteriaceae*. The genus is named after the German-Austrian physician **Theodor Escherich**, the discoverer of the type species of the genus—*Bacillus coli commune* (later named as *Escherichia coli*).

The genus includes eight species found in diverse habitats such as fresh water, soil, faecal matter, animal and human sources. *E. coli* is the most important and best known species of *Escherichia*. It is a faecal, food and water-borne bacterium.

ESCHERICHIA COLI

The species is named *Bacterium coli* (later *Escherichia coli*) because of its occurrence in the colon by **Escherich** who was the first to isolate this organism in 1885 from the faeces of healthy humans.

Escherichia coli is by far the most common and best known coliform. *E. coli* is classified into 150–220 serotypes based on somatic (O), capsular (K_1), flagellar (H) and fimbrial (F) antigens. It occurs in faecally contaminated environments (e.g., water, sediment and mud) and is prevalent in the large intestine of human beings and other warm blooded animals. The average human contains between 0.1 and 1% of *E. coli* in their intestines. It is excreted in faeces and grows massively in it for 3 days under aerobic conditions, however, remains viable in the faecal polluted water for several days, therefore, *E. coli* is used as an **indicater organism** to test environmental samples for faecal contamination. Detection of *E. coli* in drinking water is an indication of contamination with faeces.

Most strains of *E. coli* are harmless and are part of the normal microbiota of the gut benefitting their hosts by producing vitamin K2, and preventing colonization of the intestine with pathogenic bacteria, having a symbiotic relationship.

CLINICAL INFECTIONS

Most *E. coli* strains are harmless, but virulent strains can cause the following clinical syndromes:

- Urinary tract infection (UTI)
- Gasteroenterititis (diarrhoea)
- Neonatal meningitis
- Haemorrhagic colitis
- Septicaemia
- Nosocomial pneumonia

E. coli is the best known coliform and most frequently isolated bacterial species in the clinical microbiology laboratory.

MORPHOLOGY AND GRAM-REACTION

It is a Gram-negative (pink coloured), non-endosporic, straight-rod, 1–3 μm × 0.4–0.7 μm, arranged singly or in pairs (Fig. 34.1). Most strains are capsulated, motile with peritrichous flagellas and have fimbriae.

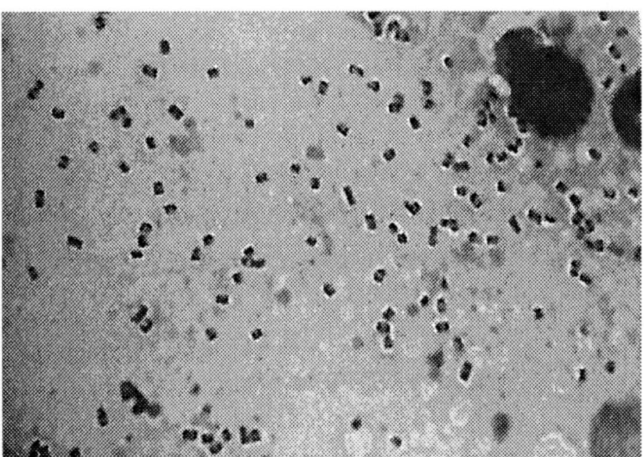

Fig. 34.1 ***Escherichia coli.*** Gram stain demonstrates safety pin shaped, pink (Gram-negative) bacilli occurring singly and in pairs.

CULTURAL CHARACTERISTICS

It is an aerobic and a facultative anaerobic bacterium that grows over a temperature range of 15–45°C (37°C optimum) and may survive 60°C for 15 minutes or 55°C for 60 minutes. *E. coli* has a rapid growth rate and a short generation or doubling time of 20 minutes at 37°C (98.6°F) i.e., at human body temperature.

On nutrient agar, the colonies are large, thick, greyish white, moist, smooth, opaque or translucent. Some strains may form **mucoid** colonies.

On MacConkey agar, the colonies are bright, pink (due to lactose fementation) dry, donut shaped and are surrounded by a dark prink area of precipitated bile salts (Fig. 34.2).

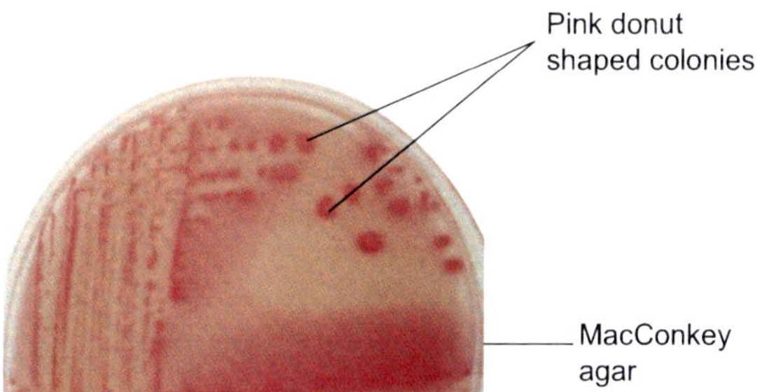

Fig. 34.2 ***Escherichia coli* on MacConkey agar.** The colonies are pink, dry, and donut shaped and are surrounded by a dark pink area of precipitated bile salts.

On blood agar, the colonies are grey, smooth and often beta-haemolytic. Aerobic growth appears within 12 to 18 hours at 35°C.

BIOCHEMICAL CHARACTERISTICS USED IN DIAGNOSIS

It ferments glucose, lactose, mannitol, maltose with acid and gas production (lactose fermented rapidly), but sucrose is not fermented.

In triple sugar iron (TSI), acid and gas are produced due to the rapid fermentation of glucose and lactose.

The four characteristic biochemical reactions (IMViC) widely used to diagnose it are: Indole (I) and methyl red (MR) positive, and Voges-Proskauer (VP) and Citrate (C) negative (Fig. 34.3).

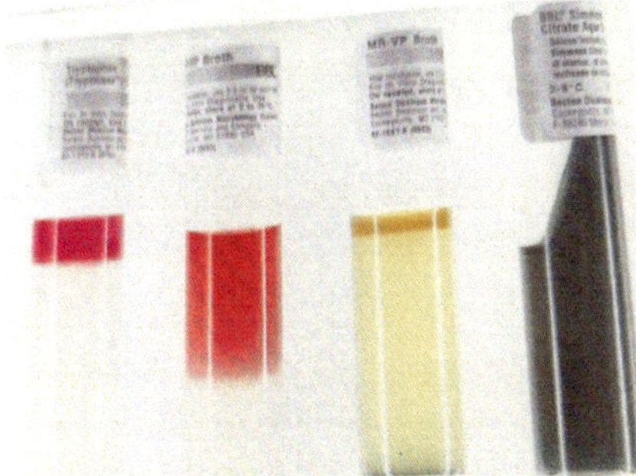

Fig. 34.3 **IMViC reactions in *Escherichia coli*.** Four characteristic reactions of *E. coli* are indole positive, methyl red positive, Voges-Proskauer negative, and citrate negative (left to right, respectively).

ANTIGENIC STRUCTURE

E. coli possesses four types of antigens:

1. **O (somatic or lipopolysaccharide) antigens:**
   There are over 175 O antigens which are heat-stable, designated as 1, 2, 3, 4, 5...
2. **H (flagellar) antigens** – 75 H antigens have been recognized which are thermolabile.
3. **K (capsular) antigens** – There are 103 K antigens which are divided into two groups: I (heat-stable), > 1,00,000 daltons (mol wt) and II (heat-labile, < 50,000 daltons).
4. **F (fimbrial) antigen**
   O, H and K antigens are used in serotyping while F antigen mediate adhesion to host cells without any role in antigenic classification.

TOXINS

Pathogenic strains of *E. coli.* produce three types of toxins:

1. **Haemolysin:** Many strains of *E. coli* play an important role in pathogensis by bringing about lysis of RBCs.
2. **Enterotoxins:** Enterotoxigenic strains of *E. coli* called **ETEC** produce two types of enterotoxins:
   - Heat-labile toxin (LT)
   - Heat-stable toxin (ST).
3. **Verocytotoxin (Shiga toxin):** *E. coli* strains (called VTEC/STEC) e.g., 0157:H7 produce either shiga toxin or shiga-like toxin (verotoxin) which are involved in food-borne illness.

URINARY TRACT INFECTIONS (UTIs)

E. coli is responsible for more than 85% of all UTIs. Worldwide, 150 million people are affected by UTIs each year. Women get UTIs up to 30 times more often than men, because the former have very short urethras. Most *E. coli* caused UTIs occur in the lower urinary tract, which includes the bladder and the urethra, causing cystitis and urethritis, respectively.

PATHOGENESIS

Pathogenic *E. coli* strains that cause UTIs often originate from the gut of the patient. Trace amounts of the faecal matter containing bacteria make their way into the urinary tract through the urethra opening, fimbriae mediating adherence to the uro-epithelial cells, and begin to multiply causing infection in an ascending manner for physiological reasons.

Sexual intercourse, improper wiping after a bowel movement, holding urine for longer duration, menopause, use of diaphragm contraceptive and condoms in brith control, diabetes, pregnancy, enlarged prostate gland, kidney stones and spinal cord injury are the factors that enhance the risk of developing a UTI.

SYMPTOMS

Common symptoms of UTI include:

- Painful and burning urination
- Strong, persistent urge to urinate
- Passing only minimal amounts of urine
- Strong-smelling, cloudy urine
- Red or pink-tinged urine due to the presence of blood
- Pain in the upper back and sides
- Fever, chills and nausea
- Pelvic pressure.

DIAGNOSIS

Diagnosis is made by microscopic examination of the clinical specimen (midstream urine) by Gram's stain method to find out the presence of pus cells, red blood cells and characteristic bacilli of *E. coli* in it, culturing of bacterium on MacConkey or other suitable media under aerobic conditions at 37°C for 18–24 hours by standard loop method (a count of $> 10^5$ per mL (CFU/mL) of urine of *E. coli* is a positive test).

TREATMENT

E. coli causing UTIs have become resistant to many of the commonly used antibiotics including ampicillin, tetracycline, ciproflaxcin and trimethoprim sulfamethoxazole (TMP–SMX).

Based on the antibiotic susceptibility testing, carbapenems class of antibiotics (e.g., imipenem, meropenem, doripenem, ertapenem) and polymyxin drugs (e.g., colistin) are considered the gold standard treatment for serious *E. coli* infection.

DIARRHOEA (DIARRHEA)

E. coli normally found in our intestine is harmless and even keep the digestive tract healthy. But some strains can cause gastrointestinal disease ranging in severity from mild, self-limiting diarrhoea to haemorrhagic colitis through consumption of contaminated food or fouled water.

The diarrhoea causing pathogenic *E. coli* strains are of five types:

- *Enteropathogenic E. coli (EPEC)* – These serotypes cause watery diarrhoea especially in infants, especially in tropical countries. Onset of disease is slow.
- *Enterotoxigenic E. coli (ETEC)* – Cause traveller's (watery) diarrhoea in areas of poor sanitation. Onset of disease is between 24 and 72 hours.
- *Enteroinvasive E.coli (EIEC)* – Cause dysentery resembling shigellosis within 24 and 72 hours of infection.
- *Verocytotoxin – producing E. coli* (VTEC) (also called shiga toxin producing *E. coli, STEC*) cause mild, watery diarrhoea to severe diarrhoea with blood in the stool (*hemorrhagic colitis*), and *hemolytic uremic syndrome* especially in children. Incubation period ranges from 24 to 72 hours.
- *Enteroaggregative E. coli (EAggEC)* – Cause chronic diarrhoeal disease in certain developing countries.

Of the various *E. coli* types, the shiga-toxin producing strain, 0157:H7, belonging to the VTEC (= STEC), is responsible for a serious food poisoning. It causes abdominal cramps, vomiting and bloody diarrhoea. It is the leading cause of acute kidney failure in children.

Infection results due to the consumption of *E. coli* contaminated undercooked ground meat, untreated (or unpasteurized) milk, and apple cider cheese, improperly washed vegetables and fruit within 2 to 5 days.

SYMPTOMS

The most common symptoms are: abdominal cramps, bloody diarrhoea, nausea, fever and constant fatigue. Some people have serious complication called hemolytic uremic syndrome, which affects the kidneys, especially in children and older people.

DIAGNOSIS

Analysis of stool sample for *E. coli* by Gram staining and culturing of the bacteria on MacConkey agar from faeces or rectal swab.

TREATMENT

Fortunately, the infection usually goes away on its own without any medication. If recovery does not happen, antibiotic therapy is needed especially in the watery traveller's diarrhoea. However, in bloody diarrhoea with fever due to shiga toxin-producing *E. coli*, antibiotics should not be given because they can actually increase the production of toxin and worsen the symptoms. It is important to rest and get plenty of fluids. When the patient starts to feel better, stick to low-fibre foods such as rice, toast, eggs and crackers. Dairy products and foods that are high in fat or fibre should be avoided.

PREVENTION

- Proper washing of hands to protect yourself and your family against *E. coli* infection, especially before preparing food, after you have used the bathroom and changed a diaper, after handling raw meat, and contact with animals.
- Cook hamburger pasties and ground beef until they're 160°F (71.1°C) inside.
- Drink only pasteurized milk, juice and cider.
- Wash fresh fruits and green leafy vegetables thoroughly.
- Holding of cooked meat between 40°F and 140°F for over 3 hours be avoided.

KEY POINTS

- *Escherichia coli* is a Gram-negative, nonspore-forming, rod-shaped, facultative aerobic bacterium.
- *E. coli* is a predominant commensal found in the intestinal tract of humans.
- Urinary tract infection and diarrhoea are the two common diseases caused by *E. coli*.
- *Escherichia coli*, the causative agent of UTI and diarrhoea, in humans has a very short generation (or doubling) time of 20 minutes (i.e., it divides in every 20 minutes).
- Serogroup 0157:H7 belonging to the VTEC (or STEC), a food-borne pathogen, is involved in haemorrhagic colitis and haemolytic uraemic syndrome.

IMPORTANT QUESTIONS

1. Write short notes on:
   (a) Diagnostic features and significance of *Escherichia coli.*
   (b) *Escherichia coli* diarrhoea.
   (c) *E. coli* urinary tract infection.

MULTIPLE-CHOICE QUESTIONS

1. The generation (or doubling) time of *Escherichia coli*, the causative agent of UTI and diarrhoea, in humans, is:
   (a) 10 minutes (b) 20 minutes
   (c) 40 minutes (d) 60 minutes.
2. Which of the following *E. coli* pathogenic group causes Traveller's diarrhoea in humans?
   (a) EHEC (b) EPEC
   (c) EIEC (d) ETEC.
3. Shigella like dysentery is caused by
   (a) EIEC (b) EPEC
   (c) ETEC (d) VTEC.
4. Significant bacteriuria represents
   (a) $> 10^2$ CFU/mL (b) $> 10^3$ CFU/mL
   (c) $> 10^4$ CFU/mL (d) $> 10^5$ CFU/mL.

ANSWERS TO MCQs

1. (b) 2. (d) 3. (a) 4. (d).

35

Klebsiella, Enterobacter, Serratia and *Citrobacter*: Coliforms other than *Escherichia*

Opportunistic pathogens: Pneumonia; Urinary tract infection; Opportunistic nosocomial infections

Klebsiella, Enterobacter, Citrobacter and *Serratia*, all members of the family *Enterobacteriaceae*, are found in the gastrointestinal tract. These belong to the coliform group of bacteria. They are aerobic or facultatively anaerobic, ferment glucose and produce catalase but not oxidase. They are commonly called **enterobacteria**. They are **opportunisitic** or **secondary pathogens** causing varied infections in hospitals, e.g., sepsis, wound infections, urinary tract infection and pneumonia.

KLEBSIELLA

Klebsiella, a member of the family *Enterobacteriaceae*, is a Gram-negative rod-shaped, non-motile and oxidase-negative, bacterium with a polysaccharide based capsule.

The genus is named after **Edwin Klebs**, a German-Swiss microbiologist. *K. pneumoniae* (also called **Friedlander's bacillus**), the type species, was first isolated from lungs in 1882 by **Carl Friedlander**, a German microbiologist and pathologist.

The genus *Klebsiella* contains 8 species which are a part of the human and animal's normal microbiota in the nose, mouth, intestine and also found in the respiratory tracts of normal individuals. *K. pneumoniae, K. oxytoca* and *K. planticoli* are of clinical significance.

KLEBSIELLA PNEUMONIAE

Klebsiella pneumoniae (originally named Friedlander's bacillus) is a Gram-negative, nonmotile, capsulated, straight rod (1-2 μm × 0.5 – 0.8 μm) occurring singly, in pairs, short chains and sometimes in clusters. Capsule appears as a clear halo in a dark background in India ink preparation.

Klebsiella grows on ordinary culture media aerobically between 15 and 40°C (37°C optimum) at neutral pH 7.0. On nutrient agar, the colonies are circular, dome shaped, greyish white, mucoid, translucent-opaque, 2-3 mm in diameter. On MacConkey agar, the colonies are 4-5 mm mucoid in appearance (due to capsule) and dark pink due to fast lactose fermentation (Figure 35.1), an important feature used to differentiate it from other bacteria present in a sample. *K. pneumoniae* can cause a primary community acquired pneumonia, hospital associated urinary tract infection, bacteremia and meningitis.

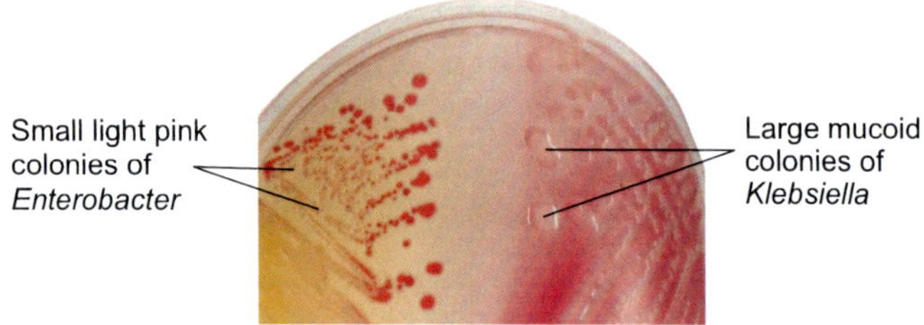

Fig. 35.1 ***Enterobacter*** and ***Klebsiella*** growth on MacConkey agar.

Pathogenic strains of *K. pneumoniae* show the following biochemical features:

- Indole negative
- Citrate positive
- Urease positive
- Methyl red (MR) negative
- Voges-Proskauer positive
- Pink colonies on MCA
- Purple colonies on EMS agar without green metallic sheen.

KLEBSIELLA PNEUMONIA

K. pneumoniae causes a severe destructive pneumonia, typically in the form of **bronchopneumonia** and also **bronchitis** leading to chronic destructive lesions, pleuritis and multiple abscess formation in the lungs (Friedländer's pneumonia). Many of the patients may develop **bacteremia** with a high mortalty rate – 50% even with antimicrobial therapy. Patients develop the following symptoms.

Cough up a characteristic sputum, fever, nausea, trachycardia and vomiting.

Microscopic examination and culturing of sputum on MCA for pink coloured colonies and biochemical tests.

Pneumonia is treated with an aminoglycoside and cephalosporin (e.g., cefotaxime), either alone or in combination, depending upon the severity of the disease.

ENTEROBACTER

Enterobacter, a motile, aerobic, Gram-negative bacillus is a member of the coilform group and family *Enterobacteriaceae*. It was discovered by **Hormache** and **Edward** in 1960. Naming of this taxon is based on Greek words: *enteron* = intestine and *bacter* = a small rod, i.e., an intestinal small rod. The members naturally inhabit soil and water, but found occasionally in human faeces.

Enterobacter species are straight, Gram-negative, non-endosporic bacilli (0.6 – 1 μm × 1.2 – 3 μm), motile by peritrichous flagella. The colonies are slightly mucoid, non-pigmented, yellow (or light pink) (Fig. 35.1). They ferment mannitol and produce gas from some sugars, but not starch.

The genus includes 36 species. *Enterobacter cloacae, E. aerogenes* and *E. agglomerans* are clinically significant. They cause a variety of nosocomial infections affecting lungs, urinary tract, abdominal cavity and intravascular devices.

Diagnosis is based on the isolation from clinical specimen and biochemical tests. Aminoglycosides, including gentamicin in combination with quinolones are the drugs of choice to treat *Enterobacter* infections.

SERRATIA

Serratia is a motile, Gram-negative, facultatively anaerobic, coccobacillus (1–5 μm). It is a coilform naturally ocurring in soil, water and intestine. Twenty species in the genus have been described.

S. marcescens is the most commonly encountered in clinical specimens. It usually causes nosocomial infections. It was named *Serratia* in honour of an Italian physicist **Serafino Serrati** by Bizio and *marcescens* because of the pigment's rapid discolouration and decay (for the Latin word). Bizio when initially observed the beautiful colony under the microscope called it **"red fungi"**. It is commonly found growing in bathrooms (especially on the tile grout, shower corners, toilet bowls, basins) forming characteristic pink to orange colonies due to the production of characteristic red pigment, **prodigiosin** and can be distinguished from other enterobactericeae by the unique production of three enzymes: DNase, lipase and gelatinase (serralysin).

It is an opportunistic pathogen which can be found on catheters, in saline irrigation and other saline solutions used in hospitals and responsible for causing serious infections in hospitals: pneumonia, lower respiratory and urinary infections, bloodstream and wound infections, meningitis, ocular infections and yellowing of teeth.

S. marcescens can grow in temperatures ranging from 5 to 40°C and pH levels ranging from 5 to 9. On MacConkey agar, at 35°C under aerobic conditions, it produces characteristic red colonies due to the pigment prodigiosin (Fig. 35.2) which is abundantly produced at lower temperature (< 30 – 37°C). It is differentiated from other Gram-negative bacteria by its ability to perform **casein hydrolysis**.

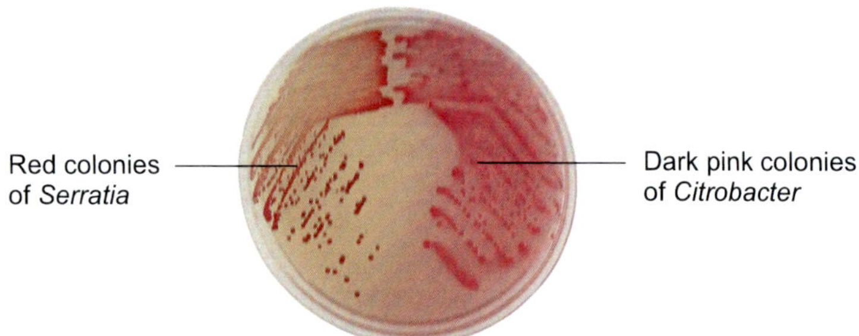

Fig. 35.2 ***Serratia marcescens*** (Left) and ***Citrobacter freundii*** (Right) growth on MacConkey agar.

Due to its multi-drug resistance (cephalosporin, ampicillin, macrolides), an aminoglycoside, such as gentamicin, is the drug of, choice. Fluoroquinolones are the alternative, as they have been found to be very active against most pathogenic strains.

CITROBACTER

Citrobacter is a Gram-negative and lactose-negative or late lactose fermenting coliform that grows well on ordinary culture media producing unpigmented colonies.

The genus *Citrobacter* was first isolated in 1932 by **Werkman** and **Gillen** and proposed the generic name after Latin words: *citrus* = lemon and *bacter* = a rod, i.e., a citrate utilizing rod. As the name suggests, it usually utilizes citrate as a sole carbon source (citrate-positive test).

Currently, *Citrobacter* contains 14 species. These bacteria are found in soil, water, human faeces and may be isolated from a variety of clinical specimens. They are rarely the source of illnesses, except for infections of the urinary tract and infant meningitis and sepsis.

Citrobacter freundii and *C. koseri* are of clinical significance. *C. freundii* is a soil organism that can be found in water, sewage and food. This bacterium plays an important role in nitrogen cycle, reducing nitrate to nitrite. It is also a common component of the gut microbiome, an opportunistic pathogen responsible for nosocomial infections of the respiratory tract, urinary tract and blood in immunocompromised patients.

On HE agar, *C. freundii* produces black colonies due to H_2S production, and if the strain is not a rapid lactose fermenter, the colonies appear green with black centres. On MacConkey agar, the colonies are dark pink (Fig. 35.2). The Gram-negative cells are long rods (1—5 µm in length) provided with several flagella for motility.

C. koseri (= *C. diversus*) occasionally causes neonatal meningitis. Surviving neonates usually reveal severe residual permanent damage of brain. Aminoglycosides, fluoroquinolnes and chloramphenicol are effective in the treatment of *C. freundii* infections, however, resistance to aminoglycosides occurs frequentey among *C. koseri* strains. Cephalosporin and meropenem are often used to treat meningitis.

KEY POINTS

- The genera *Klebsiella, Enterobacter, Citrobacter* and *Serratia,* commonly called **enterobacteria**, are opportunistic or secondary pathogens.
- *Klebsiella pneumoniae,* a Gram-negative, capsulated bacillus, causes pneumonia, and hospital associated urinary tract infection, bacteremia and meningitis.
- Pneumonia is treated with an aminoglycoside and cephalosporin used either alone or in combination.
- *Serratia marcescens,* a Gram-negative coccobacillus, characterized by a red pigment called prodigiosin, causes serious urinary and respiratory tracts infections in hospitals.
- *S. marcescens* is a nuisance acting as a weed in hospitals that is associated with contaminations of saline irrigation and other sterile solutions used in hospitals.

IMPORTANT QUESTIONS

1. Write short notes on:
   (a) *Klebsiella pneumoniae*
   (b) *Serratia marcescens.*

MULTIPLE-CHOICE QUESTIONS

1. Which of the following coliforms produces red pigment (prodigiosin) especially at low temperature?
   (a) *Escherichia* (b) *Serratia*
   (c) *Enterobacter* (d) *Klebsiella.*

2. All are coliform bacteria EXCEPT:
   (a) *Klebsiella* (b) *Enterobacter*
   (c) *Proteus* (d) *Citrobacter.*
3. All are opportunisitic enteric bacteria EXCEPT:
   (a) *Klebsiella* (b) *Enterobacter*
   (c) *Citrobacter* (d) *Salmonella.*
4. Which of the following coliform bacteria is associated with contaminations of saline irrigation and other sterile solutions used in hospitals?
   (a) *Serratia* (b) *Escherichia*
   (c) *Klebsiella* (d) *Enterobacter.*

ANSWERS TO MCQs

1. (b) 2. (c) 3. (d) 4. (a).

32

Clostridium: A Gram-positive Strictly Anaerobic Endosporic Bacillus

Tetanus; Botulism; Gas gangrene; Food-borne infection; Colitis

Clostridium is an obligately anaerobic, Gram-positive, spore-bearing, rod-shaped bacterium belonging to the family Clostridiaceae.

This bacterium was first of all reported as a cause of sausage (food) poisoning (botulism) in 1817 by the German neurologist **Justinus Kerner**. **Louis Pasteur** first named it *Vibrion butyque,* but **Adam Prazmoski** changed name to *Clostridium* in 1880. Its name is derived from the Greek word *kloster* for spindle used in cloth weaving and long sticks with a bulge at the end.

SYSTEMATIC POSITION

Domain	:	Bacteria
Phylum	:	Firmicutes
Class	:	Clostridia
Order	:	Clostridiales
Family	:	Clostridiaceae
Genus	:	*Clostridium*

This genus contains more than 100 species that normally occur in dust, soil, water, decomposing residues and in human and animal intestines. Clostridia are often described as **biological threat** but many of them play a positive role: as in natural processes of putrefaction, in cosmetics and medicines: Many clostridia are higly toxigenic.

Significant pathogens are:

- *Clostridium tetani*—tetanus
- *C. botulinum*—botulism
- *C. perfringens*—gas gangrene, food-borne infection
- C. *difficile*—colitis and serious diarrhoea

CLOSTRIDIUM TETANI

Clostridium tetani, the causative agent of **tetanus (lockjaw)**, is an obligately anaerobic, Gram-positive, endospore-forming, rod-shaped bacterium with terminal round spore resembling a drumstick. This bacterium is especially common in soil contaminated with animal faeces. Tetanus results from neurotoxin (tetanospasmin) produced by bacteria in wound.

MORPHOLOGICAL, CULTURAL AND BIOCHEMICAL CHARACTERISTICS

Motile with peritrichous flagella. Gram-positive bacilli singly and in pairs with terminal round spores (2 – 2.5 μm × 0.3 – 0.5 μm) giving a characteristic "**tennis racquet**" or "**drumstick**" appearance (Fig. 32.1). Initially, the cells appear Gram-positive but after 24 hours of incubation or upon sporulation, they stain Gram-negative.

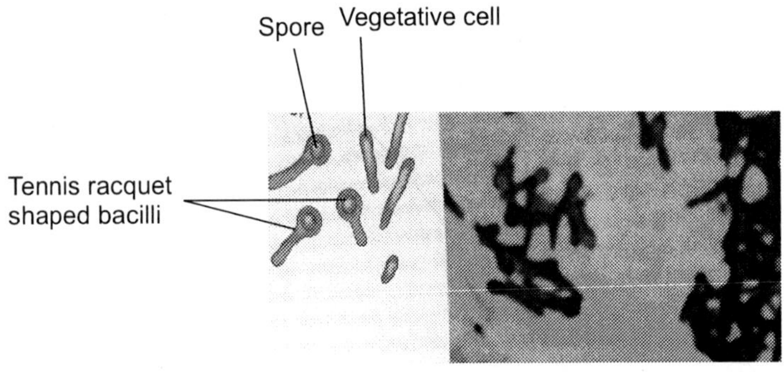

Fig. 32.1 ***Clostridium tetani.*** Bacilli with typical tennis racquet (drumstick) morphology created by terminal endospores that swell the cells (sporangia).

Grows optimally at 37°C on a variety of culture media (e.g., blood agar, cooked meat, thioglycolate casein hydrolysate) in anaerobic conditions (Fig. 32.2). A fine spreading colony—'ground glass' appearance is produced on blood agar.

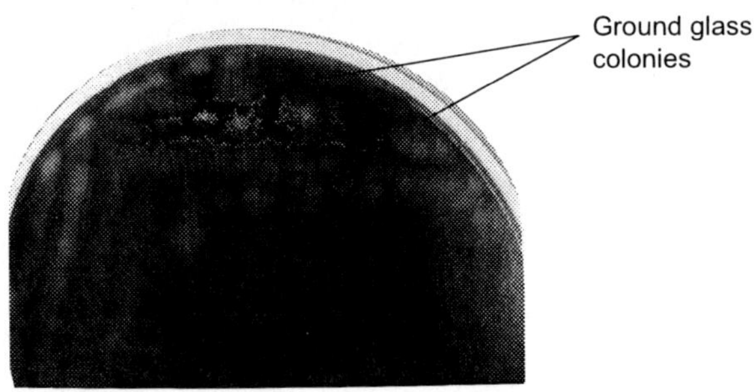

Fig. 32.2 ***Clostridium tetani.*** Colonies on CDC are 4 to 6 mm in diameter, grey, translucent, and flat with an irregular to rhizoid margin and may swarm on the agar surface. A small zone of beta-haemolysis can be observed around the colonies.

In cooked meat broth—turbidity, production of gas and meat turning black on prolonged incubation, are observed.

Biochemical tests are positive for H_2S, DNase, starch hydrolysis, lipase and lecithinase activity, and gelatin liquefaction but negative for nitrate reduction.

RESISTANCE

Endospores in soil survive for years. They are exceedingly resistant to drying, household disinfectants (e.g., ethanol, phenol, formalin), radiations, and are capable of surviving boiling but can be killed by iodine, glutaraldehyde, and autoclaving at 121°C and 103 kPa (15 psi) for 15 minutes.

TOXINS

C. tetani produces two distinct toxins:

- *Tetanospasmin* (a neuro- exotoxin)—which causes clinical tetanus.
- *Tetanolysin* (a haemolysin)—which causes local tissue destruction.

TETANUS

Tetanus (Gr. *tetanos* = to stretch) is a serious neuromuscular, noncommunicable between human hosts and is caused by the neurotoxin – *tetanospasmin*, produced by *C. tetani*. The disease is also called **lockjaw** that refers to an early effect of the disease on the jaw muscles.

CLINICAL FORMS

There are four major clinical forms of tetanus:

- *Generalised tetanus:* It is the most common and most severe form involving all skeletal muscles.
- *Neonatal tetanus:* Infection of the umblical cord in infants can cause neonatal tetanus, which kills 2 to 3 lakh infants each year worldwide.
- *Local tetanus:* It manifests with muscle spasms at or near the wound that has been infected with the tetanus bacterium.
- *Cephalic tetanus:* It manifests with a head injury or ear injury and affects muscles in the face rapidly and sometimes resulting in lockjaw.

SYMPTOMS

Spasms and stiffness in jaw muscles (trismus), stiffness of the neck and abdominal muscles, difficulty in swallowing and painful body spasms. Fever, sweating, rapid heart rate and elevated blood pressure also occur.

PATHOGENESIS

The endospores of the bacterium originate from the soil contaminated with animal faecal wastes. These enter the body through a wound/ injury and start multiplying under anaerobic conditions. Extremely potent neurotoxin, *tetanospasmin* is released upon death and lysis of the growing bacteria. It enters the CNS via peripheral nerve axons or the blood, where it binds to nerve cells that control the contraction of various skeletal muscles. The binding of tetanospasmin blocks the relaxation pathway. The result is uncontrollable muscle contractions, producing the convulsive symptoms of tetanus within an incubation period of 3–21 days, but sometimes longer.

The muscles of the jaw are affected early in the disease, preventing the mouth from opening, a condition known as *lockjaw*. In an advanced case of tetanus, spasms of the back muscles cause the head and heels to bow backward, a condition called *opisthotonus* or *opisthotonos* (especially in neonatal tetanus). Gradually, other skeletal muscles become affected, including those involved in swallowing. Eventually death (respiratory failure) results from spasms of the respiratory muscles.

Trachycardia (fast heartbeat > than 100 beats/minute, BPM) and sweating are the other symptoms that are due to the effects of the toxin on the sympathetic nervous system.

Tetanus is not contagious. In this disease, the bacteria themselves do not spread from the infection site and the disease results only when the bacterial neurotoxin reaches the CNS.

DIAGNOSIS

The diagnosis of tetanus is clinical based on the physical examination, medical and immunization history, and the signs and symptoms of muscle spams, stiffness and pains.

Laboratory test aren't helpful as *C. tetani* is no longer present in the lesion/wound by the time symptoms appear in the patient.

TREATMENT

- Administration of *tetanus immune globulin (TIG)* to neutralize unbound toxin as soon as tetanus is suspected clinically.

- *Debridement*, i.e., removal of damaged tissue to prevent growth and further toxin release by the pathogen.
- Immediate initiation of antibiotic therapy with penicillin or doxycycline that is to be taken for a week or more.

PREVENTION/IMMUNIZATION

Immunization with **tetanus vaccine (tetanus toxoid)** is used to prevent tetanus. Various kinds of tetanus vaccines available are:

- **Monovalent vaccine**. tetanus toxoid (TT)
- **Bivalent combination vaccines**:
  - Diphtheria toxoid (DT)
  - Low-dose diphtheria toxoid (DT)
- **Trivalent combination vaccines (DTP):**
  - Whole cell pertussis (WCP)—DTWP
  - Acellular pertussis (aP)—DTaP

CDC recommends DTaP vaccine to protect young children (babies) from diphtheria, **tetanus** and pertussis (whooping cough).

The WHO has recommended childhood immunization with tetanus vaccine (or TT containing vaccines) with a 5 dose schedule.

However, the national immunization schedule in Universal Immunization Program (UIP) in India, recommends 7 shots of TT in various combinations.

- Three doses of DPT in infancy administred intramuscularly, with an interval of 4-6 weeks between the first two injections and the 3rd dose 6 months later.
- Two booster doses at 16 and 24 months old baby.
- Two TTs at 10 and 16 years of age.

CLOSTRIDIUM BOTULINUM

Clostridium botulinum is a Gram-positive anaerobic, rod-shaped, spore forming, motile bacterium. It causes **botulism (paralytic disease)**, a food-borne intoxication acquired by ingesting preformed ***botulinum neurotoxins***, the most potent toxin known to humans.

The bacillus and its spores are widely distributed in nature soil, animal manure, hay and surface of vegetables. Heat-resistant endospores are able to survive under adverse conditions. The bacterium is commonly associated with bulging canned food.

MORPHOLOGY: It is a Gram-positive bacillus measuring 5 × 1 μm, motile with peritrichous flagella, producing oval subterminal endospores.

GROWTH CHARACTERISTICS: It is strictly anaerobic growing optimally at 35° C producing large surface, semitransparent, irregular colonies on blood agar. Some strains grow and produce toxin at temperatures as low as 1–5°C.

BIOCHEMICAL CHARACTERISTICS: All types ferment glucose and maltose with acid and gas.

RESISTANCE: Endospores are highly resistant to radiation and heat, withstand boiling in water (100°C) for several hours but destroyed by moist heat at 121°C within 5 minutes. Thus, insufficient heating of foods during the preservation process leads to bolulism.

BOTULINUM TOXIN: It produces *botulinum toxin,* a potent neurotoxin in food, responsible for botulism in humans. Botulinum toxin (BTX or BONT) is of seven types, designated A-G, which are antigenically distinct with pharmcologically identical actions. BTX are one of the most lethal biological substances known (i.e., 0.000,000,003 mg is the lethal dose of mice). It acts by blocking the release of **acetylcholine** by binding to nerve cells and resulting to muscle paralysis.

BOTULISM

Botulism is a serious neuroparalytic disease caused by a toxin produced by *Clostridium botulinum*. In India, it is an extremely rare disease with fewer than 5000 cases reported in a year. Botulism derives its name from the Latin word *botulus*, which means "sausage". It was coined as far back as 1793 at a time when the disease was often acquired from eating contaminated (or spoiled) sausages.

The disease occurs in four forms: **Food-borne, infant, wound**, and **inhalation**.

All forms of botulism lead to paralysis. Food-borne botulism is an intoxication caused by ingestion of preformed toxin in the food and the bacteria do not infect tissues. Infant botulism and wound botulism involve both infection and intoxication because the bacterial endospores germinate, grow in tissues and produce toxin. **Botulism is not transmitted from person-to-person**.

Food-borne Botulism

It is a serious form of botulism called **food-borne intoxication** that occurs in 90% of the cases. The disease is acquired by ingesting preformed botulinum toxin usually from preserved food - meat and meat products, canned vegetables (green beans, green peppers), fish and other seafood. The cans often bulge and bubbles appear on opening.

SYMPTOMS

Symptoms appear 12–36 hours after ingesion of toxin containing food. The toxin paralyzes muscles in a relaxed (flaccid) state—starting with small eye muscles progressing to larynx and pharynx, respiratory muscles resulting in double vision, difficulty in speaking, swallowing and breathing. Comma or delirium may occur. It ends in death due to respiratory failure within 1–7 days after onset of the disease.

The toxin, BTX, acts at junctions between neurons and muscle cells and prevents the release of neurotransmitter **acetylcholine**, the chemical that neurons release to cause muscle cells to contract, resulting in **muscle paralysis**.

DIAGNOSIS

Botulism is diagnosed:

- Based on clinical symptoms and history.
- By identifying botulinal toxin by inoculating mice with samples from patient serum, stool, vomitus or food specimen (i.e., by the mouse inoculation test). Death of the mouse within 72 hours confirms the presence of toxin.
- By finding *C. botulinum* in the patient's stool.

TREATMENT

- Mechanical ventilation for the patients who lose their ability to breathe on their own for two to eight weeks (i.e., supportive case).
- Immediate treatment with an antitoxin to neutralize the botulinum toxin in the circulatory system by passive immunization.
- Trivalent (A, B, E) botulinum antitoxin is most often used.
- Heptavalent (A, B, C, D, E, F, G) antitoxin had been approved for use for patients in 2013 by the United States FDA.

PREVENTION

Food-borne botulism is preventable by proper food preparation as the toxin is destroyed by heating at 85°C (185°F), for longer than 5 minutes, and following the 2-40-140 rule that says: Don't eat meats, dressings or salads that have been kept for more than 2 hours between 40° F (4.4°C) and 140°F (60°C).

INFANT BOTULISM

The disease is associated with feeding honey to infants. The endospores present in honey germinate and grow in the immature digestive tract of infants under 6 months of age, as the intestinal microbiota antagonistic to the bacterium, is not well established, producing the toxin. As toxin is absorbed, the infant loses the ability to suck and swallow and becomes lethargic — the disease called **"flossy baby"** syndrome. Hence, honey should not be fed to children under 12 months.

WOUND BOTULISM

The pathogen can grow in deep, crusting wounds. The endospores geminate, multiply and produce toxin under anaerobic conditions. The toxin reaches the junctions between neurons and muscles through blood causing paralysis after a week after injury.

CLOSTRIDIUM PERFRINGENS

Clostridium perfringens (formally known as *C. welchii*, *Bacillus welchii*) is a Gram-positive, rod-shaped, spore-forming, anaerobic bacterium with the shortest reported generation time of 6.3 minutes.

Major diseases caused by *C. perfringens* are **food-associated *diarrhoeal* disease** and **gas gangrene (clostridial myonecrosis)**. This bacterium is widely spread, living in a variety of common habitats, ranging from soil to the gastrointestinal tract of healthy humans and animals, fresh meat and poultry products.

MORPHOLOGY

It is a nonmotile, large Gram-positive encapsulated, spore-forming bacillus (central to terminal spores) measuring 4–6 μm in length and 1 μm in width (Fig. 32.3).

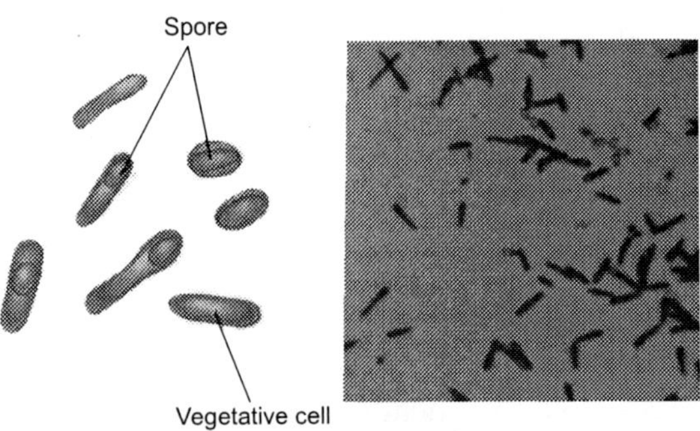

Fig. 32.3 ***Clostridium perfringens***. Gram-positive bacillus with central to terminal endospores.

CULTURAL CHARACTERISTICS

It grows rapidly on laboratory culture media under anaerobic and microaerophilic conditions, particularly at high temperatures (42°C), with the doubling time of 8 minutes. Colonies on blood agar are smooth, round, greyish, surrounded by a double zone of haemolysis.

It is a saccharolytic bacterium which causes the change of colour of the meat to pink, when grown on cooked meat medium.

BIOCHEMICAL REACTIONS

- Glucose, sucrose, maltose and lactose are fermented with the production of acid and gas.
- In litmus milk, it ferments lactose producing acid which coagulates the casein (*acid clot*), and the clotted milk is disrupted due to vigorous gas production, giving it a **strong clot appearance**.

RESISTANCE

Endospores of food poisoning strains are heat-resistant that can survive boiling for several hours, whereas those strains causing gas gangrene are inactivated within a few minutes by boiling. Autoclaving at 121°C for 15 minutes destroys the endospores.

Spores are resistant to often used antiseptics and disinfectants (e.g. formaldehydes).

STRAIN TYPES

C. perfringens is classified into five toxinotypes—A, B, C, D and E on the basis of major lethal toxins produced. Type A strains are further divided into several serotypes.

Type A bacteria → Alpha toxin
Type B bacteria → Alpha, beta and epsilon toxins
Type C bacteria → Alpha and beta toxins
Type D bacteria → Alpha and episilon toxins
Type E bacteria → Alpha and iota toxins

TOXINS

At least 12 toxins (4 major and 12 minor) are produced by the five types (A – E) of *C. perfringens* that may be involved in pathogenesis. The major toxins are *alpha, beta, epsilon* and *iota* toxin. An enterotoxin (CPE) and *neuraminidase* are also produced by certain strains.

PATHOGENICITY

The alpha toxin, produced by all the five strains (A–E) of the bacterium, causes gas gangrene and also haemolysis in infected individuals. Beta, a lethal toxin, produced by B and C strains causes enterotoxemia, a condition called **pig bel** in humans. CPE, an enterotoxin produced by this bacterium causes food poisoning in humans.

FOOD-BORNE INFECTION

Clostridium perfringens causes two forms of diarrhoeal diseases in humans and is responsible for about million cases of sickness every year.

Enterotoxin producing food-associated type A strains are a common cause of diarrhoeal infection. The infection is usually acquired by eating improperly cooked meat or poultry containing endospores. The spores germinate and multiply at room temperature. If reheating before consumption is inadequate, large number of organisms are ingested with food. The bacteria sporulate and produce enterotoxin in large intestine resulting in glucose transport inhibition, damage of intestinal epithelium and protein loss into lumen showing the watery diarrhoea symptoms within 8–24 hours of consumption.

Much more rarely, β-toxin producing type C strains produce a severe necrotizing disease called **"Pig-bel"** of the small intestine, accompanied by abdominal pain, bloody diarrhoea, ulceration and perforation of the intestine that can be fatal. This rare form of illness occurs after consumption of contaminated meat by people who are unaccustomed to a high protein diet and do not have sufficient intestinal trysin to destroy the toxin.

DIAGNOSIS

Diagnosis is made on the basis of clinical symptoms, streaking and culturing the bacteria on blood agar plates and Gram staining from the patient's stool; and by demonstrating enterotoxin production by a latex agglutination method.

PREVENTION AND TREATMENT

Antibacterial treatment is rarely required. Prevention depends on thorough reheating of food before serving, and also keeping not foods warm (generally above 60°C) and refrigerating leftovers at cold temperature (below 5°C).

In severe cases, patients can be given fluids intravenously with electrolytes for preventing dehydration from diarrhoea.

GAS GANGRENE

Gas gangrene (also called **clostridial myonecrosis** or **myonecrosis**), a fast spreading, clostridial infection of wound characterized by tissue death (gangrene) accompanied by the evolution of foul-smelling gas, is caused by several clostridia, but *Clostridium perfringens* type A (alpha toxin producer) is the most common causative agent.

It is a life-threatening disease often occurring in situations where open wounds from an injury or surgery are exposed to bacteria. The infection occurs suddenly, spreads quickly, and becomes life-threatening within 48 hours of the onset of symptoms. It is more common in people sufferring from a peripheral vascular disease (atherosclerosis) or diabetes mellitus.

PATHOGENESIS

Clostridia gain access to the surgical wounds from soil, human and animal feces. Infection develops in the areas of the body with poor blood supply (anaerobic) such as buttocks and perineum. The bacteria multiply in the subcutaneos tissues, producing gas and causing *myonecrosis* (muscle tissue death also called gangrene) and sepsis. Infection proceeds very rapidly and causes acute pain. Lecithinase (also known as α-toxin) produced by the bacterium hydrolyses the lipids in cell membranes, resulting in cell lysis and death. It can easily be noticed by the large, blackened sores and loud and distinctive crepitus (sound) caused by gas escaping the necrotic tissue.

The symptoms usally develop within 6–48 hours of initial infection. The infection may even become life threatening within 48 hours of the oneset of symptoms. Major symptoms include: increased heart rate, excessive sweating, fever, air under the skin, swollen, dark red or purple or black area with pain around the wound, and blisters with foul-smelling discharge.

DIAGNOSIS

Diagnosis is made primarily on clinical basis, followed by laboratory tests: Skin culture for the presence of *C. perfringens* from muscle fragments or necontic tissue from the affected areas; blood tests for abnormally high white blood cell count.

TREATMENT

- Immediate surgery to remove dead or infected tissues.
- High doses of antibiotics (e.g., penicillin or metronidazole) are to be used.
- Amputation of a limb may be necessary to prevent further spread of infection to rest of the body.
- Use of *hyperbaric oxygen therapy* that steadily increases the amount of oxygen in the blood thereby helping infected wounds to heal faster.

PREVENTION

The best way to prevent gas gangrene is to practise proper hygiene. In case of any injury, make sure to clean the skin thoroughly and to cover the wound with bandage.

KEY POINTS

- *Clostridium tetani*, a Gram-positive strictly anaerobic bacillus reveals a characteristic tennis racket or drumstick appearance.
- Tetanus results from *tetanospasmin* a neurotoxin, produced by *Clostridium tetani* in wound.
- Tetanus is a preventable disease and immunization with *tetanus toxoid* (TT) is a routine childhood immunization worldwide.
- Botulism is a serious neuroparalytic disease caused by botulinum toxin (BTX) produced by *Clostridium botulinum*, a Gram-positive, obligately anaerobic bacillus.
- Food-borne botulism is an *intoxication* as it is caused by preformed botulinum toxin in preserved foods spoiled by *C. botulinum* and is treated with trivalent (A, B, E) or heptavalent (A-G) botulinum antitoxin.
- Infant botulism and wound botulism involve both infection and intoxication.
- *Clostridium perfringens*, a Gram-positive, spore-producing anaerobic bacillus, often occurs in soil and gastrointestinal tracts of humans and animals.
- Two strains of *C. perfringens* cause two forms of food-borne infection: type A - common form (diarrhoea) and type C - rare form (acute necrotizing disease of small intestine called "*Pig-bel*").

- Gas gangrene (also called **clostridial myonecrosis**) a life-threatening infection of wound characterized by tissue death (called **gangrene**) and evolution of gas by *C. perfringens* type A, an alpha-toxin producer.

IMPORTANT QUESTIONS

1. Write short notes on:
   (a) Tetanus
   (b) Botulism
   (c) Gas gangrene
   (d) *Clostridium perfringens* food-borne infection (or poisoning)
   (e) How *Clostridium tetani, C. botulinum* and *C. perfringens* are distinguished?

MULTIPLE-CHOICE QUESTIONS

1. *Clostridium tetani* is an obligately anaerobic, spore-bearing, drum-stick rod-shaped, Gram-negative bacterium.
   True or False?
2. Endospore-poducing bacilli with typical tennis racquet (drumstick) morphology are produced in:
   (a) *Clostridium perfringens*
   (b) *Clostridium botulinum*
   (c) *Clostridium tetani*
   (d) *Clostridium septicum.*
3. Tetanus results from tetanospasmin, a toxin produced by *Clostridium tetani* in wound. True or False?
4. Food-borne botulism, caused by the preformed toxin in foods produced by *Clostridium botulinum*, is both an intoxication and infection. True or False?
5. All are *true* for *Clostridium botulinum* EXCEPT:
   (a) Anaerobic bacillus
   (b) Nonmotile
   (c) Treated with trivalent or heptavalent antitoxin
   (d) Human botulism is caused by A, B and E toxins.
6. Which of the following is the causative agent of gas gangrene (myonecrosis)?
   (a) *Clostridium botulinum*
   (b) *Clostridium perfringens*

(c) *Bacillus anthracis*
(d) *Clostridium septicum.*

7. *Myonecrosis* (muscle tissue death) occurs in which clostridial disease?
(a) Tetanus (b) Botulism
(c) Gas gangrene (d) Food poisoning.

8. *Opisthotonos* (head and heels to bow backward) occurs in:
(a) Tetanus (b) Botulism
(c) Gas gangrene (d) None of the above.

ANSWERS TO MCQs

1. False 2. (c) 3. True 4. False 5. (b)
6. (b) 7. (c) 8. (a).

33

Gram-negative Bacilli of Medical Importance and *Enterobacteriaceae*

WHAT ARE GRAM-NEGATIVE BACILLI?

The **Gram-negative bacilli** comprise a large group of rod-shaped, non-spore-forming bacteria that do not retain the crystal-violet stain and turn pink by taking the colour of safranin (counter-stain) when Gram-stained. They have a cell wall composed of a thin layer of *peptidoglycan* compared to their Gram-positive counterparts which appear purple.

Gram-negative bacilli are responsible for numerous diseases. The most important of these belong to the family *Enterobacteriaceae*. Some are commensal organisms present among normal intestinal flora. These commensal organisms plus others from animal or environmental reservoirs may cause disease.

UTIs, diarrhoea, typhoid fever, whooping cough, plague and blood-stream infections are commonly caused by Gram-negative bacilli.

CATEGORIES OF GRAM-NEGATIVE BACILLI

Based on their oxygen requirements, Gram-negative bacilli are grouped into three major categories:

I. **Aerobic Gram-negative nonenteric bacilli**
Pseudomonas, Brucella, Francisella, Bordetella and Lagionella.

II. **Facultative anaerobic Gram-negative bacilli**
(A) **Oxidase-negative** *(Enterobacteriaceae): Escherichia, Salmonella, Shigella, Yersinia, Klebsiella, Enterobacter, Serratia, Citrobacter, Proteus, Morganella, Providencia.*
(B) **Oxidase-positive** *(Pasteurellaceae): Pasteurella, Haemophilus.*
(C) **Genera not associated with a family:** *Gardenerella, Eikenella, Streptobacillus, Calymmatobacterium.*

III. **Obligately anaerobic Gram-negative bacilli:** *Bacteroides.*

ENTEROBACTERIACEAE

The family *Enterobacteriaceae* (classified in the order: *Enterobacteriales*, class: *Gammaproteobacteria*, phylum: *Proteobacteria*, Domain: *Bacteria*) is composed of Gram-negative bacilli that are oxidase-negative, facultative anaerobes. These rod-shaped bacteria are commonly called the **enterics** or **enterobacteria** because they are the residents of the large intestine of humans and animals.

This family is the largest and most heterogeneous collection of medically important Gram-negative bacilli that are biochemically and genetically related to each other. These bacteria are frequently isolated from clinical specimens. There are over 14 genera that have been described to cause human diseases.

Escherichia coli is by far the most important single species that causes severe invasive and toxic diseases such as infant diarrhoea and toxemia, as well as urinary tract and surgical infections.

Major characteristics of the family *Enterobacteriaceae* are:

- They are Gram-negative, non-sporing, short rods.
- They are facultative anaerobes.
- They are catalase-positive, oxidase-negative and reduce nitrates to nitrites.
- They produce acid from glucose.
- Some ferment lactose with the production of acid and gas – characteristics used to distinguish enteric from obligatly aerobic bacteria.
- Their cells contain a characteristic antigen-called the entero-bacterial common antigen (i.e., O (Outer membrane), H (flagella), K (Capsule) and Vi (Capsule of *Salmonella*).
- Some are motile by peritrichous flagella.

Tools for Identification of *Enterobacteriacecae* members:

- Motility test
- Lactose fermentation test
- Citrate utilization test
- Indole test
- Methyl red (MR) test
- Voges-Proskauer (VP) test
- Triple sugar iron (TSI) agar test
- Urease test
- Phenylalanine (PA) deaminase test.

CLASSIFICATION OF *ENTEROBACTERIACEAE*

Based on their location in the body and ability to ferment lactose, there are two informal divisions of the family:

36

Proteus, Morganella and *Providencia*: Noncoliform Enteric Bacilli

Opportunistic nosocomial infections: UTI; Urolithiasis

Proteus, Morganella and *Providencia*, are classified in the tribe *Proteae* (*Enterobacteriaceae*). These are noncoliform lactose-negative bacilli with a unique ability to oxidatively deaminate amino acids to the corresponding keto acids and ammonia (i.e., *produce phenyalanine deaminase*). They are often found in the human gastrointestinal tract as commensals not causing any harm to the host. They are saprobic organisms found in soil, manure, sewage and polluted waters.

They are opportunisitic pathogens and cause nosocomial infections that include urinary tract, wound, pneumonia, sepsis and occasionally infant diarrhoea. UTI caused by *Proteus* tends to be more serious than that caused by *Escherichia coli*.

PROTEUS

Proteus is an interesting taxon, the name referring to its pleomorphism, named after the Greek word *Proteus* who could change his shape at will.

Proteus includes five species. Three clinically significant species are: *P. mirabilis*, *P. vulgaris* and *P. penneri*. *P. mirabilis* is the most commonly isolated species, causing urinary tract and wound infections and septicaemia.

Proteus spp. can grow on ordinary culture media at 35°C under aerobic conditions productng a characteristic putrefective odour (**fishy** or **seminal**). They possess the ability to swarm (spread) on the moist agar surface due to the possession of peritrichous flagella. The wave-like swarming pattern of *P. mirabilis* is typical characterized by concentric rings of growth **bull's-eye colony** (Fig. 36.1). This pattern is one of the most striking sights in the microbiology laboratory.

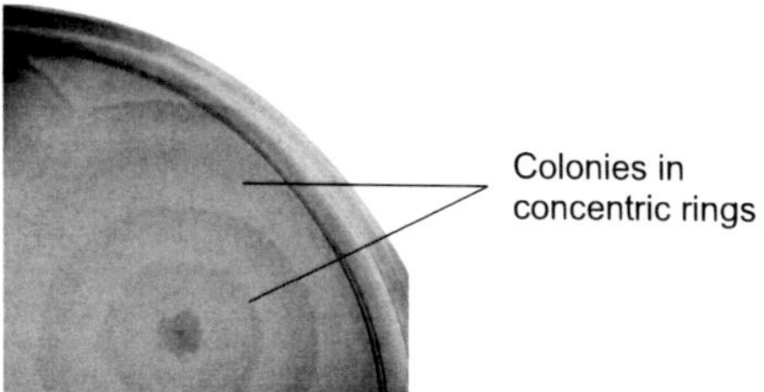

Fig. 36.1 ***Proteus mirabilis*** **on blood agar showing a wave-like swarming pattern**. Growth of the organism occurs in waves producing characterisitic concentric rings typical of the genus *Proteus*.

PROTEUS MIRABILIS

P. mirabilis, a Gram-negative, enteric bacillus is widely distributed in soil and water. Commonly found in the human digestive system, it is the cause of 90% of all *Proteus* infections. After *Escherichia coli*, *P. mirabilis* is the most frequently associated bacterium with urinary tract infection (UTI), however, the UTI caused by *P. mirabilis* is more complicated and difficult to control. 70% of kidney stones resulting from UTIs are attributed to this pathogen alone.

P. mirabilis has the following characteristic features:

- Ability to swarm on solid media
- Bull's-eye colony on an agar medium
- Positive urease test
- Ability to deaminate amino acids oxidatively (PPA test)
- Production of H_2S
- Ability to inhibit grow of related strains, as represented by **Dienes lines**.

Escherichia coli, a Gram-negative bacillus, is the commonest cause of urinary tract infection, particularly in females. *P. mirabilis*, after *E. coli*, is the prominent cause of UTI and is more complicated and associated with urinary stones (**renal calculus** or **urolithiasis** or **nephrolithiasis**). This bacterium produces high levels of a potent **urease** which acts on urea to produce ammonia $\left(\text{Urea} \xrightarrow[\text{Hydrolysis}]{\text{Urease}} NH_3\right)$ making the urine alkaline. The increased alkalinity leads to the formation of stones in the urinary tract. Once stone formation begins, bacteria can sequester within the stone making less susceptible to antibiotic treatment. Overtime, these stones may become large enough to cause obstruction and renal failure. These bacteria are highly motile with peritrichous flagella and chemotaxis may play a part in pathogenesis.

TREATMENT

UTI caused by *P. mirabilis* can be treated with ampicillin/cephalosporin or trimethorim/sulfamethoxazole (TMP/SMZ) or an oral ciprofloxacin. But renal stone associated infection is difficult to control with these medicines.

MORGANELLA

Morganella, contains a single species *Morganella morgannii*, first described and isolated in 1906 by **H. de R. Morgan**, a British bacteriologist, from stools of infants who were noted to have had summer diarrhoea. It is found in the human intestine as a commensal organism. Although a rare human pathogen, however, it may cause nosocomial urinary tract infection, wound infection and pneumonia.

It shares the characteristics with *Proteus*. It produces off-white and opaque colonies on blood agar producing Gram-negative, straight rods ($0.6 - 0.7 \times 1 - 1.7$ μm) with peritrichous flagella.

Morganella infections can be treated with ticarcill, piperacllin ciprofloxacin and cephalsporins (3rd and 4th generations).

PROVIDENCIA

Providencia (named after the place Providence, Rhode Island) is a urease producing, Gram-negative, motile bacillus of the family *Enterobacteriaceae* (tribe *Proteae*). Of the seven known species, *P. stuartii* is an opportunistic nosocomial pathogen and is involved in high incidence of urinary tract infection in catheterized patients and in patients with severe burns. This organism migrates from the urinary tract to other organs causing endocarditis, pericarditis, perifomitis and meningitis. This pathogen is ubiquitous in the environment commonly found in water, soil and animal reserviors.

P. stuartii is urease-positive. The urease activitiy contributes to the development of **urolithasis** (urinary tract stones). Specifically, *P. stuartii* and *Proteus mirabilis* co-infection contributes to the increased risk of developing urolithasis and bacteremia through synergisitic induction of urease activity during co-infection.

Similar to *Proteus*, *Providencia stuartii* deaminates amino acids oxidatively (positive PPA test). It is motile via flagella, non-sporulating, non-lactose fermenting, catalase positive and oxidase negative, grows at 37°C on nutrient agar/broth.

Infections caused by *P. stuartii* can be treated with aztreonam, an alternative to cephalosporin and aminoglycosides.

KEY POINTS

- *Proteus, Morganella* and *Providencia,* the noncoliform Gram-negative bacilli, have a unique ability to oxidatively deaminate amino acids (i.e. positive PPA test).
- A wave-like swarming pattern of the colony showing concentric rings of growth shown by *Proteus mirabilis* (typical of the genus) is one of the most striking sights in the microbiology laboratory.
- UTI caused by *Proteus mirabilis* is more severe complicated than *E. coli* and difficult to treat.
- The urease-positive *Proteus mirabilis* and *Providencia sturatii,* both the causative agents of UTI, are associated with **urolithasis** (i.e., renal stones formation) in humans.

IMPORTANT QUESTIONS

1. Write notes on:
   (a) Diagnostic features of *Proteus mirabilis* and *Providencia sturatii* and their role in urolithasis in humans.
   (b) *Proteae* genera of medical significance.

MULTIPLE-CHOICE QUESTIONS

1. All of the following deaminate amino acids oxidatively to produce keto acid and ammonia EXCEPT:
   (a) *Proteus* (b) *Escherichia*
   (c) *Morganella* (d) *Providencia.*
2. Which of the following is urease-positive and associated with urolithiasis (renal stones formation) in humans?
   (a) *Proteus* (b) *Edwardsiella*
   (c) *Morganella* (d) *Escherichia.*
3. Urinary tract infection caused by *Proteus mirabilis* is more severe and complicated as compared to that caused by *E. coli* and other enterobacteria. True or False?

ANSWERS TO MCQs

1. (b) 2. (a) 3. True.

37

Salmonella: A Gram-negative Motile, Nonsporing Enteric Bacillus

Typhoid; Gastroenteritis

Salmonella, a Gram-negative, motile, nonsporing, noncoliform, rod-shaped (bacillus), is a member of the family *Enterobacteriaceae*. Its members involve only the gastrointestinal tract and cause typhoid, gastroenteritis and septicaemia due to contaminated food and water.

The genus *Salmonella* was named after its discoverer **D.E. Salmon**, an American veterinary pathologist, in 1900 by **J.L. Lignieres**.

There are over 2600 different **antigenic types** (called **serotypes** or **serovars**) recognized as a single species (*Salmonella typimurium*) as per the **Kauffman-White** classification scheme.

Based on DNA hybridization studies, only two species are recognized in *Salmonella*: *Salmonella enterica* (found in humans and warm-blooded animals) and *Salmonella bangori* (found in cold-blooded animals, especially reptiles). *S. enterica* is classfied into six subspecies. Of these *S. enterica* subspecies *enterica* (designated subspecies 1) is clinically the most important. Salmonellae serovars are named as: *Salmonella enterica* subsp. *enterica* serovar Typhimurium can be shortened to *Salmonella* serotype typhi or *S. Typhimurium*, or just Typhimurium for use in clinical situations. It is important to note that serotype names are capitalized and not in italics. For simplicity, serovars in most of the texts are written as species, that is, *S. typhimurium*.

Major diseases caused by *Salmonella* are:

- Enteric fevers:
  - Typhoid—*Salmonella* Typhi
  - Paratyphoid—*Salmonella* Paratyphi A and B
- Gastroenteritis or food poisoning—*Salmonella* Typhimurium and *S.* Enteritidis
- Septicaemia—*Salmonella* Choleraesuis

MORPHOLOGICAL AND CULTURAL CHARACTERISTICS

Salmonellae are Gram-negative, non-sporing, non-capsulate, non-acid fast, motile (peritrichous flagella) bacilli measuring $2-5 \times 0.7-1.5$ µm.

They are facultative aerobes, capable of growing within a temperature range of 15 to 45°C (optimum 37°C) and pH between 6 and 8 on ordinary culture media. Most strains grow on nutrient agar as smooth greyish white colonies, 2 – 4 mm in diameter.

BIOCHEMICAL REACTIONS

- Produce acid and gas from glucose (except *S.* Typhi, which is anaerogenic).
- Non-fermenter of lactose.
- Production of H_2S in triple sugar iron agar except *S.* Paratyphi and *S.* Choleraesuis.
- Fail to hydrolyze urea and deaminate phenylalanine.
- They are indole-negative.

ANTIGENIC STRUCTURE

Salmonellae possess three main antigens, on the basis of which they are classified and identified. These are:

- Somatic (O) antigens
- Flagellar (H) antigens
- Surface (Vi) antigen.

RESISTANCE

- Readily killed by moist heating at 55°C in 60 minutes or at 60°C in 15 minutes and most strong disinfectants.
- Chlorination or boiling of water kills the bacilli.
- Pasteurization of milk destroys the bacilli.
- They can survive in ice for months.

TYPHOID FEVER

Typhoid fever or **typhoid** (name delived from *typhus* + *oid* means resembling typhus), an enteric fever, is a serious systemic infection marked by prolonged high fever (103°F–104°F) and intestinal inflammation. Worldwide, typhoid fever affects 21 million people annually causing over 1,61,000 deaths (WHO, 2019). It occurs through ingestion of faecal contaminated food or water predominantly in countries with poor sanitation and lack of clean drinking water.

It is caused by *Salmonella* Typhi (*S. enterica* subsp *enterica* serotype Typhi), the most virulent serotype of *Salmonella*.

On bismuth sulfite agar, the colonies are circular and discrete, surrounded by a black or brownish black zone that appears several times the size of the colony, and exhibits a distinctly characteristic metallic sheen by reflected light (Fig. 37.1). It is a strictly non-lactose fermenting bacterium. It produces a small amount of H_2S and no visible gas on TSI agar (i.e., K/A slight H_2S) (Fig. 37.2) (features used to differentiate it from other enterobacteriaceae).

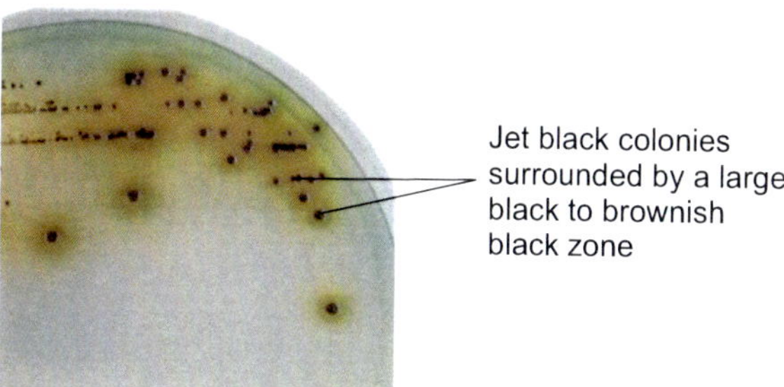

Fig. 37.1 ***Salmonella* serotype Typhi on bismuth sulfite agar.** Isolated subsurface colonies are circular, jet black, and well defined. The typical discrete surface of a colony is black which is surrounded by a black or brownish black zone that appears several times the size of the colony, as shown in this figure. By reflected light, this zone exhibits a distinctly characteristic metallic sheen.

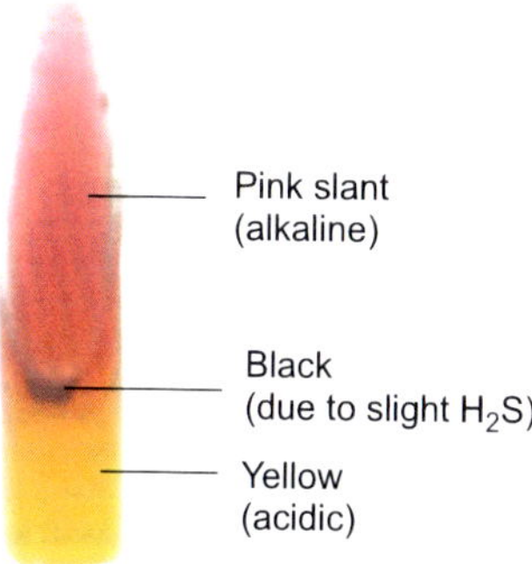

Fig. 37.2 ***Salmonella* serotype Typhi on a TSI agar slant**. Although *Salmonella* serotype Typhi ferments glucose like other *Salmonella* spp., it does not produce gas and produces only a small amount of H_2S. The resulting reaction on a TSI agar slant is K/A slight H_2S.

The disease is characterized by the sudden onset of a high fever (>40°C), severe headache, nausea and loss of appetite. Other symptoms include: constipation or diarrhoea, enlargement of the spleen, ulceration and perforation of the intestinal wall. Appearance of skin rash with rose coloured spots that fade on pressure on the skin during the 2nd or 3rd week.

Drinking water tainted by urine and faeces of infected individuals is the most common source of infection. Consumption of shellfish from polluted aquatic bodies is another source. The estimated inoculum size necessary for infection is 1,00,000 bacteria.

Transmission of *S.* Typhi, occurs only by *fecal-oral route,* often from asymptomatic individuals who act as *chronic carriers.* Some of the recoverd typhoid patients (1-3 %) harbour the pathogen in the gallbladder and continue to shed bacteria for several months and these shedded bacteria are capable of infecting others. A famous example is "**Mary Mallon**" (famous as "**Typhoid Mary**"), who worked as a cook in New York state during 1906-1907, for infecting 122 people and five deaths with typhoid.

Infection is acquired by ingestion of bacilli (10^3 to 10^6) through contaminated food or water. On reaching the gut, they multiply within the phagocytes and are disseminated into various organs, especially the liver, spleen and gallbladder . Eventually, lysis of phagocytic cells takes place and release of *S.* Typhi into the bloodstream resulting in high fever of > 40°C accompanied by headache. Onset of symptoms usually begins 6 to 30 days after exposure.

LABORATORY DIAGNOSIS

Culturing of specimens from the patient's blood, faeces or bone marrow on bismuth sulfite agar forms jet black colonies with distinctly characteristic metallic sheen of *S.* Typhi.

Widal test - Tube agglutination test to detect antibodies against *S.* Typhi antigens.

Typhidot test to detect IgM and IgG antibodies against the outer membrane protein (OMP) of *S.* Typhi. IgM reveals recent infection and IgG signifies remote infection.

PREVENTION

Chlorination of drinking water, adequate hand washing with soap and water after using the bathroom and proper food handling are important to prevent infection.

VACCINATION

Two vaccines are available:

- TAB vaccine (killed whole cell vaccine): vaccine is given in 2 doses of 0.5 mL subcutaneously at an interval of 4–6 weeks followed by a booster dose every 3 years.
- Ty 21 (typhoral): (live attenuated oral vaccine): 3 to 4 doses are given orally on alternate days to children.

TREATMENT

Typhoid is treated with chloramphenicol (introduced in 1948, is effective, however, requires long treatment of 250 capsules).

It is replaced with safer and most effective drugs: azithromycin, fluoroquinolones and third-generation cephalosporins.

SALMONELLOSIS (*SALMONELLA* GASTROENTERITIS)

Salmonellosis or ***Salmonella* gastroenteritis**, a food-borne infection caused by two serovars of *Salmonella* (*S.* Typhimurium and *S.* Enteritidis), is characterized by diarrhoea, fever, abdominal cramps, nausea and vomiting. It is one of the most common causes of diarrhoea responsible for infecting 1.4 million people and causing 1 lakh deaths every year globally.

Infection occurs by eating the contaminated meat, eggs, milk or coconut meals. Other foods contaminated with manure can also act as source of infection. A small number of salmonellae (infective dose as small as 1000 bacteria) generally found in foods cause salmonellosis. The salmonellae first invade the intestinal mucosa, multiply within the muscosal cells resulting in inflammation. After 12 to 36 hours of infection, the patient shows a moderate fever, accompanied by nausea, abdominal pain, cramps and diarrhea. During the acute phase of illness, over 1 billion salmonellae can be found in the faeces of an infected person.

Occasionally, bacilli cross the epithelial cells lining of the intestinal tract and enter the lymphatic system and bloodstream resulting in **septic shock** in infants and in the elderly, a systemic disease.

DIAGNOSIS

Diagnosis is made by isolating the pathogen from the patient's stool or from leftover food on specialized selective and differential media, as well as by serotyping. Currently, PCR-based tests are used to identify the common clinical serotypes: Typhimurium and Enteritidis, even in small numbers, within a short span of time, about 5 hours.

PREVENTION

- Follow good sanitation practices to prevent contamination at all stages of food chain- from agricultural production → processing → manufacturing → preparation of foods in both commercial establishments and at home.
- Practise good personal hygiene.

- The five keys to safer food for food handlers are:
  - Keep clean
  - Separate raw and cooked food
  - Cook thoroghly to destroy salmonellae (e.g. chicken at 76–82°C and ground beef at 71°C)
  - Proper refrigeration of foods to prevent increase in bacterial numbers
  - Use safe water and raw materials.

TREATMENT

- It is self-limiting, most people recover in 4–7 days without any medication.
- Some patients only need fluids (electrolytes), orally delivered directly into a vein (intravenous) to recover in less than a week.
- Loperamide (Imodium A–D) are used to relieve cramping.

KEY POINTS

- *Salmonella* is a Gram-negative, nonsporing, motile bacillus with more than 2600 serotypes (= serovars).
- Enteric fever includes typhoid fever and paratyphoid fever caused by *Salmonella* serotype Typhi and *Salmonella* Paratyphi A and B, respectively
- *Salmonella* gastroenteritis, caused by *Salmonella* Typimurium and *Salmonella* Enteritidis, a food-borne infection, is characterized by nausea and diarrhoea.
- Widal test, a tube agglutination test, is used to detect antibodies against *Salmonella* Typhi antigens.

IMPORTANT QUESTIONS

1. Describe briefly:
   (a) *Salmonella* taxonomy
   (b) What is the causative agent of typhoid fever? How to diagnose it? Vaccines used to prevent it.
   (c) Enteric fever
   (d) *Salmonella* gastroenteritis or food poisoning.

MULTIPLE-CHOICE QUESTIONS

1. Which of the following serotypes cause/s enteric fever in humans?
   (a) *Salmonella* Paratyphi A
   (b) *Salmonella* Paratyphi B
   (c) *Salmonella* Typhi
   (d) All of the above.
2. For detection of *carriers* in typhoid fever, which of the following specimens is most appropriate?
   (a) Faeces (b) Urine
   (c) Sputum (d) Blood.
3. Which of the following serotypes of *Salmonella* can cause gastroenteritis (food poisoning)?
   (a) *S.* Typhimurium (b) *S.* Typhi
   (c) *S. enterica* (d) All of the above.
4. Infective dose of salmonellae to cause typhoid fever is:
   (a) 10 bacilli (b) 100 bacilli
   (c) 1000 bacilli (d) 10,000–1,00,000 bacilli.
5. Recovered typhoid patients who harbour the pathogen in the gallbladder and continue to shed bacilli for several months are called:
   (a) Acute carriers (b) Chronic carriers
   (c) Permanent carries (d) All of the above.

ANSWERS TO MCQS

1. (d) 2. (a) 3. (a) 4. (d) 5. (b).

38

Shigella: A Gram-negative Bacillus

Bacillary dysentery

The genus *Shigella* (named after **Kiyoshi Shiga**, a Japanese microbiologist, who first discovered it in 1897) is a Gram-negative, notmotile, non-lactose fermenting, non-capsulated, rod-shaped bacterium. Shigellae are primarily human parasites and are the causative agents of **shigellosis** (also called **bacillary dysentery**) characterized by frequent defecation of watery stool filled with mucus and blood. *Shigella*, a typical member of *Enterobacteriaceae*, is genetically closely related to *Escherichia coli*.

MORPHOLOGY

Shigellae are nonmotile, non-encapsulated, non-endosporic, short (2–4 μm long × 0.6 μm wide), Gram-negative rods (bacilli).

CULTURAL CHARACTERISTICS

They are aerobes and facultative anaerobes, with a temperature ranging from 10°C–45°C (37°C optimum) and pH 7.4. They grow well on ordinary culture media (e.g., nutrient agar, MacConkey agar). On MacConkey agar, the colonies are colourless or pale as they are lactose-negative in contrast to pink colonies in *E. coli* (a rapid lactose-fermenter) (Fig. 38.1).

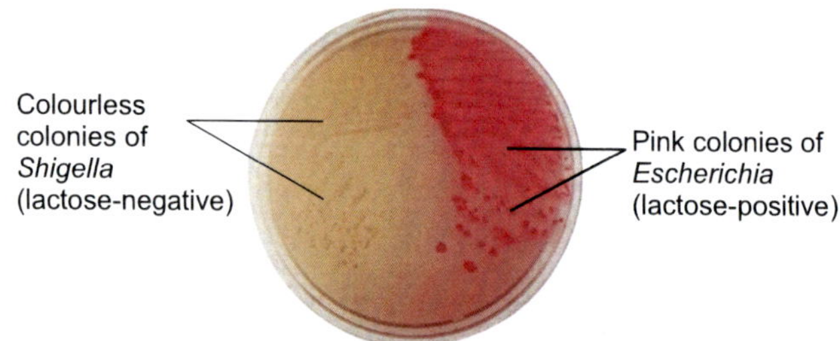

Fig. 38.1 ***Shigella*** **spp. (left) and Escherichia coli (right) growth on MacConkey agar.**

BIOCHEMICAL REACTIONS

They do not ferment lactose following overnight incubation (i.e., **lactose-negative**) with the exception of *S. sonnei*, which is a late lactose fermenter.

CLASSIFICATION

Shigellae are classified into four species or subgroups based on the combination of serological and biochemical tests.

Mannitol Nonfermenter

- Group A (*S. dysenteriae*, 12 serotypes)

Mannitol Fermenters

- Group B (*S. flexneri*, 6 serotypes)
- Group C (*S. boydii*, 18 serotypes)
- Group D (*S. sonnei*, 1 serotype)

Group A, B and C are vely similar physiologically while group D can be differentiated from other senotypes by positive β–D galactosidase and ornithine decarboxylase biochemical tests.

RESISTANCE

- Shigellae can survive in ice for 1–6 months.
- They can be killed by heating at 56°C in 60 minutes and by phenol in 30 minutes.
- In faeces, they die within hours due to the acidity produced by the most resistant species.

SHIGELLOSIS

Shigellosis, also known as **bacillary dysentry,** is a bloody diarrhoeal disease caused by *Shigella* spp. Globally, it occurs in at least 80 million people and results in about 7 lakh deaths a year, especially children. The disease is more common in the developing world. Outbreaks are most often seen in families, childcare settings and schools.

It can be caused by any of four species of *Shigella*: *S. dysenteriae*, *S. boydii*, *S. flexneri* and *S. sonnei* in descending order of severity of symptoms. *S. flexneri* is the most common species in our country, while *S. sonnei* in the United States. *S. dysenteriae* is the most serious pathogen causing severe dysentery and prostration due to the production of an exotoxin – the **shigatoxin** similar to that associated with enterohaemorrhagic *E. coli* (EHEC). Spread of shigellae takes place only from person to person by the faecal oral route. As few as 10 bacteria can initiate infection (i.e., infective dose is very low 10–100 bacteria), hence spread is easy in situations where sanitation or personal hygiene is poor.

SYMPTOMS

Frequent bouts of **watery diarrhoea** (as many as 20 bowel movements/day) with blood and mucus in stools are the main symptoms of shigellosis. Abdominal cramps, fever are the additional symptoms.

PATHOGENICITY

Shigella infection occurs by ingestion of shigellae, fewer than 100 bacterial cells are enough to cause an infection. Bacilli are not affected by stomach acidity. Although the bacteria proliferate to immense numbers in the small intestine, they generally invade the epithelial lining of the colon, causing severe inflammation and ulceration, finally death of the cells lining the colon. Dysentery is the result of damage to the intestinal wall. *Shigella* bacteria rarely invade the bloodstream.

Haemolytic-uremic syndrome (HUS), kidney failure, may occur as a complication in severe cases due to the shigatoxin produced by the bacterium.

Bacillary dysentery has a short incubation period, 24–48 hours, post-exposure.

LABORATORY DIAGNOSIS

- Diagnosis is usually based on the recovery of shigellae from diarrhoeal faecal sample (stool) or from the rectal swab taken from the ulcer by culturing on MacConkey agar or HE agar as colourless colonies.
- **Slide agglutination** with polyvalent and monovalent sera is assayed to confirm the identification of *Shigella*.

PREVENTION

- There is no vaccine to prevent shigellosis.
- Good personal hygiene, i.e., washing hands with soap and water before and after using the bathroom or change of a diaper, and before eating or preparing food.

TREATMENT

- Mild diarrhoeal infection recovers without any treatment in 5 to 7 days, however, patients should drink plenty of fluids to prevent dehydration.

- Antibiotic therapy is desired only in severe cases of diarrhoea. Ciprofloxacin, a quinolone (for adults) and azithromycin (for children) are the drugs of choice.

KEY POINTS

- Shigellae, the causative agent of bacillary dysentery, are nonmotile, Gram-negative, non-lactose fermenting bacilli.
- The **infective dose of shigellae** is small (10–100 organisms) and are unaffected by gastric acid or bile.
- *Shigella* diarrhoea usually contains blood and mucus in stool.
- Quinolones (e.g., ciprofloxacin) are the drugs of choice to treat severe bacillary dysentery.

IMPORTANT QUESTIONS

1. Briefly describe shigellosis (or bacillary dysentery).

MULTIPLE-CHOICE QUESTIONS

1. Shigellosis (bacillary dysentery) is caused by any of the four known species of *Shigella* bacteria. True or False?
2. *Shigella* bacteria invade the bloodstream and cause bacillary dysentery (shigellosis). True or False?
3. All of the following are opportunistic enteric bacteria EXCEPT:
   (a) *Proteus* (b) *Klebsiella*
   (c) *Shigella* (d) *Escherichia coli*.
4. Infective dose of *Shigella* bacilli causing bacillary dysentery is:
   (a) 1–05 bacilli
   (b) 10–100 bacilli
   (c) 1000–10,000 bacilli
   (d) 10,000 – 1,00,000 bacilli.
5. All are features of *Shigella*, the cause of bacillary dysentery, EXCEPT:
   (a) Gram-negative
   (b) Motile
   (c) Nonfermenter of lactose
   (d) Infective dose very low (10–100 bacteria).

ANSWERS TO MCQs

1. True 2. False 3. (c) 4. (b) 5. (b).

39

Pseudomonas: A Gram-negative Aerobic Motile Bacillus

Opportunistic nosocomial pathogen: Invades surgical wounds, burns, lungs

The genus *Pseudomonas* is an aerobic, Gram-negative, asporgenous, motile bacillus, belonging to the family *Pseudomonaceae*. It was named from the Greek *pseudo* (false) and *monas* ("unit") in 1894 by the German botanist **Walter Migula**. It contains 191 species occurring in soil, water and plants.

Pseudomonas aeruginosa, an opportunist pathogen, is clinically the most significant species. It is one of the most serious causes of nosocomial infections.

PSEUDOMONAS AERUGINOSA

The species name *aeruginosa* is named from Latin word *aerúgo* (= "copper rust" or verdigris, hence green) referring to the greenish - blue colour of bacterial colonies produced on the agar media. This bacterium can cause diseases in plants and animals including humans. It is the main cause of death among patients with cystic fibrosis.

MORPHOLOGY

It is a Gram-negative nonsporing, non-capsulated rod measuring 1.5 – 3.0 μm × 0.5 μm and actively motile by means of a single polar flagellum.

GROWTH CHARACTERISTICS

P. aeruginosa has very simple nutritional requirements. It is often observed *"growing in distilled water"*. It is an obligate aerobe and readily grows on ordinary culture media (e.g., nutrient agar, MacConkey agar and blood agar). Its optimum temperature for growth is 37°C, and it is able to grow at temperatures as high as 42°C and as low as 2°C (2 – 42°C). The optimum pH is between 6.6 and 7.6.

After aerobic incubation at 37°C for 24 hours, on nutrient agar, the colonies are 2-4 mm, opaque irregular, greenish, with a distinctive sweetish, earthy or grape-like smell, are characteristic features of the organism.

On MacConkey agar, colonies are non-lactose fermenting (2-3 mm) with a brownish green colouration and irregular edges.

On blood agar, the colonies are β-hemolytic, 4 mm in diameter with characteristic blue-green colour due to the pyocyanin and pyoverdin pigments and a grape-like odour due to aminoacetophenone (Fig. 39.1).

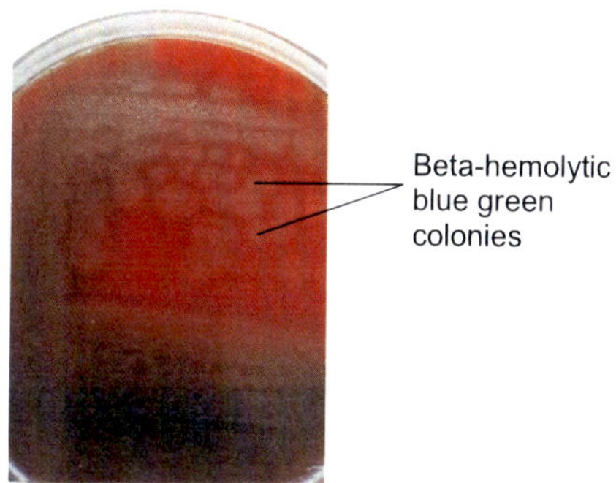

Fig. 39.1 ***Pseudomonas aeruginosa* on blood agar.** Coloines are bluish-green and beta-hemolytic and grape-like odour.

The colonies of *P. aeruginosa,* isolates recovered from respiratory secretions of patients with cystic fibrosis on blood agar, are highly mucoid, non-pigmented, usually smaller in size (2 to 3 mm in diameter) than those of the typical pigmented strains.

PIGMENTS

P. aeruginosa strains produce two types of soluble pigments:

- **Pyoverdin** (or **fluorescein**)—yellowish fluorescent pigment, sometimes detected with ultraviolet light.
- **Pyocyanin**—blue pigment produced abundantly in media. Pyocyanin (from *pyocyaneus* = blue pus) which is a characteristic of suppurative infections caused by *P. aeruginosa*.

RESISTANCE/SENSITIVITY TO PHYSICAL AND CHEMICAL AGENTS AND ANTIBIOTICS

The bacterium is resistant to high concentrations of salts and dyes, weak antiseptics and can even grow in certain types of quaternary ammonium compounds, hexachlorophane, soaps and iodine solutions.

It is resistant to many commonly used antibiotics and is, therefore, a dangerous and dreaded pathogen. However, it is tolerant to temperature and is easily killled by heating at 55°C for one hour.

DISEASES

It causes mild and superficial infections in healthy persons (i.e., community infections) and an opportunist causing more severe infections in hospitalized patients (nosocomical infections).

Community infections: Otitis externa, varicose ulcers, jacuzzi rash or whirlpool rash and industrial eye injuries.

Nosocomial infections: Urinary tract infections, pneumonia, chronic lung infections, endocarditis, dermatitis, and septicaemia.

PATHOGENESIS

Pseudomonad infections are both invasive and toxigenic. These infections are composed of three distinct stages: bacterial attachment and colonization; local invasion; and disseminated systemic disease. However, the disease process may stop at any stage.

LABORATORY DIAGNOSIS

Diagnosis depends upn the isloation of the bacterium on blood agar or MacConkey agar from the specimen (pus, wound swab, urine, sputum, CSF or blood) and its identification. It is identified on the basis of the characteristic blue-green pigments produced in the medium, Gram-negative bacillus, rod with a single polar flagellum, inability to ferment lactose, a positive oxidase reaction, its fruity odours and its ability to grow at 42°C.

TREATMENT

P. aeruginosa is a multidurg resistant organism. Although it is susceptible to gentamicin, tobramycin, colistin and fluoroquinolones, resistant forms have developed. A combination of gentamicin and carbenicillin, or imipenem and gentamicin is frequently used to treat *Pseudomonas* infections.

PREVENTION

The spread of *P. aeruginosa* can be prevented by observing:

- Aseptic techniques by thoroughly washing hands.
- Careful cleaning of respirators, catheters and other instruments in hospitals.

- By proper isolation procedures in hospitals.
- By using properly cleaned hot bath tubs and swimming pools in hotels. Removing swimming garments and shower with soap after getting out of water.

KEY POINTS

- *Pseudomonas aeruginosa*, a member of the normal flora of intestinal tract, is an aerobic, Gram-negative, oxidase-positive bacillus, motile by one single polar flagellum.
- It is an opportunistic pathogen causing nosocomial infections (UTI, bed sores, burns and eye) and community infections (otitis externa, varicose ulcers, jaczzi rash or whirlpool rash).
- *P. aeruginosa* is resistant to commonly used antibiotics, antiseptics and disinfectants.

IMPORTANT QUESTIONS

1. Briefly describe the major characteristics and human diseases caused by *Pseudomonas aeruginosa*.

MULTIPLE-CHOICE QUESTIONS

1. All are *true* for *Pseudomonas aeruginosa* EXCEPT:
   (a) Aerobic
   (b) Gram-negative bacillus
   (c) Motile by peritrichous flagella
   (d) Oxidase positive.
2. A unique feature of many isolates of *Pseudomonas* useful in identification is:
   (a) Motility
   (b) Faecal colour
   (c) Fluorescent green pigments
   (d) Drug resistance.
3. Which of the following infections can be caused by *Pseudomonas aeruginosa*?
   (a) Wound and burn infection
   (b) Urinary tract infection
   (c) Jacuzzi rash
   (d) All of the above.

4. Which bacteria can grow in distilled water and in some disinfectants?
   (a) *Salmonella enterica*
   (b) *Escherichia coli*
   (c) *Pseudomonas aeruginosa*
   (d) *Shigella dysenteriae.*
5. Which of the following is the antipseudomonal penicillin?
   (a) Amoxicillin (b) Penicillin G
   (c) Cephalexin (d) Carbenicillin.

ANSWERS TO MCQs

1. (c) 2. (c) 3. (d) 4. (c) 5. (d).

40

Brucella: A Gram-negative Aerobic Coccobacillius

Brucellosis (undulant fever)

The genus *Brucella* is an obligately aerobic, nonmotile, faintly stained Gram-negative, cocooid rods, a member of the family *Brucellaceae*. The taxon was named after **Sir David Bruce**, a Scottish physician, who first recognized the organism causing undulant (Malta) fever.

Brucella is a monospecific genus (*Brucella melitensis*, the type species, named after the Island of Malta (*Melita*) where the organism was first isolated by Bruce in 1893) with the multiple biovars. In practice, it is more useful to refer to separate species, 12 in number, which have different preferrential host specificities.

Brucellae are obligate parasites and cause **brucellosis** in humans and **abortion** in cattle, pigs and goats. Four species of *Brucella*, that are the most common human pathogens, come from different hosts:

- *B. melitensis*—sheep and goats
- *B. abortus*—cattle
- *B. canis*—dogs
- *B. suis*—pigs

B. melitensis is the most virulent and invasive species and is responsible for most human infections.

MORPHOLOGY

Brucellae are very small (0.6–1.5 μm × 0.5–0.7 μm), faintly stained Gram-negative coccoid rods (coccobacilli) with a microscopic appearance of fine sand (Fig. 40.1) The rods are noncapsulate, nonmotile and nonsporing that occur singly, in groups, or short chains.

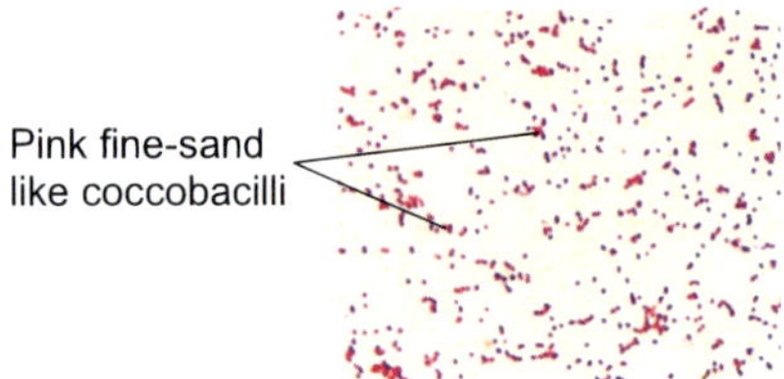

Fig. 40.1 Modified Gram stain of *Brucella*. Small Gram-negative coccobacilli showing a "fine-sand" appearance.

CULTURAL CHARACTERISTICS

Brucella spp. are strict aerobes, but some brucellae (e.g., *B. ovis* and some strains of *B. abortus*) are **capnophilic** requring 5-10% CO_2 for primary isolation. Growth *in vitro* is slow and primary isolation may require 4 weeks of incubation.

The optimum pH for growth is 6.6–7.4 and temperature 37°C (range 20–40°C). Growth does not occur on rountine media, *Brucella* agar, blood agar, chocolate agar, albumin agar and trypticase soy agar are used for their isolation. After incubation at 37°C for 48 hours, the colonies are smooth, nonpigmented, moist, transparent and glistening (honey droplet) (Fig. 40.2).

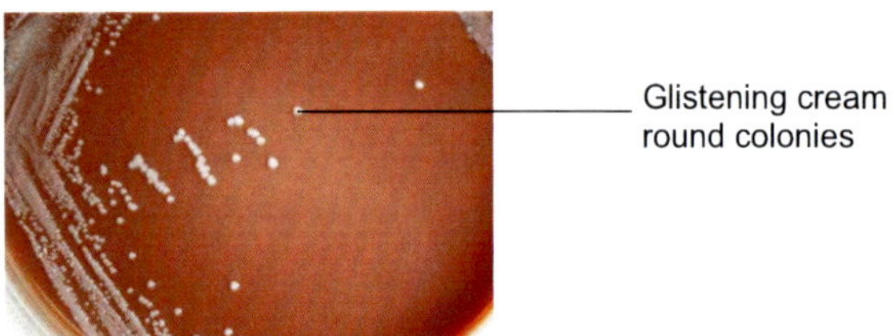

Fig. 40.2 *Brucella abortus* on chocolate agar. Colonies are small, round, raised, white to cream, and glistening at 35°C under 5 to 10% CO_2 after 7 days.

BIOCHEMICAL REACTIONS

Brucella is generally oxidase-positive and urease-positive. They ferment carbohydrates without producing acid and gas.

BRUCELLOSIS

Brucellosis is a *Brucella* caused infectious disease that spreads from animals to humans. The infection by ingestion of unpasteurized dairy products, undercooked meat from infected animals, and inhalation of infected aerosols. If affects thousands of people worldwide, fewer than 100 thousand cases per year in India. It is called by several other names: **Undulant fever**, **Malta fever**, **Mediterranen fever** and **Bang disease**.

The disease can be caused by any of the four species of ***Brucella*** (*S. melitensis, B. abortus, B canis* and *B. suis*) that come from different animal hosts. *B. melitensis* is the most virulent and invasive species causing brucellosis in humans.

Major symptoms are intermittent (recurrent) fever (38-41°C or even higher), profuse sweating, chills, fatigue, pain in muscles, joint, and/or back, in addition to swelling of the liver, heart (endocarditis), testicle and scrotum area. Brucellosis is often called **undulant fever** because of the periodic nocturnal fever that may occur over weeks, months or years, especially in untreated cases.

Eating undercooked meat or consuming unpasteurized/raw dairy products from infected animals is the most common mode of infection. Inhalation or breathing of aerosol, very few organisms (as few as 10-100), is another source of infection.

DIAGNOSIS

Culturing of *Brucella* from blood and bone marrow specimens is the gold standared in the laboratory diagnosis of brucellosis.

Blood is inoculated into trypticase soy broth or serum dextrose broth and incubated at 37°C in the presence of 5-10% CO_2. Subculturing is made on the solid medium every 3–5 days for 8 weeks, before being discarded as negative.

Biphasic blood culture bottle (*Castaneda method*), which contains both solid and liquid media (Fig. 40.3) inoculated with blood or bone marrow sample and incubated at 35–37°C for 21 days under a 5–10% CO_2. In positive case, the colonies appear on the slant. This technique is preferred due to three reasons: Frequent subculturing is not needed, reduces the chances of contamination, and risk of infection to laboratory workers.

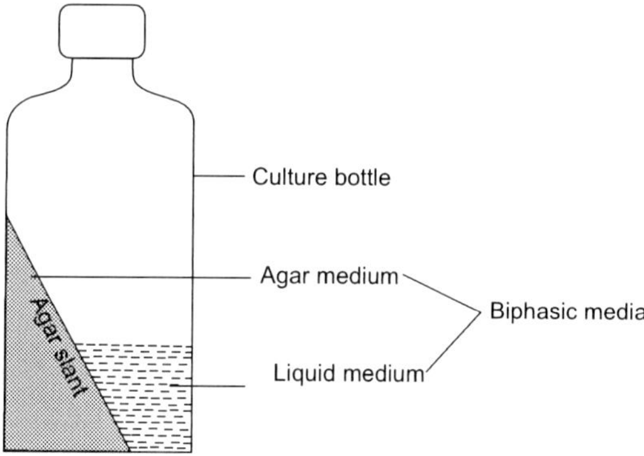

Fig. 40.3 Castaneda system for blood culture for *Brucella*. This system uses biphasic media (liquid and solid) in the same bottle. The inoculum is added to the broth and at the time of subculturing the bottle is simply tilted to allow the broth to flow over the agar slant.

Serological testing is done to detect the antibodies against the bacterium by the *standard tube agglutination test.*

TREATMENT

Brucellosis is treated by combination therapy. Two antibiotics, doxycycline or trimethoprim/sulfamethoxazole plus gentamicin, streptomycin or rifampin for prolonged period varying from 14 to 72 days.

PREVENTION

- Avoiding the consumption of undercooked/raw meat, unpasteurized milk, cheese and ice products.
- Vaccinating the domestic animals.

KEY POINTS

- **Brucellosis** is a *Brucella* caused zoonotic infection that occurs by ingestion of raw milk or undercooked meat from the infected animals.
- Brucellae are very small coccobacilli with a microscopic appearance of "fine sand".
- Of the four *Brucella* spp. causing brucellosis in humans, *B. melitensis*, pathogenic to sheep and goats, is the most virulent bacterium.
- Currently *Brucella* is recognized as a monospecific genus (*Brucella melitensis*).

IMPORTANT QUESTIONS

1. Describe in brief the causative agent, diagnosis and treatment of brucellosis in humans.

MULTIPLE-CHOICE QUESTIONS

1. Brucellosis is a zoonotic disease transmitted through unpasteurized/raw milk. True or False?
2. Which of the following organisms causes undulant fever?
   (a) *Legionella* (b) *Bordetella*
   (c) *Brucella* (d) *Yersinia.*

3. The most virulent and pathogenic species causing brucellosis in humans belongs to

(a) *Brucella canis* (b) *Brucella melitensis*

(c) *Brucella suis* (d) *Brucella abortus.*

4. Castaneda method of blood culture is used to diagnose the pathogen:

(a) *Rickettsia* (b) *Brucella*

(c) *Pseudomonas* (d) *Brukholderia.*

ANSWERS TO MCQs

1. True 2. (c) 3. (b) 4. (b).

41

Bordetella: An Aerobic Encapsulated Gram-negative Coccobacillus

Whooping cough

The genus *Bordetella* is an aerobic, Gram-negative, coccobacillus, belonging to the family *Alcaligenaceae* (*Burkholderiales*). It was named after **Jules Bordet**, who with **0. Gengou**, first isolated this organism.

Of the 14 known species, *Bordetella pertussis* is a serious pathogen which causes **pertussis**, or **whooping cough**.

BORDETELLA PERTUSSIS

B. pertussis, the type species and the causative agent of whooping cough, was first isolated from sputum of children by **Bordet** and **Gengou** and named in 1906 after Latin words: *per* = severe, extreme + *tussis* = cough, i.e., severe cough, whooping cough.

MORPHOLOGY

It is a short (0.5–2.0 μm × 0.3–0.5 μm), thin, faint, staining, Gram-negative bacillus having a "doughnut"-like appearance. The virulent strains are capsulated. The bacteria are either single or arranged in pairs or small groups. They are easier to see when carbol fuchsin is used as the counterstain instead of safranin in Gram staining.

CULTURAL CHARACTERISTICS

It is a strictly aerobic organism, grows optimally at 35–36°C. It requires rich media supplemented with blood, colonies are visible only after 3 days of incubation under 5 to 7% CO_2, *B. pertussis* being the slowest growing bacterium among the *Bordetella* species.

Bordet-Gengou (BG) agar, which incorporates potato infusion, (glycerine-potato-blood agar) is the classic medium used for its isolation.

Colonies on BG agar, after 5 days of incubation under a humid 5% CO_2 atmosphere at 35°C are small and domed, with the typical "mercury drop" appearance (Fig. 41.1). A zone of beta hemolysis is observed around the colonies with prolonged incubation.

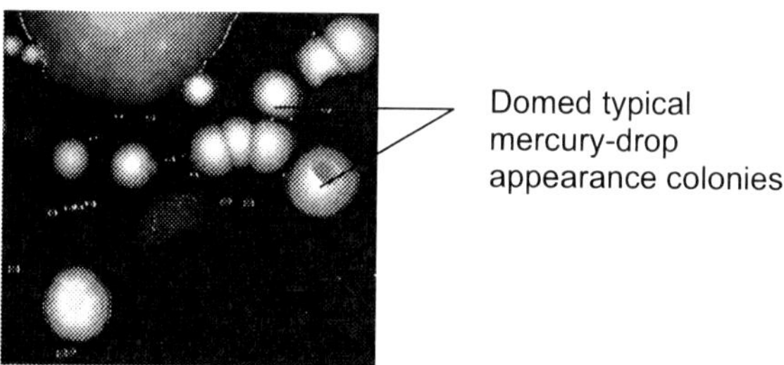

Fig. 41.1 ***Bordetella pertussis*** **on BG agar from a nosopharyngeal swab.**

BIOCHEMICAL REACTIONS

B. pertussis is catalase and oxidase-positive. It lacks the ability to ferment sugars, produce nitrate, utilize citrate (citrate –ve) or split urea (urease –ve).

SUSCEPTIBILITY TO PHYSICAL AND CHEMICAL AGENTS

It can be killed easily by mild heating (56°C for 30 minutes), drying and disinfectants. It survives on glass (5 days), cloth (3 days) and on paper (a few hours).

ANTIGENIC CONSTITUENTS AND VIRULENCE FACTORS

Antigenic constituents and virulence factors of *B. pertussis* include: heat labile toxin, tracheal toxin, lipopolysaccharide endotoxin, pertussis toxin, adenylate cyclase, haemolysin, filamentous haemagglutination and agglutinogens.

WHOOPING COUGH

Whooping cough, also called **pertussis** and **100–day cough**, caused by *Bordetella pertussis*, is a highly contagious respiratory infection associated with uncontrollable violent coughing that sounds like **whoop** and is particularly dangerous for infants. Outbreaks of the disease were first recorded in the 16th century. Millions of people are infected globally resulting in thousands of deaths each year, especially in the developing countries. If can cause serious illness in babies, children, teens and adults.

It is an air-borne pathogen which spreads easily through the cough and sneeze of an infected person. This bacterium lives in the mouth, nose and throat and is confined only to humans, hence the disease spreads from person-to-person.

The course of whooping cough follows 3 stages:

1. *Catarrhal (runny nose) stage* that lasts 2–3 weeks
2. *Paroxysmal stage:* prolonged sieges of coughing
3. *Convalescent stage:* Recovery with gradual clearing of symptoms that can last for months.

The bacteria after its entry, first colonizes the nasopharynx, grows, and spreads to the trachea, where they attach to the cialited cells, first impeding their ciliary action and then progressively destroying the ciliated cells, thereby, preventing the ciliary escalator system from moving mucus.

Two toxins: *tracheal cytotoxin,* a fixed cell wall fraction of the bacterium, damages the tracheal cells, and *pertussis toxin,* moves into the bloodstream, responsible for systemic symptoms, are involved in pathogenesis. Damage of tracheal cells and accumulation of fluid (i.e., mucus) induces the paroxysmal cough. A rapid succession of cough makes breathing difficult. Gasping for air between coughs causes a whooping sound, hence the informal name of the disease. Coughing episodes occur several times a day – lasting for 10 or more weeks, hence the phrase *"100-day cough"*.

Besides a cough that sounds like whoop, symptoms include a running nose, sneezing and nasal congestion. The first symptoms generally appear 7–10 days after infection (however, the incubation period can be as long as 21 days).

Whooping cough is a clinical diagnosis.

LABORATORY DIAGNOSIS

- Culturing of a nasopharyngeal swab on a nutrient medium (Bordet-Gengou medium or Regan-Lowe agar). Bacteria can be recovered from the patient only during the first 3 weeks of illness.
- Other methods include:
  - Polymerase chain reaction (PCR)
  - Direct fluorescent-antibody (DFA) assay
  - Serological methods (e.g., complement fixation test).

TREATMENT

Macrolides are highly effective in eradicating *B pertussis* from the nasopharynx. Erythromycin, azithromycin, clarithromycin, and trimethoprim sulfamethoxzale are the drugs used to treat whooping cough.

PREVENTION

It can be prevented with the *pertussis vaccine* which is a part of the **DTaP** (diphtheria, tetanus, acellular pertussis). DTaP immunizations are routinely given in five doses before a child's sixth birthday.

In addition to childhood vaccination, booster shot of **Tdap**, triple antigen that contains a lower quantity of diphtheria (d) acellular pertussis (ap) in the tetanus toxoid (T) adult formulation.

KEY POINTS

- *Bordetella pertussis*, the causative agent of whooping cough, is strictly aerobic, Gram-negative, oxidase-positive coccobacillus.
- Whooping cough (pertussis) consists of three stages: catarrhal (initial), paroxymal (second) and covalescence (third).
- Severe cough that sounds like a whoop, running nose, sneezing and congestion are the symptoms of pertussis.

IMPORTANT QUESTIONS

1. Write a short note on whooping cough (or pertussis).

MULTIPLE-CHOICE QUESTIONS

1. Which of the following organisms causes whooping cough?
   (a) Influenza virus (b) *Bordetella pertussis*
   (c) *Pneumocystis jirovecii* (d) *Mycoplasma pnemoniae.*
2. A contagious and potentially fatal respiratory infection associated with uncontrollable coughing and transmitted through droplets is:
   (a) Pertussis (b) Legionellosis
   (c) Brucellosis (d) Influenza.
3. The only known reservoir of *Bordetella pertussis*, the causative agent of whooping cough, is:
   (a) Cattle (b) Birds
   (c) Humans (d) Dogs.

4. Whooping cough spreads from infected animals to humans and not from humans to humans. True or False?
5. Which culture medium is employed most frequently for the isolation of *Bordetella pertussis*, the causative agent of whooping cough?
   (a) Nutrient agar
   (b) Bordet-Gengou (BG) agar
   (c) Chocolate agar
   (d) None of the above.

ANSWERS TO MCQs

1. (b) 2. (a) 3. (c) 4. False 5. (b).

42

Legionella: An Aerobic Motile Gram-negative Bacillus

Legionaires' disease; Pontiac fever

The genus *Legionella* is an aerobic, motile, pleomorphic, Gram-negative bacillus belonging to the family *Legionellaceae*. *Legionella* was discovered in 1977 that acquired its name after **America Legion**—an association of US military veterans among whom an outbreak of a "**mystery disease**" was reported for the first time in 1976 by an unknown organism.

Of the over 50 spp. recorded in varied aquatic habitats, *Lagionella pneumophila* (lung-loving) is clinically the most significant. Two main diseases caused are:

- Legionnares' disease (LD)—pneumonia-like illness.
- Pontiac fever—Flu-like mild self-limiting illness.

LEGIONELLA PNEUMOPHILA

MORPHOLOGY

It is a thin, nonspore-forming, pleomorphic, faint-staining, Gram-negative, rod-shaped bacterium varying from coccobacilli (1 – 2 μm × 0.3 – 0.9 μm) to filaments (up to 20 μm in length), motile with one or more polar or subpolar lagella (Fig. 42.1).

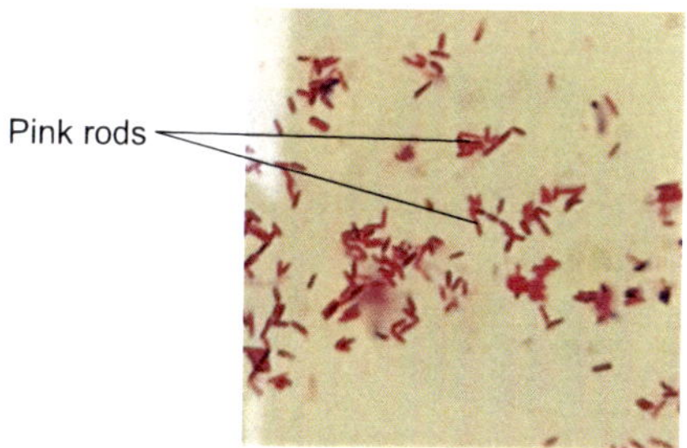

Fig. 42.1 Gram stain of *Legionella*. Faintly stained short Gram-negative bacilli.

CULTURAL CHARACTERISTICS

It is a strict aerobe growing best at 35°C (range 29 – 40°C), pH 6.9 requiring complex media such as **BCYE** (buffered charcoal yeast extract) agar. After 3–7 days incubation at 35°C, the colonies resemble cut-glass (Figure 42.2).

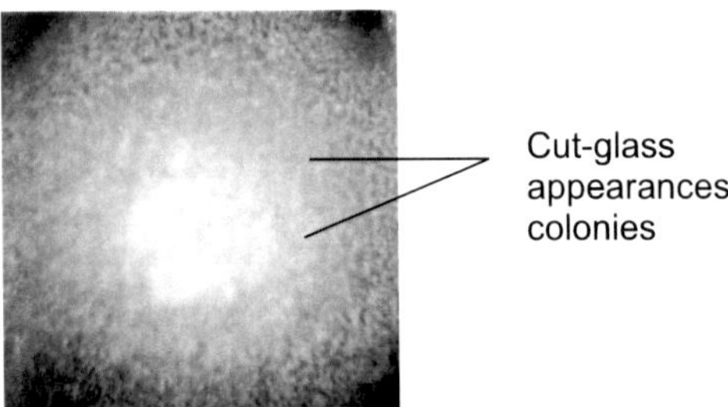

Fig. 42.2 ***Legionella pneumophila* on BCYE agar.** Colonies after 5 days of incubation at 35°C.

BIOCHEMICAL REACTIONS

It is catalase-positive and hydrolyses starch, gelatin and hippurate.

PATHOGENSIS

The natural habitat of *L. pneumophila* is water and widely distributed in varied aquatic habitats. Inhaling mist (bacteria) from these sources causes the disease.

The sources of infection include: hot and cold water taps, spa bath and spa pools, swimming pools, air-conditioning cooling towers, ice making machines, referigerated cabinets, dental equipment and water lines of hospitals.

LEGIONELLOSIS: LEGIONNARES' DISEASE, PONTAIC FEVER

The infections caused by *L. pneumophila* are called **legionellosis**. These occur in two distinct clinical forms:

1. **Legionnares' disease (LD)** is an acute infection of lungs that shows symptoms of both influenza (flu) and pneumonia, characterized by high fever (40.5°C), cough, chest pain, breathlessness. The illness may lead to respiratory failure and death.

   The disease was first recognized in 1976 after an outbreak of pneumonia at an **American Legion** convention in Philadelphia, a state of the United States.

2. **Pontaic fever** is an influenza-like mild and self-limiting illness that reveals fever, muscular aches and cough with spontaneous recovery after 2–5 days.

Infection results from inhalation of small water droplets of contaminated water sprays or mist. Incubation period ranges from 2 to 10 days though it may be longer. There is no direct person-to-person transmission.

LABORATORY DIAGNOSIS

- The best diagnostic method is to culture on a selective medium charcoal yeast extract agar at 35°C for 3-5 days from a sample of sputum (phlegum) or lung fluid.
- Other methods:
    - Microscopic examination of sputum by fluorescent antibody stain (DFA), a more sensitive method for detecting *L. pneumophila* directly than the Gram-stain method.
    - DNA probes using commercially available kit.

TREATMENT

A number of antibiotics are available to treat LD. Erythromycin and azithromycin or doxycycline are the drugs of choice.

PREVENTION

Legionellosis can be prevented by eradicating/killing the legionellae from water by the following ways:

- By managing the water system in hotels and hospitals by heating the hot water above 60°C before distribution.
- Disinfection with chlorine or other biocides of the infected water systems (e.g., cooling towers).
- No vaccine is available.

KEY POINTS

- **Legionnaires' disease** is caused by *Legionella pneumophila*, a Gram-negative, motile, pleomorphic bacillus.
- It is a noncommunicable lung infection transmitted by aerosols, from air conditioners, cooling towers and other aquatic habitats.
- LD is usually spread by breathing in mist that contains the *Legionella* bacteria.

- LD was named after the **American Legion**, Philadelphia (USA) among whom the disease "mystery disease" was first reported in 1976.

IMPORTANT QUESTIONS

1. Write short notes on:
   (a) Legionnaires' disease
   (b) *Legionella pneumophila.*

MULTIPLE-CHOICE QUESTIONS

1. The sources of infection of Legionnaires' disease (Legionellosis):
   (a) Air-conditioning cooling towers
   (b) Water taps
   (c) Ice machines
   (d) All of the above.
2. Which of the following is/are the major routes of transmission/ infection of *Legionella*?
   (a) Gastrointestinal tract
   (b) Skin
   (c) Respiratory tract
   (d) All of the above.

ANSWERS TO MCQs

1. (d) 2. (c).

43

Yersinia: A Gram-negative Pleomorphic Coccobacillus

Plague (black death); Gastroenteritis

Yersinia is a Gram-negative, pleomorphic (coccobacillus, straight rods, filamentous), nonspore-forming bacterium placed in the family *Enterobacteriaceae* (tribe *Yersiniae*).

The taxon was named for **Alexandre Yersin**, a French bacteriologist who first isolated the causative agent (in 1894) of the disease, known in Middle Ages as **Black Death**. This term comes from one of its characteristics, the dark blue areas of the skin caused by haemorrhages.

Black death (also known as the **Great Plague** or the **plague**) was one of the most devastating pandemics in human history that have killed 30% to 60% of Europe population between 1347 and 1351 and reducing the world population from 350 to 400 million in the 14th century.

Currently, *Yersinia* has 19 species, three of which are important human pathogens associated with **zoonotic** infections:

- *Yersinia pestis* – Plague
- *Yersinia pseudotuberculosis* — Gastroenteritis (Yersiniosis)
- *Yersinia enterocolitica* — Gastroenteritis (Yersiniosis)

YERSINIA PESTIS

Yersinia pestis (formerly called *Pasteurella pestis*), commonly named as the **plague bacillus**, was discovered in 1894 by **Alexandre Yersin** during an epidemic of plague.

MORPHOLOGY

It is a Gram-negative, nonmotile, stick-shaped (safety-pin appearance) bacillus (1-3 μm × 0.5 – 0.8 μm) showing a distinctive bipolar staining with an antiphagocytic slime layer (Fig. 43.1).

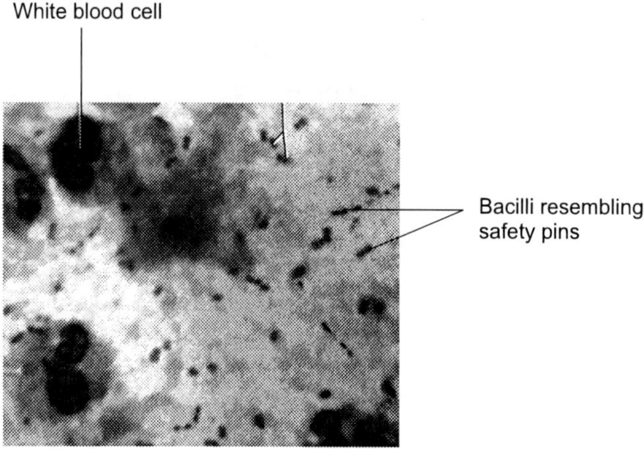

Fig. 43.1 ***Yersinia pestis*—Gram stained preparation from the blood of an infected mouse.** Gram-negative bacilli exhibiting a distinctive bipolar morphology reminiscent of a safety pin.

Under unfavourable conditions, it shows pleomorphism, the forms range from small cocci to yeast-like to safety pins and elongated filaments.

CULTURAL CHARACTERISTICS

It grows both aerobically and anaerobically at 0–37°C requiring simple nutritional requirements. Optimum temperature for growth is 27°C (14 – 37°C) and pH 7.2 (5.9 – 9.6 pH). On blood agar at 27°C after 24 hours incubation, the colonies are small, nonhemolytic, slightly viscid and translucent, however, look like fried-eggs (cauliflower-like) after prolonged incubation of 4–5 days.

On nutrient agar at 35°C, the colonies are pinpoint, and transparent.

SUSCEPTIBILITY

It is sensitive to heat (killed at 55°C in 5 minutes) and disinfectants (killed within 15 minutes in 0.5% phenol) and drying but remain viable in moist culture for many months, especially at low temperature.

BIOCHEMICAL REACTIONS

- It tests positive for catalase.
- Tests negative for oxidase, urease and indole.
- It ferments glucose, mannitol and maltose with the production of acid but no gas.

PATHOGENESIS

Y. pestis commonly called the **plague bacillus**, causes an infectious vector-borne zoonotic disease **plague** that exists in three clinical forms **bubonic, pneumonic** and **septicaemic**.

The plague bacillus is naturally parasitic in rodents (the primary host) and is transmitted by rat fleas (the vector) to humans (accidental host).

Infected humans may pass (spread) the causative agent to other humans. Symptoms develop after an incubation period of 1–7 days. These include: swollen lymph nodes which can be as large as chicken eggs in the groin, armpit or neck and may be tender and warm, fever, chills, headache, fatigue and muscle aches.

Three forms of plague are described below.

1. **Bubonic plague** is characterized by the enlarged lymph nodes or **buboes** which are formed due to the multiplication of the bacterium at the bite site. Further spread of bacilli from these primary buboes occurs to all parts of the body resulting to septicaemia, pneumonia or meningitis. It is the most common form of plague.
2. **Septicaemic plague** occurs when the bacteria enter the blood and proliferate causing septic shock. In this, the tissues turn black and die giving the skin a blackish colouration which in the past led to the name **Black Death** for plague.
3. **Pneumonic plague** is characterized by shortness of breath, cough with bloody mucus (sputum), high fever, and chest pain. Lung infection occurs by inhalation of aerosols from infected humans or animals. Incubation can be as short as 24 hours. The sputum becomes thin and blood-stained containing numerous bacilli, hence this form is highly contagious and can be fatal within 18 to 24 hours of the onset of fever.

LABORATORY DIAGNOSIS

Diagnosis is done by typically finding the bacterium in fluid/pus from a bubo (lymph node), blood or sputum by:

- Direct microscopic examination of smears of exudate or sputum stained with methylene blue or Giemsa stain for characteristic bipolar-stained coccobacilli.
- Culturing on blood agar at 27°C for identification of the bacterium is the best method.
- Rapid dipstick test that detects the specific *Y. pestis* antigens.
- PCR is the most rapid method used for diagnosis.

TREATMENT

Antibiotics used to treat plague are **streptomycin (the drug of choice)**, gentamicin, tetracycline and doxycycline.

PREVENTION

A killed or attenuated plague vaccine is available, however, WHO does not recommend vaccination, except for high-risk groups—veterinarians, laboratory and healthcare workers and military personnel.

YERSINIA ENTEROCOLITICA AND *Y. PSEUDOTUBERCULOSIS*

Yersinia enterocolitica and *Y. pseudotuberculosis* cause *Yersinia* gastroenteritis, or yersiniosis, a food-borne infection, characterized by diarrhoea, fever, headache and severe abdominal pain in the right lower part. The pain is often severe enough to cause a misdiagnosis of **appendicitis**. *Y. pseudotuberculosis* causes tuberculosis-like symptoms. These bacteria are intestinal inhabitants of many domestic animals, especially pigs and are transmitted in undercooked meat products (especially pork), unpasteurized milk and contaminated water. The symptoms generally appear 3 days after exposure.

Both these bacteria are urease-positive and oxidase-negative, Gram-negative rods and are distinctive as their ability to grow at refrigerated temperatures at 4°C. This ability increases their numbers in stored refrigerated blood, to the extent that their endotoxins can result in shock to the blood recipient.

In *Y. enterocolitica* the cells are small, plump, Gram-negative bacilli (2 μm × 0.8 μm) that appear coccoid with bipolar staining (Fig. 43.2). On blood agar at 35°C under 5% CO_2, the colonies are small (1-2 mm diameter), grey to greyish white after overnight incubation.

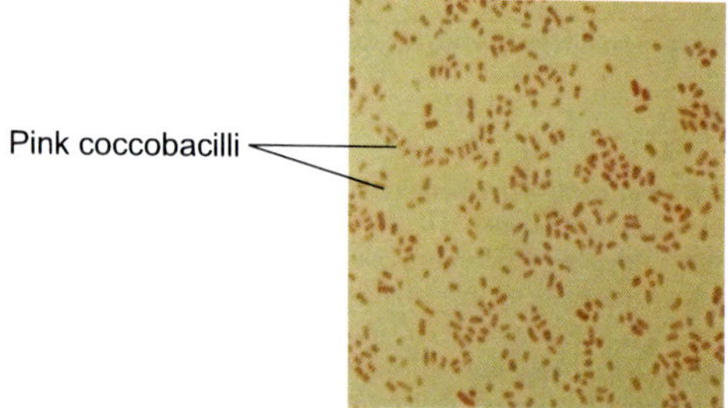

Fig. 43.2 Gram stain of *Yersinia enterocolitica*. Small, plump, Gram-negative bacilli appear coccoid with bioplar staining.

Y. pseudotuberculosis is a Gram-negative coccobacillus that grows slowly on blood and chocolate agar plates. It forms small grey and translucent colonies after 24 to 72 hours. Its growth is enhanced at a temperature lower than 28°C and shows motility at McConkey agar.

DIAGNOSIS

Laboratory diagnosis is done by culturing the organisms and demonstration of antibodies in patient's serum.

TREATMENT

Tetracycline is the drug of choice for treating *Y. enterocolitica* infection.

Y. pseudotuberculosis infection is treated with ampicillin, chloramphenicol, gentamicin or tetracycline.

KEY POINTS

- *Yersinia pestis* is a pleomorphic, capsulated, Gram-negative bacillus that appears bipolar, resembling a safety pin.
- *Yersinia pestis* shows characteristic **bipolar staining** in which the ends appear darker than the central part of rods.
- *Y. pestis* causes plague in humans that exists in three forms: bubonic plague, septicaemic plague and pneumonic plague.
- *Yersinia enterocolitica* and *Y. pseudotuberculosis* cause gastroenteritis (also called yersiniosis) and are usually acquired by ingestion of contaminated food, milk or water.

IMPORTANT QUESTIONS

1. Write short answers for the following:
   (a) How Black Death was named?
   (b) Three forms of plague.
2. Write short notes on:
   (a) Clinically important *Yersinia* spp.
   (b) Plague.

MULTIPLE-CHOICE QUESTIONS

1. Which of the following disease is named "Black Death"?
   (a) Malaria (b) Plague
   (c) Tuberculosis (d) Smallpox.

2. Bubonic plague is caused by
   (a) *Yersinia enerocolitica*
   (b) *Yersinia pseudotuberculosis*
   (c) *Yersinia pestis*
   (d) All of the above.
3. Plague is transmitted to humans by
   (a) Rat fleas (b) Ticks
   (c) Sand flies (d) Mites.
4. The primary host of *Yersinia pestis*, the causative agent of plague, is:
   (a) Rodents (b) Rat fleas
   (c) Mosquitoes (d) Humans.
5. The bubo of bubonic plague is a/an:
   (a) Infected sebaceous gland
   (b) Enlarged lymph node
   (c) Granuloma of the skin
   (d) Ulcer where the flea bite occurred.

ANSWERS TO MCQs

1. (b) 2. (c) 3. (a) 4. (a) 5. (b).

44

Haemophilus: A Gram-negative Pleomorphic Bacillius

Meningitis; Pneumonia; Epiglottitis; Chancroid

The genus *Haemophilus* is a Gram-negative, pleomorphic, facultatively anaerobic, coccobacillus belonging to the family *Pasteurellaceae*. The name *Haemophilus* **('loves heme')** is derived due to its requirement for blood during growth (Gr *haima* = blood + *philus* = love). These organisms inhabit the mucuous membranes of the upper respiratory tract, mouth, vagina and intestinal tract.

The genus contains 24 species. These bacteria are characterized by their requirement of either one or both of two accessory growth factors: X factor (haemin) and V factor (NAD) needed for respiration.

Two clinically important species that affect humans are: *Haemophilus influenzae* and *H. ducreyi*. *H. influenzae* type b (Hib) is the most virulent strain causing acute meningitis, an infection of the brain and its membranes.

HAEMOPHILUS INFLUENZAE

H. influenzae (formerly called **Pfeiffer's bacillus** or *Bacillus influenzae*) was first described in 1892 by **Richard Pfeiffer** during an influenza epidemic. It was named in 1896 by **Lehmann** and **Neumann** because of the erroneous belief that it was responsible for influenza.

MORPHOLOGY

It is a Gram-negative, pleomorphic, nonmotile, nonsporing, coccobacillus (1 μm × 0.3 μm) (Fig. 44.1). Some strains of *H. influenzae* possess a polysaccharide capsule, and these strains are serotyped into six distinct antigenic types, designated *a*, *b*, *c*, *d*, *e* and *f* based on their biochemically different capsules. The six capsular types can be identified by a polymerase chain reaction (PCR) method.

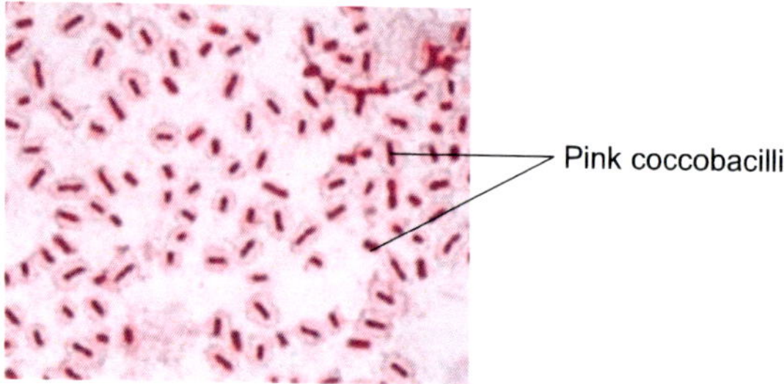

Fig. 44.1 Gram stain of *Haemophilus influenzae*. Direct smear from a sputum specimen showing small Gram-negative coccobacilli, however, long, filamentous forms are missing.

CULTURAL CHARACTERISTICS

It is a facultatively anaerobic bacterium that grows best with 5% CO_2 (or in a candle jar), optimum temperature 35–37°C (minimum 20–25°C), optimum pH 7.6, killed at 55°C within 30 minutes of heating and requires two accessory growth factors: X factor (haemin) and V factor (nicotinamide adenine dinucleotide). Both of these factors are found in chocolate agar.

On chocolate agar at 35°C under 5% CO_2 after 24 hours of incubation, the colonies are 5 mm, smooth, pale, grey or transparent, mucoid and glistening (Fig. 44.2).

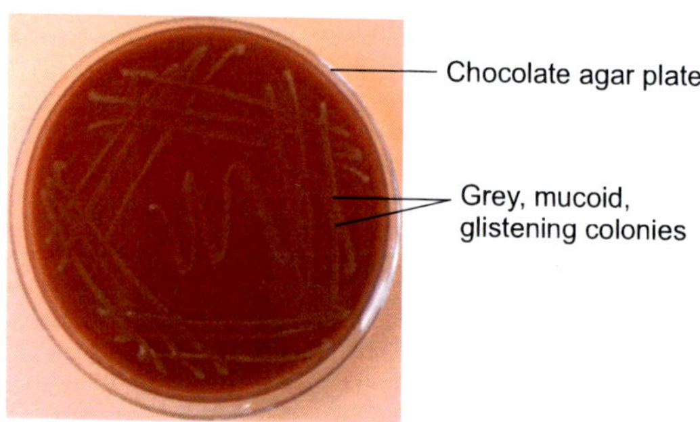

Fig. 44.2 *Haemophilus influenzae* on chocolate agar. Chocolate agar supplies both the X and V factors required for the growth of this species. The colonies are grey, mucoid, and glistening after 24 hrs. at 35°C under 5% CO_2.

SATELLITISM

On blood agar, *H. influenzae* and *H. haemolyticus* requiring X and V factors, grow around the colonies of *Staphylococcus aureus*, NAD producing organism, showing the **satellite phenomenon (satellitism)**.

BIOCHEMICAL REACTIONS

It is both catalase- and oxidase-positive and ferments the sugars: glucose, galactose and xylose but does not ferment fructose, sucrose, lactose and mannitol.

PATHOGENICITY

Capsulated Hib: Causes invasive diseases—meningitis, primary bacteremia, pneumonia, epiglottitis and arthritis, especially in children.

Non-capsulated *H. influenzae* (ncHi): Causes non-invasive diseases otitis media, conjunctivitis, sinusitis and chronic bronchitis.

MECHANISM OF PATHOGENESIS

H. influenzae is an *obligate parasite*, over 95% of infections are casued by the capsular strains. It is transmitted by direct contact and inhalation of the respiratory tract droplets. The organisms penetrate the epithelium of the nasopharynx followed by invasion of blood capillaries and resulting in infection.

SYMPTOMS OF MAJOR DISEASES

- **Pneumonia** (lung infection)—fever and chills, coughing and breathing difficulty, with excessive tiredness. Typically occurs in infants.
- **Meningitis** (serious infection of the tissue covering the brain and spinal cord)—stiff neck, headache, photophobia and nausea. It occurs in babies aged between 2 and 36 months.
- **Epiglottitis** (inflammation of the epiglottis) sore throat, drooling and breathing difficulty. It can result in death within a few hours. It is seen in children above 2 years.
- **Bacteremia** (infection of the bloodstream)—Fever and chills, pain in the belly, breathing difficulty and altered mental status.

LABORATORY DIAGNOSIS

Hib is diagnosed by direct microscopy, antigen detection, bacterial culture and molecular methods.

Direct microscopy: Microscopic examination of Gram-stained smear of clinical material will show Gram-negative coccobacilli and slender filaments.

Antigen detection: Latex agglutination test (LAT) is used to detect type b capsular antigen in patients serum, CSF, pus or urine. It is a highly sensitive method.

Bacterial culture: A sample of body fluid (e.g., blood or spinal fluid) is plated on chocolate agar with added X (hemin) and V (NAD) factors at 37°C in a CO_2-enriched incubator.

On blood agar, growth of *H. influenzae* is only achieved around colonies of *Staphylococcus aureus* that supply the needed NAD, the V factors, the phenomenon called **satellitism**. In this, *S. aureus* is streaked across the blood agar plate on which the specimen (e.g., CSF) has already been inoculated. The inoculated plate is incubated overnight at 35°C under 5% CO_2 for 24 hours. Colonies of *H. influenzae* grow only in the area surrounding the staphylococcal streak.

Biochemical tests: Catalase and oxidase tests, both of which are positive.

Molecular method: Polymerase chain reaction (PCR), a more sensitive and reliable assay, is used to diagnose, especially in case of meningitis.

Treatment

Cefotaxime and ceftriaxone are the drugs of choice to treat severe cases of meningitis and septicaemia. An association of ampicillin and sulbactam, cephalosporin (2nd and 3rd generation) or flouroquinolones are used for less severe cases.

Amoxicillin is used orally for non-invasive infections (e.g., otitis media; a middle ear infection, sinusitis, bronchitis).

Prevention

WHO recommends the use of a **pentavalent vaccine**, combining vaccines against diphtheria, tetanus, pertussis, hepatitis B and Hib.

HAEMOPHILUS DUCREYI

H. ducreyi, a Gram-nagative coccobacillus, causes a highly communicable sexually transmitted disease (STD) **chancroid** or **soft sores**, a major cause of genital ulceration in developing countries. It is characterized by painful sores with painful bleeding on penis.

Gram-negative coccobacilli are small (1 – 1.5 μm × 0.6 μm) arranged in small groups, whorls or in parallel chains giving a **"schools-of-fish"** or **"rail track"** appearance.

It grows on chocolate agar at 35–37°C in 10% CO_2 (microaerophilic conditions) producing small pin-point (0.5 mm), grey yellow or tan colonies. *H. ducreyi* requires only X factor (i.e., hemin) for its growth, hence does not show satellitism.

Symptoms and culture containing Gram-negative rods from the exudates of lesion are used for diagnosis. Antigen detection, serology and genetic amplification methods have also been reported for *H. ducreyi*, and none is commercially available. Chancroid is treated with azithromycin or ceftriaxoze.

KEY POINTS

- *Haemophilus*, a blood-loving bacterium, is a Gram-negative coccobacillus, requiring X (hemin) and V (NAD, NADP) accessory growth factors present in blood for its growth.
- *Haemophilus influenzae* type b (Hib) strains are the causative agents of meningitis, epiglottitis, pneumonia and septic arthritis.
- Noncapsulated strains of *H influenzae* are considered opportunisitic pathogens causing otitis media (middle ear infection), sinusitis, chronic bronchitis and bronchiectasis.
- *Haemophilus ducreyi*, a Gram-negative coccobacillus, causes chancroid, a sexually transmitted desease (STD).
- The phenomenon of **satellitism** is exhibited by *H. influenzae* on blood agar plates by dual culture with *Staphylococcus aureus*.

IMPORTANT QUESTIONS

1. Name *Haemophilus influenzae* infections, their diagnosis and treatment.
2. Answer briefly:
   (a) Satellitism
   (b) X and V factors
   (c) Epiglottitis
   (d) Chanchroid
   (e) How *Haemophilus influenzae* was named?

MULTIPLE CHOICE QUESTIONS

1. All of the following infections are caused by *Haemophilus influenzae* EXCEPT:
   (a) Influenza (b) Pneumonia
   (c) Meningitis (d) Epiglottitis.
2. *Haemophilus influenzae* requires .... factor/factors for growth:
   (a) Hemin (b) NAD
   (c) Blood (d) Both hemin and NAD.
3. Satellite phenomenon (satellitism) is shown by:
   (a) *Haemophilus influenzae*
   (b) *Staphylococcus aureus*
   (c) *Haemophylus ducreyi*
   (d) All of the above.
4. X and V growth factors required by *Haemophilus influenzae* stand for .... and ...., respectively.

ANSWERS TO MCQs

1. (a) 2. (d) 3. (a) 4. hemin and NAD.

45

Gardnerella: A Pleomorphic Gram-Variable Bacillus or Coccobacillus

Bacterial vaginosis

Gardnerella is a small, pleomorphic, Gram-variable, non-motile, facultative anaerobic bacillus or coccobacillus having the only species *Gardnerella vaginalis*. It belongs to the family *Bifidobacteriaceae*.

The natural habitat of *G. vaginalis* is the human vagina. It causes one of the most common forms of vaginitis called **bacteial vaginosis (BV)** characterized by abnormal vaginal odour and discharge.

GARDNERELLA VAGINALIS

Gardnerella vaginalis was previously called *Corynebacterium vaginale* and *Haemophilus vaginalis*. The genus *Gardnerella* is named after **H.L. Gardner** and the species *vaginalis* pertaining to vagina.

MORPHOLOGY

The organisms are small (1.0 – 1.5 μm in diameter), non-spore forming, non-motile, bacilli to coccobacilli. On Gram reaction, it is Gram-variable that is weakly Gram-positive to Gram-negative (Figs. 45.1 and 45.2). However, due to the presence of lipopolysaccharide in the cell wall it appears to be Gram-negative. Due to variable Gram reaction this organism was previously included in the genera *Corynebacterium* and *Haemophilus*.

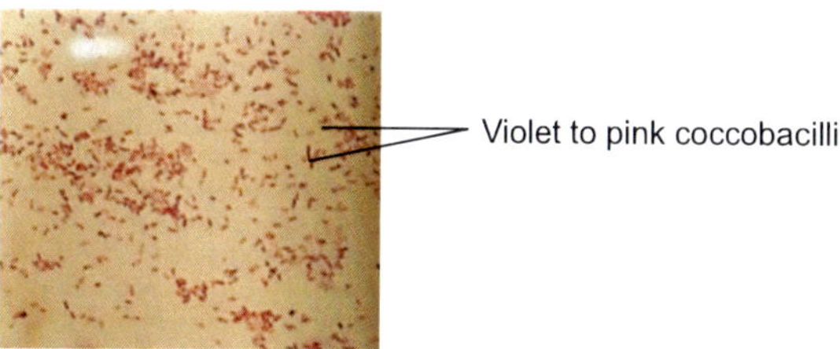

Fig. 45.1 Gram stain of *Gardnerella vaginalis*. The coccobacilli are Gram-variable.

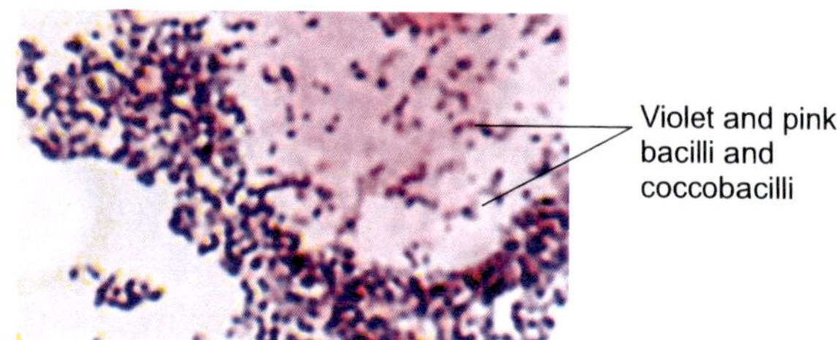

Fig. 45.2 Gram stain of Gardnerella vaginalis on clue cells from a vaginal discharge of a patient with bacterial vaginosis. The clue cell, (epithelial cell) covered with small Gram-variable and Gram-negative bacilli and coccobacilli.

CULTURAL CHARACTERISTICS

On media containing erythrocytes (human blood) such as vaginalis agar (V agar) at 37°C in an atmosphere of 5–7% of CO_2 after 48 hours are opaque, 1 mm in diameter surrounded by 3 mm of beta-haemolysis.

BIOCHEMICAL REACTIONS

It is catalase- and oxidase-negative but ferments starch and hydrolyses hippurate. These properties provide a means for presumptive identification of *G. vaginalis*.

PATHOGENESIS

G. vaginalis is a member of the endogenous vaginal flora in up to 69% of women and is the cause of **vaginosis** in females. Other bacteria are often found in association with *G. vaginalis* hence the disease is called **bacterial vaginosis** (Because there is no sign of inflammation of vagina the term *vaginosis* is preferred to *vaginitis*.)

Bacterial vaginosis is characterized by a vaginal pH above 4.5 (normal pH is less than 4.5) and a copious, frothy vaginal discharge with a characteristic **rotten fish odour** due to the amines and change in the *Lactobacillus* bacteria present in the vagina by the other types of bacteria that normally are present in smaller numbers. The vaginal discharge adheres to the vaginal wall in a thin film that varies from white to grey in colours. The discharge contains characteristic **clue cells** which are sloughed off vaginal epithelial cells covered with a biofilm of Gram-variable bacilli (Fig. 45.2). This disease has been considered more of a nuisance than a serious infection.

DIAGNOSIS

Bacterial vaginosis is diagnosed based on the gynaecological examination and laboratory tests of the vaginal fluid.

- Relative higher number of *G. vaginalis* than *Lactobacillus* spp. by direct microscopic examination of Gram-stained smear microscopic in vaginal specimens.
- pH test of vaginal discharge that shows low acidity (pH greater than 4.5).
- **Fishy odour**, when a sample of vaginal discharge is mixed with a drop of KOH (10%) on a glass slide the *whiff* test.
- Clue cells visible on microscopic examination of vaginal fluids.
- Whitish coating on the vaginal walls during the pelvic examination by a gynaecologist.

TREATMENT

- BV is treated with metronidazole and clindamycin. These can be taken either by mouth or applied as a vaginal cream or gel.

KEY POINTS

- *Gardnerella vaginalis* is a facultatively anaerobic, non-motile, non-sporing, non-encapsulated, oxidase- and catalase-negative, pleomorphic, and Gram-variable rod.
- The diagnosis of vaginosis caused by *Gardnerella vaginalis* is based on vaginal pH > 4.5; presence of clue cells in the vaginal discharge; positive whiff test and homogenous vaginal discharge.
- Metronidazole is the drug of choice to treat BV.

IMPORTANT QUESTIONS

1. Briefly describe *Gardnerella vaginalis*.
2. Answer in brief:
   (a) Is *Gardnerella vaginalis* Gram-positive or Gram-negative?
   (b) Clue cells
   (c) Diagnosis of bacterial vaginosis caused by *Gardnerella vaginalis*.

MULTIPLE-CHOICE QUESTIONS

1. The presence of clue cells in the wet unstained smear from the vaginal discharge indicates the organism:
   (a) *Trichomonas vaginalis*
   (b) *Candida albicans*
   (c) *Gardnerella vaginalis*
   (d) All of the above.
2. Diagnosis of *Gardnerella vaginalis* cause of bacterial vaginosis is based on:
   (a) Vaginal pH
   (b) Fishy odour (the whiff test)
   (c) Microscopic observation of clue cells in the discharge
   (d) All of the above.
3. All are true for *Gardnerella vaginalis* EXCEPT:
   (a) Both oxidase - and catalase-positive
   (b) Gram-variable rod
   (c) Nonmotile
   (d) Nonencapsulated.

ANSWERS TO MCQs

1. (c) 2. (d) 3. (a).

46

Mycobacterium: An Acid-fast Aerobic Bacillus

Tuberculosis; Leprosy; Mycobacteriosis

The genus *Mycobacterium* (pl. **mycobacteria**) is an acid-fast, slow growing, non-endospore-forming, aerobic bacillus (rod) surrounded by the characteristic waxy coating, classified in its own family, the *Mycobacteriaceae*. Mycobacteria resist decolorization with dilute mineral acids or alcohol, hence termed as **acid-fast bacilli (AFB)**. The name *Mycobacterium* is derived from *myco* = fungus + *bacterium* = a rod, means fungus-like bacteria.

Currently, there are 190 species in this genus. Two clinically important species causing serious diseases of humans are:

- *Mycobacterium tuberculosis:* Tuberculosis (TB)
- *Mycobacterium leprae:* Leprosy

The mycobacteria are generally classified in two groups:

- **Slow growers:** Those that form colonies in 2 to 8 weeks. Examples: obligate human pathogens: *Mycobacterium tuberculosis* and *M. leprae*.
- **Rapid growers:** Those that produce colonies in less than 7 days which include: environmental saprophytes occurring in soil and water. These are termed **nontuberculosis mycobacteria (NTM)**. Example: *Mycobacterium avium*, the avian tubercle bacillus.

TB is the world's deadliest infectious disease resulting in more than 1.6 million deaths every year, more than 75,000 deaths in South Africa alone, one of the countries with the highest number of TB cases (10 million active TB cases recorded in 2018).

MYCOBACTERIUM TUBERCULOSIS

Mycobacterium tuberculosis, called the **tubercle bacillus**, the causative agent of TB, was first of all isolated in 1882 by the German physician

Robert Koch. He proved its causative role in TB by satisfying the Koch's postulates.

MORPHOLOGY AND CELL WALL

The tubercle bacilli are straight, curved, short to long beaded rods (2–4 μm × 0.2–0.5 μm) occurring singly sometimes filamentous (Fig. 46.1). Chains of cells often form distinctive serpentine cords. They are nonmotile and do not form endospores.

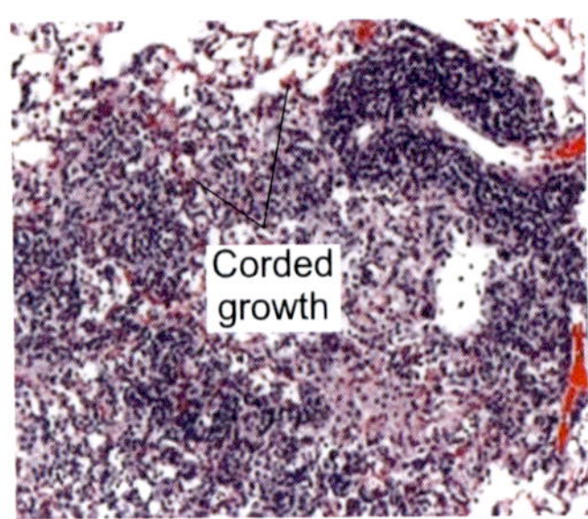

Fig. 46.1 ***Mycobacterium tuberculosis*** **from lung tissue.** The filamentous red stained fungus-like growth.

The cell wall of MTB is unique among prokaryotes, due to the presence of **mycolic acids**, a lipid (fatty acid) which are **strong hydophobic molecules** that form lipid shell around the organism. The high contents of lipids (mycolic acids, cord factor and wax-D) 60% in the cell wall of MTB are responsible for:

- Impermeability to stains and dyes
- Resistance to many antibiotics
- Resistance to killing by acidic and alkaline compounds
- Resistance to osmotic lysis
- Resistance to lethal oxidations and survival inside macrophages.

The presence of waxy coating on the wall makes them difficult to stain, as a result MTB can appear either as Gram-positive or Gram-negative. The ability of MTB to resist decolorization with up to 30% hydrochloric acid is referred to as **acid-fastness** and the bacteria (*Mycobacterium* and *Nocardia*) are classified as **acid-fast bacteria**. These bacteria retain dyes when heated and treated with acidified organic compounds.

Ziehl-Neelsen stain is the acid-fast staining method used to study MTB in smear and other clinical materials. In **Ziehl-Neelsen(ZN) staining technique**, the MTB (or sputum) smear is fixed, stained with carbol-fuchsin (a pink dye) and decolorized with acid-alcohol followed by counterstaining with methylene blue and examined microscopically (1000×). Acid-fast bacilli appear pink against a blue or green background (Fig. 46.2).

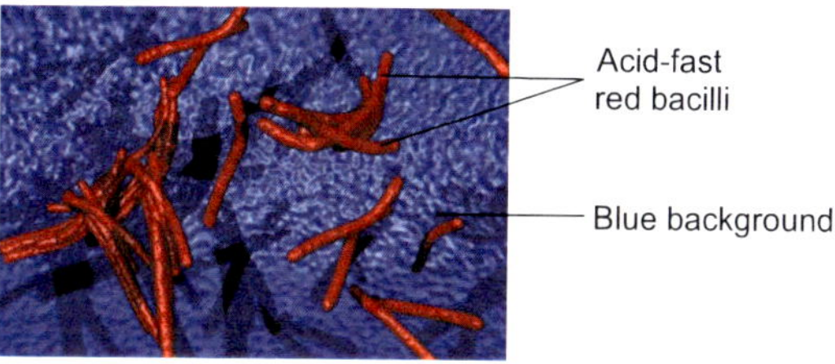

Fig. 46.2 Acid-fast stain of a sputum specimen. *Mycobacterium tuberculosis* cells appear as red against a blue background.

CULTURAL CHARACTERISTICS

MTB is an **obligate aerobe** with a slow generation time of 15–20 hours at an optimum temperature of 35–37°C (fails to grow at 25 and 41°C) and optimum pH between 6.4 and 7.0.

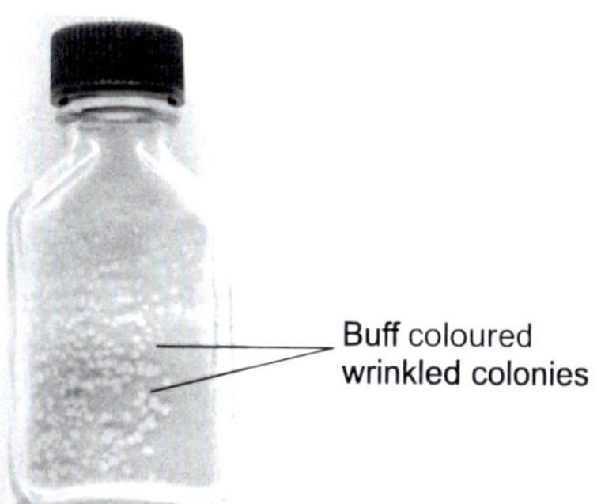

Fig. 46.3 *Mycobacterium tuberculosis* on a Löwenstein-Jensen agar slant. Colonies are dry, wrinkled, rough, thin, and fragile with an irregular periphery and buff colour.

Löwenstein-Jensen (LJ) medium, an egg based medium (salts + eggs + malachite green + glycerol), is used in which egg acts as a solidifying agent, incubated at 35–37°C under 5–10% CO_2 and inspected weekly for at least 8 weeks. MTB colonies are buff coloured, wrinkled and rough (Fig. 46.3). In liquid media, the growth forms a prominent surface pellicle.

BIOCHEMICAL REACTIONS

Key biochemical reactions used to identify MTB are:

- **Nitrate reduction**—It reduces nitrate to nitrite (positive test).
- **Niacin accumulation test**—Tubercle bacilli forms niacin as a metabolic by-product on an egg medium which accumulates in the medium. Canary yellow colour indicates a positive reaction.

- In addition to the above two positive tests, mycobacteria are positive for amidase, peroxidase and neutral red tests.

RESISTANCE

MTB is more resistant to drying and chemical disinfectants.

TUBERCULOSIS

Tuberculosis (TB), also called **white plague** of Europe, **consumption** and **Yaksma** (India), is one of the top 10 causes of death worldwide and a massive global health problem for centuries. One-third of the world's population have TB. Each year 3 million people die, and 10 million new TB cases arise.

WORLD TB DAY

World TB Day (WTBD) is celebrated each year on March 24 to educate the public about the impact of TB around the world. This annual event commemorates the date in 1882 When Dr. Robert Koch announced his discovery of *Mycobacterium tuberculosis*, the bacilius that causes TB, that still remains the world's deadliest infectious killer.

The word **tuberculosis** is derived from the Latin *tuberculum* means small swelling looking like, the encapsulated colonies of MTB, formed within the lungs. TB is transmitted through the air and acquired by inhalation of respiratory droplets or particles of dry sputum containing tubercle bacilli.

TYPES OF TUBERCULOSIS

- **Pulmonary TB**—Involvement of lungs occurs.
- **Extrapulmonary TB**—Expecting lungs, other sites of the body are involved, e.g., bones and joints, genito-urinary, gastrointestinal, lymph and CN systems.
- **Active TB (also called TB disease)**—It is contagious (i.e., spreads from one person to another) and causes symptoms like
  - Fever
  - Chills
  - Fatigue
  - Loss of appetite
  - Night sweats
  - Unexplained weight loss (hence called consumption).

Latent TB: It is not contagious and without symptoms. Tubercle bacilli are present in the body, however, these are inactive.

Miliary TB: In this potentially fatal form of TB all tissues are invaded by the MTB, producing tiny lesions (1–5 mm) that resemble millet (bajra) seeds, and hence named.

PATHOGENESIS OF TB

Pulmonary TB: TB infection spreads from person-to-person via droplets. When someone with TB infection coughs, sneezes and talks, tiny droplets (over 40,000 droplets are released by a single sneeze) of mucus or saliva are expelled into the air, which can be inhaled by another person. Single droplet of sneeze is capable to cause TB since the infectious dose of TB is fewer than 10 bacilli. The initial infection with MTB is named the **primary infection** or **primary TB**.

The infection begins when the mycobacteria are inhaled and reach the **alveoli** (small sac-like structure in the air spaces in the lungs) and are engulfed (ingested) by macrophages. The mycobacteria multiply in macrophages and the host isolates the mycobacteria in a walled-off lesion termed a **tubercle** (meaning lump or knob), a characteristic that gives the disease its name, in addition to the release of enzymes and cytokines that cause a lung-damaging inflammation.

The TB lesion formed in the middle or lower lung jones (called **primary** or **Ghon focus** or **complex**), named after **Anton Ghon** an Austrian pathologist, is characteristic of primary pulmonary TB.

After a few weeks, coughing, the more obvious symptom of the lung infection, appears as many of the macrophages die, releasing tubercle bacilli into the airways of the lungs and then the cardiovascular and lymphatic systems. Sputum may become blood stained as tissues are damaged.

In some individuals who had even inhaled the TB bacteria, the infection is arrested, the bacteria remain dormant **(latent TB)**. The lesions slowly heal and become calcified and are called **Ghon's complexes** (as visualized by X-rays and computed tomography (CT).

Extrapulmonary TB: Extrapulmonary TB (*extra* = outside of + *pulmonary* = affecting lungs) refers to TB involving other than the lungs—results from the haematogenous and lymphatic spread of tubercle bacilli.

LABORATORY DIAGNOSIS

TB is diagnosed in the laboratory by detection of tubercle bacilli in clinical specimens by microscopy, cultural techniques and by molecular methods (GeneXpert).

Various clinical specimens used for diagnosis include: Sputum (phlegm) (well coughed out early morning sputum), gastric juices, gastric lavage/washing bronchial washings, cerebrospinal fluid (CSF), pleural fluid, urine, tissue biopsies. Of these, sputum is the most usual specimen for diagnosis of pulmonary TB.

Sputum Smear Microscopy

Acid-fast mycobacteria are observed in sputum by the Ziehl–Neelsen staining technique. Visible TB germs (long, thin slender pink bacilli with beaded appearance against a blue background) indicate an active TB infection in the lungs and throat—**sputum smear positive TB** (pulmonary TB).

Cultural Methods

Sputum or sample of bodily fluid or tissue is used to grow bacteria on Löwenstein-Jensen (solid) or Middlebroke (liquid) media incubated at 35°–37°C for 8 weeks. Appearance of rough, and buff-coloured colonies on (L-J medium) and growth in the broth indicates a positive test. Bacterial growth is stained by ZN method for acid-fast bacilli.

GeneXpert (PCR test)

The GeneXpert is an automated PCR test which detects the DNA in TB bacteria from sputum samples. The method is cartridge-based, easy to use and provides results in 90 minutes. WHO in 2010 endorsed the product for use in TB in the endemic countries.

This test is mainly used to diagnose extrapulmonary TB in adults and children which are predominantly **paucibacillary samples** (i.e., having few bacilli). At the same time this list can detect the genetic mutations associated with resistance to rifampin, a major antibiotic used to treat TB.

Blood Tests (T-Spot TB and Quanti FERON TB Gold Test)

The tuberculosis blood tests are based on antigens that are more specific than the PPD used for the tuberculin skin test. These tests also called the **Interferon Gamma Release Assay (IGRA)**. T-cells in response of certain antigens of *M. tuberculosis*, are used to find out tubercle bacilli in the human body within 24 hours.

Two commercially available kits-

- **Qanti FERON-TB Gold (QFT-G)**—In this assay release of gamma interferon (IFN-γ) is detected.
- **T-SPOT-TB-** In this test T-cells are enumerated that produce IFN-γ.

Tuberculin Skin Test (Mantoux Test)

The **tuberculin skin test (TST)**—commonly called the **Mantoux test** (named after **Mantoux** who first described it) is the standard method used around the world to detect the infection of *M. tuberculosis.*

TST is based on the principle that infection with *M. tuberculosis* produces a delayed type hypersensitivity skin reaction to purified protein derivative (PPD) of the bacterium in the person infected with TB in the past (i.e., cell- mediated, immunity involving sensitized T cells).

The Mantoux test is performed by injecting a 0.1 mL of liquid containing 5 TU (**tuberculin units**) **PPD** (**purified protein derivative**) of the tuberculosis bacterium, derived by precipitation from broth cultures into the top layers of skin (intradermally on the forearm). Skin reaction is observed after 48–72 hours after the injection to detect **induration** (i.e., localized swelling of the skin)—a wheal or "bleb". The presence or absence and the amount (diameter in mm) is used to express the results of TST (Fig. 46.4).

- **Positive**—diameter > 10 mm
- **Negative**—diameter < 5 mm
- **Doubtful**—6 to 9 mm

In children it indicates active TB and in older people case of latent TB resulting from a previous infection or vaccination and a clue to further examination of patients chest by X-ray or CT examination to detect lung lesions.

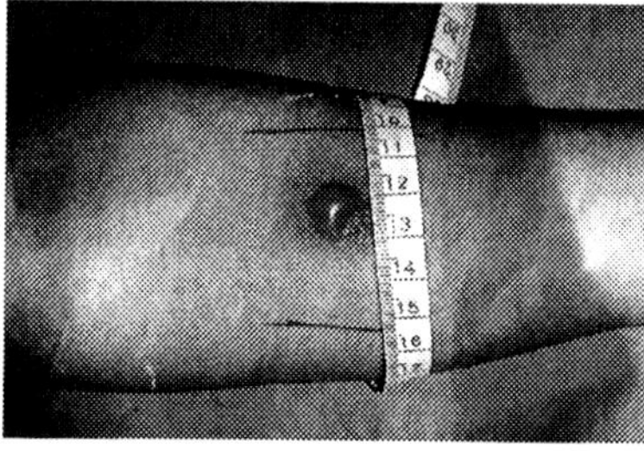

Fig. 46.4 Tuberculin skin test (= Mantoux test) on an arm. Positive test, as indicated by the area of induration more than 10 mm in diameter.

TREATMENT

- Streptomycin is the first effective antibiotic introduced in 1944 to treat TB and is still in use requiring a minimum of 6 months of treatment.
- Multidrug therapy that includes both the **bactericidal drugs** (e.g., rifampin, pyrazinamide) and **bacteriostatic drugs** (isoniazid and ethambutol) is considered the **first-line drugs** to treat TB.

DRUG RESISTANCE IN *M. TUBERCULOSIS*

These are of two types:

- **Multidrug resistant (MDR) MTB strains:** The strains resistant to the two most effective first line drugs rifampin and isoniazid, second-line drugs such as fluoroquinoline and amikacin or capreomycin (capastat) are used for 20–30 months to treat MDR strains.
- **Extensively drug resistant (XDR) TB:** Those MTB strains that are resistant to even the most effective second-line drugs. These strains are emerging globally.

New cure for deadly strains of TB:

Three-drug combination collectively known as the **BPaL regimen** that consists of bedaquiline, pretomanid and linezolid, has been recently approved by FDA (16th August 2019). The treatment involves five pills of the three drugs daily taken over just 6 months for MDRTB patients.

TUBERCULOSIS VACCINES

The **BCG vaccine** (BCG stands for bacillus of **Calmette** and **Guérin**, the French scientists who originally isolated the strain) is a live attenuated vaccine from the culture of *M. bovis*. It has been available since the 1920s and is one of the most widely used vaccines in the world.

BCG vaccine is given to babies in a dose of 0.1 mL intradermally administered soon after birth, or as early as possible thereafter, before the age of one year. Following vaccination, immunity may last for 10–15 years which is similar to the immunity following natural infection.

TUBERCULOSIS AND HIV COINFECTION

Infection with both HIV and TB is called **HIV/TB coinfection**. HIV and TB are inseparable and a close relationship exists between the two diseases. Since TB is an opportunistic infection that occurs more often or more severely in people with weak immune systems. HIV weakens the immune system, increasing the risk of TB in people with HIV.

As per WHO, 2019, the risk of developing TB is estimated to be between 16 and 27 times greater in people living with HIV than among those without HIV infection. Over 60% of the cases coinfected with TB/HIV are not diagnosed or treated.

MYCOBACTERIUM LEPRAE

Mycobacterium leprae (also called **Hansen's bacillius spirilly**) is an obligate intracellular, acid-fast, aerobic bacillus surrounded by the waxy coating of mycolic acids, unique to mycobacteria. Waxy exterior coating acts as the virulence factor.

M. leprae causes leprosy which is probably the oldest disease known to mankind. Leprosy is described as **"Kusthe"** in *Sustruta Samihita* written in India in 600 B.C. The bacterium was discovered in 1873 by **Gerhard Armauer Hansen,** a Norwegian physician, and was the first bacterium to be identified as causing disease in humans, hence leprosy was named **Hansen's disease**.

MORPHOLOGY

Leprosy bacilli resemble tubercle bacilli in general morphology, however, are not so strongly acid-fast with ZN stain.

The bacilli are straight or slightly curved rods, measuring 1 – 8 µm × 0.2 – 0.5 µm, occurring singly, in clumps or round masses known as **globi** or in groups of bacilli side by side looking like a **cigar bundle**. **It is an acid-fast Gram-positive bacterium**.

CULTURE

In vitro cultivation of *M. leprae* is not possible, however, it has been grown in mouse foot pads and more recently in nine-banded armadillos because they like humans are susceptible to leprosy. It has a doubling time of 14 days.

LEPROSY

Leprosy (from ancient Greek *Léprá* means "a disease that makes the skin scaly") is a chronic infectious decease caused by *Mycobacterium leprae* affecting the skin, mucous membranes and nerves, causing discolouration and lumps on the skin and in severe cases disfigurement and deformities, rarely a fatal disease.

Millions of people suffer from leprosy today, and over half a million new cases are reported each year. Worldwide 2–3 million people are permanently disabled because of leprosy. India has the greatest number of cases, with Brazil second and Indonesia third.

TYPES OF LEPROSY

Based on the clinical features and extent of the disease, leprosy is classified as:

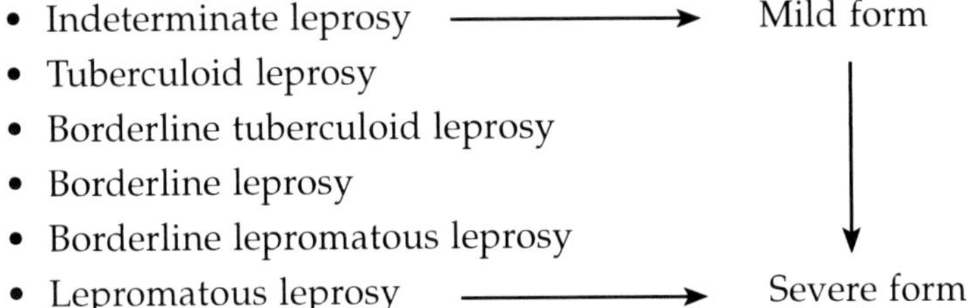

SYMPTOMS OF LEPROSY

- Skin lesions that don't heal for several weeks or months.
- Skin lesions that are lighter in colour or are less sensitive to heat, pain or touch than unaffected skin.
- Skin thickening or scarring.
- Nerve damage leading to numbness or lack of sensation in extremities.
- Weakening of muscles that get worse with passage of time.

PATHOGENESIS

Leprosy is acquired when secretions containing the pathogen contact their nasal mucosa. Infected persons shed large number of leprosy bacilli in their nasal secretions and in exudates (oozing matter) of their lesions. However, leprosy is not very contagious and is usually transmitted only between people in fairly intimate and prolonged contact.

It is an obligate intracellular bacterium which damages peripheral nerves and can affect the skin, eyes, nose and muscles. Nerve injury can cause severe disabling deformities. 30°C is the optimum growth temperature and bacilli show a preference for the outer, cooler tissues of the human body. The pathogen survives ingestion by macrophages and eventually invades cells of the myelin sheath of the peripheral nervous system, where its presence causes nerve damage from a cell-mediated immune response. *M. leprae* has a very long generation (or doubling time) of 12 days. People who develop leprosy usually incubate the infection for 3 to 5 years before manifesting illness, and they exhibit a broad spectrum of clinical and histopathological responses to the infection determined by their immunological response to *M. leprae*.

Leprosy exists in two extreme or polar forms:

- Turberculoid (neural) form
- Lepromatous (progressive) form

The **tuberculoid leprosy** (= **paucibacillary** in the WHO system) is characterized by depigmented area of the skin that have lost sensation and surrounded by a border of nodules with small numbers of bacilli. It occurs in people with effective immune reactions. Recovery sometimes occurs spontaneously.

The **lepromatous (progressive) form of leprosy** (= **multibacillary** in the WHO system) is characterized by the progressive tissue damage by forming several diffuse lesions containing many bacilli in poorly organised granulomas. Mucous membranes of the nose are affected and a lion - faced appearance is assoicated with this form of leprosy. Deformation of the hand into a clawed form and considerable tissue necrosis can also occur. The progression of the disease is unpredicatable in this form of leprosy.

M. leprae is a slow-growing bacillus, the incubation period (the time from infection to appearance of symptoms) is about 5 years (ranges from 2–10 years) and it can take as long as 20 years before the symptoms and signs of leprosy (e.g., skin lesions, nerve damage) develop in some patients. Death usually results not from the leprosy itself, but from complications, such as TB.

LABORATORY DIAGNOSIS

- **Skin biopsy sample** is used as a standard diagnostic test to diagnose leprosy. Samples are taken from margins of active patches from the earlobes, elbows and knees. Presence of acid-fast bacilli in the skin smears indicates leprosy.
- Detection of acid-fast bacilli in nasal discharges and scrapings from the nasal mucosa.
- Nerve biopsy from thickened nerves for the presence of the pathogen.
- **Slit-skin smear** is an important tool to diagnose **multibacillary leprosy** by enumerating acid-fast bacilli in the skin of an infected person.

A slit-skin smear is prepared by making superficial incisons in the skin followed by scraping out some tissue fluid and cells making smear on a glass slide followed by acid-fast staining by the ZN method. Microscopic examination under high-power objective and counting of bacilli observed in each high-power field (oil-immersion) is recorded as the **bacillary** or **bacteriological index (BI)**. Based on the number of bacilli, the smears are graded as follows:

0 zero	No bacilli in any 100 fields
1+	1–10 bacilli per 100 fields
2+	1–10 bacilli per 10 fields
3+	1–10 bacilli per field
4+	10–100 bacilli per field
5+	100–1000 bacilli per field
6+	> 1000 bacilli per field (i.e., clumps)

Patients with clinically active leprosy showing 0(zero) BI are termed **paucibacillary (PB)** and those that are positive at any site are called **multibacillary (MB)** which is used as a criterion for selection of treatmemt.

In each field of the smear, percentage of uniformly stained bacilli (i.e., live bacilli) out of the total number of bacilli (i.e., both live and dead) is calculated to find out the **morphological index** (MI), (MI = uniformly stained bacilli/total bacilli × 100). MI is used to assess the progress of patients on chemotherapy.

LEPROMIN TEST

Lepromin skin test (also called **Leprosy skin test**) (**lepromin** is an extract of human leprous tissue—an antigen), first described in 1919 by **Mitsuda**, is used to determine what type of leprosy a person has? Unfortunately this is not a diagnostic test for leprosy.

This test is performed by injecting intradermally 0.1 mL lepromin (inactivated leprosy bacillius) into the inner surface of the forearm so that a small lump pushes the skin upward. The lump indicates that the antigen has been injected at the correct depth. The injection site is labelled and examined for the reaction site, i.e., redness, swelling, nodules after 48 hours (the **Fernandez** or **early reaction**) and 3 weeks (the **Mitsuda reaction**). The palatable nodule, if develops, is measured and graded.

A positive test is a nodule more than 3–5 mm size and indicates the presence of delayed hypersensitivity to *M. laprae* antigens.

Fernandez (or early) reaction—This reaction occurs within 48 hours of inoculation to signal positive result in the lepromin skin test revealing tuberculoid form of leprosy.

Mitsuda (or late) reaction—This reaction occurs three weeks post-inoculation. The Mitsuda reaction is positive in case of tuberculoid leprosy and borderline tuberculoid leprosy and is negative lepromatous leprosy and the borderline lepromatous type and is, therefore, helpful in classification and progonsis.

TREATMENT

Multidrug therapy, consisting of dapsone (a sulfosne drug), rifampin (antibiotic) and clofazimine (a fat-soluble dye), is used in combination, for 6 months (for paucibacillary) and for 24 months (for multibacillary) to treat leprosy.

VACCINATION

- BCG vaccine for tuberculosis (caused by *M. tuberculoseis*) provides some protection against leprosy.
- MIP (*Mycobacterium indicus pranii*), the world's first vaccine for leprosy developed in our country in 1998, is used as an adjunct to chemotherapy.

NONTUBERCULOSIS MYCOBACTERIA

Nontuberculosis mycobacteria (NTM), also called **enviornmental mycobacteria, atypical mycobacteria and mycobacteria other than tuberculosis (MOTT)**, are defined as mycobacteria which do not cause tuberculosis or leprosy. However, NTM do cause pulmonary diseases that resemble tuberculosis. Any of these pulmonary disease caused by NTM is known as **mycobacteriosis**. NTM are common in the environment and can be found in water (including tap water), soil, food and on animals. NTM contains over 150 species, pulmonary infections are most commonly caused by *Mycobacterium avium* complex (MAC), *M. kansasii* and *M. abscessus*.

TAXONOMY OF NTM

Ernest Runyon, a Botanist in 1959 categorized the NTM causing human diseases into four groups based on (i) the production of pigment (yellow or orange) and (ii) the rate of growth (Runyon classification):

Group I *Photochromogens:* Those that develop pigments in or after being exposed to light.

Group II *Scotochromogens:* Those that become pigmented in darkness.

Group III *Non-chromogens:* Those that are unpigmented.

Group IV *Rapid growers:* Those that produce visible growth on Lowenstein – Jensen medium within a week on subculturing at 37°C or 25°C.

PATHOGENESIS

NTM have been implicated in causing four types of human infections:

- Localized lymphadenitis
- Skin lesions following traumatic inoculation of bacteria
- Tuberculosis-like pulmonary lesions
- Disseminated disease.

DIAGNOSIS

Isolation and identification of NTM microscopically and culturing on Löwenstein-Jensen medium from sputum or skin specimens.

- Rate and temperature of growth and pigmentation (i.e., cultural characteristics).
- Detection of sequence differences in 16S ribosomal RNA.
- Chest X-ray and high resolution CT scan (in case of lung infection).

TREATMENT

NTM infections, especially caused by *M. avium* complex, are treated by multidrug therapy that includes: Clarithomycin (or azithromycin), ribabutin, ethambutol and amikacin.

KEY POINTS

- Mycobacteria (*M. tuberculosis* and *M. leprae* and atypical) are acid-fast bacilli that are stained with **Ziehl-Neelsen stain**.
- Their cell wall contains high lipid content (40 – 60%) (**mycolic acid**) that helps them to resist phagocytosis.
- *M. tuberculosis*, the cause of tuberculosis (TB), is an aerobic, slow growing baciilus characterized by rough, tough and buff

colonies on Löwenstein – Jensen medium after 8–12 weeks of incubation.

- *M. leprae* is a non-culturable, less acid-fast bacillus, that invades both sensory and motor nerves.
- **Lepromin** used in the leprosy skin test is a preparation of the bacterium (*M. leprae*) antigen.
- **Lepromin test** (leprosy skin test) is used to classify leprosy showing biphasic response: **Early** or **Fernandez reaction** within 48 hours and **Late** or **Mitsuda reaction** after 3–4 weeks of inoculation of **lepromin** (an antigen).
- Mycobacteria other than tubercle and leprosy bacilli are called **atypical mycobacteria, environmental mycobacteria** or **mycobacteria other than typical tubercle bacilli** (MOTT).

IMPORTANT QUESTIONS

1. Answer in brief:
   (a) What are acid-fast bacilli?
   (b) How the genus *Mycobacterium* was named?
   (c) What does a positive tuberculin test indicate?
   (d) How atypical mycobacteria are classified?
   (e) Use of morphological and bacillary index in leprosy.
2. Describe the laboratory diagnosis of pulmonary tuberculosis or leprosy.
3. Write short notes on:
   (a) Mantoux test.
   (b) Pathogenesis of pulmonary tuberculosis.
   (c) Lepormin test.
   (d) Atypical mycobacteria.
   (e) How mycobacterial infections are treated?

MULTIPLE-CHOICE QUESTIONS

1. Which medium is used to culture *Mycobacterium tubeculosis*?
   (a) Blood agar
   (b) Sabouraud dextrose agar
   (c) Löwenstein-Jensen medium
   (d) Nutrient agar.
2. Rough, tough and buff colonies on Löwenstein-Jensen medium are characteristics of

(a) *Mycobacterium bovis*
(b) *Mycobacterium tuberculosis*
(c) *Mycobacterium leprae*
(d) All of the above.

3. Which of the following cannot be cultured *in vitro* (i.e., on culture media)?
(a) *Mycobacterium tuberculosis*
(b) *Mycobacterium bovis*
(c) *Mycobacterium leprae*
(d) None of the above.

4. Acid-fastness of tubercle bacilli is due to the presence of:
(a) Peptidoglycan (b) Cord factor
(c) Mycolic acid (d) All of the above.

5. Usual dose of purified protein derivative (PPD) used in Mantoux test is:
(a) 5 Iu (b) 50 Iu
(c) 100 Iu (d) 200 Iu.

6. The generation time of *Mycobacterium leprae* is:
(a) 20 minutes (b) 20 hours
(c) 12–13 days (d) 12 – 13 weeks.

7. Mitsuda reaction in lepromin test appears within:
(a) 24–48 hours (b) 3 days
(c) 2 weeks (d) 3–4 weeks.

8. Which of the following mycobacteria is a rapid grower?
(a) *Mycobacterium leprae*
(b) *Mycobacterium avium*
(c) *Mycobacterium tuberculosis*
(d) None of the above.

9. Lepromin used in the leprosy (lepromin) skin test is an:
(a) Antibody (b) Antigen
(c) Antibiotic (d) Dye.

ANSWERS TO MCQs

1. (c) 2. (b) 3. (c) 4. (c) 5. (a)
6. (c) 7. (d) 8. (b) 9. (b).

47

Spirochaetes: *Treponema, Borrelia, Leptospira*

Syphilis; Yaws; Relapsing fevers; Lyme disease; Leptospirosis

The **spirochaetes** (or **spirochetes**) are thin, Gram-negative, motile, unicellular, helical or spiral rods, resembling a metal spring. The term spirochaetes is derived from Greek words: *spiera* meaning coiled and *chaiete* meaning hair, that is, coiled hair or spring.

The most distinctive feature is their method of motility by two or more **axial filaments**, also called **endoflagella** or **periplasmic flagella** which are enclosed in the space between an outer sheath and the body of the cell that encloses them to move by a **corkscrew-like rotation**. A spirochaete can move efficiently through liquids about 100 times its body length in a second (or about 50 μm/sec). Their number ranges between 2 and > 100 per organism, a morphologic characteristic of each species (Fig. 47.1). Spirochaetes are elongated bacteria varying in size from 5 to 500 μm in length.

Spirochaetes is a group of six genera which are widespread in nature occurring either as free living saprobes or commensals of animals found in the human oral cavity. These are probably among the first microorganisms described by **van Leeuwenhoek** in the 1600s that he found in the saliva and tooth scrapings. Only a few of these cause disesase in humans and animals. These are classified in the order *Spirochaetales* in a separate phylum *Spirochaetes*. Clinically, significant genera belong to *Treponema, Borrelia* (family *Spirochaetaceae*) and *Leptospira* (family *Leptospiraceae*) each with characteristic helical form (Fig. 47.1).

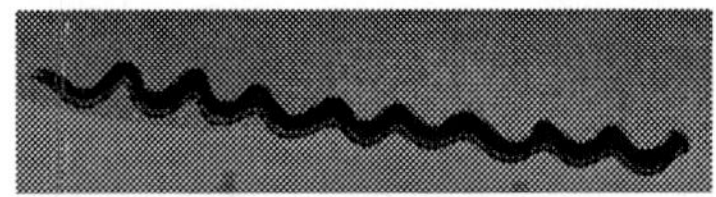

Treponema with 8–20 evenly spaced coils

Borrelia with 3–10 loose irregular coils

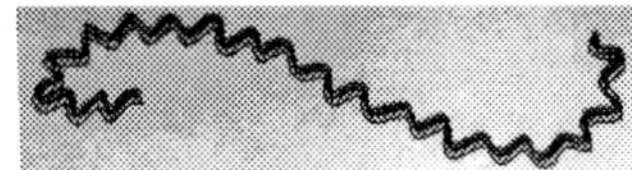

Leptospira with numerous fine regular coils and one or both ends curved

Fig. 47.1 Spirochaetes. Variations of the basic helical form as shown by major human pathogenic genera.

The principal human diseases caused are syphilis (*T. pallidum*), Lyme disease and relapsing fever (*Borrelia* spp.) and leptosporiosis (*Leptospira interrogans*).

TREPONEMA AND SYPHILIS

The genus *Treponema*, members called **treponemes**, comprises spiral-shaped, obligate parasitic, motile spirochaetes that cannot be cultured in artificial media (i.e., *in vitro*). Diseases caused by *Treponema* are called **treponematoses**.

***Treponema pallidum*:** It consists of three subspecies (previously considered as separate species), each of these causes a distinct disease:

- *T. p.* spp. *pallidum* (= *T. pallidum*): **syphilis**
- *T.p.* spp. *endemicum* (= *T. endemicum*): **bejel** or **endemic syphilis**
- *T. p.* spp. *pertenue* (= *T. pertenue*): **yaws**
- ***Treponema carateum:*** **pirnta**

Treponema pallidum

T. pallidum, the name derived from the Greek words for twisted thread and pale (*trepo* = turn + *nema* = thread; *L. pallidum* = pale), was first identified in sphilitic chancres (ulcers) in 1905 by **Fritz Schaudinn** and **Erich Hoffman**.

T. pallidum is clinically the most important spirochaete. It contains three subspecies that cause syphilis, bejal and yaws.

Morphologically, it is a helically coiled rod-shaped bacterium usually 5–15 μm long and 0.1-0.2 μm wide having a cytoplasmic and an outer membrane (i.e., double membrane, called **diderm**). The cells are best observed under dark-field microscope. Flagella at both ends of the cell (inside) give the organism its typical corkscrew motility.

The bacterium possesses Gram-negative envelope but cannot be stained by simple analine dyes or by Gram's method. By prolonged Giemsa staining, it stains pale pink.

Culturing

T. pallidum, an exclusively obligate human parasite, has not been cultured in artifical culture media (i.e., *in vitro*). Laboratory cultures are grown in rabbits for research purposes, but they grow slowly with a generation time of 30 hours or more.

A recent study published in 2018 reports a successful long-term cultivation in a tissue culture system of this pathogen.

Sensitivity to Physical and Chemical Agents

T. pallidum is a delicate, fastidious and sensitive organism, therefore, readily destroyed by heat (at 45°C for 1 hour), drying, disinfectants, soap, high oxygen tension, and pH changes. It cannot survives for long outside the body, and survives for just a few minutes to hours when protected by body secretions.

SYPHILIS

Syphilis, a **sexually transmitted infection (STI),** is caused by *T. p. pallidum*, is characterized by sores on the genitals, rectum and mouth. It was first recognized at the close of the 15th century in Europe. Worldwide, it infects over 45 million people causing over 1 lakh deaths annually. It is a rare disease in India with fewer than 1 million cases recorded per year.

Pathogenesis

Sexually transmitted syphilis is acquired through close contact with a lesion formed on gentials, rectum or mouth via skin or mucous membranes. One can also get it by sharing needles or having a blood transfusion from an infected person.

The helical structure of this bacterium allows it to move in a corkscrew motion through mucous membranes. In men, the initial lesion on the penis shaft or glans and in women it is on the labia, the walls of the vagina or the cervix. It gains access to the host blood and lymph systems through tissue and mucous membranes. In more severe cases, it infects the skeletal bones and central nervous system.

The incubation period for a *T. p. pallidum* infection is usually 21 days, but can range from 10 to 90 days.

Stages of Syphilis Infection

Based on the clinical manifestations, syphilis consists of four stages:

- Primary syphilis
- Secondary syphilis
- Latent syphilis
- Tertiary syphilis

Syphilis is most infectious in the first two stages and the tertiary is the most destructive to health.

Primary Syphilis

This stage occurs normally after 3 weeks of infection. At the site of infection (or inside the mouth, genitals or rectum), the multiplying treponemes produce a primary lesion—a small, round, hard painless sore called a **chancre**.

The sore remains between 2 and 6 weeks and disappears as the bacteria invade the blood and lymphatic system.

Secondary Syphilis

This stage sets in 1–3 months after healing of primary lesion. The appearance of a widely disseminated rash in the skin and mucous membranes and a mild fever marks the secondary stage. Spirochaetes are present in the lesions of the rash.

Latent Syphilis

The patient enters a latent period after the secondary lesions spontaneously heal. However, the bacteria remain in the body, hence called the **latent** or **hidden stage** for years before progressing to the tertiary stage.

Tertiary Syphilis

At least 10 years after the secondary lesion, this stage appears in the patients. Tertiary lesions, called **gummas** (**tumours**), appear on many organs, which have life-threatening cardiovascular and neurological effects. These include: blindness, deafness, mental illness, memory loss, heart disease, stroke, meningitis and **neurosyphilis** (i.e., infection of the brain or spinal cord).

Congenital Syphilis

In unborn foetus, congenital syphilis results from *T. pallidum* crossing the placenta (i.e., transplacentally) during the latent period, distrupting the foetal development. It causes damage to the mental development in addition to other neurological symptoms. Treating the mother with antibiotics during the first two trimesters (6 months) of pregnancy usually prevents congenital transmission of the pathogen.

Diagnosis of Syphilis

Tests to diagnose syphilis fall in two groups:

- Direct microscopic observation to detect *T. p. pallidum* from lesions or tissues for primary syphilis.
- Nontreponemal serological tests (VDRL, RPR, ELISA) for screening.
- Treponemal serological tests (EIA, FTA-ABS) for confirmation.

Microscopic Tests

Thin tightly coiled motile treponemes can be detected in exudates of lesions by microscopic examination with a dark-field microscope (because the bacteria stain poorly and are only about 0.2 μm wide). Similarly, a direct-fluorescent antibody test (DFA-TP) using monoclonal antibodies is used to see spirochaetes.

Nontreponemal Serological Tests

These serological tests are used to detect *reagin type antibodies* in the serum. A test is positive if lipoidal antigens from damaged host tissues or treponemes are present in plasma or serum. The **rapid plasma reagin (RPR)** and the **slide agglutination VDRL** (veneral disease research laboratory), are the two most widely used nontreponemal tests.

In the VDRL test, the inactivated serum (i.e., serum heated at 56°C for 30 minutes) is mixed with cardiolpin antigen on a special slide and rotated for four minutes and observed under a low-power microscope for the formation of clumps (a positive test). By testing serial dilutions, the antibody titer can be determined.

The **RPR test**, which is a modification of the VDRL test, uses the VDRL antigen containing fine carbon particles, which makes the reaction visible to the naked eye. The test can be performed with unheated serum or plasma (but not CSF). Both qualitative and quantitative results can be achieved.

Treponemal Serological Tests

These tests use the virulent Nichol's strain of *T. pallidum* grown in rabbit testes to detect antibodies and are used for confirmatory testing of syphilis. Two commonly used tests are **FTA-ABS** and **TP-PA**.

FTA-ABS (fluorescent-treponemal antibody absorption) test is an indirect fluorescent antibody test that uses *T. pallidum* fixed on a slide, as the antigen. After incubation with human serum, a tetramethylrhodamine isothiocyanate labelled anti-human immunoglobulin is added, and in individuals with specific antibodies, the spirochaetes are orange when observed under fluorscent microscope.

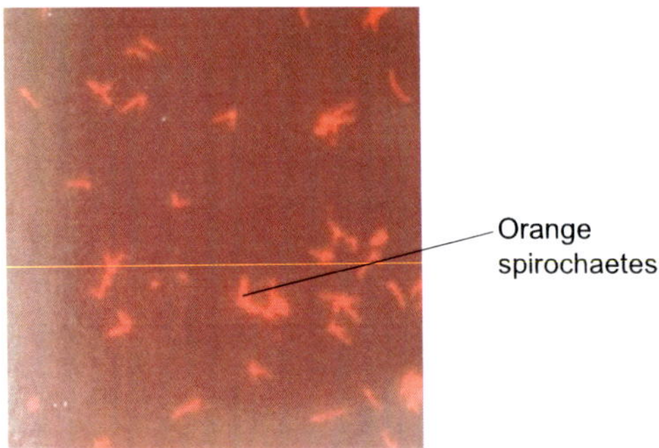

Fig. 47.2 Fluorescent treponemal antibody-absorption double-staining test. *T. pallidum* subsp. *pallidum* Nichol's is used as the antigen for the FTA-ABS DS test. The spirochaetes appear orange under fluorescence microscope.

Prevention

Syphilis can be prevented by:

- Avoiding sexual contact with an infected individual.
- Practising safe sex, i.e., use of condoms during any type of sexual activity (vaginal, anal or oral).

Treatment

Benzathine penicillin injection is the drug of choice to treat syphilis. A single dose of 2.4 million units is adequate in early cases. For late syphilis, this dose is repeated weekly for 3 weeks.

For patients allergic to penicillin, azithromycin, doxycycline or tetracycline are effective. In neurosyphilis, ceftriaxone antibiofic is effective.

NON-VENERAL TREPONEMATOSES: BEJEL, YAWS, PINTA

These are slow progressive cutaneous and bone diseases which are endemic to specific regions of tropics and subtropics, especially developing countries where hygiene is poor, little clothing is worn and due to over-crowding direct skin contact is common.

Bejel

Bejel (or **endemic syphilis**), caused by *T. p. endemicum*, is a deforming childhood infection of the mouth, nasal cavity, body, and hands. Transmission by direct person-to-person contact and by sharing contaminated eating or drinking utensils.

Yaws

Yaws (or **Frambesia**, **Rian**, **Parangi**), caused by *T. p. pertenue*, occurs from invasion of skin cut, causing a primary ulcer that crops a second crop of lesions. Flies may act as mechanical vectors.

Pinta

Pinta (also named **mal del pinto** and **carate**) is caused by *Treponema carateum*. It is characterized by superficial skin lesion that depigments and scars the skin. Transmission occurs by direct person-to-person contact with infectious lesions.

BORRELIA

The genus *Borrelia* (named after French biologist **Amédée Borrel**) comprises characteristic spirochaete (spiral shaped bacteria) that are Gram-negative and strictly anaerobic.

It contains 52 species. They are typically 20–30 µm lengthy and 0.2-0.3 µm wide, with 3–10 loose spirals with an abundance (30–40) of periplasmic flagella. The outer membrane contains outer surface proteins that play a role in their virulence. Two important diseases caused by borreliae are relapsing fevers and Lyme disease. Both are transmitted by arthropods.

RELAPSING FEVERS (RFs)

Relapsing fevers are characterized clinically by recurrent periods of fever and bacteremia. There are two forms of relapsing fever:

- The *epidemic or louse-borne relapsing fever* is caused by *Borrelia recurrentis*, an obligate human pathogen, transmitted from person-to-person by the body louse (*Pediculus humanus*). Spirochaete infects a person via mucous membranes and then invades the bloodstream.

- The *endemic* or *tick-borne relapsing fever* is caused by *B. hermsii, B parkeri* and *B. miyamotox* and is transmitted to humans from the rodents, via a tick vector.

  In both forms of RF, acute symptoms include: high fever, rigors, headache, myalgia, photophobia and cough, developing one week after infection.

  Diagnosis of RF is made by detecting borreliae in peripheral blood samples stained with Giemsa or acridine orange by dark-field illumination.

  Treatment: Tetracycline, chloramphenicol, penicillin and erythromycin are effective drugs.

LYME DISEASE

Lyme disease, also called **Lyme borreliosis**, and originally named as **Lyme arthritis** (named after **Lyme**, a town in the USA where an out-break occurred in 1975) is caused by *Borrelia burgdoferi* that is spread through the bite of one of the several types of ticks (*Ixodes*).

Characteristic **bull's-eye rash** on the skin, also known as **erythema chronicum migrans**, at the site of the tick bite is the most common symptom. Other early symptoms include fever, headache, tiredness and weight loss. Involvement of the heart joint, and central nervous system leading to facial nerve paralysis may occur at later stages of the disease. Arthritis, mainly involving the knees is the most common long-term manifestation. Onset of the disease occurs after a week of tick bite.

B. burgdorferi (named for its discoverer **Willy Burgdorfer**, who first isolated it in 1982) is a slow growing microaerophilic spirochaete with a generation (doubling) time of 24 to 48 hours. It is a Gram-negative, flat-wave shape, 5–20 µm long and 0.2–0.5 µm wide with 7–11 bundled periplasmic flagella.

Diagnosis of Lyme disease is based on characteristic ring-shaped lesions, isolation of spirochetes from the patient and testing of specific antibodies in the blood with an ELISA method, especially in the late stage of the disease since the blood tests are often negative in the early stages.

Preventive methods include: by wearing protective clothing to cover the arms, legs and using insect repellent containing N, N-Diethyl-meta-toluamide to prevent tick bites.

A human vaccine fort Lyme disease to protect high-risk population had been marketed in the USA since 1998 where about 3 lakh people are affected in a year.

A single dose of doxycycline may be used to prevent infections.

Treatment: Antibiotic therapy to treat Lyme includes: doxycycline, amoxycillin and cefuroxime. Standard treatment lasts for 2 to 3 weeks.

LEPTOSPIRA

Leptospira is a flexible, spirochete marked by tight very fine coils with characteristic hook at one or both ends (Figs. 47.1 and 47.2). It was first observed in 1907 in kidney tissue and the name proposed was *Leptospira* by **Hideyo Noguchi**, a Japanese scientist in 1917 based on its morphology from Greek words *lepto* meaing fine, thin, slender + *spira* = coil, i.e., a slender coil.

The genus contains two species: *Leptospira interrogans* which causes leptospirosis in humans and animals (dogs, rats), and *L. biflexa* is a harmless free living saprobe.

Leptospira interrogans

L. interrogans is an obligate aerobic, thin, tightly coiled rod-shaped spirochete. The species name is derived from the shape (morphology) of this organim, which is in the form of a "**question mark**" with a single hook (Fig. 47.3). More than 200 different pathogenic strains, called *serovars*, are currently recognized which are distributed among various animal groups.

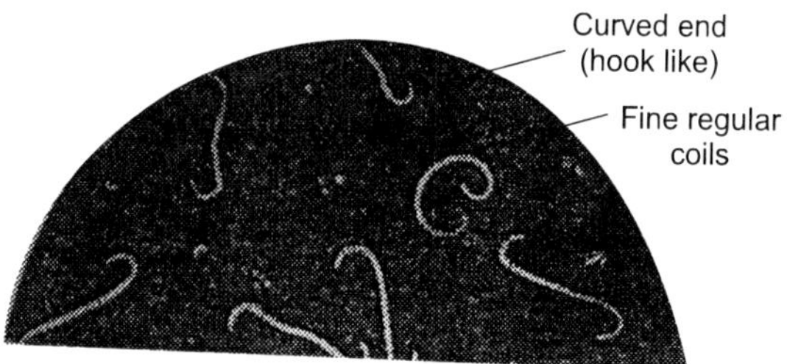

Fig. 47.3 ***Leptospira interrogans.*** Morphology of the organism in the form of a "question mark" with a single hook and numerous fine regular coils are characteristic of the bacterium.

Leptospires are very thin, delicate 6–12 μm long and 0.1 μm thick. The spirals are right handed, very close together, resulting in more than 18 coils per organism. They are faint Gram-negative organisms, actively motile, each with two subterminal periplasmic flagella with their free ends towards the middle of the bacteria.

It is difficult to culture requiring special media enriched with rabbit serum (e.g., Fletcher's, Stuart's) at 25–30°C and extended incubation period.

Leptospires are killed rapidly by desiccation, extremes of pH (e.g., gastric acid); low concentrations of chlorine; temperature above 40°C (e.g., 10 min at 50°C, within 10 seconds at 60°C); and by antibacterial substances naturally present in human and bovine milk. However, it can survive neutral or slightly alkaline water for 3 months or longer.

LEPTOSPIROSIS (WEIL'S DISEASE)

Leptospirosis, a zoonosis, usually caused by rats and cattle, also called **Weil's disease**, is attributed to **Adolf Weil** of the University of Heidelberg, Germany who first described it in 1886. It is a disease of the tropical and subtropical climate affecting 7–10 million people causing 58,900 deaths each year, woldwide.

Infection of humans usually occurs where open wounds that break the skin are immeresed in relatively stagnant water contaminated with rat or cattle urine. It does not usually result from swallowing water or rat bites.

Symptoms occur usually 7–12 days after the infection (ranges between 3 and 21 days). There can be two phases of leptospirosis:

- *The first phase:* Symptoms are similar to those of flu, including irregular high fever, headache and muscle ache. These may last 3 to 5 days before recovery.
- *The second phase:* Reoccurrence of the mild symptoms leading to severe form with bleeding from the lungs or meningitis, jaundice (yellow skin and eyes) by the 2nd or 3rd day, leading to kidney failure, the disease is then called **Weil's disease**. If it causes bleeding in the lungs, then it is known as **severe pulmonary haemorrhage syndrome**. Death can occur due to heart, liver or respiratory failure.

Diagnosis

Leptospirosis is diagnosed by:

- Demonstration of leptospires by direct wet mounts of urine or CSF by dark-field microscopy, phase-contrast microscopy or direct fluorescent antibody staining.
- Culturing of specimens of blood, **CSF** and urine on serum containing semisolid media at 28–30°C which are to examined every 3rd day for the presence of leptospires under dark ground illumination for 4 weeks.

- Serological diagnosis by microscoric agglutination test, i.e., testing blood for antibodies against the bacterium. A simple and rapid dip-stick assay is used to assay leptospira-specific antibodies in human sera.

Treatment

Penicillin, doxycycline and ceftriaxone are effective against leptospires. Penicillin is given as IV, 1-2 million units 6 hourly for 7 days in serious cases.

KEY POINTS

- **Spirochaetes** are thin, long, helical or spiral rods, highly motile by periplasmic flagella (endoflagella).
- *Treponema*, *Borrelia* and *Leptospira* are clinically important spirochaetes.
- *Treponema pallidum* subsp. *pallidum* (= *T. pallidum*) is the causative agent of syphilis, a sexually transmitted infection.
- In addition to syphilis (a veneral disease), *Treponema* causes endemic syphilis (bejel), yaws and pinta (*nonsyphilitic* or *nonveneral treponematosis*).
- *T. pallidum* is an obligate parasite that cannot be cultured on culture media and is uniformly sensitive to peniclliin.
- Diagnosis of syphilis is made by treponemes by dark field microscopy, treponemal antigens and by serological tests.
- Borrelias cause **relapsing fevers** (*B. recurrentis* and *B. hermsii*) and **Lyme disease** (*B. burgdorferi*) of humans.

  Leptospira interrogans, has a characteristic question mark morphology with a single hook, causes leptospirosis (Weil's disease) which spreads by rodent (rat) urine through contaminated water.

IMPORTANT QUESTIONS

1. Discuss the pathogensis, diagnosis and treatment of syphilis.
2. Write short notes on:
   (a) Spirochaetes morphology and three major diseases caused by them
   (b) VDRL test
   (c) Weil's disease
   (d) Lyme disease
   (e) Relapsing fevers

MULTIPLE-CHOICE QUESTIONS

1. *Treponema pallidum*, the causative agent of syphilis, an obligate parasite, is cultured in/on:
   (a) Blood agar (b) Serum broth
   (c) Animal tissue (d) Eggs.
2. The treatment of choice for syphilis is:
   (a) Sulfa drugs (b) Penicillin
   (c) Erythromycin (d) None of the above.
3. Which of the following diseases caused by *Treponema* is/are non-veneral treponematosis?
   (a) Yaws (b) Pinta
   (c) Bejal (d) All of the above.
4. Which of the following is associated with Yaw disease?
   (a) *Borrelia recurrentis*
   (b) *Borrelia hermsii*
   (c) *Borrelia burgdorferi*
   (d) All of the above.
5. Which of the following spirochaetes is transmitted by the rat urine?
   (a) *Brucella* (b) *Legionella*
   (c) *Leptospira* (d) None of the above.
6. Another name for Weil's disease is:
   (a) Lyme (b) Yaws
   (c) Leptospirosis (d) Pinta.
7. Which of the following treponematoses are *not* STDs?
   (a) Syphilis (b) Pinta
   (c) Yaws (d) Both (b) and (c).
8. Which of the following spirochaetes has a characteristic question mark morphology?
   (a) *Leptospira interrogans*
   (b) *Borrlia hermii*
   (c) *Borrelia burgdorferi*
   (d) *Treponema pallidum*.

ANSWERS TO MCQs

1. (c) 2. (b) 3. (d) 4. (c)
5. (c) 6. (c) 7. (d) 8. (a).

48

Mycoplasmas: *Mycoplasma, Ureaplasma*

Atypical (Walking) pneumonia; Genital tract infection

Mycoplasmas (also called **mollicutes**) are the smallest, wall-less, pleomorphic, nonmotile, free living bacteria. These can produce filaments that resemble fungi, hence their name (Greek: *mykes* = fungus and *plasma* = something moulded). They are so small (0.1–0.25 μm) that can pass through bacterial filters.

Albert Bernhard Frank in 1889 coined the term mycoplasma. After a decade (i.e., in 1898), *Mycoplasma mycoides* ssp. *mycoides* was isolated from cattle with pleuropneumonia. These organisms are often called **MLO (mycoplasma-like organisms)** and **PPLO (pleuropneumonia-like organisms)** because they have been found in the pleural cavities of cattle from pleuropneumonia. These organisms were originally considered to be viruses due to their very small size (0.1–0.25 μm) and simplicity.

Clinically important mycoplasmas belong to the order *Mycoplasmatales* in the class *Mollicutes* ("soft-skins").

Mycoplasma pneumoniae, the agent of atypical (walking) pneumonia that lacks typical symptoms, is clinically the most significant.

Two clinically significant genera can be differentiated:

- *Mycoplasma:* utilizes glucose or arginine, but does not hydrolyse urea. It has more than 110 named species.

  M. pneumoniae causes atypical pneumonia and *M. hominis* causes nongonococcal urethritis.
- *Ureaplasma:* Split urea. It has 6 species. *U. urealyticum* causes nongonococcal urethritis.

MYCOPLASMA PNEUMONIAE

Mycoplasma pneumoniae is a human pathogen that causes the disease **mycoplasmal pneumonia**. It is also called **primary atypical pneumoina (PAP)** because this syndrome is atypical in that its symptoms do not resemble those of pneumococcal pneumonia; and **walking pneumonia** because it is usually mild and rarely requires hospitalization.

Morphology

Mycoplasmas are the smallest known free-living organisms which can pass through bacterial filters and are surrounded only by a trilayered cell membrane which is rich in cholestrol and other lipids.

M. pneumoniae have an elongated shape, 1–2 μm (1000–2000 nm) long and 0.1–0.2 μm (100–200 nm) wide, hence cannot by examined by light microscopy. The lack of cell wall makes them undectable by Gram staining and insensitive to the activity of *β*-lactam antimicrobials.

M. pneumoniae is pleomorphic, shows unicellular small cells to filamentous growth. It reproduces by fragmentation of the filaments at the bulges (Fig. 48.1).

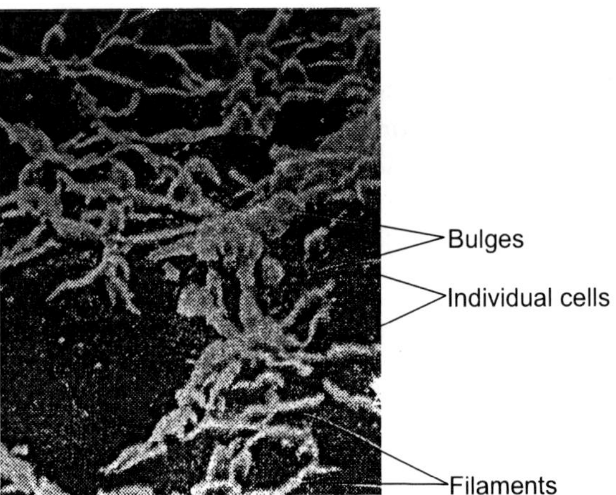

Fig. 48.1 ***Mycoplasma pneumoniae* (SEM)**. Filamentous growth like a fungus, showing fragmentation of the filaments at the bulges as a mode of reproduction.

M. pneumoniae are the only bacterial cells that possess cholestrol in their cell membranes (obtained from the host). The cells also possess an attachment organelle which is used in the gliding motility of the organism.

Cultural Characteristics

Most mycoplasmas are facultatively anaerobic growing best at 36–38°C (temperature range 22–41°C).

Mycoplasmas are cultured on media (both solid and liquid) that contain inactivated horse serum to provide cholestrol, and a source of proteins. A widely used isolation medium contains bovine heart infusion (PPLO broth) with fresh yeast extract (10%), horse serum (20%) with glucose and phenol red as a pH indicator and agar as a solidifying agent. Penicillin, ampicillin and polymyxin B as antibacterial agents, and amphotericin B as antifungal agent to inhibit bacterial and fungal contaminants.

M. pneumoniae usually is a slow grower with an incubation period of 2-3 weeks, while *M. hominis* gorws rapidly and can form colonies in 1 to 5 days (Fig. 48.2). On agar, the colonies have a typical **"fried-egg"** appearance with an opaque central zone of growth within the agar and a translucent peripheral zone on the surface, measuring 10–600 μm in diameter, visualized with a hand lens.

M. pneumoniae produces clear zones of β-hemolysis.

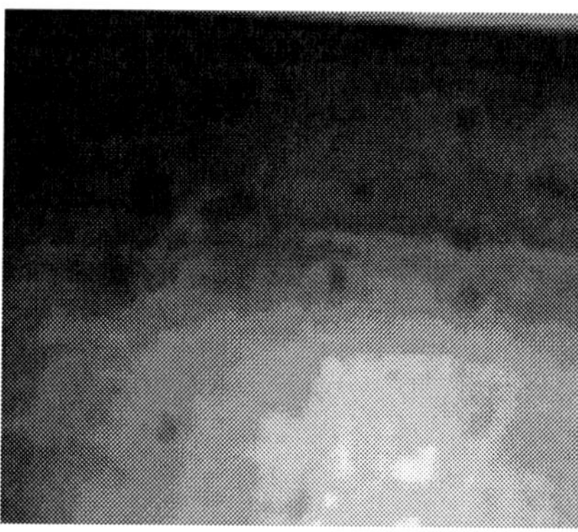

Fig. 48.2 ***Mycoplasma hominis on A7 agar***. Colonies have a typical "fried-egg" appearance.

Resistance: They are resistant to penicillin and cephalosporin as well as to lysozymes that act on the bacterial cell walls but are susceptible to tetracycline and many other antibiotics.

MYCOPLASMAL PNEUMONIA

M. pneumoniae produces "atypical pneumonia" also called walking pneumonia, that accounts for 10 to 20% of the reported pneumonias. Transmission is by aerosol droplets of nasopharyngeal secretions, and most of the cases occur in the fall and winter.

The disease more frequently occurs among young children, older people, and those living in closed-in groups such as military personnel and labour class families.

Most infections are asymptomatic, mild following an incubation period of 2-3 weeks, nonproductive cough, fever, headache, running nose, pharyngitis and ear pain.

Laboratory Diagnosis

Diagnosis can be made using culture, serology or nucleic acid amplification methods:

Culture: Throat swabs or respiratory secretions are inoculated into mycoplasma medium at 35°C for 1–2 weeks for the appearance of small β-haemolytic, homogenous granular (multiberry shaped) colonies. **Polymerase chain reaction (PCR)** assay is used for rapid detection.

Serological diagnosis is made by using mycoplasmal antigens: Immunofluorescence or haemagglutination inhibition for detection of antibodies to *M. pneumoniae* are the most sensitive tests.

Non-specific Serological Tests

- **Cold agglutination test**, a non-specific serological test, has been used for many years to diagnose mycoplasmal pneumonia that is performed by demonstration of cold agglutinins to human red blood cells at a titre greater than 32. Formation of cold agglutinins is the first humoral response to *M. pneumoniae* within 6 weeks. After infection, the cold agglutinins titre declines toward the pre-existing level. Demonstration of these antibodies is fast and simple to perform.

  In this test, serial dilutions of the patient's serum are mixed with an equal volume of 0.2% washed human O group erythrocytes and observed for clumping after overnight incubation of the mixture at low temperature. Clumping is dissociated at 37°C, i.e., reversal of the test. A litre of 1:32 or more is suggestive, but demonstration of rise in titre in paired serum samples is more reliable.
- **Streptococcus MG test:** Serial dilutions of the patient's unheated serum is mixed with a heat killed *Streptococcus* MG suspension and incubated over night at 37°C. A titre of 1:20 or more is considered suggestive of *M. pneumoniae* infection.

MYCOPLASMA HOMINIS

M. hominis (from Latin *hominis* meaning of man), a weak sexually transmitted pathogen, is often associated with polymicrobial infections, mainly vaginitis, pelvic inflammatory disease and kidney inflammation. It can also cause fever and infection in new born baby.

It grows rapidly on Mycoplasma media producing colonies in 2 days at 37°C which measure 50–300 μm in diameter with a typical "fried egg" appearance (Fig. 48.2). The typical colony morphology and the orginine positivity of *M. hominis* are usually the adequate criteria for identification.

Doxycycline (tetracycline family) is the antibiotic of choice to treat the patients.

UREAPLASMA UREALYTICUM

U. urealyticum, originally called for tiny mycoplasma, associated with infections of the urogenitial tract, is present in cervix or vagina in most healthy women and urethra in males. It spreads during sex. In females, it causes pain, odour or discharge from the vagina, and discharge and swelling at the opening of urethra. In males, it causes urethritis (i.e., inflammation of the urethra).

In the A 7 agar, which contains calcium chloride and urea, it produces very small colonies from 15–30 μm, in addition to black precipitate of calcium ammonium chloride.

It can be readily identified by urea test. It rapidly hydrolyzes urea, turning the colour of the medium from yellow to red-purple as a result of the change in the pH in the presence of phenol red in the medium as an indicatior.

Maxifloxacin, azithromycin and doxycycline are used to treat the infection.

KEY POINTS

- **Mycoplasmas** are the smallest, wall-less, pleomorphic, non-motile bacteria.
- **Mycoplasmal pneumonia** (atypical or walking pneumonia) is caused by *Mycoplasma pneumoniae.*
- Demonstration of cold agglutinins to human red blood cells at titre greater than 32 (**cold agglutination test**) is usually used to diagnose mycoplasmal pneumonia.
- *Mycoplasma hominis* and *Ureaplasma urealyticum* are normal colonists of most persons, however, these may cause sexually transmitted diseses.

IMPORTANT QUESTIONS

1. Write short notes on:
   (a) Diagnostic features and pathogenicity of *Mycoplasma pneumoniae.*
   (b) Name major mycoplasmal diseases with their causative agents.

MULTIPLE-CHOICE QUESTIONS

1. All are true for mycoplasmas EXCEPT:
   (a) Smallest prokaryotic organisms
   (b) Cell wall made of peptidioglycan
   (c) Fried-egg appearance
   (d) Pleomorphic.
2. Colonies of *Mycoplasma pneumoniae* have the characteristic feature:
   (a) Caron coil appearance
   (b) Fried-egg appearance
   (c) Medusa head appearance
   (d) None.
3. Mycoplasma refers to the filamentous (fungus-like) nature of the organisms. True or False?
4. *Mycoplasma pneumoniae* reproduces by fragmentation of the filaments at the bulges. True or False?

ANSWERS TO MCQs

1. (b) 2. (b) 3. True 4. True.

49

Rickettsia and *Coxiella*

Rocky Mountain spotted fever; Typhus; Q Fever

Rickettsiae (**Rickettsias**) are tiny, Gram-negative, highly pleomorphic obligate intracellular parasites transmitted by arthropod vectors.

Rickettisiae include three genera: *Rickettsia*, *Orientia* and *Ehrlichia* classfied in the family *Rickettsiaceae* (order *Rickettsiales*). The diseases caused by these are called **rickettsioses** and **spotted fever group** (e.g., typhus, Rocky Mountain spotted fever and ehrichioses) which are usually transmitted by tick bite or tick faeces.

Rickettsiae are **obligate intracellular parasites** and are able to grow and multiply (reproduce) only in cell culture, animals (guinea pigs, mice), and chick embryos, they were therefore originally considered to be viruses.

RICKETTSIA

Rickettsia consists of small, nonmotile pleomorphic coccobacilli 0.3–0.6 µm × 0.8–2 µm. They are Gram-negative, though they do not take the stain well.

The bacterial genus *Rickettsia* was named after an American bacteriologist **Howard Taylor Ricketts**, in honour of his pioneering work on tick-borne spotted fever.

Being obligate intracellular parasites, the species cannot grow in artificial culture media and are grown either in tissue or embryo cultures, typically chick embryo following a method developed by **Ernest William Goodpasture** and his colleagues at Vanderbilt University in the early 1930s.

Diseases

Most common infections caused by *Rickettsia* are:

- Rocky Mountain spotted fever—*R. tickettsii* (Ticks)
- Rickettsialpox—*R. akari* (Mites)
- Mediterranean spotted fever—*R. conorii* (Ticks)
- Murine typhus—*R. typhi* (Fleas)
- Epidemic typhus—*R. prowazekii* (Lice)

Pathogenesis

Rickettsiae normally enter the human body by the arthropod vectors through their bite or faeces.

These bacteria primarily target the microvascular endothelial cells, resulting in endothelial dysfunction. Bacteria after entering the endothelial cells multiply leading to enlargement, degeneration and thrombosis, with occlusion of the vascular lumen.

The pathologic effects are mainfested by: skin rash, oedema, hypotension and gangrene. Mental changes and other neurological symptoms may occur due to intravascular clotting in the brain.

Based on their clinical features, two main groups of human infections are recognized:

- Spotted fever (e.g., RMSF, Rickettsialpox)
- Typhus (e.g., Epidemic typus, Murine typhus)

ROCKY MOUNTAIN SPOTTED FEVER (RMSF)

RMSF caused by the bacterium *Rickettsia rickettsii* spreads through the bite of an infected tick.

The disease was named for the place it was first seen in the 1800s in the Rocky Mountains of Montana (USA).

It is the most serious type of spotted fever (also called **black measles** because of the characteristics spotted (petechial) rash. Fewer than 5000 cases are reported a year in the United States (most often in June to July). In India, 100 thousand cases are recorded every year.

RMSF typically begins with a fever and headache within 2 to 14 days after a person is bitten by a tick harbouring *R. rickettsii*, which is followed a few days later with the development of a **rash**—frequently with blackened and crashed skin at the site of tick bite. The rash has a centripetal or "inward" pattern of spread that usually starts in the extremities involving the palms and soles, and spreads to the trunk. Early lesions are sligthly mottled like measles but later petechial, and severe cases necrotic, predisposing to gangrene of the toes or fingertips. Long-term complications following recovery may include hearing loss.

DIAGNOSIS

Serology testing and skin biopsy are considered to be the best methods of diagnosis. Heparinized blood should be collected early in the course of infection for isolation and serological testing.

- The **Weil-Felix** (WF) test which employs *Proteus* antigens (OX2, OX19, OXK), is the most widely used serological test for the presumptive diagnosis of rickettsial diseases. This test can be done either a slide or a tube test.
- **ELISA** test to detect rickettsial antibodies by a change in serum titer is a reliable test to confirm a presumptive diagnosis.
- Staining rickettsias directly in a tissue biopsy using fluorescent antibodies is a very useful method for early diagnosis.
- Rickettsiae can be isolated in embryonated chicken eggs, cell culture, mice or guinea pigs followed by the Giemsa stained examination.

Treatment

The drug of choice to treat RMSF (both suspected and known cases) is **doxycycline** (a tetracycline) that is administered for one week.

THYPUS GROUP OF DISEASES

Typhus, also called **typhus fever**, is a group of infectious diseases, characterized by fever, headache and rashes. The name comes from the Greek *typhos* meaning hazy, describes the state of mind (i.e., altered mental status) of those infected.

Girolamo Fracastoro, a Florentine physician, first described typhus in his famous treatise in 1546. It was a devastating disease for humans that was responsible for hundreds of thousands of deaths during World War II.

Typhus is of three types:

Epidemic typhus (also called **louse-borne typhus**)—caused by *Rickettsia prowazekii* is transmiited by the humans body louse (*Pediculus humans corporis*). It often causes **epidemics** (rapid spread of a disease affecting a very large number of people) following wars and natural disasters, hence named epidemic typhus.

The initial symptoms are similar to those described for RMSF, i.e., high fever (102°F), headache and muscular pain. Rash on the chest begins after 5 days fever and spreads to the trunk and extremities. The patients may develop mycocarditis and involvement of the CNS. A mild recurring form of the disease called **Brill – Zinsser disease** can occur after several years.

Endemic typhus (or **murine typhus** or **flea-borne typhus**) is caused by *Rickettsia typhi* (= *R. mooseri*) and spreads by fleas. It is endemic in tropical and subtropical areas of the world. The rash is restricted to the chest and abdomen.

Scrub typhus is caused by *Orientia tsutsugamus* (formerly *Rickettsia tsutsugamushi*), and spreads by chiggers. The disease occurs mainly in Asia, Australia and Japan. Rash starts to the trunk and spreads to the extremities. Involvement of the reticuloendothelial system, with cardiovascular and CNG complications, can occur.

Doxycycline is used to treat typhus.

COXIELLA

Coxiella is an obligate intracellular Gram-negative pleomorphic coccobacillus, a member of the family *Coxiellaceae* (order *Legionellales*). It is named after **Hearld Rea Cox**, an American bacteriologist, who in association with **Davis** first isolated the pathogen from ticks in Montana in 1938. *Coxiella burnetii,* the causative agent of Q-fever, is the only member of this genus, and can be misused as a biological warfare agent.

This bacteriun naturally infects some animals, such as goats, sheep and cattle. It is an intracellular bacterium and survives in the phagolysosomes of its host. It is highly resistant to envionmental stresses such as high temperature, ultraviolet light and osmotic pressure due to the presence of unique endospores that are released when the cell disintegrates. Free spores survive outside the host and are important in transmission. This organism is difficult to study because it cannot be cultured *in vitro* on culture media. However, scientists succeeded in axenic culturing of this pathogen in 2009.

The disease caused by the organism is called **Q-fever** because the causative agent was not known when the illness was first described (Q stands for *query* meaning to *question* or of *unknown origin*). **Q-fever** is an extremely rare disease, fewer than five thousand cases recorded annually in India. It is mild and self-limiting. Humans typically contract Q-fever by inhaling aerosols from contaminated environment (air and dust), consuming unpasteurized milk and meat. *C. burnetti* is one of the most infectious known organisms since it requires an extremely low infectious dose (only 1–10 organisms). Lungs are the main organs involved. Disease occurs in two stages:

An acute stage that presents with headache, chills and respiratory symptoms and is self-limiting.

Chronic stage that presents as endocarditis.

Laboratory diagnosis. By serology, indirect immunoflouresence assay or ELISA.

Treatment. Doxycycline is the drug of choice.

Prevention. Q-VAX vaccine is effective to prevent Q-fever. It is administered by injection under the skin, usually in the upper arm.

KEY POINTS

- **Rickettsias** are tiny obligate intracellular bacteria that live in the bodies of ticks and lice and grow only within a host cell.
- The genus *Rickettsia* is the causative agent of Rocky Mountain spotted fever and typhus (epidemic and endemic).
- All rickettsial infections are characterized by fever and rashes and treated by doxycycline (tetracycline).
- Q-fever, a self-limiting infection, is caused by *Coxiella burnetii.*
- *Coxiella burnetii* can be misused in bioterrorism.
- *C. burnetii* is unqiue in producing endospores that help in survival and transmission.

IMPORTANT QUESTIONS

1. Write notes on:
   (a) Rocky Mountain spotted fever
   (b) Q-fever
   (c) Laboratory diagnosis of rickettsial infections
   (d) Typhus fever.

MULTIPLE-CHOICE QUESTIONS

1. Rocky Mountain spotted fever is caused by
   (a) *Rickettsia prowazekii* (b) *Rickettsia typhi*
   (c) *Rickettsia rickettsii* (d) *Coixella burnetii.*

2. Epidemic typhus caused by *Rickettsia prowazekii* is transmitted by (or vector);
   (a) body louse (b) Ticks
   (c) Flea (d) Mite.

3. Weil-Felix, a serological test, is used for the diagnosis of:
   (a) Scrub typhus (b) Plague
   (c) Q-fever (d) Brucellosis.

4. Which of the following is *not* an arthropod vector of rickettioses?
   (a) Tick (b) Louse
   (c) Mosquito (d) Flea.

ANSWERS TO MCQs

1. (c) 2. (a) 3. (a) 4. (c).

50

Chlamydiae: *Chlamydia*

Trachoma; Inclusion conjunctivitis; STDs; Atypical pneumonia; Ornithosis

Chlamydiae (or **chlamydias**) are small obligate intracellular Gram-negative bacteria with a unique biphasic life cycle that is adaptable to both intracellular and extracellular environments and quite distinct from that of other bacteria. They are as small as or smaller than many viruses and cannot be cultured *in vitro*.

They are widely distributed in nature and are responsible for a variety of ocular, genito-urinary and respiratory diseases in humans.

Two genera: *Chlamydia* and *Chlamydophila* were recognized in the family *Chlamydiaceae* (order *Chlamdiales*, phylum *Chlamydiae*).

However, *Chlamydophila* is a controversial genus hence *Chlamydia* is the only valid genus in the family.

The clinically important human pathogenic species of *Chlamydia* are: *C. trachomatis*, *C. pneumoniae* and *C. psittaci*.

Morphology

Chlamydiae are small, non-motile bacteria having the typical LPS of Gram-negative bacteria, although they stain poorly with Gram's stain. They exhibit a unique **dimorphic growth cycle** which consists of two morphologically distinct forms:

- **Elementary body (EB):** The infectious non-dividing very small, spherical (200–300 nm), extracellular metabolic inert environmentally resistant structure that initiates the infection in the host.
- **Reticulated body (RB):** The large (500–1000 nm) non-infectious intracellularly proliferative structure that has pathologic effects.

Growth (or Reproductive) Cycle

Chlamydial growth or reproductive or infectious cycle (Fig. 50.1) is unique which conists of two alternating cellular forms: EB and RB. The cycle is initiated with the attachment (or adhesion) of infectious EBs to the surface of host's epithelial cell followed by its entry into the cell by phagocytosis. EBs reside and replicate within an intracellular host membrane-bound cytoplasmic compartment called the **chlamydial inclusion**. In about 6–8 hours, the EBs undergo differentiation to reticulate bodies (RBs), the latter divide by binary fission with a doubling time of about 2 hours. Later, the daughter cells are converted to EBs. The developing chlamydial microcolony consisting binary of RBs, EBs and various intermediate forms, is called the **inclusion body**. There are 100–500 infective EBs in a mature inclusion body which are ultimately released from the host cell and can initiate another round of infections.

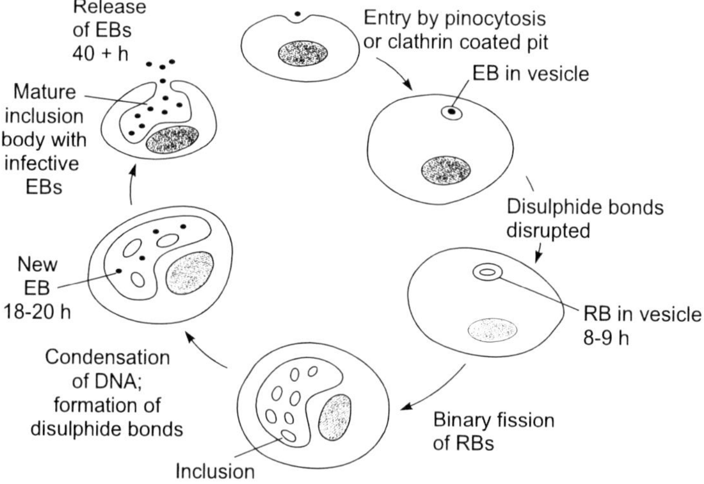

Figure 50.1 The chlamydia growth cycle showing alternation of two cellular forms: EB and RB, a unique biphasic (dimorphic) cycle.

Laboratory Propagation

Chlamydias are propagated in cell culture, chick or mouse embryo for the lab diagnosis. Commonly used host cells for cell culturing include He La 229 cells and McCoy cells contained in shell vials or microtiter plates. These are inoculated with cervical specimens. The presence of chlamydial inclusions is determined after 48 hours incubated at 37°C by fluorsescent microscopy with labelled monoclonal antibody.

Large apple-green fluoresent intracytoplasmic inclusions against the red background of the Evans blue counter-stain in infected cells is a positive cell culture for *C. trachomatis*.

CHLAMYDIA TRACHOMATIS

Chlamydia trachomatis, clinically the most significant chlamydiae, is an obligate intracellular human pathogen that infects epithelial cells of the eyes, oropharynx, urogenital and anorectal mucosa. It is a leading cause of oculogenital infections:

- **Trachoma** (blindness) and **inclusion conjunitivitis** of eye.
- **STDs:** NGU (nongonococcals), **pelvic inflammatory disease** and **lymphogranuloma venereum**.

C. trachomitis (Gr. *chlamys* = a clock + *trachoma* = rougness) was first described in 1907 by **Stanislaus von Prowazek** and **Ludwig Halberstädter** in scrapings from trachoma cases and named it "Chlamdozoa" from the Greek "*chlamys* meaning mantle, a mantled protozoan". **Tang Fei-fan** and coworkers in 1957 first isolated and cultured this organism in yolk sac of eggs. Based on the presence of DNA, RNA and ribosomes and electron microscopic studies it was proved to be a bacterium in 1966. Unlike the cell walls of most of other bacteria, it lacks muramic acid which hinders staining of the cell wall, however, this bacterium is still classified as Gram-negative.

In *C. trachomatis*, a Gram-negative bacterium, the infective EBs are 200–400 nm in diameter surrounded by a rigid cell wall that can initiate new infection when it comes in contact with a susceptible host. The RBs are 600–1500 nm which are found only in host cells. Most strains carry a plasmid that contains 8 genes.

CHLAMYDIAL DISEASES OF THE EYE

TRACHOMA (OCULAR TRACHOMA)

Trachoma is an infectious disease of the eye caused by *Chlamydia trachomatis*. It is the leading cause of blindness in the world today. It is a public health problem in 44 countries, and is responsible for the blindness or visual impairment of about 1.9 million people. India has become free of trachoma, overall prevalence is of only 0.7% (National Trachoma Survery Report 2014–2017).

It's very contagious and infection spreads easily through personal contacts (via contaminated hands, clothes and bedding) and by flies that have been in contact with discharge from the eyes or nose of an infected person.

The pathogen infects epithelial cells of the eye causing a roughing of the inner surface of the eyelids leading to pain in the eyes. With repeated episodes of infection over many years, the eyelashes may be drawn in so that they rub on the outer surface of the eye, with pain and discomfort and permanent damage to the cornea and eventual blurred vision or blindness (advanced blinding stage is called **trichiasis**).

Trachoma is usually clinically diagnosed: people are examined for clinical signs through the use of magnifiers (coupes).

Treatment

Azithromycin (single oral dose) and topical tetracycline are effective to treat early infection. Surgical repair of in-turned eyelid and eyelashes is required in later stages of trachoma.

INCLUSION CONJUNCTIVITIS (NEONATAL AND ADULT)

Inculsion conjunctivitis is an inflammation of the conjunctiva, or white of the eye. In newborns (**opthalmia neonatrum**), within 5–6 days, there is an abundant ocular water discharge with swollen eyelids. It is usually acquired through contact with secretions of the infected gentiourinary tract and appears 5–14 days after birth.

Adult inclusion conjunctivitis (**paratrachoma**) is usually transmitted sexually and is most prevalent in sexually active young people. It develops when the eye is infected by the urogenital secretions of *Chlamydia* infected person and eye-to-eye contact. Symptoms appear 2–19 days after contact. These include a foreign body sensation, watery eyes, and eyelids that stick together upon awakening. Large follicles on the lower lid and swollen preauricular nodes (lymph nodes near the ear) may be seen.

Diagnosis: Based on clinical symptoms obsevered by the eye care provider.

Laboratory testing of the swabbed sample from inside of the eyelids to test for the presence of characteristic inclusion bodies made only by *Chlamydia* by Giemsa stain. Immunofluoresence monocolonal antibody testing, enzyme immunoassays, serum antibodies tests and DNA probes.

Treatment: Erythromycin 4 times a day for 2 weeks is the standard treatment for an infant younger than 4 months. The eye may be irrigated with saline to remove the mucus discharge.

Prevention: The incidence of neonatal conjunctivitis can be reduced by applying erythromycin ointment to the newborn's eyes shortly after delivery. Sliver nitrate is not effective against chlamydia.

SEXUALLY TRANSMITTED CHLAMYDIAL INFECTIONS

NON-SPECIFIC URETHRITIS (NSU)

C. trachomatis (serovars D-K) is responsible for about 30% of NSU in men. Globally, NSU is one of the commonest STDs and repeated infections are common. This infection ranges from asymptomatic to mucopurulent discharge which progresses to epididymitis or prostatis, especially in aged less than 35 years. Chronic epididymitis leads to occlusion of the tube and infertility due to azoospermia.

Anal intercourse may cause **chlamydia proctitis** in either sex. Associated symptoms include rectal pain and bleeding, mucopurulent discharge and diarrhoea.

PELVIC INFLAMMATORY DISEASE (PID)

C. trachomatis serovars D-K infections in women cause **mucopurulent cervicitis (MPC)** (white discharge), **endometritis** (inflammation of the endometrial lining of uterus), and **salpingitis** (infection of the fallopian tubes leading to infertility). Endometritis is and salpingitis are collectively called **pelvic inflammatory disease**. Chlamydia often coexist with gonococcus and other genitourinary pathogens, thereby greatly complicating treatment.

LYMPHOGRANULOMA VENEREUM (LGV)

Lymphogranuloma venereum (also called **tropical bubo** and **lymphogranuloma inginuale**) an STD, is a disfiguring disease of the external genitalia and pelvic lymphatics. It is caused by the L1, L2, and L3 serovars of *C. trachomitis*. It is a long-term (chronic) infection of the lymphatic system characterized by small genital or rectal lesion which can ulcerate at the site of infection within 3 to 30 days followed by lymphadenopathy of the regional lymph nodes. These nodes or buboes can cause lymphatic obstruction (blockage) that leads to chronic, deforming oedema of the genitalia and anus.

CHLAMYDIA PNEUMONIAE

Chlamydia pneumoniae also known as ***Chlamydophila pneumoniae***, was originally named **Taiwan acute respiratory agent (TWAR)**, from the names of the original isolates—Taiwan (TW-183) isolated in 1950 and AR-39 (acute respiratory isolate). It infects respiratory tract (lungs) and is a common cause of pneumonia around the world. It is a serious complication in asthma patients. The bacteria cause illness by damaging the lining of the respiratory tract including the throat and windpipe. It is one of the commonest causes of community-acquired pneumonia. 60–80% of people worldwide become infected with this pathogen during their life cycle.

In addition to pneumonia (also called atypical pneumonia), the bacterium also causes pharyngitis, bronchitis and coronary artery disease.

CHLAMYDIA PSITTACI

Chlamydia psittaci (also called *Chlamydophila psittaci*), a lethal intracellular chlamydiae, is the cause of **psittacosis** (*psittacos* means parrot hence also called **parrot fever**) or **ornithosis** (derived from the Greek word *ornithos* for bird in humans). The disease was first reported in 1879 in Switzerland and the causative agent was identified 61 years later in 1930. The incubation period is about 10 days. The disease starts with flu-like (influenza-like) symptoms with fever, sore throat, headache, lung congestion to a severe life-threatening pneumonia. The infection is acquired from birds, i.e., a zoonosis. The organism is blood-borne through the body producing severe complications resembling enteric and Q-fevers.

LABORATORY DETECTION OF *CHLAMYDIA* INFECTIONS

Several laboratory methods are available to diagnose *Chlamydia* infections and nucleic acid amplication tests are the most sensitive tests. The samples used for various tests are conjunctival scrapings, sputum, throat swab, bubo pus, genital swabs, urine (firstly void) and blood.

- **Demonstration of inclusion or elementary bodies in infected cells:** Direct microscopic examination of Giemsa stain smears prepared from conjunctival scrapings and bubo pus show characteristic inclusion bodies in infected cells.
- **Demonstration of characteristic inclusions in cell culture:** Cell culture of *C. trachomatis* in McCoy cell tissue is considered to be gold standard method for its diagnosis. Presence of dark purple with a halo, a distinct intracytoplasmic inclusion, is a positive test to diagnose *Chlamydia* infection.
- **Chlamydial antigen detection by direct fluorescent antobodies stain (DFA):** DFA is a specific, sensitive and one of the first commercially available tests to identify *C. trachomatis*. In this test, smears of the infected exudate are fixed and stained with fluroscent-labelled monoclonal antibodies. Apple-green fluorescing EBs or RBs by fluorescence microscopy is a positive DFA test.

- **Enzyme immunoassay (EIA) to detect chlamydial antigen:** EIA is a commercially available antigen based rapid assay for the direct detection of *C. trachomatis* from genital specimens. This test detects and measures antibodies in the blood. It is a rapid and simple test.
- **Serological testing:** The **microimmunofluorescence assay (MIF)** is the gold standard for *Clamydia* serological testing and is used as an epidemiological tool to investigate various infections caused by the major serotypes of *Chlamydia trachomatis, C. pneumoniae* and *C. psittaci*. In the MIF assay, purified preparation of formalin fixed EBs are used as the antigens. Presence of distinct and fluorescent EBs examined under 400× magnification is a positive MIF assay. Serially diluted patient's serum is applied to the wells of a multiwell microscope slide.
- **Nucleic acid detection: Nucleic acid amplification tests (NAATs)** are now the methods of choice for clinical specimens. Urine or vaginal tampons are used for *C. trachomatis* DNA amplification. Alternatively, chlamydial mRNA can be dectected in infected cells. However, NAATs are expensive and are not widely available.

TREATMENT OF CHLAMYDIAL INFECTIONS

A single dose of azithromycin, or doxycycline twice daily for 7 days are the antibiotics of choice. Oral erythromycin is used to treat babies.

KEY POINTS

- **Chlamydiae** (or **chlamydias**) are obligate intracellular Gram-negative bacteria with a unique biphasic cycle.
- **Biphasic (or dimorphic) cycle** consists of two distinct forms: elementary body (EB) and reticulate body (RB).
- The cytoplasmic compartment in which EBs reside and replicate is called **chlamydial inclusion** (or simply **inclusion**).
- *Chlamydia trachomatis,* clinically the most significant species, causes a prevalent STD that can damage the reproductive tract and can cause blindness.
- *Chlamydia pneumoniae* is a community acquired pathogen that causes pneumonia and *C. psittaci* causes a zoonotic disease called **ornithosis** (also called **psittacosis**).
- Visual loss (blindness) occurs in trachoma, an ocular infection, caused by *Chlamydia trachomatis.*

IMPORTANT QUESTIONS

1. What are chlamydiae? Discuss laboratory diagnosis of chlamydial infections.
2. Write short notes on:
   (a) Unique life cycle of chlamydiae.
   (b) Sexually transmitted chlamydial infections.
   (c) Chlamydial diseases of eye.

MULTIPLE-CHOICE QUESTIONS

1. All are true for chlamydias EXCEPT:
   (a) Form infective elementary bodies
   (b) Intracellular parasite
   (c) Can be grown on culture media
   (d) Have dimorphic growth cycle.
2. All are true for reticulate bodies produced in chlamydia EXCEPT:
   (a) They are infectious
   (b) They are larger than elementary bodies
   (c) They are inracellular proliferative
   (d) They are responsible for pathologic effects.
3. Ornithosis (psittacosis) is a .... infection associated with:
   (a) Chlamydial, mice (b) Rickettsial, parrots
   (c) Chlamydial, birds (d) Rickettsial, flies.
4. Lymphogranuloma venereum is caused by
   (a) *Chlamydia psittaci*
   (b) *Chlamydia trachomatis*
   (c) *Chlamydia pneumoniae*
   (d) All of these.
5. *Chlamydia trachomatis* causes visual loss (blindness) in which ocular infection?
   (a) Trachoma
   (b) Paratrachoma
   (c) Chlamydial ophthalmia neonatarum (inclusion conjuntivitis)
   (d) All of the above.

ANSWER TO MCQs

1. (c) 2. (a) 3. (c) 4. (b)
5. (a).

51

Vibrio: Curved Gram-negative Motile Rods

Cholera; Gastroenteritis

Vibrio is a Gram-negative, curved (comma-shaped) rod that is actively motile by a single polar flagellum. It is classified in the family *Vibrionaceae*. The name is derived from the characteristic vibratory motility from the Latin word *vibrare* meaning to *vibrate* or *shake*. **Vibrios** are facultative anaerobes that test positive for oxidase and are found in salty water. They typically possess **two chromosomes**, unusual for bacteria.

Vibrio cholerae, V. parahaemolyticus and *V. vulnificus* are the most important human pathogens that cause cholera, gastroenteritis, wound infection and cellulitis.

VIBRIO CHOLERAE

Vibrio cholerae was first isolated and identified in 1854 by the Italian scientist **Filippo Pacini** from the cholera patients naming it "**choleigenic vibrios**" based on their motility. **Robert Koch** in 1884 carried out extensive work on this bacterium naming it **Kommabacillus** due to the characteristic comma-shaped morphology. International Committee on Nomenclature in 1965 adopted *Vibrio cholerae* (Gr. *chole* = bile) as the correct name of the cholera causing organism.

Morphology

It is a short, curved, Gram-negative bacillus measuring 1.5–2.5 μm long and 0.5–0.8 μm wide (Fig. 51.1). The bacterium is typically comma-shaped, hence once named *Vibrio comma* (Fig. 51.1). It is actively motile by a single polar flagellum. The motility is characteristically of the **darting type**.

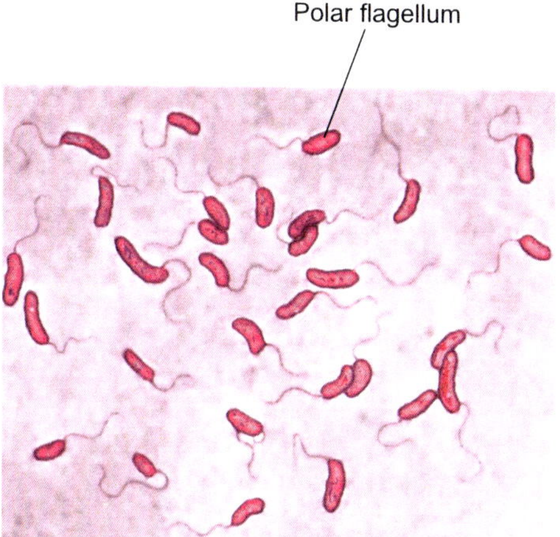

Fig. 51.1 ***Vibrio cholerae* curved rods looking like comma**, a characteristic feature of the genus (SEM).

CULTURAL CHARACTERISTICS

It is strongly aerobic, best growth occurring when abundant oxygen is present at 35–37°C (range 16–42°C) in an alkaline medium in the pH range 7.4–9.6 (optimum pH 8.2).

It is a **non-halophilic** species that grows on ordinary media without added salt (e.g., nutrient agar, MacConkey agar, blood agar, peptone water). On nutrient agar, the colonies are translucent, round disk (1–2 mm) with a bluish tinge in transmitted light. On blood agar, the colonies are 1-3 mm in diameter, nonhaemolytic opaque with a greenish hue.

TCBS (Thiosulphate-citrate-bile sucrose) agar is a selective medium used for *V. cholerae* isolation from faecal specimems. Characteristic yellow colonies are produced at 35°C under aerobic conditions (Fig. 51.2) because it ferments sucrose whereas most other *Vibrio* spp. causing gastroenteritis are sucrose-negative and appear as green colonies.

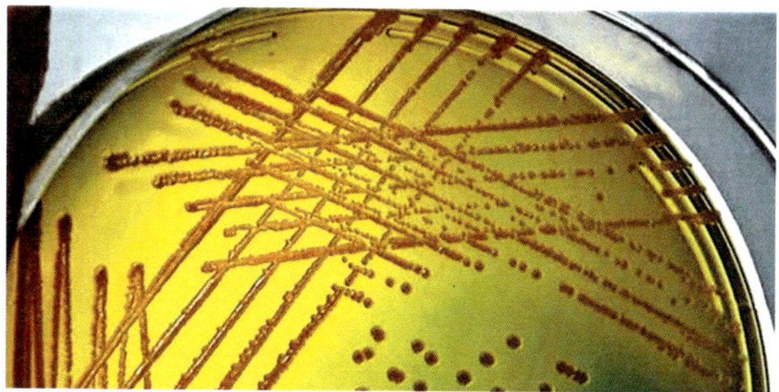

Fig. 51.2 ***Vibrio cholerae*** yellow colonies on TCBS agar, a selective medium.

String test: String test is used to distinguish *Vibrio* spp. In this test, a loopful of growth (colony) is suspended in a drop of sodium deoxycholate (0.5%) on a glass slide. Lysis of bacteria results when mixed with this reagent forming a viscous suspension. A string of viscous material appears when the suspension is drawn away from the test surface with a loop (Fig. 51.3).

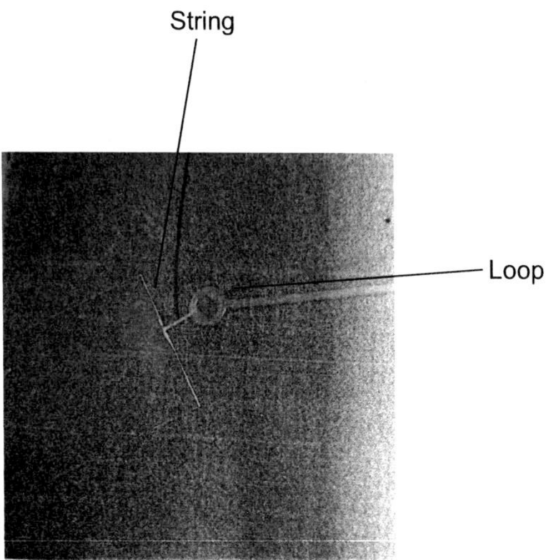

Fig. 51.3 String test used for the identification of *Vibrio* spp. A string of viscous material appears on pulling away the bacterial suspension from the test surface with a loop.

Biochemical Characteristics

- It is *oxidase* and *catalase-positive*
- It is *methyl red* and *urease-negative*
- It is strongly indole-positive and reduces nitrites to nitrates.

  These two properties contribute to the **cholera-red reaction** due to the formation of red coloured compound, **nitrosoindole**.
- *Sugar fermentation:* It ferments glucose, sucrose, mannitol, maltose and mannose producing acid without gas. Fermentation of lactose occurs only after several days (i.e., late lactose fermenter).
- *Gelatin is liquefied.*
- It *decarboxylates lysin* and *ornithine* but not arginine.

Susceptibility to Physical and Chemical Agents

- Killed by heating at 56°C within 30 minutes.

- Sensitive to common disinfectants, drying and a pH less than 5.
- Killed by normal gastric juices within minutes.

Antigenic Structure

V. cholerae possesses unique **O (somatic) antigens** that confer serologic specificity and has been divided into corresponding number of serogroups or serovars. All strains share a single heat-labile **flagellar antigen (H antigens)**.

Two serogroups of *V. cholerae* associated with epidemic chloera: serogroups 01 and 0139 Bengal, are the most important pathogens, that have the heat-labile cholera toxin (CT) and produce chloera.

V. cholerae contains **two biogroups:** old or classical and Eltor. The Eltor biotype is responsible for virtually all cholera cases throughout the world while the classical cases have been encountered in Bangladesh.

Based on the variations in minor O antigens (A, B, C), *V. cholerae* 1 is further subdivided into 3 **subtypes**:

- **Ogawa** (A and B antigens)
- **Inaba** (A and C antigens)
- **Hikojima** (A, B and C antigens)

An updated classification of the genus *Vibrio* as suggested by **Gardner** and **Venkataraman** is given in Fig. 51.4.

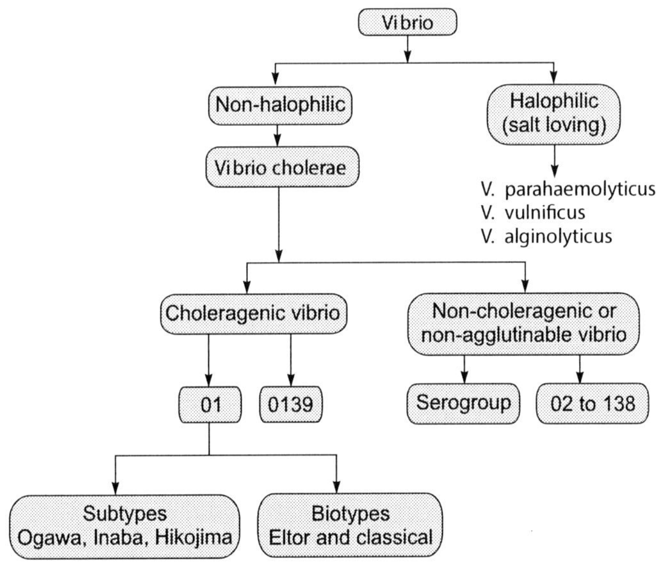

Fig. 51.4 Classification of *Vibrio cholerae*, the causative agent of cholera based on somatic (O) antigen.

CHOLERA

Cholera (from Greek: *kholera* means bile), an acute diarrhoeal disease, is caused by *Vibrio cholerae* (especially serogroups 01 and 0139) by eating contaminated food or drinking water. It is a terrifying illness characterized by profuse pain-less watery diarrhoea and copious effortless vomiting that may lead to hypovolemic shock and death in less than 24 hours. Cholera remains a global threat to public health. It affects an estimated 3–5 million people worldwide and causes 28800–130000 deaths every year. The disease likely has its origin in the Indian subcontinent, the first cholera pandemic occurred in Kolkata (WB) during 1817–1824.

It is an illness of the small intestine characterized by large amounts of watery diarrhoea and copious effortless vomiting that may lead to dehydration causing sunken eyes and wrinkling of hands and feet and skin to turn bluish and death in less than 24 hours.

V. cholerae is an exclusive human pathogen without any animal reservoirs. Infection is acquired orally from contaminated water (usually) or food. After passing the acid barrier of stomach, the bacteria begin to multiply in the alkaline environment of the small intestine. Cholera toxin (CT), a protein, is produced by the bacteria on the intestinal epithelium that causes profuse, watery diarrhoea, known as **"rice-water stools"**, with a fluid loss of 500 to 1000 mL/ hour. CT acts by interruping regulation of adenyl cyclase inside the cell causing efflux of water and sodium into the intestinal lumen. The incubation period varies from less than 24 hours to about 2–3 days. The rapid loss of fluid and electrolytes leads to profound dehydration and resulting in death in a few hours to days in untreated children. Cholera can occur in many forms: sporadic, endemic, epidemic or pandemic.

Laboratory Diagnosis

Diagnosis is based on the identification of the bacteria in a stool sample, biochemical tests and rapid cholera dipsitck tests. A fresh specimen of the stool that have 10^6 to 10^9 vibrios per mL collected in the acute stage of the disease before the administration of antibiotics is the most suitable and useful for lab diagnosis.

- ***Microscopy:*** For rapid diagnosis, demonstration of the characteristics motility of the vibrio and its inhibition by antiserum using cholera stool from acute cases by dark field microscopy.
- ***Culturing on TCBS agar:*** Stool specimens are inoculated into alkaline peptone water in which vibrios grow rapidly and

accumulate on the surface within 3 to 6 hours of incubation. A loopful taken from the surface is inoculated on TCBS agar and observed for **yellow colonies** at 35°C after 24 hours, is suggestive of infection.

Vibrios should be picked up with a straight wire and tested for the enzyme oxidase and slide agglutination with cholera 01 serum (rabbit antibodies specific for the 01 lipopolysaccharide antigens).

- ***Biochemical tests:*** Other biochemical tests, such as fermentation of sugars, utilization of amino acids and cholera red reaction, are used.
- ***Confirmation of the Identification and Record:*** The strain of *V. cholerae* may be sent to the reference centre for phage typing at the NICED (National Institute of Cholera and Enteric Disease) at Kolkata (WB) for their record and confirmatory results.

Treatment

- **Rehydration:** Immediate administration of ORS (oral rehydrate salts) dissolved in boiled or bottled water to replace the lost fluids and electrolytes is of prime importance.
- **Intravenous fluids:** Severely dehydrated patients are treated with intravenous fluids.
- **Antibacterial therapy:** Oral tetracycline or doxycycline is recommeded only for shortening symptoms, number of *Vibrio* excretion and preventing further spread of cholera.
- **Zinc supplements:** Zinc supplements decrease and shorten the duration of diarrhoea in children with cholera.

Prevention

- Provision of a clean (chlorinated) water supply and the proper sewage (faeces) disposal.

Vaccines

Vaccines prevent to cholera are of two types:

- **Whole cell killed vaccines:** Currently there are three WHO pre-qualified oral cholera vaccines (OCV): **Dukoral**, **Shanchol** and **Fuvichol**. All three vaccines require two doses for full protection. Dukroral is admistered with a buffer solution, that for adults requires 150 mL of clean water.

- **Live oral vaccine:** CVD 103 – HgR (Vaxchora, Paxvax) for the prevention of cholera for adult travellers aged 18 to 64 years (approved in June 2016 by FDA, USA).

VIBRIO PARAHAEMOLYTICUS AND GASTROENTERITIS

Vibrio parahaemolyticus is a Gram-negative halophilic (salt requiring) curved, rod-shaped bacterium found in marine aquatic ecosystems (saltwater). It causes seafood-borne gastroenteritis following the consumption of contaminated shell fish (usually oysters). The incubation period is 24 hours. The infection is self-limited with explosive watery (sometimes bloody) diarrhea accompanied by nausea, vomiting abdominal cramps, sometime fever. It usually causes hemolysis of human red cells (erythrocytes) due to the production of thermostable hemolysin.

Laboratory diagnosis is made by the production of green colonies on TCBS agar (Fig. 51.5). On blood agar, the colonies of *V. parahaemolyticus* are with a darker greenish coloration measuring 2-4 mm in diameter (slightly larger to *V. cholerae*). On TSI agar slant, the slant is alkaline (pink) due to nonfermentation of lactose and sucrose. On blood agar, it exhibits beta-haemolysis.

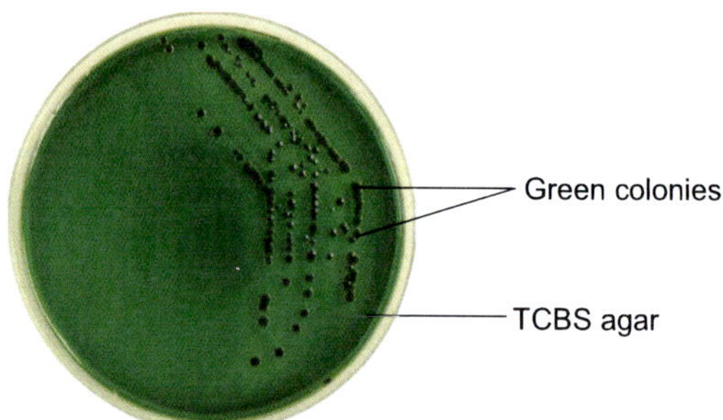

Fig. 51.5 ***Vibrio parahaemolyticus* on TCBS agar**. Characteristic green colonies are produced on this medium, a feature used to distinguish it from *V. cholerae*.

This food infection is self-limiting, however, in severe cases, fluid and electrolyte replacement is required.

VIBRIO VULNIFICUS AND GASTROENTERITIS

V. vulnificus is a halophilic, Gram-negative, curved bacillus associated with about 95% of all seafood related deaths. It lives in salt and brackish water and can cause serious, potentially fatal diseases: gastroenteritis, wound infections and primary septicaemia which occurs when the bacterium eneters host's blood and causes infection throughout the body.

John L. Reichelt in 1976 described this halophilic species under the genus *Beneckea* and 3 years later (i.e., in 1979) to the genus *Vibrio* by **J.J. Farmer**.

It enters the body via ingestion through consumption of raw oysters, symptoms occur after 24 hours.

Tetracycline in combination with gentamicin or chloramphenicol is the best therapy to treat *V. vulnificus* infections.

KEY POINTS

- **Vibrios** are Gram-negative, comma-shaped, oxdiase and catalse-positive bacteria that prefer an alkaline environment.
- *Vibrio cholerae*, the most important species in the genus, causes cholera.
- **Epidemic cholera** is caused by two serogroups: *V. cholerae* 01 and *V. cholerae* 0139, hence are clinically most important pathogens.
- *Vibrio cholerae* is comma-shaped, Gram-negative, facultative anaerobic bacillus, highly motile by a single polar flagellum.
- **Vibrios contaminated water** acts as the major source of human infections.
- **Cholera** is characterized by multiple episodes of **watery diarrhoea (rice-water stools)** leading to rapid dehydration.
- Fluid and electrolyte replacement (oral rehydration therapy, ORT or IV fluids) is the best treatment.
- *Vibrio parahaemolyticus* and *V. vulnificus* are Gram-negative halophilic seafood-borne pathogens causing gastroenteritis in humans.

IMPORTANT QUESTIONS

1. Discuss in brief the morphology, classification, pathogenesis, laboratory diagnosis and vaccines for *Vibrio cholerae*.
2. Write a short note on cholera.

MULTIPLE-CHOICE QUESTIONS

1. All are true for *Vibrio cholerae* EXCEPT:
   (a) Comma-shaped
   (b) Gram-negative
   (c) Motile by a single polar flagellum
   (d) Halophilic.

2. The primary habitat of *Vibrio cholerae* is
   (a) Aquatic (natural waters)
   (b) Exoskeleton of crustaceans
   (c) Intestine of animals
   (d) Intestine of humans.
3. The best therapy for cholera is:
   (a) Antiserum injection
   (b) Oral vaccine
   (c) Oral rehydration therapy
   (d) Oral tetracycline.
4. Which of the following bacteria show darting motility?
   (a) *Escherichia coli*
   (b) *Salmonella Typhi*
   (c) *Proteus mirabilis*
   (d) *Vibrio cholerae.*
5. Which of the media is used to differentiate colonies of *Vibrio cholerae* and *Vibrio parahaemolyticus*?
   (a) Nutrient agar
   (b) Thiosulphate-citrate-bile sucrose (TCBS) agar
   (c) MacConkey agar
   (d) Alkaline bile salt agar.
6. All of the following bacteria are halophilic EXCEPT:
   (a) *Vibrio parahaemolyticus*
   (b) *Vibrio cholerae*
   (c) *Vibrio vulnificus*
   (d) *Vibrio alginolyticus.*
7. Cholera is characterized by bloody diarrhoea. True or False?

ANSWER TO MCQs

1. (d)	2. (a)	3. (c)	4. (d)
5. (b)	6. (b)	7. False.	

52

Campylobacter and *Helicobacter*: Gram-negative Curved Flagellated Rods

Infective diarrhoea; Gastritis; Peptic ulcer

Campylobacter and *Helicobacter* are spiral-shaped flagellate bacteria, earlier called **vibrios**, are classified in the families *Campylobacteriaceae* and *Helicobacteriaceae*, respectively. Members of both these genera are especially adapted to colonize mucous membranes and are of great medical significance causing acute infective diarrhoea and peptic ulcer.

CAMPYLOBACTER

Campylobacter is a Gram-negative, nonspore forming, curved "seagull wing-shaped" microaerophilic motile bacillus with a single polar flagellum having a special darting motility, once classified as vibrios. The name is derived from Greek: *kampulos* (= curved) and *baktron* (= rod) means curved rod, because it typically appears comma- or S-shaped. In 1963, **Sebald** and **Veron** proposed *Campylobacter* on the grounds that the microaerophilic vibrios were different biochemically and serologically from the classical cholera and halophilic vibiros. These are adapted to the intestines of many animals (especially poultry) and humans. It includes 34 species classified in the family *Campylobacteriaceae*. *C. jejuni* and *C. coli* commonly cause enteritis in humans.

CAMPYLOBACTER JEJUNI

C. jejuni (*C. jejuni* subsp. *jejuni*) named after Latin word: *jejunum*, the small section of the intestine between duodenum and ileum.

Morphology

It is a curved, Gram-negative, motile bacillus showing a typical "seagull-wing-shaped" appearance. The bacilli measure 0.5–5 µm long and 0.2–0.9 μm wide. In Gram stain, fuchsin in place of safranin as a counterstain gives better results. Under phase-contrast microscopy, a typical "darting" motility is observed.

Cultural Characteristics

It is a **microaerophilic** requiring an atmosphere with decreased oxygen (5%), grows best at 42-43°C. Colonies of *C. jejuni* on *Campylobacter* blood agar (Compy BAP) grown in a microaerophilic environment at 42°C for 48 hours, are grey-white, raised or flat, moist "runny looking" like water drops and spreading along the streak lines. When exposed to atmospheric oxygen, it changes from bacillus to a coccal form.

Biochemical Reactions

It is a strongly oxidase (+ve) and catalase (+ve), reduces nitrates to nitrites, hippurate and does not ferment carbohydrates.

CAMPYLOBACTERIOSIS—ACUTE INFECTIVE DIARRHOEA

It is a food-borne infection mainly acquired by ingestion via undercooked meat and meat products, contaminated water and milk. Chicken acts as the main source. *C. jejuni* is present in high numbers in diarrhoea stools of infected individuals and animal faeces that can contaminate the various sources. The average incubation period is 3 days, with a range of 1–7 days. It takes a small amount of bacteria as few as 500–800 organisms, to cause infection. The organisms are invasive causing destruction of gut mucosa along with cytotoxin. Severe abdominal pain, watery diarrhoea (frequently bloody), nausea and fever are the main symptoms. The illness is self-limited usually lasting 5–7 days, but excretion of bacteria may continue for several weeks.

Complications may include reactive arthritis (painful inflammation of the joints) and neurological disorders such as Guillain-Barré syndrome, a polio-like form of paralysis.

Laboratory Diagnosis

Faecal specimen containing blood, pus and mucus are used for direct examination and specimen should be refrigerated pending delivery to the lab.

- **Direct microscopy** of Gram stained stool smears (counterstained with carbol fuchsin rather than safranin) for typical seagull wing-shaped rods of campylobacters.

- **Dark-field microscopy** of stool wet mounts for typical darting or tumbling motility of the spiral rods.
- **Culture:** Isolation of campylobacters from faeces on selective media at 42°C under microaerophilc conditions for 48 hours. Flat and effuse colonies with a tendency to spread on moist agar.
- **Biochemical tests:** Positive oxidase, catalase campylobacters and nitrate reduction.
- **Serology:** Recent infection can be detected by complement fixation test and ELISA.

Treatment: Severe complicated infections are to be treated with erythromycin or ciprofloxacin.

HELICOBACTER

Helicobacter (*Helico* means spiral) is a Gram-negative motile bacterium possessing a characteristic helical shape (Fig. 52.1). Initially, it was considered to be a member of the genus *Campylobacter* but in 1989, **Goodwin** and **coworkers** gave it the new genus name. Currently, it contains 35 species classified in the family *Helicobacteriacae*.

H. pylori is clinically the most important species that lives in or on the lining of the stomach and is the major cause of peptic ulcer disease (PUD) in humans. It was earlier thought that the disease was caused by the spicy food, acid, stress and life style.

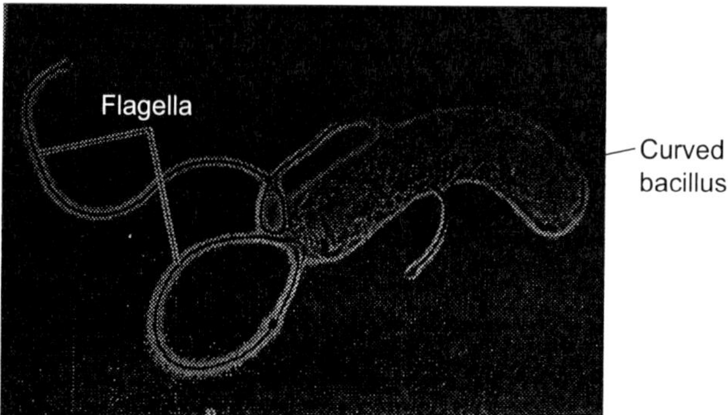

Fig. 52.1 ***Helicobacter pylori*, the cause of peptic ulcer**. Curved rod with multiple flagella.

HELICOBACTER PYLORI

H. pylori, earlier known as *Campylobacter pylori*, was first discovered in 1982 by two Australian scientists **Barry J. Marshall** and **J. Robin Warren**. These researchers also found that it causes peptic ulcer disease. They got the 2005 Noble Prize in medicine for this contribution.

Morphology

It is a Gram-negative, helical (spiral) shaped, flagellated microaerophilic bacillus measuring 2–4 μm long and 0.5–0.9 μm wide.

Cultural Characteristics

It requires complex media for growth. Chocolate agar, brain heart infusion and bucella agar, supplemented with horse or rabbit blood are good nonselective media. Tayer-Martin agar serves as the selective medium for its isolation. Gastric biopsy is the typical specimen for its culture. Colonies after 4 to 7 days of incubation at 37°C under microaerophilic conditions are small (1–2 mm in diameter), round, translucent and nonhemolytic.

Biochemical Reactions

- **Urease production:** It produces an exceptionally powerful urease (the enzyme that hydrolyzes urea yielding NH_3 that changes the colour of the indicator) that is 100 times more active than *Proteus vulgaris*, is used for its diagnosis.
- It is positive for oxidase, catalase, phosphatase and H_2S production.

PEPTIC ULCER

Pathogenesis

H. pylori can be found in stool, saliva, and plaque of teeth. It is the main cause of peptic ulcers, and can also cause gastritis and certain types of stomach cancer. Infection is very common and increases with age. By age 60, about 50% of people are infected worldwide. **Peptic ulcers** are open sores on the lining of stomach or upper part of small intestine.

Gastritis: (the inflammation of the stomach lining) and **adenocarcinoma** (a common type of stomach cancer) are also caused.

H. pylori is usually found in the stomach and is probably transmitted from person to person by the oral-oral or oral-faecal route. The infection is acquired during early childhood and carried asymptomatically until its activities begin on the digestive mucosa. Of the several ways, production of virulence factors, i.e., toxins (vaculating toxin and a cytotoxin) is one factor involved in damage. *H. pylori* produces ammonia by the powerful urease, which helps to protect it from stomach acid and enables it to distrupt and penetrate the mucosal layer.

Breath test and upper **endoscopy** (examination of stomach using a flexible viewing tube) help a physician (doctor) to diagnose PUD.

Laboratory Diagnosis

Lab diagnosis is made by two ways:

1. **Invasive tests:** By finding the pathogen in biopsy specimens of the stomach lining (gastric mucosa), upper endoscopy, biopsy urease test, histopathology, microscopy and culture.
2. **Non-invasive test:** (serology, urea breath test, fecal antigen test, PCR).

The major tests are:

- **Urea breath test:** Swallowing carbon labelled (C-14 or -13) urea capsule by the patient and the emission of the radioactive CO_2 exhaled in breath is a positive test. This test detects bacterial urease activity, i.e., splitting of urea into CO_2 and NH_3 in the stomach.
- **Biopsy urea test:** The biopsy specimen is placed in urea containing gel with an indicator and incubated at 37°C and examined for change in colour of pH indicator from yellow to magenta (pink), due to production of ammonia by the urease activity of the organism.
- **Histological examination of gastric biopsy specimens:** It is a gold standard for the diagnosis. Bluish, slender, curved bacilli are observed in specimens stained with haematoxylin and eosin, or Warthin-Starry silver stain.
- **Culture:** Isolation of the pathogen from biopsy specimens on selective meida. Thayer-Martin medium under microaerophilic conditions at 37°C for 4-7 days.

  The bacterium is identified based on the colonial morophology, Gram staining, positive catalase, oxidase and rapid urease reactions.
- **Enzyme immunoassay (EIA)-Serological test:** *H. pylori* antigen can be detected from stool specimens by an enzyme immounassay, a highly specific, sensitive and promising new test for diagnosis.
- **ELISA-Serological test:** ELISA principle is used to detect antibodies to *H. pylori*. Rapid bedside test kits are available in the market. In India, *H. pylori* antigen rapid test-kit ELISA kit

for the qualitative detection of antibodies of all isotypes (IgG, IgM, IgA) specific to *H. pylori* in human serum or plasma, test results in 10 minutes, is available.

- **PCR:** Direct detection of *H. pylori* by PCR in gastric juices, stool, dental pleques and water supply.

Treatment

It is treated with a combination of

- Omeprazole, amoxicillin and clarithromycin for 10 days;
- Bismuth subsalicyclate, metronidazole and tetracycline for 14 days.
- Lansoprazole, amoxicillin and clarithromycin for 10 to 14 days.

KEY POINTS

- The genera *Vibrio, Campylobacter* and *Helicobacter* are curved and short spiral-shaped, Gram-negative bacteria that were earlier included in **vibrios**.
- *Campylobacter jejuni*, named after Latin *jejunum*, is the common cause of severe gastroenteritis.
- *Helicobacter pylori*, a helical microaerophile with multiple flagella, causes peptic ulcer, gastritis and stomach cancer in humans.

IMPORTANT QUESTIONS

1. Write short notes on:
   (a) Differentiate between *Campylobacter* and *Helicobacter*.
   (b) *Helicobacter pylori*
   (c) Diagnosis is of *Helicobacter pylori*.

MULTIPLE-CHOICE QUESTIONS

1. All are vibrios EXCEPT:
   (a) *Escherichia* (b) *Vibrio*
   (c) *Helicobacater* (d) *Campylobacter.*
2. Peptic ulcer disease of humans is caused by:
   (a) *Campylobacter jejuni*
   (b) *Helicobacter pylori*
   (c) *Treponema pallidum*
   (d) *Chlamydia trachomatis.*

3. The Australian workers Marshall and Warren, got the 2005 Medicine Nobel Prize for their work on:

(a) *Campylobacter jejuni*

(b) *Helicobacter pylori*

(c) *Chlamydia trachomatis*

(d) *Neurospora sitophila*.

ANSWERS TO MCQs

1. (a) 2. (b) 3. (b).

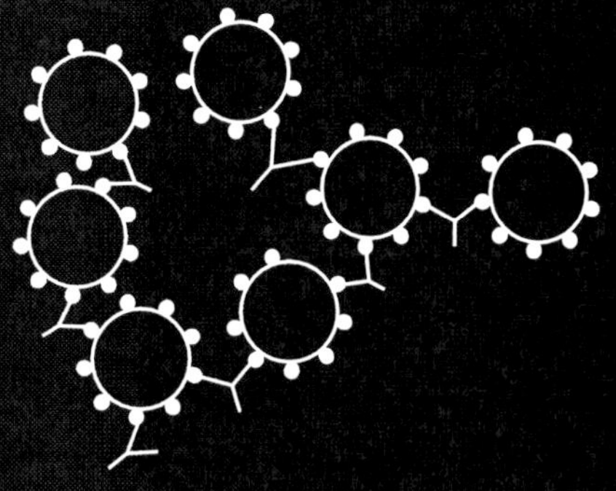

Unit IV B

VIRUSES-MEDICAL VIROLOGY

- General Properties of Viruses
- Nomenclature and Classification (Taxonomy) of Viruses
- Cultivation, Isolation and Diagnosis of Animal Viruses
- Influenza (Flu) Viruses: Enveloped Segmented RNA Viruses
- Hepatitis Viruses: RNA and DNA Viruses
- Human Immunodeficiency Virus: An RNA Retrovirus
- Poliovirus: An RNA Picornavirus
- Rabies lyssavirus: A Bullet-shaped RNA Virus
- Coronaviruses: Corona (Crown)-shaped RNA Viruses
- Arbo and other RNA Viruses of Medical Importance
- DNA Viruses: Double and Single Stranded

53

General Properties of Viruses

WHAT IS A VIRUS?

Viruses (sing. **virus**) (Latin word: *virus* refers to poison or venom) are small infectious particles of genetic material (either DNA or RNA) that are surrounded by a protein coat. Some viruses also have a fatty "envelope" covering. The extracellular infectious particle of a virus is called a **virion** (pl. **virions**). These are too small to be seen with a light microscope, hence they can be visualized with an electron microscope (i.e., ultramicroscopic).

DISCOVERY OF VIRUSES

The credit for the discovery of viruses goes to **D.J. Iwanowski**, a Russian botanist, who in 1892 first discovered a virus, in an infected tobacco plant. However, **W.M. Beijerinck**, a Dutch microbiologist and botanist demonstrated that the extract of an infected plant causes infection in a healthy plant. He founded the discipline of virology and in 1898 coined the term virus. **W.M. Stanley**, an American chemist in 1935 isolated pure crystlas of Tobacco Mosaic Virus (TMV) and concluded that viruses are made of **nucleoproteins**.

VIRAL DIVERSITY

Viruses are among the most common and diverse entities in the biosphere. They are found in almost every ecosystem of earth. Only a small diversity of viruses has been studied. Although there are millions of types and only 4958 virus species have been described so far (ICTV, 2018).

Viruses infect every form of life that is — invertebrates, vertebrates, plants, protists, fungi and bacteria. However, most viruses are able to infect specific types of cells of only one host species.

The diseases caused by them range from minor ailments such as the common cold, influenza, chicken pox, to serious diseases of humans such as polio, AIDS, rabies, COVID-19, and viral hepatitis which is one of the most common infectious diseases in the world. They may cause sporadic outbreaks, endemic diseases or even epidemics and pandemics. Some viruses can even cause cancer in humans by inserting their genetic material into human genome.

VIROLOGY

The study of viruses and the diseases caused by them is called **virology**, a branch/subspeciality of medicine/microbiology, **M. Beijerinck**, a Dutch microbiologist, is considered the **father of virology**.

UNIQUE FEATURES OF VIRUSES

Viruses (or virions) are the most primitive entities with the following distinctive features:

- Viruses exist at a level between living organisms and nonliving molecules.
- They are **acellular** (i.e., not cells) infectious agents called **virions**.
- They are **ultramicroscopic** (20 nm to 450 nm), pass through bacteriological filters and crystalizable.
- They are made up of protein shell (capsid) surrounding the nucleic acid core (i.e., **nucleocapsid**).
- Their genome consists of either DNA or RNA, not both.
- Some viruses have unique nucleic acid structure (single-stranded DNA and single-stranded RNA).
- They are **obligately intracellular parasites** and connot be cultured on nutrient cultured media.
- They are highly host-specific, specificity is imparted by molecules on virus surface.
- Viral replication inside a cell usually causes death or disease of the cell.

BIOLOGICAL POSITION OF VIRUSES

Viruses lack a cytoplasmic membrane and do not have the basic component of a cell, hence called acellular entities. They can only replicate (multiply) inside the host cell. Outside the host cell, they are non-living. Thus, viruses show characters of both living and non-living. Differences between these are:

(I) Non-living Characteristics of Viruses:

- They can be crystallized and precipitated.
- Outside the host, they behave like inert chemicals.
- They have no enzymes and do not show growth, development and reproduction of their own.

(II) Living Characteristics of Viruses:

- They possess genetic material (DNA or RNA).
- They multiply within host cells.
- They exhibit mutations.
- There are definite races or strains.

Because of the above reasons, viruses form a bridge between the non-living things and living organisms.

SIZE OF VIRUSES

Viruses are submicroscopic ranging in size from 20 to 450 nanometers in diameter (1 nanometer = 10^{-9} meter). Most viruses are smaller than bacteria, some of the largest viruses (e.g., pithovirus, vaccinia virus, mimi virus) are about the same size and same smallest bacteria (e.g. mycoplasmas, rickettsias and chlamydias). The comparative size of several viruses is shown in Fig. 53.1.

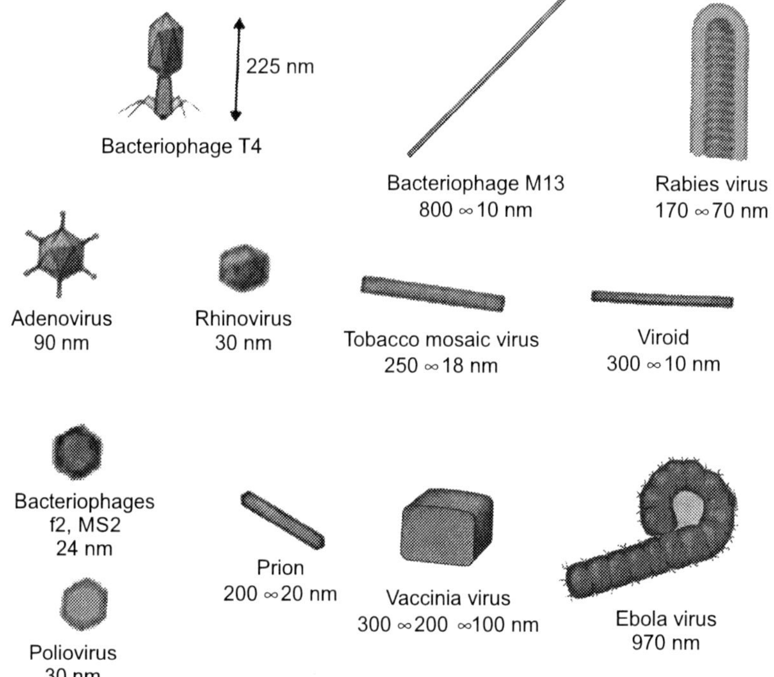

Fig. 53.1 Size of viruses. Dimensions (diameters or length) are given in nanometers (nm) and are either diameters or length by width.

VIRAL STRUCTURE

A virus is a kind of nanoparticle found in nature. Viruses are acellular, that is, they are biological entities that do not have a cellular structure.

They contain the following two components: a **nucleic acid genome**; and a **protein capsid** that covers the genome together this is called the *nucleocapsid* (Fig. 53.2) and the viruses are called **naked viruses** (Fig. 53.2). In addition, many animal viruses contain a **lipid envelope** and viruses are known as **enveloped viruses** (Fig. 53.2).

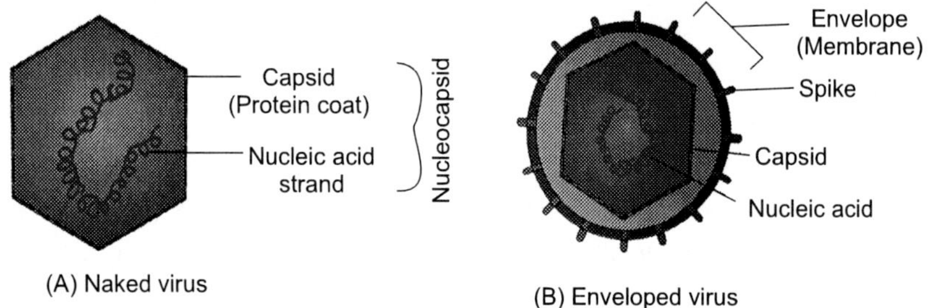

Fig. 53.2 Generalized structure of viruses. (A) A naked virus (nucleocapsid) consisting of a geometric capsid assembled around a nucleic acid strand or strands. (B) An enveloped virus is composed of a nucleocapsid surrounded by a flexible membrane called an envelope. The envelope usually has special receptor spikes inserted into it.

VIRAL GENOME

The genomes of viruses are comprised of only one type of nucleic acid either DNA or RNA, never both, in the form of single-stranded (ss) or double-stranded (ds), linear or circular. They vary greatly in size–from 5 – 10 kb to greater than 100 – 200 kb.

PROTEIN CAPSID

Viral genome is surrounded by a protein coat (shell) known as **capsid** (Fig. 53.2). The capsid is composed of subunits called **capsomeres** (Fig. 53.3), which can be a single type of protein or of several types. The arrangement of the individual capsomeres around the nucleic acid determines the *symmetry* of the virion. Symmetry or shapes of viruses can be icosahedral, helical or complex.

The capsid protects the genome from agents in the enviornment, and helps making contact, sticking or adsorbing to host cells.

VIRAL ENVELOPE

In some animal viruses, the nucleocapsid is surrounded by an **outer envelope** or **membrane** (Fig. 53.2). This envelope is generally a **lipid bilayer** of host cell origin into which virus proteins and glycoproteins are inserted. Some envelopes are covered with carbohydrate-protein complexes called **spikes** (Fig. 53.3).

MORPHOLOGY (SYMMETRY) OF VIRUSES

Viruses display a wide diversity of shapes and sizes called **morphology**. They are much smaller than bacteria and are ultramicroscopic. They range in size from 20 to 1000 nm in length (nanometer, nm is the unit of measurement). The smallest among viruses is poliovirus (30 nm) and the largest among them is vaccinia virus (300 nm) (Fig. 53.1). Pithovirus sibericum (1500 nm 1.5 μm in length) is physically the largest virus, which is even larger than some bacteria known today. The arrangement of capsomeres (protein subunits) around its nucleic acid determines the symmetry of the virion. Based on the capsid architecture, viruses have been classified into four morphological types.

Helical viruses: They resemble long rods. Their nucleic acid is found within a hollow, cylindrical capsid that has a helical structure (Fig. 53.3).

Examples include: Rabies and Ebola virus.

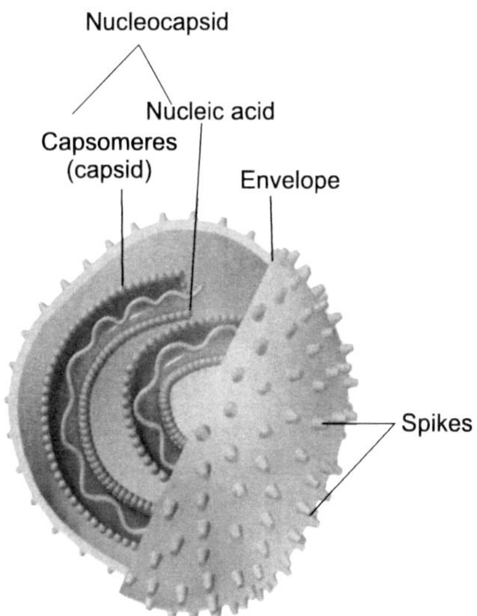

Fig. 53.3 Morphology of an enveloped helical virus as seen in *influenza virus* A2.

Polyhedral viruses: They are polyhedral or many-sided viruses. Their capsid is in the shape of an **icosahedron**.

Examples include: Adenovirus and poliovirus.

Enveloped viruses: They are covered with an envelope and are roughly spherical. They are of two types:

Enveloped helical viruses (e.g., influenza virus) (Fig. 53.3).

Enveloped polyhedral viruses (e.g., simplex virus)

Complex viruses: These have complicated (or complex) structures. ***Examples are:*** vaccinia virus (a pox virus), a large DNA virus and bacteriophage. Many bacteriophages have a polyhedral capsid with a helical tail attached to it.

VIRAL SUSCEPTIBILITY TO DISINFECTANTS AND PHYSICAL AGENTS

The viruses are usually more resistant than bacteria to chemical disinfectants. Most viruses are relatively resistant to phenol. The oxidizing agents, such as H_2O_2, potassium permanganate, hypochlorite, and organic/inorganic iodine compounds, are the most active antiviral disinfectants. Formaldehyde and β-propiolactone are active **virucidal** agents, which are commonly used for killed viral vaccines preparation.

The chlorination of drinking water is useful for killing most of the common viruses with the exception of hepatitis-A and polioviruses which are relatively resistant to chlorination.

Ether chloroform, and detergents (lipid solution) inactivate the enveloped viruses, however, the naked viruses are not affected by them.

Most viruses are easily killed by heat. They are inactivated within seconds at 56°C, within minutes at 37°C and within days at 4°C. However, hapatitis-B shows resistance to heating at 60°C for 60 minutes and scrapie virus resistant to autoclaving at 121°C for 15 minutes. The viruses are readily inactivated by sunlight, UV radiations and ionizing radiations.

MULTIPLICATION (REPLICATION) OF VIRUSES

The formation of viruses during the infection process in target host cells is called **viral replication**. Viral populations do not grow through cell division because they are acellular. Instead, they use the machinery and metabolism of a host cell to produce multiple copies of themselves, as they assemble in the cell. There are six basic stages in the replication ((life) cycle of viruses to produce more virions:

1. **Adsorption or attachment:** Specific binding between viral capsid protein and specific receptors on the host cellular system.
2. **Penetration:** The entry of virions (or their genomes) into host cells.

3. **Uncoating:** Loss of the capsid leading to the release of the viral genomic nucleic acid and its incorporation into host cell.
4. **Biosynthesis:** The synthesis of new nucleic acid molecules, capsid proteins and other viral components within host cells using the metabolic machinery of these cells.
5. **Maturation:** The assembly of the viral particles.
6. **Release:** Release of new virions can occur through direct lysis of the host cell or by budding through the host membrane.

Synthesis and maturation differ in RNA and DNA viruses.

CHEMOTHERAPY OF VIRAL INFECTIONS

Many viral infections resolve on their own without treatment. Other times, treatment of viral infections simply focusses on symptoms relief, not fighting the virus. For example, medicine for cold helps alleviate the pain and congestion associated with the cold, but it does not act directly on the cold virus.

There are some drugs that act directly on the viruses. These are known as antiviral medications/agents. Major modes of action of antiviral drugs are:

- By inhibiting the production of virus particles.
- Interfering with the production of viral DNA.
- Preventing viruses from entering host cells.

In general, antiviral medications are most effective when they are taken early in the course of an initial viral infection or a recurrent outbreak. A few examples of the common antiviral drugs are:

- **Ribavirin (Virazole)** – A wide spectrum antiviral drug
- **Zidovudine (AZT or Retrovar)** – An anti-AIDS (HIV) drug
- **Amantidine** – An anti-influenza A virus drug.

IMMUNOENHANCERS OF VIRAL INFECTIONS

Certain medicines act as antiviral agents by stimulating the production of antiviral proteins in normal cells (e.g., **interferons**) to treat influenza, hepatitis, herpes, colds or by stimulating the immune system to resist viral infections (e.g., **Levamisole** to cure chronic upper resipiratory infections and **Inosiplex** to resist infection from cold and influenza virus).

PROPHYLAXIS TO PREVENT VIRAL ILLNESSES

Immunoprophylaxis of viral infections is by active and passive immunization.

Active immunization. Active immunization by vaccines can reduce the risk of acquring some viral illnesses. Vaccines vary in effectiveness and in the number of doses required to confer protection. Some vaccines require booster shots to maintain immunity. Vaccines commercially available are of three types:

- **Live-viral vaccines** – Smallpox, yellow fever, poliomyelitis (sabin type) measles, mumps, rubella and varicella.
- **Inactivated viral vaccines** – Poliomyelitis, rabies, influenza, hepatitis A and B, Japanese encephalitis.
- **Anti-idio type DNA vaccines.**

Passive immunization: Passive immunization with human gamma globulin, convalescent serum or specific immune globulin provides temporary protection against several viral infections.

KEY POINTS

- **Viruses** are ultramicroscopic infectious particles of genetic material (either DNA or RNA) surrounded by a protein coat, together called the **nucleocapsid**.
- Extracellular infectious particle of a virus is called a **virion**.
- Viruses cannot be cultured outside their hosts on a nutrient medium.
- Viruses range in size from 18 nm (human parvovirus) to 450 nm in length (vaccinia virus) to even 1500 nm in length (pithovirus).
- Protein subunits forming the viral capsid are called **capsomers**.
- Viruses are usually more resistant than bacteria to chemical disinfectants.
- Morphologically viruses are classified as **helical**, **polyhedral**, **enveloped** and **complex viruses**.
- **Adsorption** (or **attachment**), **penetration, uncoating**, **biosynthesis**, **maturation** and **release** are the six basic stages in the replication cycle of viruses.
- Ribavirin, zidovudine and amantidine are few examples of antiviral medications.
- Vaccination (or active immunization) by vaccines and passive immunization are used to prevent viral illnesses.

IMPORTANT QUESTIONS

1. Answer in brief:
   (a) What is a virus?

(b) What are capsomeres?
(c) Genome of a virus.

2. Write short notes on:
   (a) Unique characteristics of viruses.
   (b) Living and non-living characteristics of viruses.
   (c) Structure of a virus.
   (d) Name the six steps in the replication of animal viruses.
   (e) Chemotherapy and prophylaxis of viral infections.

MULTIPLE-CHOICE QUESTIONS

1. Extracellular infectious particle of a virus is called a capsid. True or false?
2. All are true for viruses EXCEPT:
   (a) Obligate intracellular parasites
   (b) Don't have cellular organization
   (c) A virus particle is called a virion
   (d) Viral genome is made up of DNA similar to bacteria.
3. All are true for viral genome EXCEPT:
   (a) Single stranded DNA
   (b) Double stranded RNA
   (c) Both DNA and RNA
   (d) Either DNA or RNA.
4. Which of the following scientists is called the father of virology?
   (a) M. Beijernick (b) W.M. Stanley
   (c) D.J. Iwanowski (d) Edward Jenner.
5. Symmetry of influenza virus is:
   (a) Spiral (b) Icosahedral
   (c) Helical (d) Round.
6. Which of the following is virucidal in action?
   (a) Formaldehyde
   (b) Chlorine
   (c) Potassium permanganate
   (d) Hydrogen peroxide.
7. In animal viruses, release of nucleic acid and its incorporation into host cells occurs at which stage of replication?
   (a) Biosynthesis (b) Adsorption
   (c) Uncoating (d) Penetration.

8. Which of the following viruses is relatively resistant to chlorination?
   (a) Hepatitis A virus
   (b) Flavivirus
   (c) Rotavirus
   (d) Hantavirus.
9. Dimensions of viruses are taken in:
   (a) Micrometers (μm)
   (b) Nanometers (nm)
   (c) Millimeters (mm)
   (d) None of these.
10. Which of the following is the smallest virus?
   (a) Adenovirus (b) Poliovirus
   (c) Rabies virus (d) Vaccinia virus.

ANSWERS TO MCQs

1. False	2. (d)	3. (c)	4. (a)
5. (c)	6. (a)	7. (c)	8. (a)
9. (b)	10. (b).		

54

Nomenclature and Classification (Taxonomy) of Viruses

Virus classification is the process of naming viruses (i.e., nomenclature) and placing them into a taxonomic system. Species form the basis for any biological classification system.

VIRUS SPECIES

A **viral species** is a group of viruses sharing the same genetic information and ecological niche (host range). Specific epithets for viruses are not used. Thus, viral species are designated by descriptive common names, such as human immunodeficiency virus (HIV),with subspecies (if any) designated by a number (HIV – 1).

The complete set of viruses in an organism or habitat is called the **virome**. For example, all human viruses constitute the **human virome**.

CLASSIFICATION

Due to the pseudo-living nature of viruses, they do not fit neatly into the established biological classification used for cellular organisms, and the virus classification is in a state of flux. Seven to eight schemes of classification for viruses have been proposed. Nomenclature and classification are now the official responsibility of the **International Committee on Taxonomy of viruses** (ICTV), which authorizes and organizes the taxonomic classification of viruses.

Major criteria used to classify viruses include:

- Phenotypic characteristics (e.g., morphology)
- Type of nucleic acid
- Mode of replication

- Host organisms
- Type of disease caused by them.

Until 1950 little was known about the viruses. On the basis of their affinity to different systems or organs of the body, they were classified into four groups:

- Those producing the skin lesions (e.g., smallpox, chickenpox)
- Those affecting the nervous system (e.g., polio, rabies)
- Those affecting the respiratory system (influenza viruses)
- Causing visceral lesions (yellow fever)

Viruses are classified into two main divisions, depending upon the type of nucleic acid they possess:

- *Deoxyriboviruses* – Contain DNA
- *Riboviruses* – Contain RNA

Of the various systems of virus classification, **the Baltimore virus classification** is named after **David Baltimore**, an American virologist and Nobel Prize-winning biologist, is the most widely accepted system. The Baltimore classification of viruses is based on the type of genome and their method of replication (i.e., mRNA). According to this system of classification, viruses are classified into seven groups (I – VII):

- **I ds DNA viruses:** Adenoviruses, Herpesviruses, Poxviruses
- **II ss DNA viruses** (+ strand or sense): Parvoviruses
- **III ds RNA viruses** Reoviruses
- **IV (+) ss RNA viruses** (+ strand or sense): Picornaviruses, Togaviruses
- **V (–) ss RNA viruses** (– strand or antisense): Orthomyxoviruses, Rhabdoviruses
- **VI ss RNA RT viruses** (+ strand or sense): Retroviruses
  RNA with DNA intermediate in life cycle
- **VII ds DNA RT viruses:** Hepadnaviruses DNA with RNA intermediate in life cycle

In modern classification, the ICTV classification system is used in conjunction with the Baltimore classification system. As per this system the chickenpox virus, *Varicella zoster* (VZV) belongs to the order *Herpesvirales*, family *Herpesviridae*, sub-family *Alphaherpesvirinae*, and genus *Varicellovirus*. VZV is in Group I of the Baltimore classification because it is a dsDNA virus that does not use reverse transcriptase.

ICTV CLASSIFICATION

A **unified taxonomy** – a universal system for classifying viruses was established in November 2018 by the International Committee on Taxonomy of Viruses (ICTV). A total of 4958 viral species have been classified in 846 genera, 64 subfamilies, 143 families and 14 orders.

Classification of Viruses that Affect Humans

Families of viruses, based on the viral genome, with examples of human pathogenic viruses are summarized in Tables 54.1 and 54.2.

Table 54.1 Families of DNA viruses (deoxyriboviruses) affecting humans

Characteristics/ Dimensions	Viral family	Important genera	Clinical or special features
Single-Stranded DNA, Nonenveloped			
18 – 25 nm	Parvoviridae	Human parvovirus B19	Fifth disease; anemia in immunocompromised patients.
Double-Stranded DNA, Nonenveloped			
70 – 90 nm	Adenoviridae	*Mastadenovirus*	Medium-sized viruses that cause various respiratory infections in humans; some cause tumors in animals.
40–57 nm	Papovaviridae	*Papillomavirus* (human wart virus) *Polyomavirus*	Small viruses that cause warts and cervical and anal cancer in humans.
Double-Stranded DNA, Enveloped			
200–350 nm	Poxviridae	*Orthopoxvirus* (vaccinia and smallpox viruses) *Molluscipoxvirus*	Very large, complex, brick-shaped viruses that cause smallpox (variola), molluscum contagiosum (wartlike skin lesion), and cowpox.

Contd.

Table 54.1 Contd.

150–200 nm	Herpesviridae	*Simplexvirus* (HHV-1 and -2) *Varicellovirus* (HHV-3) *Lymphocryptovirus* (HHV-4) *Cytomegalovirus* (HHV-5) *Roseolovirus* (HHV-6 and HHV-7) *Rhadinovirus* (HHV-8)	Medium-sized viruses that cause various human diseases: fever blisters, chickenpox, shingles, and infectious mononucleosis; cause a type of human cancer called Burkitt's lymphoma.
42 nm	Hepadnaviridae	*Hepadnavirus* (hepatitis B virus)	After protein synthesis, hepatitis B virus uses reverse transcriptase to produce its DNA from mRNA; causes hepatitis B and liver tumors.

Table 54.2 Families of RNA viruses (riboviruses) that affect humans

Characteristics/ Dimensions	Viral family	Important genera	Clinical or special features
Single-Stranded RNA, + Strand, Nonenveloped			
28–30 nm	Picornaviridae	*Enterovirus* *Rhinovirus* (common cold virus) Hepatitis A virus	At least 70 human enteroviruses are known, including the polio-, coxsackie-, and echoviruses; more than 100 rhinoviruses exist and are the most common cause of colds.
35–40 nm	Caliciviridae	Hepatitis E virus *Norovirus*	Includes causes of gastroenteritis and one cause of human hepatitis.
Single-Stranded RNA, + Strand, Enveloped			
60–70 nm	Togaviridae	*Alphavirus* *Rubivirus* (rubella virus)	Included are many viruses transmitted by arthropods (*Alphavirus*); diseases include eastern equine encephalitis (EEE), western equine encephalitis (WEE) and chikungunya. Rubella virus is transmitted by the respiratory route.

Contd.

Table 54.2 Contd.

40–50 nm	Flaviviridae	*Flavivirus* *Pestivirus* Hepatitis C virus	Can replicate in arthropods that transmit them; diseases include yellow fever, dengue and St. Louis and West Nile encephalitis.
80–160 nm	Coronaviridae	*Coronavirus*	Associated with upper respiratory tract infections and the common cold; SARS and COVID-19 virus.
–Strand, One Strand of RNA			
70–180 nm	Rhabdoviridae	*Vesiculovirus* (vesicular stomatatis virus) *Lyssavirus* (rabies virus)	Bullet-shaped viruses with a spiked envelope; cause rabies and numerous animal diseases.
80–14000 nm	Filoviridae	*Filovirus*	Enveloped, helical viruses; Ebola and Marbug viruses
150–300 nm	Paramyxoviridae	*Paramyxovirus* *Morbilli virus* (measles virus)	Paramyxoviruses cause parainfluenza, mumps, and Newcastle disease in chickens.
32 nm	Deltaviridae	Hepatitis D	Depend on coinfection with hepadnavirus.
–Strand, Multiple Strand of RNA			
80–200 nm	Orthomyxoviridae	Influenza virus A, B, and C	Envelope spikes can agglutinate red blood cells.
90–120 nm	Bunyaviridae	*Bunyavirus* (California encephalitis virus) *Hantavirus*	Hantaviruses cause hemorrhagic fevers such as Korean hemorrhagic fever and *Hantavirus* pulmonary syndrome; associated with rodents.
110–130 nm	Arenaviridae	*Arenavirus*	Helical capsids contain RNA-containing granules; cause lymphocytic choriomeningitis, Venezuelan hemorrhagic fever, and Lassa fever.

Contd.

Table 54.2 Contd.

Produce DNA			
100–120 nm	Retroviridae	Oncoviruses *Lentivirus* (HIV)	Includes all RNA tumor viruses. Oncoviruses cause leukemia and tumors in animals; the *Lentivirus* HIV causes AIDS.
Double-Stranded RNA, Nonenveloped			
60–80 nm	Reoviridae	*Reovirus* *Rotavirus*	Generally mild respiratory infections transmitted by arthropods; Colorado tick fever is the best known.

KEY POINTS

- A viral species is a group of viruses sharing the same genetic information and ecological niche.
- A total of 4958 viral species have been defined by ICTV.
- Classification of viruses is based on the type of nucleic acid (DNA or RNA), morphology, mode of replication, host organism and type of disease caused.
- Baltimore viral classification system is based on viral genome and mode of replication.

IMPORTANT QUESTIONS

1. Answer in brief:
   (a) Define a viral species.
   (b) International Committee on Taxonomy of Viruses.
2. Briefly describe the Baltimore classification system for viruses.

MULTIPLE-CHOICE QUESTIONS

1. A viral species is defined on the basis of the disease symptoms it causes. True or False?
2. All are DNA viruses EXCEPT:
   (a) Reoviruses (b) Adenoviruses
   (c) Herpesviruses (d) Poxviruses.

3. All are RNA viruses EXCEPT:
   (a) Rhabdoviruses
   (b) Reoviruses
   (c) Orthomyxoviruses
   (d) Poxviruses.

4. All of the following features are used to classify viruses EXCEPT:
   (a) Type of nucleic acid
   (b) Symmetry
   (c) Host organism
   (d) Cellular organization.

ANSWERS TO MCQs

1. False   2. (a)   3. (d)   4. (d).

55

Cultivation, Isolation and Diagnosis of Animal Viruses

Viruses cannot be grown in non-living culture media or agar plates alone. They can be grown in living cells *in vivo* (within living animals and embryonic bird tissue) and *in vitro* outside a living organism in animal cells/tissue in an artificial environment such as a test tube, cell culture flask or agar plate.

The primary purposes of viral cultivation are:

- to isolate and identify viruses in clinical specimens for diagnosis;
- production of vaccines; and
- for basic research on their structure, multiplication cycles, genetics and effects of viruses on host cells.

The methods employed for cultivation of animal viruses in the laboratory include:

- Inoculation of laboratory animals
- Inoculation of bird embryos
- Inoculation of animal tissue (i.e., organ, explant and cell culture).

ANIMAL INOCULATION

A viral preparation or specimen is injected/inoculated into the brain, blood, muscle, body cavity, skin, or footpads of the experimental healthy animal. Specially bored strains of white mice, rats, monkeys guinea pigs, and rabbits are used for isolation of human pathogenic viruses. Suckling mice (less than 48 hours old) are most commonly used. After inoculation, virus multiplies in the host and develops disease.

The viral growth in inoculated animals is indicated by symptoms of a disease and death. Then the virus is isolated and purified from the tissue of these animals.

EMBRYONATED EGGS (BIRD'S EMBRYOS) INOCULATION

Developing bird's embryos within the closed protective case of an egg (called embryonated egg) is nearly a perfect system with its own sterile environment and nourishment for viral propagation. Chicken, duck and turkey eggs are often used for inoculation. **Goodpasture,** an American pathologist, was the first scientist to use embryonated (fertile) hen's egg for cultivation of viruses in 1931.

Viruses are inoculated into chick embryo of 2 – 12 days old (Fig. 55.1). To inoculate a virus, the egg shell is first disinfected with iodine and perforated with a small sterile drill making a hole or small window and a virus preparation is injected. After inoculation of the virus, the opening is sealed with gelatin or paraffin and incubated at 36°C for 2 – 3 days. The egg is broken and virus is isolated from tissue of the egg. Viral growth is observed by the death and cell damage of the embryo, or by formation of typical pocks, or lesions on the egg membranes.

Viruses can be inoculated in one of the four sites of the egg embryos: allantoic cavity, chorioallantoic cavity, chorioallantoic membrane or yolk sac (Fig. 55.1), depending on the type of virus being grown and goal of the experiment:

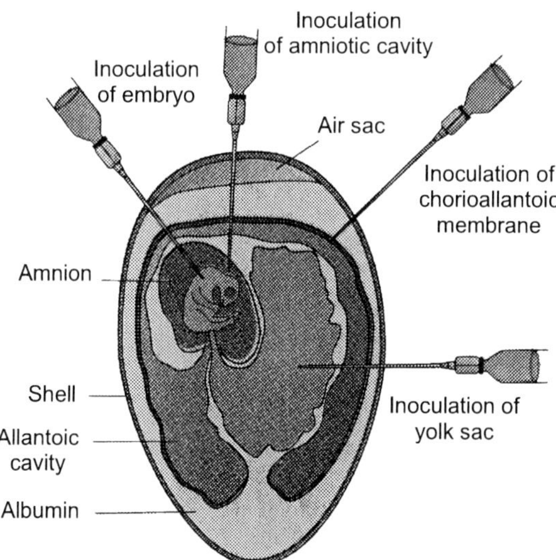

Fig. 55.1 Embryonated egg of a bird showing its structure and different routes of inoculation for cultivating (growing) animal viruses.

- **Allantoic cavity** (a fluid-filled sac) – employed for cultivation of influenza virus and some paramyxoviruses for vaccine production. It produces a rich yield of virus.

- **Amniotic cavity** (a sac that cushions and protects the embryo itself) is used for the primary isolation of the influenza and mumps viruses.
- **Chorioallantoic membrane (CAM)** (functions in the embryonic gas exchange) produces visible opaque spots (pocks). Pock morphology is different in different viruses. Used for poxvirus and herpes simplex virus.
- **Yolk sac** (a membrane that mobilizes yolk for embryo nourishment) is used for cultivation of some viruses (e.g. pseudorabies virus).

The signs of viral growth include: formation of pocks, death of embryo and defects in the development of embryo.

TISSUE CULTURE

There are three types of tissue culture: organ culture, explant culture and cell culture.

Organ culture: This is mainly used for isolation of highly specialized parasites of certain organs. Tracheal ring organ culture is done for isolation of coronavirus, a respiratory pathogen.

Explant culture: Fragments of minced tissue can be grown as **explants** (or embedded in plasma clots) and then viruses can be grown in them. This method is rarely used.

Cell culture: Cell culture is considered gold standard for isolation and diagnosis of viruses. Cell culture of animal viruses growing animal cells under controlled aseptic conditions on glass or plastic surfaces (Petri dishes) using broth media containing growth factors. The medium, a balanced salt solution containing 13 amino acids, sugar, proteins, salt, calf serum, buffers, antibiotics and phenol red, and inoculated with host cells in suspension prepared from animal tissues by enzymatic method using trypsin enzyme and gentle shaking in flasks. On incubation, the cell divides and spread out on the glass surface to form a confluent monolayer sheet of cells within a weak, called **cell lines**.

The patient's specimens (i.e., virus) are inoculated into cell lines and incubated at 37°C and observed for the virus produced changes in the cells, called the **cytopathic effects**.

Types of cell culture: Three basic types of cell culture are widely used in clinical and research virology:

(1) Primary cell culture

(2) Diploid cell strains

(3) Continuous cell culture

Primary cell culture: These are normal cells directly derived from animals or humans. They are able to grow only for limited time and cannot be maintained in serial culture.

They are used for the primary isolation of viruses and vaccine production. Monkey kidney cell culture and human aminion cell culture are the examples.

Diploid cell strains (Semi-continuous cell lines): They are diploid and are derived from subcultured primary cell culture and produce stable culture that can be maintained for years. They are used for the isolation of some fastidious viral pathogens and to produce viral vaccines. Examples: Human embryonic lung strain, Rhesus embryo cell strain.

Continuous cell lines (heteroploid cultures): They are derived from cancer cells and can be serially cultured indefinitely so named as **continuous cell lines** (or **immortal cell lines**) and can be maintained by storing in deep freeze at -70°C. These lines are **heteroploid** (have different number of chromosomes) and are therefore genetically diverse. Examples: Hela (human epithelial cell line of cervical carcinoma), adenovirus; vero (monkey kidney cell line); MDCK (dog kidney cell line): oral and killed polio vaccine production.

ISOLATION OF VIRUSES

Unlike bacteria, most of which can be grown/cultured on an artificial nutrient medium, viruses require a living host cell for replication. Infected host cells can be cultured and grown, and then the growth medium can be harvested as a source of virus. Virions in the liquid medium (broth) can be separated from the host cells by either centrifugation or filtration. Membrane filters with pore size of 200 nm (0.2 μm) with pores small enough to allow viruses to pass through can physically remove anything present in the solution that is larger than the virions; the viruses can then be collected in the filtrate.

Detection/Identification of Growing Virus in Cell Cultures

Viruses can be detected/identified in cell cultures by cytopathic effects and haemadorption changes.

Cytopathic effect (CPE): Micoscopically visible virus-induced cellular changes in the monolayer cells is called a **cytopathic effect**. These changes include: plaques (well-defined patches), swelling and shrinkage of cells, formation of multinucleated giant cells (syncytia), production of inclusions in the nucleus or cytoplasm, change in the cell shape from flat to round, vacuolation (holes) in the cytoplasm, formation of malignant cells, clumping, and complete lysis of the infected cells. Some viruses produce characteristic CPEs that aid in the presumptive identification of the infecting virus. For example, human adenoviruses and herpesviruses characterized by swallowing of infected cells (due to fluid accumulation); paramyxoviruses cause syncytia; and picornaviruses cause lysis of cells.

Haemadorption: Cells acquire the ability to stick to mammalian red blood cells, called **haemdorption**. It is mainly used for the detection of influenza and parainfluenza viruses.

LABORATORY DETECTION OF VIRAL INFECTIONS

The six common approaches to diagnose viral diseases, often used together, include:

1. Detection of virus particles (virions) in clinical specimens taken from appropriate sites.
2. Detection of viral antigens (Ag) in blood and body fluids.
3. Serological procedures to detect specific antiviral antibodies (rise in antibody titre or presence of IgM antibody)/detection of presence of a cell-mediated immune response.
4. Detection of viral genome in the blood or body cells of a patient.
5. Culture of infectious virus from appropriate clinical specimen.
6. Cytological examination of cells for characteristics CPE.

1. **Microscope Examination of Viruses**

   Clinical specimens such as skin lesions or biopsy materials are examined by direct microscopic examination by three types of microscopy:

   - **Electron Microscopy (EM)**

     It is an important tool to identify viruses that cannot be cultured and with new viruses based on their size and morphology. EM is used for the detection of rotavirus and hepatitis A virus in faecal specimens, poxviruses in vesicle fluid, and herpesvirus in brain biopsy tissue.

     Light Microscopy: It reveals characteristic inclusion bodies or multinucleated giant cells. MGCs, for example, herpes-virus induced MGCs in vesicular skin lesions can be easily observed in Tzanck smear under LM.

Fluorescence Microscopy

Virions or viral antigens can be detected in frozen tissue sections, cells from virus infected cultures or vesicles fluid by direct or indirect fluorescent antibody technique. It is used to diagnose herpesvirus, rabiesvirus, paramyxovirus, orthomyxovirus and adenovirus.

2. **Detection of Viral Antigens**

Antigen detection is successfully used **directly in clinical specimens** for rapid diagnosis of many viral infections. Various tests (e.g., ELISA, radioimmunoassay and latex agglutination) are useful for detecting viral antigens in the patient's blood and biopsy materials. For the diagnosis of Hepatitis virus infection, HBsAg (surface antigen of HBV), HBeAg (the hepatitis "*e*" antigen), and for HIV infection (AIDS), p24 viral antigen can be detected in serum. The COVID-19 antigen test detects coronavirus surface proteins in the mouth or throat which is performed on a sample that is taken by swabbing inside your nose. This test determines whether a patient is currently infected with COVID-19 or not. **Coviself** is India's first COVID-19 rapid antigen test kit for self-use.

3. **Detection of Nucleic Acids (Viral Genome)**

Detection of viral genome (DNA or RNA) requires the use of **polymerase chain reaction (PCR)** technique to amplify the viral genome present in the sample and detection of specific gene sequence of that particular virus by the use of a specific primer (while performing PCR) and labelled nucleic acid probe (while detecting the specific sequence). For the detection of viral RNA, it is first converted into DNA by reverse transcriptase.

PCR can be used for the diagnosis of infections caused by SARS-CoV-2, HIV-1, HIV-2, HLV-1, human papillomavirus, herpes simplex viruses, HBV, HCV, HDV, HEV, rubella virus, Epstein-Barr virus, varicellazoster virus, human herpes virus 6 and 7, parvovirus B 19, enteroviruses, coxsackie viruses, echoviruses, rhinoviruses, measles virus and rotavirus.

PCR, a highly specific tool with rapid results, is becoming the "gold standard" in viral diagnosis.

4. **Serological Tests to Detect Specific Antiviral Antibodies**

A rise in antibody titre to the virus during the course of a disease is a strong evidence that it is the etiological agent. For this it is essential to examine paired zero samples collected during the *acute phase* (as soon as viral etiology is suspected) and second in the *convalescent phase* (10 – 14 days later). If the antibody titre in the convalescent phase is at least **4-fold higher** than the titre in the acute phase sample, the patient is considered to be infected.

IgM specific antibodies tests on sera samples are done to diagnose constant viral infections that generally indicates a recent viral infection.

Various tests used to determine antibody titre are ELISA, RIA, Western blot, latex agglutination, haemagglutination inhibition, immunofluorescence, immunodifusion and complement fixation.

5. **Identification in Cell Culture**

   The growth of viruses in cell culture/tissue culture produces characteristic **cytopathic effect** which helps a virologist in presumptive diagnosis. *Hemadorption* and decrease in acid production in infected culture cells aid in identification in some viruses.

6. **Cytological/Histological Examination**

   Examination of human cells from the site of infection by light microscopy for virus-induced multinucleate giant cells and inclusion bodies help to diagnose some viral diseases, for example, measle virus (inclusion bodies), vaccinia (Guarnieri's bodies), herpes simplex and varicella-zoster virus (Cowdry Type-A, intranuclear bodies seen in infected cells, named after **Edmund Cowdry**).

KEY POINTS

- Cultivation of viruses is important for diagnosing viral infections.
- Growing animal viruses in the laboratory requires the presence of some form of host cell (whole animal, embryo or cell culture).
- Cell culture is the method of choice for culturing viruses.
- Viruses can be isolated from samples by filtration using filters of pore size (0.2 μm).
- Virus growth in cell (tissue) culture is detected by the **cytopathic effects** (e.g., plaques).
- Viruses are identified/detected by cytopathic effects in cell culture, serological assays and nucleic acid amplification assays (PCR, RT-PCR).

IMPORTANT QUESTIONS

1. Briefly explain the various methods of culturing animal viruses.
2. How are the human viruses diagnosed?

MULTIPLE-CHOICE QUESTIONS

1. Viruses can be diagnosed and observed using *a*(*n*) ——— microscope.
2. Which of the following cannot be used to culture animal viruses?
   (a) Tissue culture
   (b) Bird embryos
   (c) Liquid medium only
   (d) Live animals.
3. The signs of viral growth in the inoculated tissue/cell culture is detected by:
   (a) Pocks (b) Colonies
   (c) Plaques (d) All of these.
4. Examples of cytopathic effects of animal viruses in cell culture is/are
   (a) Multiple nuclei
   (b) Giant cells
   (c) Inclusion bodies
   (d) All of these.
5. What size of litre pore is needed to collect a virus through filtration?
   (a) 0.2 μm (b) 2.0 μm
   (c) 5.0 μm (d) All of these.

ANSWERS TO MCQs

1. Electron microscope 2. (c) 3. (c)
4. (d) 5. (a).

56

Influenza (Flu) Viruses: Enveloped Segmented RNA Viruses

Avian Flu; Swine Flu; Spanish Flu

Influenza, commonly called **flu,** is an infectious respiratory disease characterized by high fever, running nose, chills, headache and muscular aches which is caused by influenza viruses. Although influenza can be mistaken for *common cold* it is a much more severe disease. These viruses cause endemic, epidemic and pandemic influenza.

According to WHO, the annual seasonal influenza epidemics result in about 3 – 5 million cases of severe illness and about 2.5 to 5 lakh deaths. Influenza viruses are enveloped viruses having single-stranded segmented RNA genome and belong to the family Orthomyxoviridae. These viruses constantly undergo genetic changes. On the basis of their core protein, ribonucleoprotein (RNP), the influenza viruses are classified into four types/genera with one species each:

Genus	Species	
• *Influenza virus* A	• *Influenza* A virus	Infect humans
• *Influenza virus* B	• *Influenza* B virus	
• *Influenza virus* C	• *Influenza* C virus	
• *Influenza virus* D	• *Influenza* D virus	– Identified in 2016 infects pigs and cattle, and not humans

Influenza A virus is further subdivided into 28 subtypes (strains) according to their envelope glycoproteins (antigens) with hemagglutinin (HA) and neuraminidase (NA) activity. The different forms of antigens are assigned different numbers, for example, H1, H2, H3, … and N1, N2, …. There are 18 sub types of HA antigens (H1 → H18) and 11 of NA (1–11).

Four major pandemics known in the human history are:

- **1918 Spanish influenza**: H_1N_1 20-50 million deaths
- **1957-58 Asian flu** H_2N_2 2 million deaths
- **1968 Hong Kong flu** H_3N_2 1 million deaths
- **2004 Avian influenza (bird flu)** H_5N_1 32 deaths, millions of poultry deaths

Pandemic human influenza viruses belong to the infleriza A virus, such as A/H1N1 (Spanish and Swine flu), H2N2 (Asian flu). H3N2 (Hong Kong) and H5N1 (bird flu) responsible for 20th and 21st century pandemics. Worldwide, 3 – 5 million cases of severe illness and 2,90,000 to 6,50,000 human deaths occur every year due to influenza.

INFLUENZA A VIRUS

Influenza A viruses (IAVs) constitute a major threat to human health. Strains of all subtypes of influenza A virus circulate among wild birds which are considered their natural host. They are very similar in structure to influenza viruses type B, C and D.

STRUCTURE

Structurally, a virion is typically spherical 80–120 nm in diameter. Pleomorphism is common and produces filamentous forms. It is covered in an envelope made of a lipid bilayer with spikes of glycoproteins called **haemagglutinin** and **neuraminidase** (Fig. 56.1). These proteins enable the virus to effectively find a host cell and function as **antigens** that trigger an immune response.

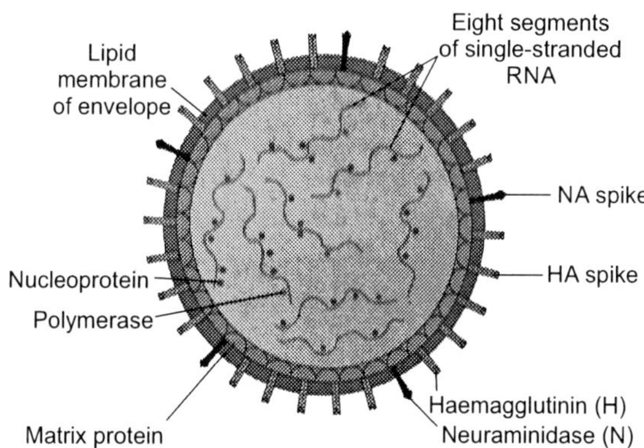

Fig. 56.1 Detailed structure of the influenza A virus. The virus particle shows two types of spikes: HA and NA (haemagglutinin and neuraminidase, type specific antigens) and genome comprised of 8 segments of single-stranted RNA. Nucleoprotein and polymerase proteins are closely associated with RNA segments to form ribonucleoproein (RNP).

The genome is composed of eight separate segments of single-stranded RNA, a unique characteristic, enclosed in a helical nucleocapsid (Figure 56.1).

ANTIGENIC VARIABILITY

An influenza virus is able to change frequently H and N proteins on its surface, therefore, changing its antigenic properties. This change can occur in two different ways.

- **Antigenic Drift**

Antigenic drift occurs more commonly and refers to minor gradual changes that occur through mutations in the genetic material that cause small changes in the surface proteins. Antigenic drift is seen in all influenza viruses.

- **Antigenic Shift**

This process involves a sudden major change, referred to as **shift,** in the antigenicity of the H or N antigens that produces a new influenza subtype. It involves only type A influenza viruses. Antigens shift is based on recombination between different virus strains when they infect the same cell (for example in 2009 swine flu virus). The new types of viral strains produced set the basis for the epidemic or pandemic outbreaks that happen every now and then.

DIAGNOSIS

The demonstration of **viral antigens** in respiratory tract secretions of the **antibodies** specific for H proteins are two widely performed tests.

AVIAN INFLUENZA (BIRD FLU)

Avian influenza (also known as **avian flu** or **bird flu**) is caused due to a variety of viruses adopted by birds such as A(H5N1), A(H7N9).

In humans, it is characterised by flu-like symptoms. Highly pathogenic avian influenza (HPAI) causes severe illness and results in high death rate, nearly 60% of those infected with A(H5N1).

The name H5N1 refers to the subtypes of surface antigens present on the influenza A virus: **haemagglutinin** type 5 and **neuraminidase** type 1. It is endemic in birds in South-East Asia and represents a long-term pandemic threat. It has 11 genes in 8 separate RNA molecules.

HISTORY

Influenza A/H5N1 was first isolated in 1996 from a goose in China and the first outbreak of avian influenza with HPAI A(H5N1) in human was reported in 1997 in Hong Kong (China) which was linked to handling infected poultry. Since 2003, this virus has spread from Asia to Europe and Africa, and has become endemic in poultry populations in some countries resulting in millions of poultry infections. Eleven outbreaks of H5N1 were reported worldwide in June 2008 in five countries (China, Egypt, Indonesia, Pakistan and Vietnam) compared to 65 outbreaks in June 2006 and 55 in June 2007. As per WHO over 40 countries have been affected with influenza H/H5N1. In 2013, human infections with another strain of HPAI virus-A/H7N9 was reported for the first time in China. Between 2013 and 2017, 916 lab confirmed human cases were reported to the WHO.

CLINICAL FEATURES

The **inubation period** following exposure to infection in humans for A (H5N1) virus is 2 to 5 days but ranging up to 17 days and for A(H7N9) virus averages 5 days and ranging from 1 to 10 days. For both viruses, the average incubation period is longer to seasonal influenza (2 days).

Clinical presentation of avian influenza ranges from flu-like symptoms with high fever (over 100.4°F or 38°C), cough, muscle aches to severe respiratory illness. Gastrointestinal symptoms (e.g., nausea, vomiting and diarrhea) may also occur. Virulent forms of the virus can result in respiratory failure to multiple-organ failure and even death.

MODE OF TRANSMISSION

Wild aquatic bird such as waterfowl is the natural reservoir of the virus and has the ability to spread easily to domestic poultry. The route of transmission of virus is via bird-to-human. The disease is transmitted to humans through direct or indirect contact with infected live or dead birds or virus contaminated surfaces. Birds infected with H5N1 continue to release the virus infections and saliva for as long as 10 days and the virus has the ability to survive for extended periods of time. Human-to-human transmission is not known to occur.

DIAGNOSIS

Avian influenza in humans is diagnosed by:

- Molecular methods (e.g., RT-PCR)

- Viral culture
- Rapid influenza diagnostic tests (RIDTs), however, these cannot provide subtype information.
- Finding a fourfold rise in H5-specific antibody levels in paired serum samples.

TREATMENT

Antiviral drugs like oseltamivir (Tamilflu), zenamivir (Relenza) and peramivir (Rapivab) are recommended in the early stages of infection.

PREVENTION

- **Handling poultry:** Avoid touching poultry, birds, animals and their droppings.

  Wash eggs with detergent if soiled with fecal matter and cook and consume them immediately.
- **Maintain good personal hygiene:** Perform hand hygiene frequently, cover your mouth and nose and use personal protective equipment (PPE) during outbreaks in poultry.
- **Maintain good environmental hygiene:** Regularly clean and disinfect frequently touched surfaces (e.g., furniture) with 1:99 diluted household bleach and metallic surfaces with 70% alcohol; maintain good indoor ventilation; and maintain drainage pipes properly.
- **Vaccination:** At present, only vaccine against A/H5N1 is available on the market and is only recommended for specific workers at higher risk of exposure to this virus.
- **Antiviral drugs:** People who have had contact with infectious birds may be given Tamilflu prevently.

SWINE FLU (H1N1 FLU)

Swine flu (also called **swine influenza, H1N1 flu**) is a human respiratory infection caused by the H1N1 swine influenza A virus. It's called swine flu because in the past, the people who caught and had direct contact with pigs. It was responsible for a global flu outbreak called a **2009 swine flu pandemic** that lasted for 20 months (from January **2009** to August 2010) and the second of the two pandemics, the first being the **1918 Spanish flu pandemic** (that occurred between 1918 and 1920).

HISTORY

The first human case was a 5-year-old boy in La Glooria, Mexico, a rural town in Veracruz on March 9, 2009 followed by an outbreak (widespread H1N1 infection) in the state of Veracruz and spread rapidly to the US, Canada and other parts of the world as a result of air travel. The virus was identified in April 2009 as a new strain of H1N1 (pandemic H1N1/09 virus) called a **quadruple assortment virus** which was found to have two genes from flu viruses that normally circulate in pigs in Europe and Asia, and two other genes, one of avian origin and other of human origin. This virus appeared to spread by human-to-human resulting in widespread community transmission. The WHO on June 11, 2009 declared it as pandemic. Around 700 million to 1.4 billion people contracted the illness with 12000 – 18000 deaths globally. However, as per CDC 2019, there were more than 284000 deaths. Subsequent cases of swine flu were reported in India in 2015 with over 31156 positive test cases and 1841 deaths up to March 2015.

STRUCTURE AND VIROLOGY OF H1N1 VIRUS

Structure is the same as described under influenza A virus (Fig. 56.1) the designation H1N1 indicates the surface proteins: Haemagglutinin and neuraminidase that have unique tracts which exhibit characteristics that identify the virus to the immune system and allows for attachment and replication of the virus.

The incubation period is 24 – 48 hours (ranges 2 to 7 days). The shedding stage of the virus is during the first 4-5 days of illness. The period (human-to-human viral infections) for swine influenza in adults usually begins one day before the symptoms develop in a patient (which means you can pass on the H1N1 virus without even knowing you have it) and can last 5 – 7 days after they get sick. It is different from avian flu virus in its mode of transmission: swine virus is transmitted readily from human-to-human while avian flu virus cannot.

Symptons of swine flu are similar to normal human flu that include chills, fever (100°C or 37.8°F), cough, sore throat and stiff nose. Swine flu is more likely to include diarrhea and vomiting. The most serious implication of flu is pneumonia and respiratory failure especially among pregnant women and aged individuals.

LABORATORY DIAGNOSIS

Diagnosis is made by **real-time RT-PCR** test that differentiates between pandemic H1N1 and regular seasonal flu. Other widely used tests include **rapid influenza diagnostic tests** (RIDT) which yield results in 30 minutes, and direct and indirect immunofluorescence assays (DFAIFA) which take 2 to 4 hours. Nasopharyngeal, nasal or oropharyngeal tissue swabs are used as specimens which are to be collected within the first 4 or 5 days of illness (the most infectious period of the disease).

TREATMENT

Two antiviral drugs used for treatment are:

- Oseltamivir (Tamilflu) oral administration.
- Zanamivir (Relenza) which is inhaled.

  These should be initiated in the first 24 hours to lessen the cause and severity of infection.

PREVENTION

- The best way to prevent swine flu is to get a yearly flu vaccination.
- Frequently washing hands with soap or hand sanitizer.
- Avoid touching your nose, mouth or eyes (since the virus can survive on surfaces like telephones and table tops).
- Avoiding of close contact with people to prevent transmission of illness.

THE 1918 SPANISH FLU PANDEMIC

The **Spanish flu**, also known as the **1918 flu pandemic**, caused by H1N1 influenza A virus, was the most severe and deadliest influenza pandemic in human history. The virion of the Spanish flu name stems from the pandemic spread to Spain from France in 1918, the first newspaper report publishing the outbreak of the disease lasting more than 12 months from January 1918 to early summer 1999. Between 50 and 100 million people died including more than 5 lakh Americans of the 500 million people infected worldwide about a third of the world's people at the time.

Today as the world grinds to a halt in response to the Coronavirus COVID-19, scientists and historians are studying the 1918 outbreak for clues to the most effective way to stop a global pandemic. Moreover, in any discussion of influenza, the great pandemic of 1918-1919 must be mentioned.

The 1918 spanish flu was the first of two pandemics caused by H1N1 influenza A virus, the second was the 2009 swine flu pandemic.

In India, the 1918 flu pandemic broke out in Bombay in June 1918 via ships carrying troops returning from the First World War (1914-1918) in Europe, hence also referred as the **Bombay influenza** or **the Bombay Fever** in India. The outbreak most severely affected younger people in the age group of 20 to 40, with women suffering disproportionately. The pandemic is believed to have killed up to 14 – 17 million people in the country, the most among all countries of the world. A recent study by David Arnold (2019) published in the Transactions to the Royal Historical Society estimates at least 12 million dead, about 50% of the population.

KEY POINTS

- **Influenza (flu)**, characterized by fever chills, headache and general muscular aches, is caused by *influenza viruses*.
- Influenza is transmitted by droplet inhalation.
- Severe influenza outbreaks recorded during the 20th century include: Spanish flu (1918-19), Asian flu (1957), Hong Kong flu (1968), Bird flu (2004) and Swine flu (2009).
- The influenza viruses are characterized by single-stranded segmented RNA genome enclosed in a helical nuucleocapsid.
- The **internal ribonucleoprotein (RNP)**, a group specific antigen, is used to classify influenza A, B, C and D viruses.
- Antigenic differences in the surface proteins: (haemagglutinin (HA)) and neuraminidase (NA) are used to identify subtypes (strains) of influenza A virus.
- Multivalent vaccines are available to prevent influenza for older adults and other high- risk groups.
- Antiviral agents rimantadine and amantadine are effective prophylactic and curative drugs against influenza A virus.

IMPORTANT QUESTIONS

1. Write short notes on:
   (a) Influenza A virus
   (b) Avian (bird) flu
   (c) Swine flu.

MULTIPLE-CHOICE QUESTIONS

1. All are true for influenza A virus EXCEPT:
   (a) Segmented RNA genome
   (b) Transmitted by droplet inhalation

(c) Nonenveloped

(d) Lipid bilayer with two types of spikes.

2. Which of the following subtypes of influenza A virus caused Spanish flu (1918 pandemic)?

(a) H_1N_1 (b) H_5N_1

(c) H_3N_2 (d) H_2N_2.

3. Influenza A viruses are divided into subtypes on the basis of:

(a) Surface proteins

(b) Segmented RNA geneome

(c) Influenza ribonucleoprotein (RNP)

(d) All of the above.

4. Which of the following causes swine flu?

(a) A/H_1N_1 (b) A/H_2N_2

(c) A/H_3N_2 (d) A/H_5N_1.

5. Which of the following subtype of the influenza A virus causes avian (bird) flu?

(a) H_3N_1 (b) H_1N_1

(c) H_2N_2 (d) H_5N_1.

ANSWERS TO MCQs

1. (c) 2. (a) 3. (a) 4. (a)
5. (a).

57

Hepatitis Viruses: RNA and DNA Viruses

Viral hepatitis (Jaundice)

Hepatitis refers to a liver disease characterized by inflammation of liver tissue, yellow discoloration of the skin and whites of eyes (jaundice), fibrosis (scarring), cirrhosis or liver cancer. The word is derived from the Greek *hepar* meaning liver and *atis* meaning inflammation.

Hepatitis is often caused by viruses (called **viral** hepatitis) and is of five types, i.e., hepatitis A, B, C, D and E based on the virus involved. Other causes include heavy alcohol use, certain drugs, other infections and autoimmune disorders.

Currently, about 2.3 billion people of the world are infected with one or more of the hepatitis viruses and results in 1.4 million deaths each year. Hepatitis B's prevalence is highest (257 million people living with chronic hepatitis) followed by hepatitis C (71 million people), these two are responsible for 90% of the facilities worldwide.

World Hepatitis Day (WHD) observed on July 28 every year, aims to raise global awareness of hepatitis, a serious disease of liver and encourage its prevention, diagnosis and treatment.

HEPATITIS VIRUSES

Viruses that cause hepatitis are called **hepatitis viruses** or **hepatotrophic viruses** which currently consists of types A, B, C, D and E. Their genome is made of RNA or DNA. Except for type B, which is a DNA virus, the rest are RNA viruses.

Two common features shared by these viruses are:

- Ability to infect liver tissue (hepatocytes);
- Cause a similar, icteric illness (*icterus* = jaundice)

Two common modes of transmission are:

- **Fecal-oral route**, i.e., contaminated food and water (Hepatitis A and E)
- **Blood** (Hepatitis B, C and D)

Serology (viral antigens, anti-viral antibodies) and molecular markers are used to differentiate these viruses.

HEPATITIS AND HEPATITIS A VIRUS

Hepatitis A (in short **Hep A**) is an infectious acute illness of the liver (acute viral hepatitis) caused by the HAV. At one time, it was referred to as "**infectious hepatitis**" because it could be spread easily from person-to-person like other viral infections.

Hep A occurs worldwide, more common in regions of the world with poor sanitation. Globally, around 114 million infections, occur each year mainly among children below age 10. It is the most common cause of acute hepatitis in children.

STRUCTURE

Hepatovirus A (= *Hepatitis A virus*), a picornavirus, is an icosahedral (27 nm), non-enveloped, single-strain positive sense, RNA virus. Only one serotype is known. It is usually spread by eating food or drinking water with contaminated feces and by dirty hands (i.e., by fecal-oral route).

CLINICAL FEATURES

The onset of the disease (i.e., appearance of symptoms) occurs between two and six weeks after infection. Following infection, HAV enters the blood streams through epithelium of the oropharynx or intestine. Blood carries the virus to the liver, where it multiplies in hepatocytes and kupffer cells (liver macrophages). Virions exit the host cells by lysis and viroporins and are secreted into bile and released in stool.

The clinical disease occurs in two stages: the **prodormal** (or **preicteric**) and **icteric** stage. Symtoms typically appear 2 to 6 weeks after the initial infections (the **incubation period**). Major symptoms of Hap are nausea, fever, fatigue, jaundice, dark urine (due to bile), clay-colored faeces (alcholic faeces) and pain in the abdomens.

Hepatitis A occurs sporadically or as outbreaks.

LABORATORY DIAGNOSIS

- Detection of the virus in stool specimens by electron microscopy two weeks before clinical illness develops.

- Detection of HAV specific IGM antibodies in the serum (blood) which are detectable from 1 – 2 weeks after the initial infection and persist for up to 14 weeks.

TREATMENT

No specific treatment for hepatitis A is known.

PREVENTION

It can be prevented by good hygiene, good sanitation and vaccination: either inactivated *Hepatovirus* A or a live but attenuated virus that provides active immunity for over 20 years.

No vaccination is required for persons who had experienced HAV infection since he/she becomes immune for the rest of life.

HEPATITIS B (SERUM HEPATITIS) AND HBV

Hepatitis B (HB) is originally called **serum hapatitis** (due to the presumption that it could only spread through serum). It is a life-threatening infectious disease caused by the **hepatitis B virus (HBV)** causing both acute and chronic hepatitis, cirrhosis and liver cancer caused in 25% of the chronic patients. Based on the evidence obtained from 4500 year old human remains, the HBV has infected humans since the Bronze Age. Currently, it is a major health problem and most important of the five types of hepatitis A, B, C, D and E. At present there are 390 million population, i.e., 5% of the world's population as HBV carriers, causing 7,50,000 deaths every year worldwide. In our country it is a serious infection with more than one million cases recorded each year.

TREATMENT

Antiviral drugs to suppress the level of virus replication and slow its ability to damage the liver include: entecavir (Baraclude), tenofovir (Viread), adefovir (Hepsera), lamivudine (Epivir) and telbivudine (Tyzeka).

PREVENTION

Vaccination: *Hepatitis B vaccine*, a safe and effective vaccine that provides lifetime protection is available. This vaccine is also known as the first anti-cancer vaccine because it prevents hepatitis B, the casue of cancer worldwide.

Engerix - B, Heplisav - B and Recombivax (HB) (all trade names) are examples of hepatitis B vaccine. WHO recommends that all infants and children up to age of 18 years should receive their first dose of vaccine as soon as possible after birth preferably within 24 hours. The birth dose should be followed by 2 or 3 more doses to complete the primary series, vaccine will provide a lifetime protection.

Three dose schedule:

- 1st shot at any given time in the delivery room within 12 hours.
- 2nd shot 28 days after the 1st shot.
- 3rd shot 16 weeks (4 months) after the 1st shot (minimun age of infants should be 24 weeks).

General Preventive Measures

In addition to vaccination, other simple ways to stop the spread of hepatitis B are:

- Avoid direct contact with blood and bodily fluids, sharing sharp items (e.g., razors, nail clippers, tooth brush, earrings, body rings) of patients and carriers.
- Avoid injectable antiviral drugs.
- Use condoms with soap and water after any potential exposure to blood.
- Use condoms with sexual partners.

HEPATITIS B VIRUS

Hepatitis B virus (HBV), a partially double-stranded DNA virus, is a species of the genus *Orthopadnavirus*, a member of the family *Hepadnaviridae*. The virus (virion) was originally referred to as the **Dane particle** based on its first discovery by **David Dane,** a British pathologist and clinical virologist with his colleagues in 1970.

STRUCTURE

HBV (Dane particle) is an enveloped virus (42 nm diameter) consisting of an outer lipid envelope and an iosahedral core (27 nm diameter) composed of proteins (Fig. 57.1). The virus is one of the smallest enveloped animal viruses. But pleomorphic forms exist, including filamentous and spherical bodies lacking a core (Fig. 57.1). These particles are not infectious. The viral envelope contains hepatitis B surface antigen (HBsAg).

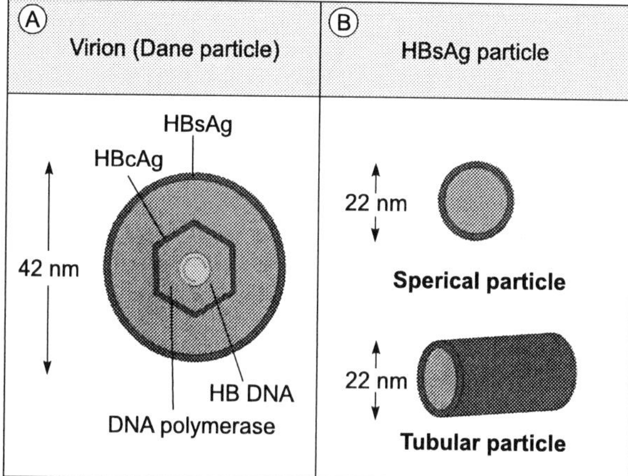

Fig. 57.1 Hepatitis B virus particles. (A) Dane particle. (B) spherical and tubular (filamentous) particles. During acute infection and in some carriers there are $10^6 - 10^7$ infectious (Dane) particles and as many as 10^{12} HB surface antigen (HBsAg) particles/ml of serum (B).

The **genome** of HBV enclosed by nucleocapsid is made of unusual circular DNA, that is not fully double-stranded (hence called partially ds). One end of the full length strand is linked to the viral DNA polymerase (Fig. 57.1).

MULTIPLICATION

HBV multiplies inside the liver cells. Synthesis of DNA takes place from an RNA template by reverse transcriptase activity similar to retroviruses.

PHYSICAL AND CHEMICAL SUSCEPTIBILTY

HBV is a relatively heat stable virus (such as 10 hours heat leading at 60°C does not kill the virus but reduces infectivity). It remains alive at room temperature for long periods.

HBV is susceptible to chemical agents. Exposure to hypochlorite (10,000 ppm available chlorine) and 2% glutaraldehyde inactivates infectivity, though HBsAg may not be inactivated by such treatment.

ANTIGENIC STRUCTURE

- **Hepatitis B surface antigen (HBsAg):** HBV protein present on the viral envelope, the first to be discovered, produces antibodies when infected.
- **Hepatitis B core antigen (HBcAg):** The antigen expressed on the core is used as marker of infection.

- **Hepatitis B antigen (HBeAg):** It is primarily secreted into the serum.

CLINICAL MANIFESTATIONS

Clinical symptoms in hepatitis B develop between 30 and 180 days after HBV infection which are similar to that of type A but it tends to be more severe and prolonged (chronic). The structure and clinical manifestations varies in both acute and chronic infections:

Acute Infection

1. ***Preicteric phase:*** Fever and anorexia followed by nausea, vomiting, abdominal pain and chills.
2. ***Icteric phase:*** Liver damage (jaundice, dark urine, pale stools).
3. ***Convalescent phase:*** Recovery within 1-2 months of onset (90 – 95%).

CHRONIC INFECTION

One to ten percent of hepatitis B cases remain chronically infected as asymptomatic carriers. In chronic cases, liver failure, cancer or scarring can occur.

MODE OF TRANSMISSION

HBV, a blood borne virus, is commonly transmitted via body fluids such as blood, semen and vaginal secretions by the following routes:

- ***Perinatal transmission:*** From mother to baby during pregnancy, labour and nursing.
- ***Parenteral transmission:*** By blood products, unclean needles and unscreaned blood transfusion.
- ***Sexual transmission:*** By having unprotected vaginal, anal and oral sex.

LABORATORY DIAGNOSIS

For diagnosis, clinical signs of liver damage (e.g., yellowing skin or belly pain), liver ultrasound (transient elastography) are not specific for hepatitis B infection. Hence, microbiological investigations are done by serological tests for detection of HBV antigens and antibodies, using radio-immuno assays (RIA), enzyme-linked immunosorbent assays (ELISAs), and HBV DNA by PCR, biochemical tests and isolation of the virus from the blood or liver tissues.

1. **HBsAg (Hepatitis B surface antigen)**

   Presence of HBsAg in the serum indicates case of a recent acute infection or a carrier of HBV. It is a standard screening test used to diagnose hepatitis B.
2. **Polymerase chain reaction:** PCR tests are used to detect and measure the amount of HBV DNA, called the **viral load**, in clinical specimens. These tests are significant to assess a person's infection status and to monitor treatment.

   Individuals with high viral loads, characteristically have **ground glass hepatocytes on biopsy**.
3. **Biochemical tests:** Serum bilirubin levels may rise up to 25-fold.

HEPATITIS C AND HCV

Hepatitis C (Hep C), caused by the hepatitis C virus (HCV), causes liver inflammation, sometimes leading to serious liver damage.

Globally, an estimated 7.1 million people have chronic hepatitis C virus infection. Approximately 4 lakh people died from Hep C in 2016, mostly from cirrhosis and hepatocellular carcinoma (primary liver cancer). More than one million cases are recorded every year in India.

STRUCTURE

Hepatitis C virus (= HCV) is a member of the genus *Hepacivirus* (family *Flaviviridae*). It has a small (55-65 nm), enveloped, positive-sense single-stranded RNA genome.

MODE OF TRANSMISSION

The virus mainly spreads by blood transfusion, contact with contaminated blood and blood products by sharing needles and can also occur from mother to baby.

CLINICAL FEATURES

The incubation period is long which ranges from 15 – 160 days (most often 50 days).

Most people have no symptoms. The acute illness is usually mild showing fatigue, nausea, fever and muscle aches. In some patients, progress to chronic hepatitis developing cirrhosis and hepatocellular carcinoma (cancer).

LABORATORY DIAGNOSIS

- **Serological antibody assays:** These assays measure human antibodies generated in response to HCV infection. These can be performed by:

- **Rapid immunoassays:** The oral quick rapid antibody test can detect the antibodies in whole blood obtained by finger stick or venipuncture. This test is used for initial HCV antibodies. The results are available within 40 minutes.
- **Molecular HCV RNA tests:** These tests directly detect RNA of the virus and the process is commonly referred to as a **nucleic acid test (NAT)** or **nucleic acid amplification test (NAAT).**

TREATMENT

α-Interferon combined with ribavirion is used to treat chronic hepatitis.

PREVENTION

Screening of blood donors to prevent transmission of HCV infection through blood transfusion.

HEPATITIS D (DELTA) AND HDV

Hepatitis D (also called **delta hepatitis**) is a liver disease in both acute and chronic forms caused by the hepatitis delta virus (HDV). HDV can only infect people already infected with hepatitis B. It occurs only simultaneously (i.e., coinfection) or as superinfection with HBV.

HDV-HBV coinfection is considered the most severe form of chronic viral hepatitis due to more rapid progression towards liver related death and hepatocellular carcinoma. Globally, 5% of people with chronic HBV infection are coinfected with HDV, resulting in a total of 15 – 20 million persons infected with HDV worldwide.

Hepatits delta virus (HDV) (Fig. 57.2) is a small spherical (36 nm) enveloped virus. It is considered to be a **subviral satellite** because it can propagate only in the presence of *Hepatitis B virus*.

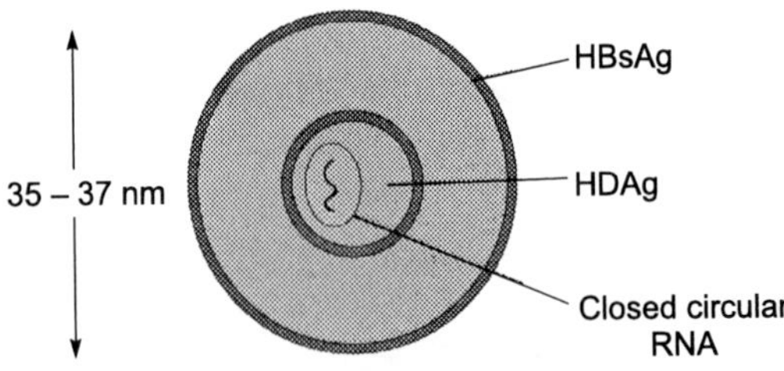

Fig. 57.2 Structure of hepatitis D virus in serum. Ag = antigen.

The genome is composed of negative sense single-stranded, closed circular RNA of 1679 nucleotides. The hepatitis D circular genome is unique among animal viruses because of its high GC nucleotide content. HDV is the smallest virus known to infect animals. It has been proposed that HDV may have originated from viroids (small single-stranded RNAs without a protein coat plant pathogens) which are much smaller than viruses.

TRANSMISSION

The mode of transmission of HDV is similar to HBV. Transmission of HDV occurs either via simultaneous infection with HBV (coinfection) or superimposed on chronic hepatitis B or hepatitis B carrier state (superinfection).

Symptoms observed are feeling tired, nausea and vomiting leading to liver cirrhosis.

Laboratory Diagnosis

By detecting delta antigen or antibodies by ELISA and radiommuno assay procedures.

TREATMENT

Chronic hepatitis D is treated with interferons (e.g., Pegylated interferon alfa, **PEG-IFN-α**).

PREVENTION

No specific prophylaxis exists, however, human immunization with the HBV vaccine can prevent HDV infection.

HEPATITIS E AND HEV

Hepatitis E, a water-borne viral disease, is caused by *hepatitis E virus* **(HEV)**, a public health problem in many developing countries, especially in East and South Asia.

There are over 20 million HEV infections worldwide, causing 44,000 deaths in 2015 alone.

Hepatitis E virus is a spherical, nonenveloped virus (32 – 34 nm diameter) having a single-stranded RNA genome. It is classified in the genus ***Hepevirus*** under the family ***Hepeviridae***.

HEV has four different types 1 and 2 (found only in humans) and 3 and 4 in animals (e.g., pigs, wild boars and deer).

TRANSMISSION

HEV is transmitted via the fecal-oral-route through fecal contaminated water.

CLINICAL FEATURES

The virus is shed in the stools of infected persons and enters the human body through the intestines. The incubation period ranges from 2 to 10 weeks with an average of 5 to 6 weeks, producing the symptoms.

- An initial phase of mild fever, reduced appetite (anorexia), nausea and vomiting lasting for a few days.
- Jaundice with dark urine and pale stools.
- A slightly enlarged, tender liver (hepatomegaly).

These symptoms are often indistinguishable from other liver illnesses and typically last for 1 – 6 weeks.

In rare cases, acute hepatitis can be severe, and results in *fulminant hepatitis* (acute liver failure), finally leading to death.

LABORATORY DIAGNOSIS

- Detection of specific IgM antibodies to HEV in person's blood by ELISA tests, western blot blood assay.
- **PCR** – Reverse transcriptase polymerase chain reaction (RT-PCR) is used to detect the HEV RNA in blood and/or stool.
- **Immunoelectron microscopy:** For aggregated calcivirus-like particles using monoclonal antibodies in feces.

TREATMENT

No specific treatment is required as the disease is self-limiting.

PREVENTION

- Maintaining clean water supplies and proper disposal systems for human feces and maintaning hygenic panties.
- A recombinant vaccine to prevent HEV infection was developed in China in 2011, however, WHO has not approved its use in other countries.

GB VIRUS C

GB virus C **(GBV-C)** formerly known as *hepatitis G virus* **(HGV)** also known as human **pegivirus (HPgV),** is a member of the genus *Pegivirus* (Family *Flaviviridae*) is known to infect humans. Worldwide, it currently infects around a sixth of the world's population, but is not known to cause any human disease.

GBVC has a single stranded, positive sense RNA genome. It is phylogenetically related to *hepatitis C virus*, but replicates primarily in lymphocytes.

KEY POINTS

- **Hepatitis** refers to inflammation of the liver tissue that can lead to yellow discoloration of the skin (jaundice, fibrosis (scarring), cirrhosis or liver cancer.
- **Hepatitis viruses** (viruses causing hepatitis in humans) have been identified by the letters A, B, C, D and E.
- All the hepatitis viruses are RNA viruses (A, C, D, E and G) except the hepatitis B virus (HBV), which is a DNA virus.
- Hepatitis B, C and D are transmitted through blood and blood products and hepatitis A and E are feco-orally transmitted viruses.
- Except for hepatitis A and B there are no vaccines for these infections, HBV vaccine also protects against delta infection.
- **Hepatitis delta virus (HDV)**, smallest virus to infect animals via a subviral satellite, propagates only in the presence of HBV.
- **G B virus** (= **Hepatitis G virus**), an RNA virus, infects a sixth of the world population without causing a disease.
- **Hepatitis B virus** is unique in having three different forms of viral particles, i.e., pleomorphic (HBV or Dane particle two subvirion forms spherical particle and tubular particle) secreted from an HBV infected cell.
- Hepatitis B, with over 350 million carriers worldwide, is prevented with hepatitis B vaccine and treated with Ramividine, adefovir and interferon alpha.

IMPORTANT QUESTIONS

1. What is hepatitis? Describe hepatitis B, HBV, diagnosis, vaccines and treatment of hepatitis B infection.

2. Write short notes on:
   (a) Pleomorphism in hepatitis B virus
   (b) Virus contaminated food hepatitis
   (c) Infectious hepatitis
   (d) Hepatitis D virus
   (e) Blood transfusion associated hepatitis.

MULTIPLE-CHOICE QUESTIONS

1. Which one of the following is a DNA virus?
   (a) Hepatitis A virus (b) Hepatitis V virus
   (c) Hepatitis D virus (d) Hepatitis E virus.
2. Which of the following is a defective satellite virus?
   (a) Hepatitis A virus (b) Hepatitis C virus
   (c) Hepatitis D virus (d) Hepatitis E virus.
3. Which of the following virus hepatitis is most serious?
   (a) Hepatitis A (b) Hepatitis B
   (c) Hepatitis C (d) Hepatitis E.
4. Hepatitis E virus is mainly transmitted by:
   (a) Sexual intercourse
   (b) Infected syringes and needles
   (c) Fecally contaminated drinking water
   (d) From mother to child.
5. Fecal-oral route is the mode of transmission in which hepatitis viruses?
   (a) Hepatitis A and E virus (b) Hepatitis A and B virus
   (c) Hepatitis B and C virus (d) Hepatitis D and E virus.
6. In addition to hepatitis B, HBV vaccine provides protection aganist which viral hepatitis?
   (a) Hepatitis A (b) Hepatitis C
   (c) Hepatitis D (d) Hepatitis E.
7. All the following viruses are transmitted via blood EXCEPT:
   (a) Hepatitis A (b) Hepatitis B
   (c) Hepatitis C (d) Hepatitis D.
8. Hepatitis D cannot occur in the absence of hepatitis B virus infection because HDV requires HBV for its multiplication.
   True or False?

ANSWERS TO MCQs

1. (b)	2. (c)	3. (b)	4. (c)
5. (a)	6. (c)	7. (a)	8. True.

58

Human Immunodeficiency Virus: An RNA Retrovirus

AIDS/HIV Infection

Human immunodeficiency virus (HIV), the etiologic agent of AIDS, that harms the immune system by destroying the white blood cells (CD4 cells). It is a **retrovirus**, an RNA virus that has an enzyme reverse transcriptase and has the unique property of transcribing its RNA into DNA after entering a cell (Latin *re* = reverse, backwards and *tre* transcriptase). The AIDS virus was identified in 1983 by an American **Rolert Gallo** or French scientists **Luc Montagnier** and **Francoise Sarre-Sinoussi. Acquired Immunodeficiency Syndrome** (AIDS) is a chronic potentially life threatening condition where the immune system is severely weakened (compromised). It is one of the world's most fatal infectious diseases and has had the greatest global impact on society (both as a source of illness and as a source of discrimination) and economy.

HISTORY OF AIDS/HIV INFECTION

It is widely believed that HIV originated in Kinshara, the Democratic Republic of Congo around 1920 when HIV crossed species from Chimpanzees to humans. However, it was first recognized in 1981 in the United States among the intravenous drug users and a year later in 1982 among the homosexuals. Its epidemic subsequently occurred in San Francisco, New York and other cities of the USA and a few years later in the UK and other European countries.

Currently, AIDS is one of the world's most fatal infectious diseases. According to the global Recap from UNAIDS/WHO, globally 37.9 million people (36.2 million adults and 1.7 million children, 15 year old) were living with HIV infection at the end of 2020. In 2020, 1,80,000

(4,80,000–1.0 million) people died from HIV related causes and 1.5 million people acquired HIV. Swaziland, a country of the sub-Saharan Africa has the highest prevalence of HIV with a death rate of 27.3 per cent.

HIV/AIDS is an epidemic in India and is home to the world's 3rd largest population suffering from this disease with under 60,000 deaths occurring every year. The NACO (National AIDS Control Organization) estimated that 2.11 million people currently live with HIV/AIDS in India.

WORLD AIDS DAY

World AIDS Day, a global health day, introduced by WHO in 1988, is an international day observed on 1 December every year. It is dedicated to raising awarness of the AIDS pandemic caused by the spread of HIV infection and mourning those who died of this disease.

HUMAN IMMUNODEFICIENCY VIRUS

HIV, a retrovirus causative agent of AIDS, was isolated in 1983 from blood lymphocytes (a kind of WBC that provides immunity) by two research groups independently led by **Robert Gallo** (American), and **Francoise Barrè-Sinoussi** and **Luc Montagnier** (French) in 1984. In the same year another American scientist **Jay Levy,** at the University of California, identified a retrovirus as the cause of AIDS. Each group called the virus by a different name: HTLV-III, LAV and ARV respectively.

The International Committee on Virus Nomenclature (ICVN) decided the name **Human Immunodeficiency Virus** (in short **HIV**) for these viruses. HIV belonged to the genus *Lentivirus* (slow virus), a subgroup of *Retrovirus* that infects humans.

On the basis of genetic characteristics and differences in the viral antigens, two types (also called species) have been characterized:

- **HIV-1:** Originally discovered (initially referred to as LAV or HTLV-III), more virulent, more infective, global, origin from Chimpanzee, pandemic and presence of UPU (viral protein U).
- **HIV-2:** Lower infectivity, poor capacity for transmission, largely confined to West Africa, origin from sooty mangaey; and presence of VPx (viral protein *x*).

  HIV attacks the body's immune system, specifically the white blood cells (WBC's) called **CD4 cells** (also called **T-cells, T-lymphocytes** or **helper cells**) that fight infection and play an important role in the body's immune system. **CD 4** (cluster of differentiation 4) is a glycoprotein found on the surface of immune cells in humans (hence also called *CD4 T cells*).

STRUCTURE OF HIV

It is a spherical enveloped virus (100 nm in diameter). It has two identical strands of single-stranded RNA (i.e., diploid genome), the enzyme reverse transcriptase (characteristic feature of retrovirus) and an envelope of phospholipid (Fig. 58.1). The envelope has glycoprotein spikes termed gp 120 (the notation for a glycoprotein with a molcular weight 1,20,000) and transmembrane glycoprotein termed gp 41. These two glycoproteins are involved in attachment to a receptor on the $CD4^+$ cell and fusion of the HIV with the cell, respectively.

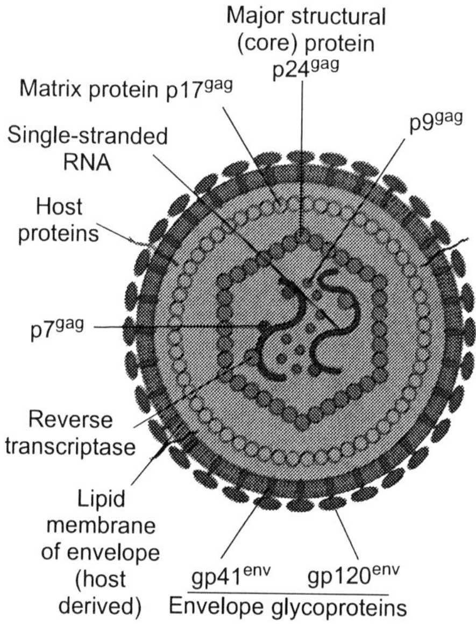

Fig. 58.1 Structure of HIV, the causative agent of AIDS.

VIRAL GENES

The genome of HIV contains seven structural landmarks and nine genes encoding 19 proteins. Of the nine genes, three are **structural genes** (*gag, pol* and *env*) present in all retroviruses that contain information needed to make structural proteins for new virus particles. The remaining six genes (*tat, rev, nef, vif, vpr* and *vpu*) are **regulatory genes** for proteins that control the ability of HIV to infect cells, replicate and cause disease.

RESISTANCE

HIV is a delicate thermolabile virus that can be inactivated at 56°C in 30 minutes, at 60°C in 10 minutes, and at 77°C in just fraction of a second (0.006 sec). In dried blood, it may survive at room temperature for 7 days at 20 – 25°C and for 10 – 15 days at 37°C.

It is susceptible to common disinfections:

- At room temperature, inactivation occurs in 10 minutes when treated with 70% ethyl alcohol, 35% isopropyl alcohol, 1% lysol, 5% formaldehyde, 2% glutaraldehyde and household bleach or bleaching powder (undiluted). Full strength bleach is more effective than diluted bleach in killing HIV in syringes. To treat contaminated medical instruments 2% solution of glutaraldehyde is more useful.
- It is highly susceptible to detergents.

ROUTES OF TRANSMISSION

The virus can be transmitted through contact with infected blood, semen or vaginal fluids. It can be acquired by three routes:

- **Sexual:** AIDS is primarily a sexually transmitted infection (STD). It can be acquired by unprotected sex-vaginal, anal and oral sex. The anal sex is riskier than the vaginal sex. Both the partners are equally affected.
- **Parenteral (blood and blood products):** Uncleaned needles, needle sharing, unscreened blood transfusions or products.
- **Perinatal (vertical transmission from mother to baby).** Infection from mother to child can occur across the placenta during pregnancy, and delivery, and breast feeding.

  Remember: Individuals cannot become infected through ordinary day-to-day contact such as kissing, hugging, shaking hands, or sharing personal objects, food or water.

PATHOGENESIS

HIV enters a host with infected blood, semen and vaginal fluids. It is often spread by dendritic cells which pick up the virus and carry it to the lymphoid organs where it contacts the activated T cells, the cells of the immune systems.

The infective process goes through four steps of attachment, fusion, entry and infection (latent and active) as shown diagrammatically in Figure 58.2.

1. **Attachment:** HIV gp 120 spike attaches to a CD4$^+$ and coreceptors (CCR5 or CXCR4) on the host cell (T helper cells, macrophages and dendritic cells).

↓

2. **Fusion:** HIV fuses with the cell (which is facilitated by gp41 transmembrane glycoprotein of the virus).

↓

3. **Entry:** An entry pore is created and viral RNA is released into the cell, leaving the viral envelop behind.

↓

4. **Latent infection:** Viral RNA is transcribed to DNA by reverse transcriptase, and DNA is integrated into the host chromosome (DNA) via integrase enzyme and forms new viruses (latent provirus), HIV evades the immuno system in latency, and vacuoles by using cell-cell fusion, and by antigenic change, and remain as *latent virions*.
5. **Active infection:** The provirus (DNA) is activated, allowing it to control the synthesis of new viruses, which bud from the host cell. Final viral assembly takes place at the cell membrane, taking up the viral envelope proteins as the viral buds from the cell (progeny HIV).

   Categories of infection: By symptoms, HIV infection is categorized into three phases:
   - Phase 1 (asymptomatic or chronic lymphadenopathy)
   - Phase 2 (symptomatic: early indications of immune failure)
   - Phase 3 (AIDS indicator conditions) CD4$^+$ cell population drops to 200 cells/ml.

Fig. 58.2 Steps involved in HIV infection in humans.

The period from the infection of the cell to the release of new virus particels is called the **latent period** and incubation period of HIV infection. Following infection, the virus often enters a dormant stage lasting 2 to 15 years. Clinical manifestations in HIV infection are primarily due to failure of immune response resulting from the destruction of T cells essential for the body's defenses against infectious diseases and cancer.

Acquired Immunodeficiency Syndrome (AIDS)

AIDS is the final stage of HIV infection representing the irrversible breakdown of immune defense mechanisms, leaving the patient prey to progressive opportunisitic infections and maliginancies (e.g., Kapsoi's sarcoma).

As per classification of WHO (1986, 2007), stages of HIV infection are categorized as follows:

- **Primary HIV infection:** A person may not have any symptoms or experiences a brief period of flu-like symptoms.

- **Stage I:** Infection is asymptomatic with a CD 4 count greater than 500 per µl (microlitre) of blood. May show enlargement of lymph node.
- **Stage II:** Mild symptoms – minor mucocutaneus manifestation and recurrent upper respiratory infections. A CD 4 count of less than 500 µl.
- **Stage III:** Advanced symptoms – chronic diarrhea, severe tuberculosis of lungs and a CD count of less than 350 µl.
- **Stage IV or AIDS:** Severe symptoms – toxoplasmosis of brain, candidiasis of esophagus, trachea, bronchi or lungs, and Kaposi's sacroma. A CD count of less than 200 µl.

  The US Center for Disease Control and Prevention (2008, 2014) created a classification systems for HIV based on CD 4 count and clinical symptoms into five groups.

LABORATORY DIAGNOSIS

HIV infection/AIDS is diagnosed by two types of tests: tests for immunodeficiency and specific tests for HIV infection (demonstration of antigens/antibodies in blood, isolation of virus). As per WHO, HIV antigen-antibody combination assay is helpful in closing the **window period** (the time between HIV infection and appearance of antibodies to HIV) as HIV antigen is present in the blood before antibodies to HIV can be detected.

I. *Immunodeficieny tests*

(a) **Total leukocyte (WBC) and lymphocyte counts:** Leukopenia (low level of WBC in blood) and a lymphocyte count below 2000/mm^3.

(b) **Platelet count:** Thromocytopenia (low level of platelets in the blood).

(c) **T cell subset assays:** Low CD 4 and reversed T4:T8 ratio.

(d) **IgG and IgA:** Raised levels.

II. *Specific tests for HIV infection*

(a) **Antigen detection:** ELISA is used to detect p 24, the major virus core antigen, the earliest virus marker to appear in blood. This can be used in screening blood donors for early infection of HIV.

(b) **Virus isolation:** The virus can be is isolated from the peripheral lymphocytes, however, not suitable as a routine diagnostic test.

(c) **Polymerase chain reaction:** RT-PCR technique is used to detect viral RNA, that can be detected as early as 72 hours post-infection. PCR can be used for diagnosis and for monitoring the level of viraema. This, test is **gold standard** to diagnose HIV at any stage of infection.

(d) **Antibody detection:** Simplest and most widely used technique to diagnose HIV infection by detecting antibodies in the blood is by ELISA test. Anti-HIV antibodies appear in the individual's blood in 2 – 8 weeks.

Western blot test is another test used for detection of antibodies. If an ELISA test is positive, the Western blot test is usually adminstered to confirm the diagnosis.

III. Combined antigens/antibody tests (4th generation HIV test)

These tests detect HIV antibodies as well as p24 antigens and are useful to detect HIV from one's mouth after infection. These are performed by rapid HIV tests and self-testing at home can be done.

Rapid HIV testing has become the mainstay of the most HIV screening programs. Rapid HIV test kits, which can provide results in 20 mintues or less, have been developed and three are currently available in the United States.

Ora Quick Advance Rapid HIV-1/2 Antibody Test is the first rapid HIV test that got approval from the FDA in 2004. The assay strip detects antibodies to both HIV-1 and HIV-2 in 20 minutes in whole blood (from a fingerstick or venipunture sample) plasma, or oral fluid samples during an acute infection window period (20 – 25 days after infection).

Oral fluid testing procedure consists of:

- Step 1: Collection of sample: swab between the teeth and upper and lower gums once.
- Step 2: Insert the device into the buffer.
- Step 3: Read the results between 20 and 40 minutes.
  - Appearance of line in the zone – **non-reactive**.
  - Appearance of line in the C and T zones – **preliminary positive HIV.**

TREATMENT

Currently, there's no vaccine and no cure for HIV/AIDS. The progression of HIV infection and the life of an AIDS patient can be prolonged by using proper chemotherapy.

Highly active antiretroviral therapy (HAART), i.e., adminisering drug combinations of 2 or more taken together daily, commonly combined into a single pill. Based on the mode of action, HAART are grouped into six classes:

- *Nucleoside reverse transcriptase inhibitors (NRTIs)*
- *Non-nucleoside reverse transcriptase inhibitors (NNRTIs)*
- *Protease inhibitors*
- *Fusion inhibitors*
- *Cell entry inhibitors (CCR 5 antagonists)*
- *Integrase strand transfer inhibitors*

Two commonly used drugs (combined into a single pill) are:

- **Truvada:** *tenofovir + emtricitabrine* (both NRTIs)
- **Atripla:** *tenofovir + emtricitabrine* (NRTIs) + *afavirenz* (NNRTI)

As per WHO recommendations of 15 Nov. 2019, *ralteguavir* should be included in antiretroviral therapy (ART).

Chemotherapy has been successful to reduce the chances of transmission from an infected mother to her newborn.

PREVENTION

Currently, there is no licensed vaccine. In 2009, **RV 144** vaccine was found partially effective for HIV/AIDS.

Preventive measures include:

- Health education regarding the danger of promiscuity and other high risk sexual activities.
- Safe sex: use of condoms and vaginal antiseptics, avoiding oral sex.
- Screening of blood and blood products for HIV before blood transfusion.
- Avoid sharing needles.
- Antiretroviral medication of HIV infected mothers in later stages of pregnancy and to the baby after birth, use of bottle feeding rather than breast feeding.
- Use of newer HIV prevention tools like PrEP (pre-exposure prophylaxis) and **TasP** (treatment prevention) which offer greater protection.

KEY POINTS

- **HIV, (human immunodeficiency virus)** the causative agent of AIDS, is a virus that infects and kills CD4 cells causing immunodeficiency.

- **HIV** is an enveloped retrovirus with two identical copies of single-stranded RNA (diploid RNA genome), reverse transcriptase, and phospholipid envelope with gp 120 spikes.
- **AIDS** (acquired immunodeficiency syndrome or acquired immunodeficiency syndrome) denotes the final (advanced) stage of a 'long' HIV infection.
- A person with a CD4 count below 200 per cubic millimeter (200 cells/µl) is considered to have AIDS.
- The progression from HIV infection to AIDS takes between 10 and 15 years.
- **AIDS** pandemic has resulted in 32 million deaths worldwide between 1981 and 2018, currently 37.7 million people are living with HIV worldwide and causing 68000 deaths in a single year, 2020.
- HIV-1 (a type or species of HIV) is responsible for the devastating pandemic worldwide.
- HIV infection can be acquired by sexual contact, needle sharing, blood transfusion or products, and transfer across the placenta from mother to foetus and breast milk.
- Currently, there is no vaccine to prevent or treat HIV/AIDS.
- It is treated/managed through antiretroviral therapy—using a regimen of three medicines combined in one pill.

IMPORTANT QUESTIONS

1. Describe in brief:
   (a) Human immunodeficiency virus (HIV).
   (b) Describe the stages of HIV infection.
   (c) The routes of HIV transmission.
   (d) Differentiate between HIV infection and AIDS.
   (e) How HIV infection is diagnosed?
   (f) Current methods of preventing and treating HIV infection.

MULTIPLE-CHOICE QUESTIONS

1. Which cells are infected by HIV most often and leads to AIDS?
   (a) B cells
   (b) CD8 cells (lymphocytes)
   (c) CD4 cells (lymphocytes)
   (d) Null cells.

2. Viruses that contain two complete copies of positive strand RNA and the enzyme reverse transcriptase are:
   (a) Reoviruses (b) Togaviruses
   (c) Retroviruses (d) None of the above.
3. The commonest mode of transmission of HIV, the causative agent of AIDS, is:
   (a) Oral (b) Perinatal
   (c) Parenteral (d) Sexual.
4. HIV is transmitted by the following routes EXCEPT:
   (a) Shaking hands
   (b) Sexual
   (c) Contaminated blood and blood products
   (d) Mother to child.
5. Which is correct in the laboratory diagnosis of HIV?
   (a) Elevated platelets
   (b) Decreased CD4 counts
   (c) Decreased IgG and IgA levles
   (d) Elevated WBC counts.
6. Antiretroviral therapy for HIV should be initiated when CD4 counts is
   (a) < 200 cells/cu mm
   (b) < 250 cells/cu mm
   (c) < 350 cells/cu mm
   (d) < 500 cells/cu mm.
7. AIDS denotes only the final stage of a long HIV infection.
   True or False?
8. HIV infection/AIDS can be prevented by a vaccine.
   True or False?
9. Human immunodeficiency virus (HIV), the causative agent of AIDS, is a retrovirus composed of double stranded DNA.
   True or False?

ANSWERS TO MCQs

1. (c) 2. (c) 3. (d) 4. (a)
5. (b) 6. (c) 7. True 8. False
9. False.

59

Poliovirus: An RNA Picornavirus

Poliomyelitis (Polio)

Picornaviruses are smallest known viruses (27–30 nm) having a single-stranded plus-sense RNA genome classified in the family *Picornaviridae* (*pico* referring to extremely small + RNA). They are found in mammals and birds.

The family includes 80 species divided among 35 genera. Poliovirus, a well-known and most studied picornavirus, causes poliomyelitis, a paralytic disease of children revealed by muscle weakness and inability to move.

PULSE POLIO DAY

Pulse polio is an immunization programme which was launched by the Government of India in 1995 to eliminate polio from the country. Hence, every year every child under 5 years of age gets polio drops every time to fight polio. India is now a polio free country since 2014, as declared by the WHO on March 27, 2014.

POLIOVIRUS

Poliovirus, a picornavirus, is a member of the genus *Enterovirus* that causes polio in humans. There are three serologic (antigenic) types of poliovirus.

- **Poliovirus 1 (PV-1):** Most common and is the cause of most epidemics globally.
- **Poliovirus 2 (PV-2):** Causes endemic infections.
- **Poliovirus 3 (PV-3):** Causes less epidemics.

It was an Austrian immunologist **Karl Landsteiner,** the discoverer of blood groups, who first isolated and identified the poliovirus in 1908. Its genome was studied in 1981 by two different teams of researchers; **David Baltimore** and **Vincent Racaniells** of MIT and **Naomi Kitamura** and **Eckard Wimmer** at Stong Brook University. It is now one of the most well-characterised viruses and a useful model system for understanding the biology of RNA viruses.

STRUCTURE

It is a very small (27–30 nm, diameter) nonenveloped RNA virus with protein capsid having icosahedral symmetry. It's genome is a single-stranded of positive sense RNA that is 7500 nucleotides long.

SUSCEPTIBILITY OF POLIOVIRUSES

The poliovirus is rapidly inactivated by heat (pasteurization), chlorine and ultraviolet light.

POLIOMYELITIS (POLIO)

Poliomyelitis (also called **polio**) is an acute disease of the central nervous system resulting in paralysis (can't move parts of the body). The word was coined by **Adolph Kussmaul**; a German physician, in 1874 from Greek words *polio* = grey or pale + *myelos* = marrow + *itis* = inflammation because the gray matter in the spinal cord is inflammed, which causes paralysis.

The disease has existed for thousands of years, with depictions of it in ancient art. It was first recognized as a distinct condition in 1789 by **Michael Underwood**, an English physician. Polio made its first appearance in the United States in 1894. Major outbreaks started to occur in the late 19th century and in the United States it was the most worrying childhood disease in the 20th century.

PATHOGENESIS

Poliovirus is strictly a human pathogen that lives in infected person's throat and intestines. Infection is more common in infants and young children and occurs via the **fecal-oral route**. It enters the body through the mouth by contact with the feces (poop) of an infected person and fecal contaminated water.

After entering the oropharynx, the virus multiplies locally in the tonsils and lymph nodes of the neck and subsequently in Peyer's patches and small intestine. From lymph nodes, it enters the blood resulting in **minor** or **primary viremia**. Through the capillary walls it reaches motor nerve cells in the upper spinal cord, multiplies there producing **secondary viremia**. The cells die resulting in paralysis and finally death due to respiratory failure.

SYMPTOMS

Most people infected with poliovirus (72%) will not have visible symptoms (**asymptomatic**). About 1 out of 4 people (25%) have flu-like symptoms (fever, fatigue, headache) that usually last for 2 to 5 days, then go away on their own. About 1% of people will have stiffness of neck, pain and weakness or paralysis in their arms, legs or both. The paralysis can lead to permanent disability (**paralytic poliomyelitis**). About 2 – 10 of paralysed patients from polio die because the virus affects the muscles (immobilized muscles that help them breathe) due to respiratory failure.

The incubation period of nonparalytic poliomyelitis is 3 to 6 days. For the onset of paralysis in paralytic poliomyelitis, the incubation period is usually 7 to 21 days.

LABORATORY DIAGNOSIS

Diagnosis of polio is made by PCR (polymerase chain reaction) and isolation of the virus on cell culture lines. Two stool specimens and two throat swab specimens at least 24 hours apart, ideally within 14 days of symptom onset, should be collected.

Isolation of the virus: Currently human cell culture (e.g., human amnion cell line and human embryo cell line) are used for poliovirus cell culture inoculation (in place of monkey kidney cell cultures). Viral growth is detected by its **cytopathic effects** within 7 days of inoculation.

TREATMENT

No cure for polio exists. Physical therapy and portable ventilators are used as supporting treatments.

POLIO VACCINE

Polio is prevented by polio vaccines that provide protection to a child for life by stimulating the immune system by vaccination. Two types of vaccines are used:

1. **Inactivated polio vaccine (IPV):** The first polio vaccine, known as the **inactivated polio vaccine** because it consists of inactivated (killed) strains of all three virus types. **Jonas Edward Salk,** an American physician, in 1952 developed this vaccine, hence, it is named the **Salk vaccine**. It is given by intramuscular injection in the leg or arm, depending upon the patient's age. It is the only vaccine that has been given in the United States since 2000.
2. **Oral polio vaccine (OPV):** It consists of live attenuated (weakened) poliovirus strains and is given orally. It was developed in 1957 by **Albert Bruce Sabin**, an American physician and microbiologist, hence named **Sabin vaccine**. OPV came into commercial use in 1961 and became the vaccine of choice for most national immunization programmes globally.

Three types of OPV exist:

- Monovalent OPV 1 (m OPV 1) — for serotype PV 1
- Bivalent OPV (b OPV) — for serotypes PV 1 and PV 2
- Trivalent OPV (t OPV) — for all three types

The inactivated polio vaccines are very safe, however, OPV are more effective. OPV mimics an actual infection and induces excellent and probably life-long immunity by producing antibodies in the blood (humoral or serum immunity) to all three types of poliovirus and the mucosal immune response at the site of infection. **OPV is the vaccine of choice for poliomyelitis eradication programmes globally.**

Children are given four doses of polio vaccine: at ages 2 months, 4 months, 6 – 18 months, with a booster dose between 4 and 6 years.

KEY POINTS

- **Poliomyelitis** (or **polio**) caused by a poliovirus is a paralytic diease of children revealed by muscle weakness and inability to move.
- **Poliovirus** the causative agent of polio an *Enterovirus* is the smallest known animal virus having a single-stranded RNA genome with protein capsid.
- Of the three poliovirus subtypes (PV-1, PV-2 and PV-3), human poliovirus 1 (PV-1) is the most common and causes of epidemic.
- Polio is transmitted via the fecal-oral-route, infecting human through fecal contaminted water.
- Laboratory diagnosis of poliovirus is made by the cytopathic effect on human cell culture lines, PCR and the clinical symptoms.

- Globally, OPV is the vaccine of choice for polio eradication programme which is given to children in 4 doses at 2nd, 4th and 6 – 8 months of age and a booster dose between 4 and 6 years.
- Since 2014, India is a polio-free country.

IMPORTANT QUESTIONS

1. Write short notes on:
   (a) Compare the salk and Sabin polio vaccines.
   (b) Polio.

MULTIPLE-CHOICE QUESTIONS

1. All are true for poliovirus EXCEPT:
   (a) An enterovirus
   (b) Single-stranded RNA genome
   (c) In is an enveloped virus
   (d) Sabin vaccine is used for prevention.
2. Which of the following serotypes is/are usually associated with endemic polio infection?
   (a) Poliovirus subtype - 1 (b) Poliovirus subtype - 2
   (c) Poliovirus subtype - 3 (d) All of the above.
3. All are true for salk vaccine EXCEPT:
   (a) Inactivated poliovirus vaccine
   (b) Oral polio vaccine
   (c) First poliovirus vaccine
   (d) Large scale use of SPV begin in 1954.
4. The main route of poliovirus transmission is:
   (a) Respiratory route (b) Sexual contact
   (c) Fecal-oral-route (d) None of the above.
5. All are true for oral polio vaccine EXCEPT:
   (a) Live attenuated vaccine
   (b) Discovered by Jones Salk
   (c) Come into commercial use in 1961
   (d) Used in most polio eradication programmes.
6. In which year India became polio free?
   (a) 1988 (b) 1995
   (c) 2014 (d) 2019.

ANSWERS TO MCQs

1. (c) 2. (b) 3. (b) 4. (c)
5. (b) 6. (c).

60

Rabies lyssavirus: A Bullet-Shaped RNA Virus

Rabies (Hydrophobia)

Rabies lyssavirus (syn. *Rabies virus*), the causative agent of **rabies** is an enveloped, bullet or rod-shaped, RNA virus, a member of the family *Rhabdoviridae*.

Worldwide, humans are infected with the rabies virus from the bite of an infected animal, especially dogs (hence a zoonotic disease). Nearly 60,000 people die annually in over 150 countries, India has the highest annual rate of deaths in Asia-20,000, the majority of victims are under 15.

In 1804 **George Gottfried Zinke** demonstrated that rabies was caused by germs via a rabid dog and 73 years later in 1881, **Louis Pasteur** established that the causative agent, rabies virus was present in the brain of infected animals. To save the humanity, he carried out work on the vaccine and in 1885 the first rabies vaccine was developed by **Louis Pasteur** and **Emile Roux**.

India is the hot bed of human rabies with over 36% (20,000 – 30,000) of the world's rabies death annually, over 97% due to dogs bite.

WORLD RABIES DAY

World Rabies Day is celebrated annually on 28th September to raise awareness about rabies prevention. 28th September is the anniversary of Louis Pasture's death who developed first rabies vaccine and laid the foundation of rabies prevention.

RABIES LYSSAVIRUS

Rabies lyssavirus (derived from Greek word *lyssa* for violent or furious), formerly called *Rabies virus,* is a species of the genus, *Lyssavirus*. The members are commonly called *rhabdo viruses* (from the Greek *rhabdo* meaning rod) based on the rod-shaped morphology.

STRUCTURE

Shape: The virion has a cylindrical **bullet-like** morphology (180 nm × 75 nm) with one end conical and other plane (or concave) (Fig. 60.1).

It has a lipoprotein envelope that contains glycosylated G-protein spikes embedded in lipid membrane derived from host cell. This envelope does not cover the planer end. Beneath the envelope lies membrane or matrix (M) protein.

Nucleocapsid tightly binds the RNA to form the **helical nucleocapsid** core that lies inside the M protein. The genome is single-stranded, negative sense RNA (12 kb) of 50 nucleotides followed by N, P, M, G and L genes. RNA is highly cased by the nucleoprotein (Fig. 60.1)

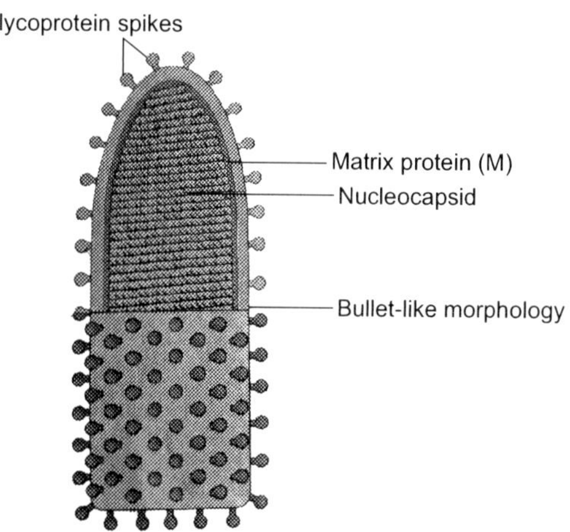

Fig. 60.1 The structure of the rabies virus with bullet-like characteristic shape.

ANTIGENIC PROPERTIES

There is a single sero type of rabies virus, but there are strain differences among viruses isolated from different species.

SUSCEPTIBILITY/RESISTANCE

- The virus survives at 4°C for weeks and at 70°C for years.
- Sensitive to ethanol, iodine preparations, NH_4^+ compounds, soaps, detergents and lipid solvents (acetone, ether, chloroform).
- It is inactivated by:
    - UV and sunlight
    - Heat at 60°C in 5 minutes, at 50°C in 60 minutes
    - Phenol, formalin and B propiolactone (BPL)
    - CO_2 (For storage in dry ice, it should be sealed in glass vials)

RABIES

Rabies is a zoonotic viral disease of the nervous system that often results in fatal encephalitis. The origin of the word rabies is either from the Sanskrit word *rabhas* (to do violence) or the Latin *rabidus* (mad) as observed in a virus infected dog (rabid dog).

In humans, the disease is called **hydrophobia** (Gr. *hundro* = water + *phobos* = fear, meaning a psychological fear of water) because the patient panics when presented with liquids to drink and cannot quench his thirst.

Rabies has been known since around 3000 B.C. from india. The first written record of rabies is in Mesopotamian Codex of Eshnunna (Circa 1930 BC). Rabies appears to have originated in the Old World, the first epizootic in the New World occurring in Boston in 1768.

PATHOGENESIS

Rabies is spread when an infected animal bites or scratches a human or other animal. Globally, humans usually are infected with the virus from the dog bites (over 99%). In India, dogs are responsible for 97% of human rabies followed by cats (2%), jackals, mangoose and others (1%).

The virus is often present in the salivary glands of rabid dog and is secreted in the saliva. Infection of human results from the bite that introduces the virus into a fresh wound (Fig. 60.2).

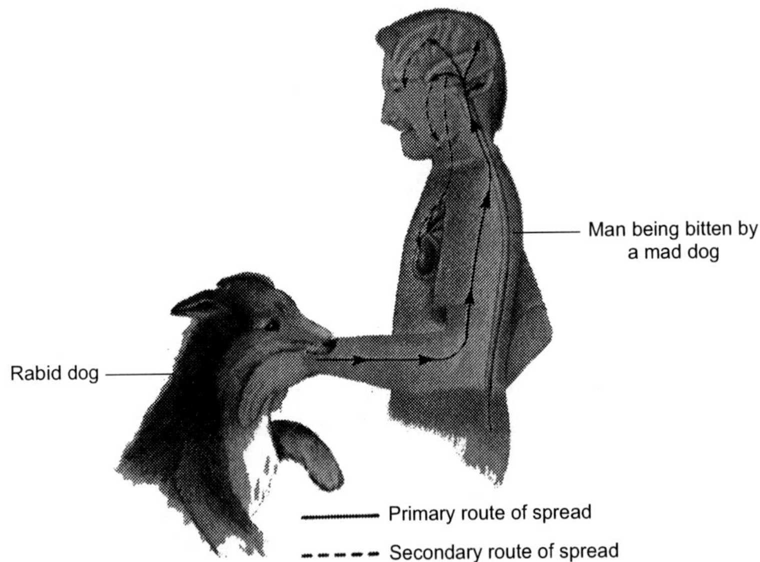

Fig. 60.2 A pathologic picture of rabies. After an initial bite by the rabid dog, the virus spreads to the nervous system of the host and multiplies. From there it moves to the salivary glands and other organs.

The virus usually propagates initially on the muscle cells where it replicates. As new progeny of virions produced. They enter peripheral nerve cells by way of acetylcholine receptors and make their way to central nervous system. The virus then replicates in motor neurons and eventually makes its way to the brain and causes fatal encephalitis. From the brain, it travels to the salivary glands and other organs of the victim.

CLINICAL MANIFESTATIONS AND SYMPTOMS IN HUMANS AND DOGS

The usual incubation period in humans is one to three months, however, it can be as short as 4 days or longer than 6 years depending upon the location of virus entry (i.e., animal bite site) and viral load. It is usually short in persons bitten on the face and head and longer in those bitten on the legs, and usually shorter in children.

There are four phases of the disease: a short predormal phase, an acute neurologic (or encephalic) phase, coma, and death.

Initial symptoms are fever with pain, an unusual or unexplained tingling, pricking and burning sensation **(para-aesthesia)** at the wound site. These are followed by: excess salivation, violet movements, uncontrolled excitment, fear of water **(hydrophobia)** and inability to move parts of body **(paralysis)**, mental confusion, loss of consciousness, delirium coma and finally death usually occurring within 2 and 10 days post first symptoms.

Two clinical forms of human rabies are:

- **Furious rabies:** It occurs in 80% of the patients. The infected individuals experience **hydrophobia** that is caused by the inability to swallow. Sometimes **aerophobia** (fear of droplets of fresh air) also occurs.
- **Paralytic rabies:** It occurs in 2% of the patients. Muscle weakness and paralysis occurs.

Clinical Forms of Rabies in Dogs

In dogs incubation period ranges from 2 to 4 months. The first phase called **prodromal** phase that lasts for 2-3 days. The dog undergoes a marked change in temperament:

- quite dogs become agitated, and
- active dogs become nervous or shy.

Following this, there are two recognized forms of the clinical disease:

- **Furious rabies:** The rabid dog becomes aggressive, highly excitable, displays evidence of a decreased appetite, eating and chewing stones, earth and rubbish (pica). Finally, paralysis and unable to eat and drink, and ultimately death in a violet seizure. Hydrophobia does not occur in dogs.

- **Dumb rabies:** It is more common in dogs. There is progressive paralysis involving the limbs, distortion of the face and a similar difficulty in swallowing. Finally, the dog becomes comatose and dies.

  There is no treatment for a dog with rabies.

LABORATORY DIAGNOSIS

Diagnosis of rabies in humans can be made by four methods: (i) rabies antigens; (ii) virus RNA; (iii) antibodies; and (iv) isolation of virus by inoculation. For post-mortem diagnosis, **DFA test is the gold-standard technique**.

- **Rabies antigens by direct fluorescent-antibody test (DFA or FAT)**

FAT is an accurate, sensitive and rapid test for rabies diagnosis. In FAT impression smears prepared from a composite sample of brain tissue are treated with antirabies serum or globulin labelled with fluorescein isothiocyanate (FITC). Specific aggregates of rabies virus antigen are detected by their fluorescence using a reflected light (incident light) fluorescence microscope.

A direct rapid immunohistochemical test (dRIT) Similar to FAT, it is used when flourescence microscope is not available. The principle of dRIT is similar to FAT except that the dRIT uses streptavidin-biotin peroxidase staining.

- **Detection of rabies virus replication by inoculation test**

Samples of brain tissue, saliva, CSF or urine are injected cerebrally into newborn mice (i.e., mouse inoculation) and examined at signs of illness and their brains are examined at 28 days after inoculation for **Negri bodies** or by immunofluorescence rabies antigen.

Isolation of virus on living substrates, i.e., cell culture is tried.

- **Detection of nucleic acid (RNA) of rabies virus**

Reverse transcriptase polymerase chain reaction (RTPCR) is used to amplify a certain fragment of viral RNA and is used as a confirmatroy test.

Recently, **real-time PCR** has been developed to increase sensitivity and to obtain results even faster.

- **Serological Tests**

ELISA—a rapid serological test that detects antibodies that can specifically bind to rabies virus antigens (viral glycoprotein and mucleoprotein) in serum and CSF.

ANIMAL RABIES

Diagnosis of animal rabies can be made by histopathogical examination of brain by the presence of **Negri bodies** (named after **Adelehi Negri**): cellular inclusions (2 – 10 µm) found in the cytoplasm of nerve cells, especially in the pyramidal cells of Ammon's horn of the hippocampus, that consist of ribonuclear proteins produced by the rabies virus.

TREATMENT

Rabies is fatal if left untreated, hence all cases of suspected exposure should be treated immediately to prevent the onset of clinical symtoms and death.

Treatment for people bitten by animals with rabies requires postexposure prophylaxis (PEP) that consists of wound treatment, passive immunization with rabies immune globulin and active immunization with series of antirabies vaccines. Rabies is one of the few infectious diseases for which a combination of passive and active post-exposure immunization is used.

- **Wound treatment:** Local treatment of the wound includes thorough washing of bites (wounds for 15 minutes with soaping water for 15 minutes followed by application of an antiseptic (e.g., alcohol or peroxide or poidine iodine) of the bitten person.
- **Passive immunization:** This is done by injecting a fast-acting dose of human rabies immune globulin(HRIG) close to the wound, to prevent the virus from infecting the individual.
- **Active immunization:** This includes a full course of vaccination with **human diploid cell vaccine (HDCV)** in a series of four injections at intervals during a 14-day period. In addition to HDCV, two other cell culture vaccines, purified chick embryo cell (PCEV) and purified vero cell rabies vaccine (PVRC), are equally safe and effective.

Rabies was initially treated with vaccines developed in 1885 by **Louis Pasteur** and **Emile Roux** (the Pasteur treatment) in which virus was attenuated (weakened) by drying for 5 – 10 days in the dissected spinal cords of rabies infected rabbits.

Do not consume alcohol while on medication.

Pre-exposure treatment of rabies consists of vaccination with three doses of HDCV to protect against possible exposure to rabies especially for high-risk individuals (e.g., veterinarians, animal control professionals and laboratory workers).

CONTROL

The risk of contracting rabies can be reduced by

- Vaccinating dogs, cats and ferrets against rabies
- Keeping pets under supervision to monitor their activities
- Not handling wild animals or strays.

KEY POINTS

- The *rabies virus* (syn *Rabies lyssavirus*), is a **rhabdovirus** that is bullet-shaped, enveloped, RNA virus.
- **Rabies** (also called **hydrophobia**), a viral disease of nervous system, is a 100% fatal infection, transmitted through the saliva of an infected animal, mainly dogs.
- DFA tests that detect rabies antigen is the gold standard technique for rabies diagnosis.
- Post-exposure treatment of rabies is done by cleaning of wound, passive immunization with human rabies immune globulin simultaneously with human diploid cell vaccine or chick-embryo grown vaccines.
- **World rabies** day is celebrated every year on 28th September to raise awareness about rabies' prevention.

IMPORTANT QUESTIONS

1. Write short notes on:
   (a) Rabies virus.
   (b) Post-exposure treatment for rabies.
   (c) Clinical forms of rabies and pathology of rabies infection.

MULTIPLE-CHOICE QUESTIONS

1. All are true for rabies virus EXCEPT:
   (a) RNA virus (b) Bullet-shaped to cylindrical
   (c) Non-enveloped (d) Rhabdovirus.
2. Rabies is spread by
   (a) Blood (b) Saliva
   (c) Tears (d) All of these.

3. What should you do if you are bitten by a dog?
   (a) Put a bandage on the bite and wait to see if you start to feel bad
   (b) Take your temperature every hour
   (c) Wash out the bite really well and go to the doctor
   (d) All of these.

4. What causes rabies?
   (a) A bacterium (b) A worm
   (c) A virus (d) A dog.

5. If someone is bitten by an animal with rabies, how long before rabies develops?
   (a) One to two days
   (b) Two to three weeks
   (c) One to three months
   (d) One to two years.

6. For which disease are active and passive immunization given simultaneously?
   (a) Measles (b) Yellow fever
   (c) Rabies (d) Influenza.

ANSWERS TO MCQs

1. (c)	2. (b)	3. (c)	4. (c)
5. (c)	6. (c).		

61

Coronaviruses: Corona (Crown)-Shaped RNA Viruses

Severe respiratory tract infections: COVID-19; SARS; MERS

Coronaviruses are solar corona or crown-shaped, spherical, enveloped RNA viruses, belonging to the family *Coronoviridae*. These viruses have club-like spiky projections on their surface that look like crowns (Fig. 61.1).

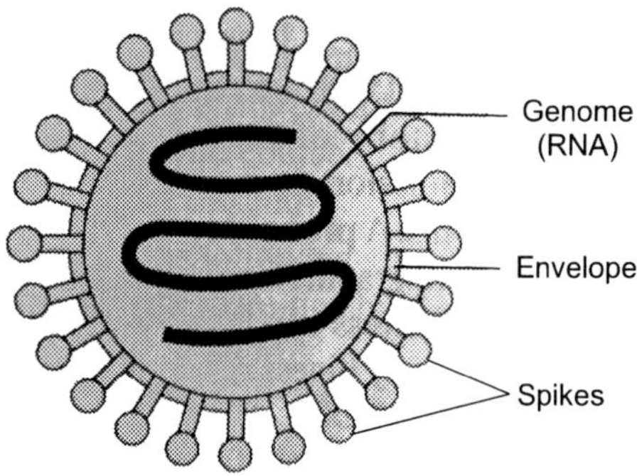

Fig. 61.1 Structure of a *Coronavirus.*

Corona means crown in Latin—and that's how they got their name (Fig. 61.1). The term was coined by **June Almeida** and **David Tyrrell** in 1960 who first observed and studied human coronaviruses. Coronaviruses were first observed causing respiratory infection in chickens in North Dakota by **Arthrur Schalk** and **M.C. Hawn** in 1931. First human coronavirus was isolated in 1960 from a boy by **E.C. Kendall**, **Malcon Byone** and **David Terrell** who were working at the Common Cold Unit of the British Medical Research Council.

Coronaviruses cause diseases in mammals and birds. These viruses in humans cause mild to lethal respiratory tract infections of epithelial cells by inhalation of droplets or aerosols.

Seven different kinds/species of coronavirus can infect humans. Four of these are common causing mild symptoms especially in the temperate climates, most people will experience at least one of them during their life.

The three coronaviruses responsible for causing severe respiratory syndromes are:

- SARS (2002 – 2004) → SARS-CoV-1
- MERS (2012, 2015, 2018) → MERS-CoV
- COVID-19 (2019) → SARS-CoV-2

The coronaviruses are divided into four subtypes/genera. *Alpha* and *Beta* (infect animals) and *Gamma* and *Delta* coronavirus (primarily infect birds).

STRUCTURE OF A CORONAVIRUS

Coronaviruses (Caps) are enveloped spherical (125 nm diameter) and pleomorphic with characteristics 20 nm long bulbous surface projections, the **spikes** which look-like **solar corona** from which their name derives. The viral envelope consists of a lipid bilayer in which the membrane, envelope and spike structural proteins are anchored (Fig. 61.1).

Their genome is composed of single-stranded (positive-sense) RNA. Coronaviruses possess the largest genome (26.4-31.7 kb) among all known RNA viruses; with G + C contents varying from 32% to 43%.

The lipid bilayer envelope, membrane proteins and nucleocapsid protect the virus when it is outside the host cell.

SEVERE ACUTE RESPIRATORY SYNDROME (SARS)

Severe acute respiratory syndrome or **SARS** caused by a coronavirus (SARS-CoV now called SARS-CoV-1), was a contagious and potentially fatal respiratory illness. An outbreak of SARS occurred between 2002 and 2003, but the disease is not occurring at present, although it could reappear one day.

SARS was a zoonotic viral disease that has been traced through the intermediatory of Asian palm civets to cave-dwelling horse shoe bats by Chinese scientists in late 2017. It first appeared in China (Guandong provice) in November 2002 and by February 2003 it had spread to Hong Kong and subsequently to 24 other countries of the region resulting in 774 deaths of the 8098 cases worldwide from 2002 to 2003 before health authorities managed to contain it. No known transmission of SARS has occurred since 2004 globally.

THE VIRUS

SARS was caused by a coronavirus that was identified in Feb. 2003 and named **severe acute respiratory syndrome coronavirus (SARS-CoV or SARS-CoV-1)**, related to the virus that has caused COVID-19 infection. It is an enveloped, positive-sense, single-strained RNA virus which infects the epithelial cells within the lungs. It infects humans, bats and palm civets.

This virus can survive after drying on plastic surfaces for up to 48 hours. It can survive in urine for up to 24 hours and in feces for 2 days.

TRANSMISSION

The primary route of transmission is contact of the mucous membranes with respiratory droplets or fomites. It spreads most often by close person-to-person contact involving exposure to infectious droplets and possibly by touching contaminated surfaces, kissing, and skin-to-skin contact (handshakes or hugs).

The incubation period is usually 2 to 7 days but may extend up to 10 days.

A fever of more than 100.4 °F (38.0°C) with lower respiratory tract illness such as dry cough, shortness of breath and hypoxia and difficulty in breathing are the initial symptoms.

LABORATORY DIAGNOSIS

Specimens used include: Blood, stool, nasal secretions, and throat swab.

- Detection of virus by RT-PCR
- Antibody detect tests by ELISA and immunofluoresence assay (IFA)
- Virus culture on vero cell lines.

TREATMENT

Treatment of SARS is supportive with antipyretics, supplemental oxygen and mechanical ventilation. Ribavirin, an antiviral drug, has been used. Use of corticosteroids is recommended.

PREVENTION

There is no vaccine for SARS. Clinical isolation and quarantine are the most effective means to prevent the spread. Hand hygiene and isolating oneself are the other means.

MIDDLE EAST RESPIRATORY SYNDROME (MERS)

Middle east respiratory syndrome (MERS), also known as **camel flu**, is a severe lung infection caused by the **MERS-coronavirus (MERS-CoV)**, posing a global threat to human health. MERS, characterized by severe acute respiratory illness, including fever, cough, and shortness of breath, was first reported in Saudi Arabia in September 2012 and has since spread to 27 countries (by January 2020). Globally, WHO has confirmed 2519 cases of MERS and 866 deaths. Larger outbreaks have occurred in South Korea in 2015 and in Saudi Arabia in 2018.

MERS-CoV

MERS-CoV, believed to be originated from bats, humans are typically infected from dromedary camels, either during direct contact or indirectly (hence also called camel flu). The virus does not seem to pass easily from person-to-person unless there is close contact, as in a healthcare setting.

MERS-CoV with a single-stranded RNA, belongs to the genus *Betacoronavirus* which is distinct from SARS-CoV and the common cold coronavirus. The virus grows readily on vero cells and LLC-MK2 cells.

SYMPTOMS

The symptoms usually appear 5 to 6 days after exposure to the virus, but they may take 2 to 14 days to arise. MERS can range from asymptomatic disease to severe pneumonia leading to acute respiratory distress syndrome (ARDS). Fever, cough, expectoration and shortness of breath are the major symptoms.

DIAGNOSIS

Polymerase chain reaction tests (rRT-PCR) can be used in a confirmatory test for the presence of the virus.

TREATMENT

Treatment includes rest, fluids, pain relievers and oxygen therapy in severe cases.

PREVENTION

There is currently no vaccine to protect against MERS. Virus transmission can be by frequently washing the hands with soap and water for 20 seconds; washing fruit and vegetables thoroughly; wearing a medical mask and avoiding/minimizing close contact with an infected person.

COVID-19 PANDEMIC

The **COVID-19 (Coronavirus disease 2019)** is a highly contagious respiratory illness caused by a **novel coronavirus 2019** (n **CoV**), named as **severe acute respiratory syndrome coronavirus** 2 **(SARS-CoV-2).** The disease got the name COVID-19 from the coronavirus disease that appeared in 2019. COVID-19 is several times deadlier than previously pandemic viruses, such as H1N1. As it is a disease caused by a new virus, no body has prior immunity, which means the entire human population is potentially susceptible to SARS-CoV-2 infection.

The first confirmed case of this disease was traced back to 17 November 2019 in **Hubei**. COVID-19 outbreak was first identified in **Wuhan** (Hubei, China) on December 31, 2019. Initially, superspreading events, a cruise ship in Japan, mass gathering of a religious group in South Korea, Skiing resorts in Italy and Austria, and a popular pilgrimage city (Iran) contributed to its rapid dissemination globally. Since then the rate of global spread has accelerated and a widespread epidemic has occurred in numerous countries. The WHO declared COVID-19 outbreak a **Public Health Emergency of International Concern** on 30 January 2020 and a **pandemic** on March 11, 2020. In spite of imposing lockdowns around the world to **"flatten the curve"** of the COVID-19 infection, globally, these have been 2,29,37,963 confirmed cases of COVID-19 including 47,05,111 deaths, reported to WHO by 22 September 2021 (between, December 2019 and 22 September 2021).

The highest total cases have been recorded in the US (42,034,347) followed by India (33,531,498) Brazil (21,247,667) UK (7,496,547), Russia (7,333,557), Turkey (6,904,285) and France (6,753,865).

SOCIAL AND ECONOMIC IMPACT

COVID-19 pandemic has caused global social and economic disruption including the largest global recession. It has caused a great academic loss and depression among the student community due to closing of schools, colleges and universities in 172 countries either on a nationwide or local basis, affecting 98.5% of the world's student population. It has also caused a global famine affecting 265 million people. According to IMF the global economy is expected to shrink by over 3% in 2020. The pandemic has also led to the postponement and even cancellation of sporting, religious, and political activities.

Due to movement restriction and a significant slow down of social and economic activities, air quality has improved due to decreased emissions of pollutants and greenhouse gases, and improving the quality of water due to decreased soil pollution around the world.

However, the increased use of PPE (e.g., face mask hand glores, etc.), their haphazarad disposal, and generation of a large amount of hospital waste has negative impacts on the environment.

THE VIRUS

Severe acute respiratory syndrome coronavirus 2 (SARS-CoV-2) is a novel virus, a species of the genus *Betacoronavirus*, first isolated from three people with pneumonia connected to the cluster of acute respiratory illness cases in Wuhan, was named by the ICTV on 11 February 2020, because it is genetically closely related to SARS-CoV responsible for the SARS outbreak of 2003, and is thought to have a zoonotic origin (bats). All features of this virus occur in related coronaviruses in nature.

It is a round or elliptic, single-stranded RNA enveloped virus having mushroom-shaped proteins called spikes protruding from the surface give a virion, a crown-like appearance (Fig. 61.2).

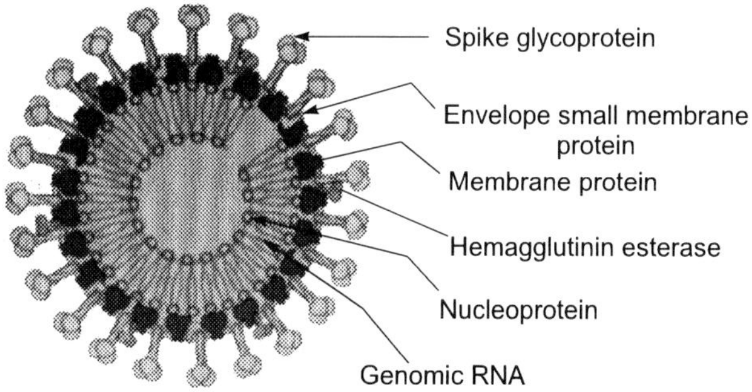

Fig. 61.2 Schematic representation of SARS-CoV-2, the causative agent of COVID-19 (Source. Mousavizadeh L., and S. Ghasemi. J.M.I.I. 2020. 03. 022).

SENSITIVITY TO PHYSICAL AND CHEMICAL AGENTS

Like other CoVs, COVID-19 virus is sensitive to ultraviolet rays and heat, however, it resists cold even below 0°C. It can effectively be inactivated by lipid solvents including ether (75%), ethanol, chlorine-containing disinfectant, peroxyacetic acid and chloroform except for chlorhexidine.

TRANSMISSION

COVID-19 spreads primarily from person-to-person when people are in close contact with one another (within about 6 ft) through small respiratory droplets produced by an infected person (symptomatic or not) during coughing, sneezing, talking, singing, or laughing. The droplets usually fall to the ground or onto surfaces rather than travelling through air and long distances. Transmission may also occur through smaller droplets that are suspended in the air for longer period of time. Less commonly, people may become infected by touching a contaminated surface and then contacting their faces. People are most infectious when they show symptoms (even mild), and remain infectious 7 to 12 days in moderate cases and for two weeks in severe cases. Sputum and saliva carry large amounts of virus.

Contaminated droplets that fall to floors or surfaces can, though less commonly, remain infectious for different durations on different surfaces: up to 4 hours on copper, 24 hours on cardboard. 72 hours on plastic (polyproplene) and stainless steel.

Airborne spread may also occur as the virus can survive in aerosol up to 3 hours. Aerosol transmission also occurs in health facilities and inadequately ventilator indoor locations where infected patients spend long periods of time (such as restaurants and night clubs).

SYMPTOMS

The typical incubation period for COVID-19 is 5 days, but it can range from 2 to 14 days. Common symptoms include fever, cough with sputums, loss of appetite, fatigue, shortness of breath, and loss of smell and taste; sometimes no symptoms at all (i.e., asymptomatic). Mostly the symptoms are mild, some progress to **acute respiratory distress syndrome (ARDS)** possibly precipitated by cytokine release syndrome, septic shock, multiorgan failure, and blood clots, resulting in death.

Less common symtpoms include, sneezing, runny nose, sore throat and skin lesions.

DIAGNOSIS

Diagnosis is made by:

- **COVID-19 antigen test:** This is a rapid test that provides result within 15 minutes. In most cases, the test sample is taken and analyzed at the same location (this is called point-of-care testing). Kits are available for at home COVID-19 antigen testing. This test is performed on a sample that is taken by swabbing into the nose. It is obtained by inserting a cotton-tipped swab into the nostrils on gently rotating the swab and immediately analyzed to detect viral antigens (positive or negative to SARS-CoV-2).

- **Molecular or PCR testing:** Real-time reverse transcription polymerase chain reaction (rRT-PCR) from a nasopharyngeal swab, a positive nucleic acid amplification test (NAAT) is used to confirm the diagnosis of COVID-19 (SARS-CoV-2).
- **Chest CT Imaging** with severe symptoms is used as a clinical diagnosis.

TREATMENT

Management involves: isolation, supportive care at relieving symptoms and may include a pain reliever (ibuprofen or acetaminophen), cough syrup, rest and fluid intake. **Remdesivir**, an intravenously administared antiviral drug, and **dexmethasone**, a steroid; and **blood thinners** are all proving beneficial; each under specific circumstance and for critically sick patients who require supplementary oxygen or mechanical ventilation.

VACCINES FOR COVID-19

Globally, a number of vaccines are available for preventing COVID-19. Commonly used are Pfizer-Biontech (mRNA Vaccine), Moderna (mRNA vaccine), Johnsons Johnson (Virus vector vaccine), Oxford-Astrazeneca (carrier vaccine), Novavox (protein adjuvant vaccine), Covishield (recombinant vaccine) and Covaxin (inactivated vaccine). Over 83 crore Indians had been vaccinated by 23 September 2021 by the two indigenously produced vaccines (Covishield and Covaxin). More than 4.52 billion people worldwide have received a dose of a COVID-19 vaccine, equal to 58.9% of the world population (as of December 26, 2021).

PREVENTION

Preventive measures include:

- Staying at home.
- Wearing a face mask or cloth face covering in public.
- Avoiding close contact by keeping a distance from others at least 6 ft.

- Avoiding crowded places.
- Washing hands with soap and water for at least 20 seconds.
- Use of hand sanitiser with at least 60% alcohol.
- Follow quarantine (i.e., isolation of the patients) rule for the patients.
- Avoiding touching the eyes, nose or mouth with unwashed hands.
- Practising good respiratory hygiene.
- Sanitizing the frequently touched surfaces.

KEY POINTS

- **Coronaviruses** are solar-corona or crown-like RNA viruses that cause fatal respiratory tract infections in humans.
- The name **coronavirus** is derived from crown (solar corona) appearance of the virus.
- **Human coronaviruses** infect the respiratory tract by inhalation of droplets or aerosols generated by cough and sneezes of infected individuals.
- SARS outbreak (2002-2003) caused by SARS-CoV-1 is no longer in existence since 2004.
- **Middle east respiratory syndrome (MERS)** was caused by the coronavirus: **MERS-CoV** that was transmitted to humans from camels.
- **COVID-19** (novel coronavirus disease 2019) is a highly contagious human disease that spreads through close contact with an infected person through droplets (sneezing, coughing, talking, laughing) and constant touching of face, eyes or mouth in public place.
- Physical distancing of 6 ft (2 metres) is the best method to prevent COVID-19.
- More than 4.52 billion people worldwide have received a dose of a COVID-19 vaccine, equal to 58.9% of the world population.

IMPORTANT QUESTIONS

1. Write notes on:
   (a) What are coronaviruses? Name three major respiratory coronaviruses infections of humans?
   (b) COVID-19 pandemic.
   (c) Epidemiological, social and economic impact of COVID-19.
   (d) Prevention of COVID-19.

MULTIPLE-CHOICE QUESTIONS

1. All are true for coronaviruses EXCEPT:
   (a) Club-shaped spikes
   (b) Positive-stranded RNA
   (c) Cause respiratory infections
   (d) Non-enveloped (naked).

2. Which of the following coronavirus disease had its origin from bats (*chamgadar*)?
   (a) COVID-19 (b) MERS
   (c) SARS (d) None of the above.

3. SARS virus is spread by
   (a) Close contact with camels
   (b) Respiratory route
   (c) Mosquito bite
   (d) Bats.

4. The genome of coronaviruses is made up of:
   (a) Positive-sense single-stranded RNA
   (b) Negative-sense single-stranded RNA
   (c) Double-stranded DNA
   (d) Single-stranded DNA.

5. Which of the following virus/viruses has/have club-shaped peplomers (spikes) and infect/s the respiratory tract?
   (a) SARS-CoV-1 (b) MERS-CoV
   (c) SARS-CoV-2 (d) All of the above.

6. What is COVID-19?
   (a) Name of the virus
   (b) Name of the disease
   (c) Name of a drug
   (d) All of the above.

7. In which country was COVID-19 first reported?
   (a) Italy (b) America
   (c) China (d) Iran.

8. Which virus causes COVID-19 disease?
   (a) SARS-CoV-1
   (b) MERS-CoV
   (c) SARS-CoV-2
   (d) NIPAH.

9. What are the most common symptoms of COVID-19?
(a) Dry cough
(b) Fever
(c) Tiredness
(d) All of the above.

10. When was the COVID-19 declared pandemic by WHO?
(a) December 31, 2019
(b) January 30, 2020
(c) March 11, 2020
(d) None of the above.

11. Is there a vaccine, drug or treatment for COVID-19?
(a) Yes (b) No

12. Which of the following disease is no longer in circulation now?
(a) MERS (b) SARS
(c) COVID-19 (d) None of these.

13. Which of the following is an indigenously produced COVID-19 vaccine?
(a) Covaxin (b) Pfizer-BioNTech vaccine
(c) Moderna vaccine (d) Novavax.

ANSWERS TO MCQs

1. (d)	2. (a)	3. (b)	4. (a)
5. (d)	6. (b)	7. (c)	8. (c)
9. (d)	10. (c)	11. (b)	12. (b)
13. (a).			

62

Arbo and other RNA Viruses of Medical Importance

Chikungunya; Yellow fever; West nile fever; Dengue; Kyasanur forest disease. HFRS; Lassa fever; Mumps; Measles; Rubella; Marburg hemorrhagic fever; Ebola; Rotavirus severe diarrhoea.

An **RNA virus** (also called **a ribovirus**) is a virus in which the genetic material is RNA (ribonucleic acid). This RNA is usually single-stranded (ssRNA) but one group (e.g., Reoviruses, Rotavirus) has double stranded (dsRNA), and may be enveloped or not (i.e., naked). **Ribovirus** (*ribo + virus*) – an RNA virus other than a retrovirus, is the another term used for RNA virus. Notable human diseases caused by RNA viruses are COVID-19, AIDS, common cold, influenza, SARS, hepatitis, CNE, polio, rabies, mumps, measles, Ebola and West fever.

ARBOVIRUSES AND VECTOR-BORNE DISEASES

Arboviruses (From *ar* for athropod + *bo* for borne, carried by + virus, i.e., arthropod-borne virus) are the RNA viruses that are transmitted to humans by blood-sucking arthropod vectors. (e.g. mosquitoes and ticks). *Alphavirus, Flavivirus* and *Hantavirus* are the common examples of arboviruses. The most common clinical features of infection are fever, headache, or malaize, but encephalitis and viral hemorrhagic fever may also occur. Notable examples of these viruses and the diseases caused by each are as follows:

Disease	Vector
• Chikungunya virus (CHIKV)	– *Aedes aegypti* (Mosquito)
• Yellow fever virus	– *Aedes aegypti* (Mosquito)
• Japanese ancphalitis virus	– *Culex* (Mosquito)
• Dengue virus	– *Aedes aegypti* (Mosquito)
• West Nile virus (WE virus)	– *Culex* (Mosquito)
• Kyasanur forest disease virus	– *Haemphysatis spingera* (Tick)

Hantavirus (orottho hantavirus): Enveloped, single-stranded RNA rodent-borne viruses are categorized into two types:

- New World Hantavirdae (under Buntaviruses): Antaviruses- in Nombre orthohantavirus
- Old World hantaviruses- Hantaan.

CHIKUNGUNYA (CHIKF) AND CHIKUNGUNYA VIRUS

The term "**chikungunya**" often refers to both the virus Chikungunya virus (CHIKV) and the illness of fever - CHIKF caused by this virus. It is derived from the African dialect Swahili or Makonde and translates as that "which bends up" due to the "stooped-over posture" exhibited by the patients due to severe pain.

Chikungunya virus (CHIKV), mosquito-transmitted *Alphavirus*, was first isolated from human patients and *Aedes aegypti* mosquitoes from Tanzania (Africa) in 1955. Currently, CHIKF is found worldwide, particularly in Asia and Africa. Outbreaks have been reproted in Europe and the Americas since 2000s. More than one million cases have been reported globally in 2014. Death rate is very-low, around 1 in 1000. The **symptoms** include a sudden high fever and severe, crippling joint pains—especially in the fingers and ankels—that can persist for weeks, months or years. There is often a rash and massive blisters. Symptoms typically occur 2 to 12 days (most often a week) after exposure to the virus.

DIAGNOSIS

Laboratory criteria include:

- A decreased lympocyte count.
- Virus isolation from whole blood on specific cell lines.
- Identification of the virus by RT-PCR from blood.
- Serological analysis: ELISA assay for specific IgM levels in the blood serum.

PREVENTION

The best preventive measure is overall mosquito control and avoidance of mosquito (*Aedes*) bites, especially during the daytime.

TREATMENT

Treatment is aimed at relieving pain, joint iswelling and fever by non-steroidal anti-inflammatory drugs such as naproxen, paracetamol and fluids (Aspirin and corticosteroids are not to be used due to increased rick of bleeding).

YELLOW FEVER VIRUS

Yellow fever (also called yellow jack, yellow plaque, bronze john) is a serious, potentially deadly hemorrhagic fever caused by **yellow fever virus**—an arbovirus of the *Flavivirus* genus (family *Flaviviridae*).

The virus is injected into the skin by a mosquito, *Aedes aegypti* and symptoms occur 3 to 6 days post-exposure.

Symptoms include fever, chills, headache, nausea, rashes, bleeding and jaundice, a yellowing of skin that gave the disease its name. This colouration indicates liver damage which results in bile pigments deposited in the skin and mucous membranes. The morality rate for yellow fever is high, about 20%.

Since the 17th century several major outbreaks of yellow fever have occurred in the Americas, Africa and Europe. In 2013, 1,27,000 severe infections and 45,000 deaths occurred due to this disease. Interestingly, in 1927, in the human's history, yellow fever virus became the first human virus to be isolated.

DIAGNOSIS

Diagnosed by the isolation of the virus and its growth in cell culture using blood plasma, identification by RT-PCR and serologically by IgM-ELISA and a fourfold increase in IgG.

TREATMENT

Rehydration and pain relief with paracetamol is the only treatment. Hospitalization is advisable and intensive care may be necessary because of rapid deterioration in some cases.

PREVENTION

Yellow fever vaccine – an attenuated live viral strain – 17D, developed in 1937 by **Max Theiler** is available. As per WHO, a single dose of vaccine confers life long immunity, to be administered between 9th and 12 months after birth, for people living in affected areas. Mosquito control and avoidance of mosquito bites is the best preventive measure.

WEST NILE FEVER AND THE VIRUS

West Nile Virus (WNV), the causative agent of a fatal neurological disease in humans, is a culex mosquito transmitted *Flavivirus* that causes **West Nile fever**. This virus was first isolated in the West Nile district of Uganda in 1937 and since then it has been reported in Europe, Africa, Australia, North America and Asia (including India).

Symptoms include fever, headache, vomiting, skin rash and swollen lymph glands. In a few patients (< 1%) encephalitis or meningitis occurs, with associated neck stiffness, confusion or seizures, resulting in 10% of the patients.

In 2012, United States experienced one of its worst epidemics in which 286 people died, Texas State being hard hit it by this virus.

WNV is usually spread by *Culex* mosquitoes that become infected when they feed on infected birds, which often carry the disease. Onset of the disease occurs 2 to 14 days after exposure. The disease does not spread directly between people.

Diagnosis of WNV infection includes:

- Lymphocytic pleocytosis, elevated protein level, reference glucose and lactic acid levels, and no erythrocytes.
- Serology: Detection of virus specific IgM and neutralizing antibodies.
- Viral RNA in serum or CSF by PCR.
- Elevated level of white blood cells in CFS.

TREATMENT

Disease is self-limiting and treatment is symptomatic. In severe cases, hospitalization with supportive treatment (intravenous fluids, pain injection and nursing care) is advised. Preventing measures require control of mosquitoes.

JAPANESE ENCEPHALITIS AND THE VIRUS

Japanese encephalitis (JE) is an infection of the brain caused by *Culex* mosquito-borne, *Japanese encephalitis virus (JEV)*, a *Flavivirus.*

The disease was first described in Japan in 1871, hence named JE. JE occurs in Southeast Asia and the Western Pecific, and is a major health problem in India. It causes annually 17,000 deaths of the over 68,000 symptomatic cases recorded, especially during the outbreaks.

JE is characterized by the inflammation of the brain with headache, high fever (38 – 41°C = 100.4 – 105.6 °F), vomiting, confusion and seizures. The symptoms usually appear 5 to 15 days after infection (incubation period). Mental retardation usually occurs in half of the survivors.

DIAGNOSIS

It is based on blood and cereborospinal fluid testing by commercially available kits that detect JE virus-specific IgM antibodies. Viral antigen can be detected in tissues by indirect antibody staining. Virus culturing and PCR are used in fatal cases for confirmatory tests.

TREATMENT

It is supportive with assistance given for feeding, breathing and seizure control as per need.

PREVENTION

It consists of avoiding mosquito bites.

Immunization by JE vaccines: JE vaccines first became available in the 1930s (e.g., JE-VAX-inactivated mouse-brain derived vaccine). Currently three vaccines licensed for use around the world are:

1. **Live-attenuated SA 14-14-2** (introduced in China in 1988).
2. **IC51-Inactivated, vero-cell derived based** on **SA 14-14-2** (marketed as **JESPECT** in Australia and New Zealand and **IXIARO** in the USA, Australia and Europe in 2009) and in 2012 in India.
3. **ChimeriVax-JE** (Marketed IMOJEV)- Live attenuated yellow-fever—Japanese encephalitis chimeric vaccine (Licensed for use in Australia (in August 2010) and Thailand (in December 2012).

Current status: As of 2015, 15 different vaccines (based on recombinant DNA techniques, weakened virus and inactivated virus) are available.

DENGUE AND THE DENGUE VIRUS

Dengue, also known as **dengue fever** and **breakbone fever**, an *Aedes aegypti* mosquito-borne tropical disease, is caused by the ***dengue virus* (DENV)**, a member of the genus *Flavivirus* (Arbovirus). There are four DENV serotypes (DENV-1, DENV-2, DENV-3 and DENV-4) that cause dengue. The term **dengue** is derived from the African Swahili phrase "**ka-dinga pepo**" meaning "scram-like seizure" caused by an evil spirit.

Outbreak of dengue is known since 1779 while its viral cause and spread were understood by the early 20th century. The global incidence of dengue has grown dramatically in recent decades. Current estimates are that as many as 390 million infections occur each year, including the 40,000 annual deaths.

The characteristic symptoms of dengue are sudden onset of high fever (40°C/104°F), headache (typically located behind the eyes), a characteristic skin rash (described as islands of white in a sea of red) and severe muscle and joint pain. The disease was named **breakbone** (break + bone) by **Benjamin Rush** in 1789 because it makes the bones ache as if breaking at the joints. The incubation period ranges from 5 to 14 days (but most often it is 4 to 7 days).

In a few patients, the disease develops into **severe dengue**, also known as **dengue hemorrhagic fever (DHF)**, resulting in bleeding, low level of blood platelets and blood plasma leakage, or into **dengue shock syndrome**, where dangerously low blood pressure occurs, resulting in death in a few hours; the leading cause of death among Southeast Asian children.

DIAGNOSIS

Isolation of virus from blood by cell cultures, nucleic acid detection by RT-PCR, viral antigen detection or virus-specific antibodies-IgG or IgM by ELISA, the presence of IgM anti-dengue antibody is indicative of recent virus infection.

Low white blood count and positive tourniquet test that is performed by inflating a blood pressure cuff on the upper arm to midway between diastolic and systolic blood pressure for 5 minutes. More than 20 petechiae/in^2 on the skin area that was under pressure is a positive test for dengue.

TREATMENT

Administration of fluids and pain killers such as acetaminophen or paracetamol is used to treat dengue patients. Severe dengue cases require hospital care.

PREVENTION

Mosquito-control and prevention of mosquito bites is the best strategy.

Vaccine: Currently, a vaccine for dengue is available. Therefore those individuals who have been previously infected or, in populations with a high rate of prior infection by age nine (WHO 2018).

Dengvaxia (CYD-TDV)- It is a live attenuated dengue vaccine developed by Sanoti Pasteur, a French Pharma, in 2015. CDC has given its approval for use in the United States in 2019.

KYASANUR FOREST DISEASE AND THE VIRUS

Kyasanur forest disease virus (KFDV), a tick-borne *Flavivirus*, causes **kyasanur forest disease (KFD),** a hemorrhagic fever pandemic to Karnataka, (formally Mysore) the South-Western part of India.

KFDV was identified in 1957 when it was isolated from the patients and sick (dead) also called monkey fever is in the Kyasanur Forest in Karnataka state (hence the name). KFDV is transmitted to humans and Monkey through the bite of infected hard ticks *(Haemaphysalis spinigera)* which act as a reservoir of the virus.

The symptoms of KFD after an incubation period of 3 to 8 days, begin suddenly with chills, high fever and headache. Severe muscle pain with vomiting, gastrointestinal symptoms and bleeding may occur 3-4 days after initial symptoms. Patients may experience abnormally low B.P and low platelet, red blood cell and white blood cell counts.

The disease has a fatality rate of 3 – 10 %, and it affects 400 – 500 people every year. The disease now occurs in the adjacent states of Karnataka—Kerala, Goa, Maharashtra, T.N and Gujarat.

DIGNOSIS

In the early stage of illness KFD is diagnosed by

- Molecular detection of RNA by PCR and virus isolation from blood by *in vivo* inoculation
- Later, serologically by using ELISA.

TREATMENT

No specific anti-viral drug therapy for KFD is available. **Supportive treatment** with maintenance of proper hydration and circulation by transfusion of intravenous fluids or blood products for the patients with bleeding disorders, is the mainstay of treatment.

HANTAVIRUSES AND HANTAVIRUS PULMONARY SYNDROME

Hantaviruses or **orthohantavirus** are rodent-borne enveloped RNA viruses. The genome consists of three single-stranded RNA segments: designated S (small), M (medium) and L (large). The name is derived from the Greek word *ortho*-meaning "straight "or" true" and for the Hantan River in South Korea, where the first member species (Hantaan virus) was identified and isolated in 1976 by **Ho Wang Lee**. They are natural pathogens of rodents (mice and rats). Several hantavirus serotypes are known and each serotype has a specific rodents species and is spread to people via aerosolized virus that is shed in urine, feces (dropping) and saliva. They are not transmitted by a vector. Two major types of hantaviruses are:

- Hantaviruses in the Americas, are called **"New World" hantaviruses**, that cause **hantavirus pulmonary syndrome (HPS)**
- Hantaviruses found mostly in Europe and Asia are known as **"Old World" hantaviruses**, that cause **hemorrhagia fever with renal syndrome (HFRS)**, the milder form of which is called **nephropathia epidemica (EN).**

HFRS

HFRS is caused by five hantaviruses : Hantaan, Dobrava, Saaremaa, Seoul and Puumala, named after the place of its occurrence. Symptoms develop within 1 to 2 weeks after exposure to infectious meterial. The disease begins with sudden intense headaches, back and abdominal pain, fever, chills, nausea and blurred vision. Later symptoms include low blood pressure, acute shock, vascular leakage and acute kidney failure, which can cause severe fluid overload.

DIAGNOSIS

- Demonstration of virus specific IgM antibody in serum by IgM capture ELISA.
- Evidence of hantavirus antigen in tissue by immunohistochemical staining and microscopic examination.
- Detection of viral RNA in serum or CSF by PCR.

TREATMENT

Supportive treatment – management of the patient's blood (hydration) and electrolyte (e.g., Sodium, potassium and chloride) levels, and maintenance of oxygen and B.P, dialysis may be required in severe cases. Intravenuos administration of antiviral drug – ribavirin, is successful.

HPS

HPS was first recognized during the 1993 outbreak in the four-corner regions of the South Western United States by **Dr. Bruce Tempest** and the disease was termed **four corners disease**. Since 1993, the disease has been identified throughout the USA. It is a severe sometimes fatal respiratory disease caused by the **Sin Nombre orthohantavirus (SNV)** that is spread by the deer mouse rodent. The disease is characterized by *flu-like symptoms* – nausea, fever and chills, headache, muscle aches, vomiting, diarrhea or abdominal pain, that can progress rapidly to potentially life threatening breathing problems resulting in respiratory and cardiac failure.

TREATMENT

It involves supportive therapy, including mechanical ventilation with supplemental oxygen during the critical respiratory failure stage of illness.

ARENAVIRUSES

Arenavirus (Latin *arena* = sandy from the grany particles present in virion) is a bisegmented RNA virus, spread by rodent secretions, droppings, member of the family *Arenaviridae*. At least eight arenaviruses are known to cause human diseases. Two important diseases caused are:

- **Lymphocytic choriomeningitis (LCM)** – Influenza-like febrile illness; but can also cause meningitis, characteristically accompanied by large number of lymphocytes (as the CSF in the name LCM suggests). It is caused by lymphocytic choriomeningitic viruses.
- **Lassa fever also known as Lassa hemorrhagic fever** – A severe fatal hemorrhagic fever caused by Lassa virus. It is characterized by high fever, severe myalgic, hemorrhagic skin rash and coagulopathy. Lassa virus was first isolated in 1969 from Americans stationed in the village of Lassa, Nigeria endemic in West Africa.

Diagnosis: Laboratory diagnosis is made by direct isolation of the virus from blood or tissue specimens. Cell culture on vero or BHK cell lines; antigen and antibody detection from blood by ELISA; and viral RNA by RT-PCR.

TREATMENT

It consists of supportive treatment and immunotherapy by convalescent plasma.

PARAMYXOVIRUSES

Paramyxoviruses are enveloped single-stranded RNA viruses (150 – 200 nm) assigned to the family *Paramyxoviridae*. These cause acute respiratory diseases and are usually transmitted by airborne droplets. They include the agents of mumps, measles (rubeola), respiratory syncytial, parainfluenza and Newcastle disease. The term paramyxovirus has its origin from Greek *para* = by the side of, beyond, *myxo* = mucus or slime and latin *virus* = poison.

MUMPS AND MUMPS VIRUS

Mumps (also called **parotitis**), is a contagious viral disease that primarily affects saliva – producing (salivary) glands that are located near the ears. It is caused by the mumps virus, a **Paramyxovirus** and is characterized by painful swelling of the salivary glands. The disease was described by Hippocrates in the 5th century BCE. The term **mumps** ("grimace") given by Circa 1600, refers to the painful difficulty in swallowing. Mumps is more common in the developing world.

CLINICAL FEATURES

Humans are the only natural hosts, having the mumps virions in its saliva. The virus spreads from person-to-person with respiratory secretions such as saliva from an infected person. When an infected person coughs or sneezes, the droplets aerosolize which can enter the eyes, nose or mouth of a healthy person. Mumps can also spread by sharing eating utensils and cups. The incubation period varies from 12 to 25 days, but is typically 16 to 18 days in adults. Clinical symptoms start with fever, muscle ache, headache, tiredness and loss of appetite. This is followed by painful swelling of the one or both parotid salivary glands, causing the puffy cheeks and a tender swollen jaw. Skin over the enlarged glands may be stretched, red and hot. It can lead to serious complications like hearing loss (deafness).

DIAGNOSIS

- Clinically diagnosed on the basis of swollen glands.
- Elevated level of the enzyme amylase.
- Isolation of the virus from the saliva, CSF or urine on cell lines.
- Testing for the mumps IgM antibodies in serum samples.

TREATMENT

Treatment consists of symptoms relief in: use of pain relievers such as acetaminophen, ibuprofen to bring down fever; soothe swollen glands by applying ice packs; and drink plenty of fluids to avoid dehydration due to fever. Infection usually passes within a week or two.

PREVENTION

Getting vaccinated is the best way to prevent infection. Two live, attenuated vaccines that can prevent mumps are:

- **MMR vaccine** protects children and adults from measles, mumps and rubella.
- **MMRV vaccine** protects children from mumps measles, rubella and chickenpox.

MEASLES (RUBEOLA) VIRUS AND MEASLES

Measles (also called **rubeola** and **Khasra**) is a highly cantagious systemic disease caused by the **rubeola virus**, species of the genus *Morbillivirus* classified in the family *Paramyxoviridae*. It is one of the leading causes of death and disability among young children. It affects about 20 million people globally. Worldwide, there were for many years 1 million annual deaths from measles. The number of deaths (2.6 million in 1980) had reduced to 1,40,000 (in 2018) due to the global vaccination programs. The name measles is derived from the characteristic spots on the face and body, skin to Middle Dutch masel spot.

CLINICAL FEATURES

It is an air-borne disease which spreads easily from person-to-person through the coughs and sneezes and through direct contact with mouth or nasal secretion. The first symptom of measles is usually a high fever (>40°/104 °F) which begins after 10 to 12 days after exposure to the virus, along with cough, running nose, inflammed and watery red eyes, and a red blotchy skin rash (called also **rubeola**). Appearance of small bluish white spot on a bright red background called **Koplik's spot**, on the inside lining of the cheek 2 to 3 days after the start of the symptoms is a diagnostic symptom. Death due to measles results by the complications associated with the disease like blindness, encephalitis, pneumonia and severe diarrhea.

DIAGNOSIS

- Presence of skin rash on the body. Koplik's spot on the oral cavity is diagnostic feature of measles.
- Significant rise in measles IgM by enzyme-linked immunoassay. (IA).
- Viral RNA by real-time polymerase chain reaction (RT-PCR)
- Isolation of measles virus from urine, nasopharynx, blood, and throat.

TREATMENT

Use of fever reducers, such as acetaminophen or ibuprofen or naproxen sodium, in addition to vitamin A supplements as symptoms usually go away within 7 to 10 days.

PREVENTION BY VACCINATION

WHO recommends immunization for all children with 2 doses of measles vaccine, either alone, or in a measles-rubella (MR), or measles-mumps-rubella (MMR) combination.

In India measles vaccination is given under Universal Immunization Programme at 9 – 12 months of age (Ist dose) and 2nd dose at 16 – 24 months of age.

MEASLES IMMUNIZATION DAY

Measles (Khasra) is a highly contagious viral disease that kills more than 380 children every day. To make people aware about this deadly disease and how it can be prevented through vaccination, every year 16th March is celebrated as the **Measles Immunization Day**.

RUBELLA VIRUS AND RUBELLA

Rubella, also called **German measles** and **three-day measles**, best known by its distinctive red rash, is caused by the **rubella virus**, a **Togavirus.** It is a single-stranded RNA enveloped virus. The name rubella is derived from Latin that means *little red*. It was first described in 1814 by German physicians, hence named German measles. The disease lasts for 3 days, hence called 3-day measles.

Rubella occurs worldwide. It causes mild fever and rash in children and adults. However, infection during pregnancy may cause the birth of an infant with **congenital rubella syndrome (CRS),** an important cause of severe birth defects. Of the over 1,00,000 cases of CRS reported globally, 30,000 cases are reported in India each year.

CLINICAL FEATURES

Rubella is an infectious disease that usually spreads from person-to-person through the air via coughs of infected people. A rash may start around two weeks after exposure to the virus (i.e., incubation period is 2 weeks). It is mild illness with the symptoms: a low grade fever, sore throat and as a rash on the face and spreads to the rest of the body. The rash is sometimes itchy and is not as bright (i.e., less intensely red) as that of measles. Symptoms usually last for 3 days, hence, called 3-day measles.

Infection during early pregnancy may result in a miscarriage or a child borne with serious birth defects (such as deafness, cataracts, effect on brain and heart) referred to a congenital rubella syndrome (CRS) that occurs in over lakh women each year.

Rubella infection gives life lasting immunity as there is no antigenic type of the rubella virus.

DIAGNOSIS

- Serology: Testing the blood for the presence of rubella virus specific IgM antibodies.
- Isolation of the virus from the blood, throat or urine.

TREATMENT

- Mild symptoms can be managed with bed rest and acetaminophen to reduce fever.

PREVENTION

Rubella is prevented with **MMR vaccine** that protects against three diseases: measles, mumps and rubella. Two doses of vaccine are given to each child.

FILOVIRUSES

Filoviruses (*filo*, from the Latin for thread) are filamentous, enveloped, non-segmented, negative-single-stranded RNA viruses. Marburg virus and Ebola virus, the causative agent of severe hemorrhagic fevers, are the two well-known filoviruses.

MARBURG VIRUS AND MARBURG HEMJRRHAGIC FEVER

Marburg virus (MARV) is a single-stranded RNA virus (genus ***Marburgvirus,*** family *Filoviridae*), considered to be extremely dangerous, as a Risk Group 4 (WHO) as well as **category A Bioterrorism Agent.** It is the causative agent of a severe and highly fatal **Marburg virus disease (MVD)** also named **Marburg hemorrhagic fever**, **MHF** in humans with a fatality ratio of up to 88%. The virus was first described in 1967 during small outbreaks of hemorrhagic fever that occurred simultaneously in Marburg and Frankfurt (Germany) and in Belgrade, Yugoslavia (now Serbia). African green monkey is considered to be the natural reservoir, hence named **green monkey virus**. The name of the virus is derived from Marburg, the site of outbreak. Between 1967 and 2017 several outbreaks have been found around the globe.

The virus is filamentous (filovirus) that appears as shepherd's crook or a "U" or a "S" and may be coiled, toroid or branched, 80 nm in width but ranging in length from 795 to 828 nm. The genome is made up of linear non-segmented, single-stranded RNA.

CLINICAL FEATURES

The symptoms of WVD are initially mild headache with muscle pain. After a few days, the patient suffers from high fever and begins vomiting blood and bleeding profusely, both internally and from external openings such as nose and eyes. Death results in a few days from shock and organ failure.

DIAGNOSIS

The IgM-capture ELISA is the best assay for diseased persons. Isolation of the virus, viral RNA by PCR from blood from tissue specimens and immunohistochemistry are used to diagnose MHF.

TREATMENT

Only supportive hospital therapy is utilized which includes maintaining the patient's fluids , electrolytes, oxygen status and blood pressure, and replacing lost blood and clotting factors.

EBOLA VIRUS AND EBOLA VIRUS DISEASE

Ebola virus (Zaire ebola virus), is one of six known species in the genus ***Ebolavirus,*** a member of the family ***Filoviridae***). It causes **Ebola virus disease (EVD)**, also known an **Ebola hemorrhagic fever (EHF)**, a rare but severe, often fatal illness in humans.

Ebola virus and its genus were both originally named for **Zaire** (now the Democratic Republic of the Congo), the country and for a regional river—the **Ebola river** where it was first described in 1976. The natural reservoir of the virus is fruit bats and it is primarily transmitted between humans and from animals to humans through body fluids. Since the first outbreak recorded on 26 August 1976 in Yambuku, more than 24 outbreaks of EVD (1976 – 2018) have been recorded in Africa, the worst being the 2013 – 2016 epidemic in Western Africa which resulted in 11,323 deaths of the 28,646 cases. In July 2019 the WHO declared the Congo Ebola outbreak (May 2017 – 2018) a world health emergency.

CLINICAL FEATURES

The virus enters through direct contact with infected bodily fluids such as blood or saliva or uncleaned reused needle. The local custom of washing the body before burial often triggers new infections. Incubation period ranges from 2 to 3 weeks. EVD begins with sudden onset of fever, fatigue, sore throat, muscular pain and headaches. This is followed by vomiting, diarrhea, and rash, along with the decreased function of the liver and kidneys. The walls of the blood vessels are damaged, the virus disrupt the blood clotting system and the blood continues to leak into the surrounding tissue, hence called **Ebola hemorrhagic fever**, with mortality rate approaching 90%. This is often due to low blood pressure from fluid loss, and typically follows 6 to 16 days.

DIAGNOSIS

- Low platelet count, elevated levels of liver enzymes (e.g., ALT or AST) and abnormalities in blood clotting.
- Unique filamentous shapes of the virus in cell cultures examined with electron microscopy
- Isolating the virus by cell culture, detecting viral RNA by PCR, and detecting antibodies in the blood.
- Rapid antigent test which gives results in 15 minutes (approved by WHO in 2015)

TREATMENT

Treatment is supportive that consists of intravenous fluids (IV), and balancing electolytes (body salts), maintaining oxygen status and B.P.

PREVENTION

The first Ebola **vaccine-rVSV-ZEBOV** (trade name Ervebo), a single dose vaccine, approved by USFDA on Dec 19, 2019 for use to prevent Ebola.

ROTAVIRUSES AND STOMACH FLU

Rotaviruses are double-stranded RNA viruses displaying sharp-edged double-shelled capsids which like - spokes grouped around the hub of a wheel, in the family *Reoviridae*. The name is derived from *rota*, in Latin meaning wheel. Rotavirus is the most common cause of severe diarrhea among infants and children causing over 5 lakh deaths worldwide annually. The genus *Rotavirus* was discovered in 1937 by **Ruth Bishop** and collegues. It consists of ten species, referred to as A, B, C, D, E, F, G, H, I and J and *Rotavirus A*, is the most common species that causes more than 90% of the rotavirus infections in humans.

CLINICAL FEATURES

Rotaviruses are the most common cause of severe watery diarrheal disease which is often called **"stomach flu"** in young children throughout the world resulting in over 2 million infections and 2,15,000 deaths annually, especially in the developing countries. Symptoms can start within 2 days post-exposure to the rotavirus. Severe diarrhea accompanied by vomiting, a high fever (> 104°F/40°C), dehydration, abdominal pain and severe fatigue. Symptoms of dehydration observed in infant are dry mouth, cool skin, lack of tears when crying, reduced urination and sunken eyes. Transmission occurs through fecal-oral route i.e., by stool contaminated hands. The virus can also remain on contaminated surfaces for several days to weeks. The disease is self-limiting and patients recover within 5 to 10 days.

LABORATORY DIAGNOSIS

- **Demonstration of the virus in stool** by immunoelectron microscopy, latex agglutination tests, and ELISA. Presence of 10^{11} virus particles per ml of feces indicates the disease at its peak.
- **Detection of RNA by PCR**
- **Serological test** for antibody detection by ELISA.

TREATMENT

Rehydration by drinking plenty of fluids, eating broth-based soups, pedialyte or other fluids with electrolyte. Administration of intravenous (IV) fluids to prevent life-threatening complications, in case of severe dehydration.

PREVENTION

Vaccination: Since 2006, rotavirus oral vaccine for infants (6-32 weeks old) is available in two forms:

- **Rotarix** – Two-dose vaccine, with an interval of 4 weeks between the doses.
- **Rota Teq** – Three-dose vaccine with an interval of 4 – 10 weeks between the doses.

Hand hygiene: Washing your hands frequently, particularly before eating, is the best way to prevent the transmission of infection.

KEY POINTS

- A virus in which the genetic material is RNA is called an **RNA virus** (or **ribovirus**)

- RNA viruses mainly consist of single-stranded RNA (ssRNA) as their genetic material (except reoviruses).
- **Retroviruses** (e.g., HIV) are unusual viruses that can use ssRNA to synthesize dsDNA using a reverse transcriptase enzyme.
- **Rotavirus** (a **reovirus**), the common cause of diarrhea in infants and children, is the only **dsRNA virus.**
- Yellow fever, dengue, Marburg, Ebola, Lassa, *Hantavirus* pulmonary syndrome, and the viral hemorrhagic fever, are diagnosed by serology, nucleic acids (RT-PCR) and virus culture.
- **Zoonotic RNA viruses** (arboviruses, arenaviruses and lantaviruses) are spread by animal vectors.
- If the RNA of the virus is in a form ready to be translated by the host's machinery, it is considered a **positive-sense genome** (RNA); and if it is not directly translatable by the host, it is a **negative-sense genome**.
- Vaccine-preventable RNA viral human diseases include: Japanese encephalitis, dengue, mumps, measles, rubella, Ebola and rotavirus.

IMPORTANT QUESTIONS

1. Write short notes on:
   (a) Arboviruses.
   (b) Chickengunya virus.
   (c) Yellow fever.
   (d) Japanese encephalitis virus.
   (e) Breakbone fever.
   (f) Hantaviruses.
   (g) Mumps virus.
   (h) Measles (rubeola) virus.
   (i) Rubella virus.
   (j) Ebola virus.
   (k) Viral hemorrhagic fevers.

MULTIPLE-CHOICE QUESTIONS

1. All are single-stranded RNA viruses EXCEPT
   (a) Dengue fever virus
   (b) Rotavirus
   (c) Rubella virus
   (d) Ebola virus.

2. A common, highly diagnostic sign of measles is
   (a) Red rash
   (b) Sore throat
   (c) Koplik's spot
   (d) Inflammatory salivary glands.
3. Chikungunya and dengue are transmitted by:
   (a) Red flea
   (b) *Culex*
   (c) *Anopheles*
   (d) *Aedes ageypti.*
4. The name Ebola (virus and disease) is derived from
   (a) Name of a Scientist
   (b) Name of a River
   (c) Name of a State
   (d) Greek word.
5. All of the following RNA viruses cause hemorrhagic fevers EXCEPT:
   (a) Morburg virus
   (b) Ebola virus
   (c) Dengue virus
   (d) Paramyxovirus.
6. Which of the following are spread by arthropod vectors?
   (a) Arboviruses
   (b) Arenaviruses
   (c) Hantaviruses
   (d) Rotaviruses.
7. All are preventable by MMR-vaccine EXCEPT:
   (a) Rotavirus
   (b) German measles
   (c) Measles
   (d) Mumps.

ANSWERS TO MCQs

1. (b)	2. (c)	3. (d)	4. (b)
5. (d)	6. (a)	7. (a).	

63

DNA Viruses: Double and Single Stranded

Smallpox; Herpes; Chickenpox; Shingles; Infectious mononucleosis; Burkitt's lymphoma; Nasophargngeal carcinoma; Cytomegallic inculsion; Roseala infantium; Kaposis's sarcoma; Cervical cancer; Fifth disease.

A **DNA virus** is a virus in which the genetic material or genome is DNA rather than RNA. All DNA viruses are double-stranded (dsDNA) except for parvoviruses which have ssDNA. Based on the type of DNA; these viruses are classified into two classes: **dsDNA viruses** and **ssDNA viruses**. Based on the nature of genome and envelope, the DNA viruses are grouped as shown in Figure 63.1.

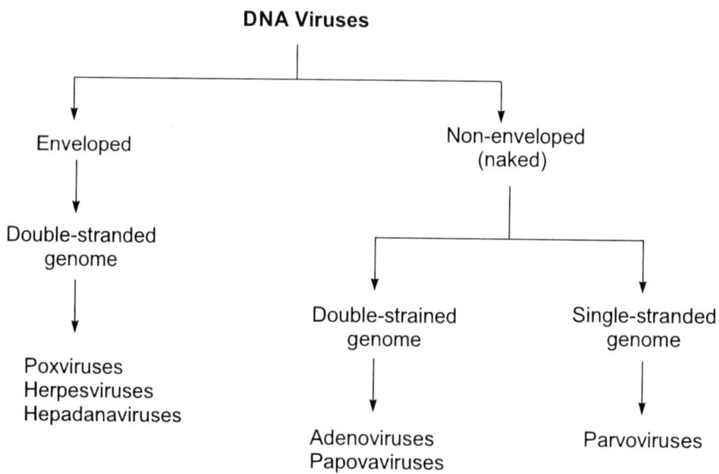

Fig. 6.31 DNA virus groups with examples.

POXVIRUSES

The **poxviruses** (members of the family **Poxviridae**) are the largest known brick-shaped (240 nm × 300 nm) dsDNA enveloped viruses that produce eruptive skin pustules called **pox** or **pocks** that leave scars. These have the largest genome of all viruses and multiply in the cytoplasm.

The common examples of poxviruses are:

- Smallpox virus (variola) – The causative agent of smallpox.
- Vaccinia virus – Agent used for smallpox vaccination.
- Molluscum contagiosum virus (MCV) – The cause of waxy nodules on skin.
- Monkeypox virus – May infect humans causing a disease similar to smallpox.

SMALLPOX (VARIOLA)

Smallpox, (also called **variola**) now a disease of the past, is a serious, contagious, and sometimes fatal infectious disease caused by the smallpox (Variola) virus. The disease gets its name from the Latin word for "spotted" and refers to the small pus-filled blisters that appear on the face and body of an infected person. About 30% of people who become infected with smallpox die from their illness.

Forms of Smallpox

There are two basic forms of smallpox:

- **Variola major**, with a mortality rate of > 20%.
- **Variola minor,** with a mortality rate of < 1%

TRANSMISSION

Humans are the only host for the smallpox virus. Smallpox is spread from person-to-person by the respiratory route and direct face-to-face, and fairly prolonged contact with an infected person.

PATHOGENESIS

Variola viruses may enter through mucosa of the upper respiratory tract, infect many internal organs before they eventually move into the bloodstream, infecting the skin and producing more recognizble symptoms. The growth of the virus in the epidermal layers causes lesions (pocks) that become pustular after exposure between 7 and 17 days (incubation period).

SYMPTOMS

The patients initially show fever, headache, vomiting, mouth sores backache and general fatigue (pre-eruptive phase). The telltale sign is the development of a unique skin rash, which has an indentation (hollow area) at its center, covering the entire body. The rash progresses to a raised bump, then to a pus-filled blister that crusts and scabs over before finally falling off about 3 weeks, leaving behind a pitted scar.

DIAGNOSIS

Smallpox is diagnosed based on the symptoms and PCR is used as the confirmatory test.

PROPHYLAXIS

The preventive measures include immunization with smallpox vaccine prepared from vaccinia virus, and chemoprophylaxis.

Smallpox was the first disease to which immunity was artificially induced through the **Edward Jenner's** 1798 vaccination work on this disease and the first disease to be eradicated from the human population globally as certified by WHO in 1980. The last naturally occurring case was diagnosed in October 1977 in Somalia.

HERPESVIRUSES

Herpesviruses are enveloped dsDNA latent viruses that cause recurrent infections of the skin, mucous membranes, glands and are potentially carcinogenic. The name herpesvirus is derived from Greek word *herpein* (= to creep) for the tendency of some herpes infections to produce a creeping rash (spreading cutaneous lesions). Examples of the common herpesvirus diseases are cold sores, genital herpes, chickenpox, shingles, mononucleosis and roseola. They also cause cancers in humans such as lymphomas.

Herpesviruses are calssified in the family *Herpesviridae*. In 2020, the International Committee on Taxonomy of Viruses recognized 107 species types in herpesviruses. Nine herpesvirus types are known to infect humans. They are now called **human herpesviruses (HHV)**.

- Herpes simplex virus 1 and 2 (HSV-1 and HSV-2)
- Varicella-zostervirus (VZV)
- Entomegalovirus (CMV)
- Epstein-Barr virus (EBV)
- Human cytomegalovirus (HCMV)

- Human herpesvirus 6A and 6B (HHV-6)
- Human herpesvirus 7 (HHV-7)
- Kaposi's sarcoma—associated herpesvirus (KSHV)

STRUCTURE

Herpesviruses are among the larger viruses, with a diameter between 150 nm and 200 nm (Fig. 63.2). They have a uniqne four-layered structure.

A **core** contianing the large, linear double-stranded DNA genome enveloped by an icosahedral protein cage, the **capsid** which is composed of 162 capsomeres.

The capsid is surrounded by an amorphous protein coat called the **tegument**. It is encased in a glycoprotein-bearing lipid bilayer membrane called the **envelope** (Fig. 63.2).

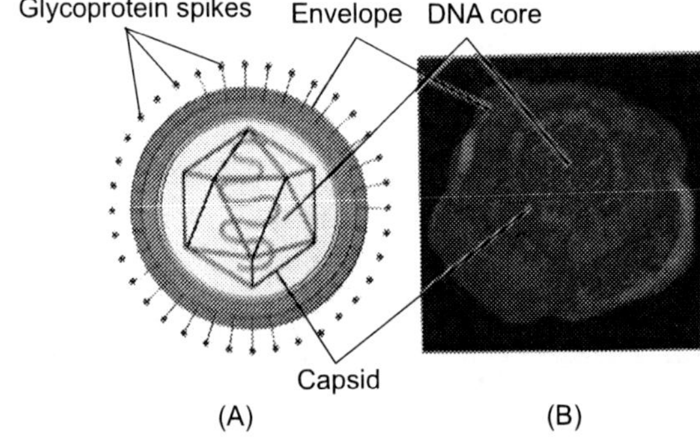

Fig. 63.2 Morphology and structure of an enveloped DNA virus. (A) Schematic view of a herpesvirus. (B) A color enhanced view of cytomegalovirus.

Susceptibility to Organic Solvents

Herpesviruses are prone to deactivation by organic solvents and detergents and are unstable outside the host's body.

HERPES SIMPLEX VIRUS

Herpes simple virus (HSV) is categorized into two types: HSV-1 and HSV-2. The official names for these are: **human herpesvirus 1** and **2** (**HHV-1** and **HHV-2**).

These viruses cause intermittent episodes of reactivation of **herpes** (painful, fluid-filled blisters) on major parts of the body. The main diseases include: **facial herpes** (oral, optic and pharyngeal) and **genital herpes**.

HSV 1 DISEASES

HSV-1 is transmitted mainly by oral-to-oral contact mainly infecting lips to cause **oral herpes** that includes symptoms called **herpes labialis**, **cold sores** or fever **blisters**. These are painful short lived vesicles that are located mainly at the margin of the red areas of the lips. The infection is acquired during childhood and is life long. Globally, 3.7 million people under age 50 have HSV-1 infection, highly prevalent in Africa.

Occasionally, HSV-1 infects oropharynx causing herpetic **gingivostomatis** involving the inflammation of the entire oral mucosa, tongue, cheeks and lips. HSV-1 can also cause **gential herpes**, which can be asymptomatic or can have mild symptoms: one or more genital or anal blisters or ulcers. However, this does not recur frequently unlike gential herpes caused by HSV-2.

Most of these infections have been reported to occur in the Americas, Europe and Western Pacific.

Herpetic whitlow infection of fingers (causing small blisters on fleshy areas around the finger tips) of nurses, physicians and dentists, who carelessly touch lesions. It is characterized by painful deep-set vesicles that become inflammed and necrotic, which are difficult to treat. **Herpes gladuatorum** (**mat herpes**) characterizing cluster of clear fluid filled blisters that are typically surrounded by red skin, is seen among wrestlers are caused by skin contact with HSV-1 lesions.

Herpetic keratitis (also called **ocular herpes**), an infective inflammation of the eye involving **cornea** – the clear dome that covers the coloured part of the eye, occurs when the HSV-1 travels to the opthalmic nerve. Gritting feeling of the eye, conjunctivitis, sharp pain and sensitivity to light are the symptoms observed.

HSV 2 DISEASES

HSV-2 is the usual cause of **genital herpes** (**herpeo genitalis**), a disease primarily transmitted by sexual contact. The vesicles start out separate, but become confluent and ulcerate into painful red erosions. The chief symptoms are urethritis, painful urination, cervicitis and itching.

HSV-2 rarely spreads to the brain.

LABORATORY DIAGNOSIS

- Oral and genital herpes is usually diagnosed based on the symptoms: appearance and distribution of sores.

Laboratory tests include:

- **Direct cytologic examination** of scrapings from base of lesions stained with Giemsa, Wright or Papanicolarou (Pap smear) methods for multinucleate gaint cells and multinucleate inclusions.
- **Culture of the virus** on chorioallantoic membrane of the chick embryo by the appearance of typical pocks within 24 to 48 hours; culturing in rabbit kidney and human amnion tissue culture and identification by typical intranuclear inclusion bodies.
- **Direct fluorescent antibody (DFA)** on specimens or cell cultures that identifies and differentiates HSV-1 and HSV-2.
- **Polymerase chain reaction** (PCR) – To detect viral DNA in fluid from blisters.

TREATMENT

Aciclovir (zovirax) is the most effective and specific antiviral drug for HSV.

Paracetamol (acetaminophen) and topical lidocaine is used to relieve symptoms.

PREVENTION

There is no available vaccine.

The most effective method of avoiding genital infections is by avoiding vaginal, oral and anal sex.

VARICELLA-ZOSTER VIRUS AND CHICKENPOX AND SHINGLES

Varicella-zoster virus (VZV) causes **chickenpox** and **herpes zoster** (**shingles**). This virus is known by a composite name: **varcella-zoster virus** because the same virus causes two clinical forms of disease. Other names used for VZV are **chickenpox virus, zoster virus** and **human alphavirus** 3.

CHICKENPOX

Chickenpox (the term drived from chickpeas, based on the resemblance of rash's lesions to chickpeas and/or from the rash resembling chicken pecks) is also called **varicella**. The term chickenpox was first used in 1658. It is a highly contagious mild childhood disease, result of an initial infection with VZV characterized by small, red, itchy, vesicular rashes. Encephalitis (infection of brain) and Reye's syndrome are the complications of chickenpox. Duration of the disease is 5 to 10 days and people usually only get chickenpox once in their life. There were 140 million cases of chickenpox and singles in 2013 worldwide. Death occurs in about 1 per 60,000 cases.

Pathogenesis: Chickenpox spreads easily from person to person by the respiratory route through the coughs and sneezes of an infected person. The disease is acquired when the virus enters the respiratory system. Symptoms begin 10 to 21 days after exposure to virus (incubation period) and the infection localizes in skin cells after about 2 weeks. For 3 to 4 days, the infected skin is vesicular: the red vesicles (lesions) full with puss, eventually becoming pustules that rupture and form scabs before healing. The lesions individually occur on the face, scalp, trunk and throat followed by lower back and shoulders. The number of lesions varies from a few to hundreds and are more abundant in adolescents and adults compared to young children.

SHINGLES

Shingles (is derived from the Latin *cingulus* = "girdle or belt"after the belt-like dermatonatal rash or **herpes zoster** (from the Gr. *zoster* = girdle) also called **zoster** and **zona** characterized by a painful skin rash with blisters occurring in a single wide stripe on the chest and back. It is caused due to a reactivation of the latent VZV in a persons's body.

The latent virus found in the nerve cells, usually in late adulthood, becomes reactivated, caused by stress or weakening of the immune system causing shingles. It is usually limited to one side of the body at a time because these nerves are unilateral. Severe burning or stringing pain is a frequent symptom, which occasionally persists for months or years, a condition called **postherpetic neuralgia.**

DIAGNOSIS

- Clinical diagnosis is made by cutaneous lesions and distribution pattern on the body.
- Presence of multinucleate giant cells in Giemsa stained smears of vesicle scrapings characteristic for shingles.
- Fluorescent antibody detection of viral antigens in skin lesions.
- Culturing (isolation) of the virus from the fluid sample.
- PCR testing of the blister fluid scabs is used for confirmation.
- Blood tests can be used to identify a response to acute infection (IgM) or previous infection and subsequent immunity (IgG).

TREATMENT

Treatment mainly consists of easing the symptoms.

- Topical application of a calamine lotion.
- Use of paracetamol (acetaminophen) (but not aspirin) to reduce fever.
- Acyclovir, an antiviral intravenous drug, is effective to treat systemic infection.

PREVENTION

- An attenuated live **varicella vaccine** is available which is given to child at one year age. This chickenpox vaccine not only protects against chickenpox, it also reduces the risks of shingles (i.e., two-for-one).

  Currently two vaccines exist against shingles:
- **Zostavax** for adults age 60 and older.
- **Shingrix** is the vaccine of choice for adults age 50 and older. It got approval for use in 2017.

EPSTEIN-BARR VIRUS AND INFECTIOUS MONONUCLEOSIS

Epstein-Barr viruse (EBV), a double-stranted DNA virus, also known as **human herpes virus 4** (**HHV-4**), a member of the *Herpesviridae,* is one of the most common viruses in humans. The virus was named after its discoverers; Sir **Michael Anthony Epstein** a British virologist and his student **Yvonne Barr** in 1964 in cells from a common tumor (lymphoma) in African children studied by **Denis Burkitt** an Irish physician (hence the disease called **Burkitt's lymphoma**). EBV was the first human cancer virus to be isolated. Humans are the natural host of EBV. It is the causative agent of **infectious mononucleosis** and associated with several human malignancies (e.g., Burkitt's lymphoma and nasopharyngeal carcinoma).

INFECTIOUS MONONUCLEOSIS

The name of the disease **infectious mononuclosis, IM** (also called **glandular fever, kissing disease** and **mono**) (Gr. *mono* = one + *nucleco* = nucleus *sis* = state) is derived from the increased level of atypical lymphocytes (WBCs) with unusual lobed nuclei in the blood which resembled **monotypes** when they were first discovered. The infection spreads through saliva by kissing which is why some people refer it as the **kissing disease**.

EBV infection occurs early in childhood without any symptoms (asymptomatic). In young adults, it causes high fever, enalrged lymph nodes in the neck, tiredness, sore throat with swollen tonsils, a gray-white exudate and rash on the palate that can be of some use in diagnosis. Swelling of the liver or spleen may occur in some patients.

The symptoms develop after a long incubation period of 30 to 50 days. The epithelium of the oropharynx is the portal of entry for EBV during the primary infection and from there the virus moves to the parotid gland and replicates in the resting memory B cells and persist in the dormant state and reactivated later by some ill-defined mechanism.

DIAGNOSIS

- Differential blood count that shows increased blood lymphocytes (50% with atleast 10% atypical).
- Microscopic examination of blood smear for abnormally large lymphocytes containing indented nuclei with light discolorations.
- Elevated hepatic transaminase level is suggestive of IM (occurring in 50% people).
- Serology blood tests for specific antibodies against the EBV. Positive IgG reflects a past infectious whereas IgM mainly reflects a recent infection.

TREATMENT

IM is generally **self-limiting**, hence most people recover in 2 to 4 weeks without any medication.

- Paracetamol (acetaminophen) or ibuprofen is used to relieve pain and fever.
- Antibacterial antibiotics are sometimes used to stop/treat/prevent secondary infections of the throat (such as *Streptococcus*).

BURKITT'S LYMPHOMA

Burkitt's lymphoma, an EBV-associated cancer of the lymphatic system, particularly B lymphocytes found in the germinal center. It is characterized by swelling and distortion of the facial bones and a rapid growth of lymph nodes. It is reconized as a fast growing human tumor which is the most common childhood cancer prevalent in African children.

It is named after **Denis Parsons Burkitt**, an Irish surgeon who first described the disease in 1958 while working in eastern Africa.

EBV infection at an early age is accompanied by chronic immunosuppression due to endemic malaria and proceeds to a highly aggressive tumor.

Biopsy of tumors and physical examination of patients is used to diagnose it. It is treated with combination chemotherapy (e.g., cytorabine cyclophosphamide, doxorubicin).

NASOPHARYNGEAL CARCINOMA

Nasopharyngeal carcinoma (NPC), also called **nasopharyngeal cancer**, is the most common cancer (especially in South-East Asia and China) originating from the epithelum of the nasopharynx, which is located behind the nose and above the back of the throat. It is by far the most common cancer of nasopharynx.

NPC has been strongly linked to EBV. The change in DNA causes cells to grow and divide abnormally, causing cancer. Lump in the neck is the most common symptom indicating that the cancer is spreading to the lymph nodes. Other symptoms include: double vision, ear infection, face pain, headache, sore throat, stuffy nose and hearing loss.

Treatment consists of radiation therapy, chemotherapy and surgical removal of tumor.

CYTOMEGALOVIRUS AND CYTOMEGALOVIRUS DISEASE

Cytomegalovirus (CMV), (Figure 63.2) a genus belonging to herpesviruses, is named for its tendency to produce enlarged cells, a condition called **cytomegaly** (Gr. *cyto* = cella, *megalo* = large, i.e., swollen state of infected cells) as seen in culture and in infected tissues. The nuclei of productively infected cells contain a large distinctive inclusion body, giving a typical **"Owl's eye"** appearance under a microscope, a feature useful in diagnosis. It was first observed in 1881 by **Hugo Ribbert**, a German pathologist in the cells of an infant.

The genus contains 11 species. Humans and monkeys act as the natural hosts. Of these, *human herpesvirus* 5 HHV-5 (= *human cytomegalovirus* 5, *human beta herpes virus* 5, CMV) only infects humans.

Diseases: The diseases caused by HHV-5 are:

- Cytomegalic inclusion disease (ID) (cytomegalovirus disease) in newborns.
- Mononucleosis syndrome

In immunocompromised patients, it causes life-threatening (pneumonitis), cytomegalvirus retinitis (an eye infection), hepatitis, encephalitis, colitis, hepatitis and pancreatitis.

Transmission: CMV spreads from person-to-person through body fluids, such as saliva, urine, blood, semen, tears and breast milk.

Symptoms: Most people with CMV infection show no symptoms, a few feel ill and have a fever, sore throat, swollen glands and fatigue.

DIAGNOSIS

Diagnosis is made by histopathology, culturing virus, detecting DNA by PCR and enzyme immunoassay for CMV IgG. Samples to diagnose CMV include: urine, saliva, broncho-alveolar salvage fluid and biopsy tissue.

- Histopathological studies of tissue biopsy is done for the **characteristic owl's eye effect** in the infected cells.
- **Detection of virus** can be made by any one of the following:
  - Infected sample by PCR
  - Hybridization assay
  - CMV early antigen in cell culture (human embryo fibroblasts) 24 hours post-inoculation by immunofluorescence.
- **Detection of CMV IgG antibodies** in the serum by enzyme immunoassay.

TREATMENT

Ganciclovir (cytovene) is the drug of choice, to treat serious CMV illness, which is administered intravenously twice daily.

PREVENTION

No vaccine exists to prevent CMV infection. VB-1 1501 A and V 160 are the probable vaccine candidates under clinical human trial.

HUMAN HERPESVIRUS 6 AND ROSEOLA INFANTUM

Human herpesvirus 6 (HHV-6) is a set of two closely related enveloped dsDNA herpesviruses known as **HHV-6A** and **HHV-6B**. These were recognized as two distinct species of the genus ***Roselovirus***. These infect 100% of the human populations. **Roseola inflantum**, also called **exanthem subitum** and 6th disease is caused by HHV 6, espeually HHV6B in infants: HHV6A is a neuro virulent pathogen infecting the patients with multiple sclerosis.

HHV-6 was first isolated in 1986 by **Salahuddin** and coworkers from the blood of patients with lymphoproliferative disorders. Some of whom had AIDS. Roseola inflantum, HHV-6B virus transmitted by infected bloods, found in children under 2 years of age initiates with a sudden onset of fever that may reach 105°F followed by a rash–many small, pink spots on the stomach that may spread to the face, arms and legs. The virus enters the body through the nose and mouth through coughs, sneezes, talks or laughs of infected persons. Very common disease in India, affecting over 10 million children each year.

DIAGNOSIS is made by clinical symptoms (rash and high fever), serology (antibodies to roseola) and detection of viral DNA by PCR.

TREATMENT Consists of administration of acetaminophen or ibuprofen to relieve fever and discomfort and plenty of rest and fluids to the child. Gaciclovir (cytovene) is given in severe cases.

HUMAN HERPESVIRUS 7

Human herpesvirus 7 also called **human betaherpesvirus** 7) **(HHV-7)** was first isolated in 1990 from CD4+ T cells taken from the peripheral blood by **Frenkel** and colleagues and classified in the genus *Roseoelovirus* HHV-7 often acts together with HHV-6 and causes primary infection in most individuals during childhood before the age of 2 and 5. The clinical mainfestations include: **pityrasis rosea** and **roseola infantum**, followed by a lifelong latent state with prossible reactivation in case of immunodeficiency causing **encephalitis**.

Detection of HHV-7 DNA in serum or plasma by PCR is used to diagnose infection. No specific treatment is known.

HUMAN HERPESVIRUS 8 AND KAPOSI'S SARCOMA

Human herpesvirus 8 (HHV 8) (also known as **Kaposi's sarcoma associated herpesvirus, KSHV**) belongs to the genus **Rhadinovirus,** a member of the family Herpesviridae. The scientists in 1984 reported the presence of this virus in KS tumors in AIDS patients and ten years later in 1998 it was identified by **Yuan Chang** and **Patrick S.,** a wife and husband team at Cloumbia University. It is one of seven currently known cancer viruses, or oncon viruses. This virus causes Kaposi's sarcoma and primary effusion lymphoma.

Kaposi's sarcoma (KS), named after **Mortiz Kaposi** who first described it in 1872, as a type of cancer especially caused in AIDS patient. It is characterized by abnormal cells forming purple, red or brown blotches (lesions) or tumors on the skin. Lesions can also develop on other parts of the body (e.g., inside the mouth, lymph nodes, lungs or digestive tract. KS can cause serious problems or even become life threatening when the lesions are in the lungs (trumble breathing) or in digestive tract (cause bleeding).

KS is commonly found in people with HIV/AIDS and patients following organ transplant. In 2017, over 35% of AIDS patients were affected with this cancer.

Diagnosis is made only by biopsy and microscopic examination. Detection of the KSHV protein LANA in tumor cells confirms the diagnosis.

TREATMENT

Five kinds of treatment generally used to treat KS:

- KS is usually a localized tumor that can be treated either surgically through cytotherapy (scraping to remove a lesion) or through local irradiation (i.e., radiation therapy)
- Systemic chemo by liposomal doxorubfin (Doxil R), anthracyclines or paclitaxel.
- Intralesional (local) chemotherapy
- HIV antiviral therapy.

ADENOVIRUSES

Adenoviruses are nonenveloped, medium-sized (90 – 100 nm), dsDNA viruses with an icosahedral nucleocapsid. Their name is derived from their initial isolation from human adonoids in 1953. They have been described as the **weeds** on the virological garden.

They are heat sensitive and destroyed within minutes at 56°C, and killed in objects by heat and bleach.

Adenoviruses are the common infectious agents of upper respiratory tract, eyes and lymphoid organs causing mild infection. They spread through close personnel contact such as touching or shaking hands, through aerosols by coughing and sneezing. Major diseases caused by adenoviruses are:

- **Common cold** (or flu-like symptoms with fever and sore throats)
- **Acute bronchitis** (inflammation of the airways of the lungs, sometimes called a chest cold).
- **Pneumonia** (infection of the lungs).
- **Pink eye** (conjunctivitis)
- **Acute gastroenteritis** (inflammation of the stomach or intestine causing diarrhea, vomiting, and nausea.

DIAGNOSIS

- Demonstration of virus particles in stool extracts by electron microscopy
- Viral antigen assay of nasopharynx by immunofluorescence
- Detection of viral DNA by PCR
- Virus culturing from respiratory specimens, eye swabs, feces and urine
- Serology – A rise in antibody levels in blood indicates recent infection.

TREATMENT

Most infections are mild and may require only cure to help symptoms such as pain medicines and fever reducers.

Cidofavir is used to treat severe adenovirus infections in immunocompromised patients.

PAPOVAVIRUSES

Papovaviruses are small (45–55 nm) nonenveloped, icosahedral, dsDNA viruses. It consists of two genera *Papillomavirus* and *Polyomavirus* classified in the class *Papovaviricetes*. The term **papova** is derived from the names of the viruses includied: Pa, papilloma; po, polyoma; va, vaculating virus (SV40 which is now included in the genus *Polyomavirus*). These viruses cause warts, cervical and anal cancer in humans.

PAPILLOMAVIRUS AND CERVICAL CANCER

Human papillomavirus (HPV), with over 40 different strains is the cause of most common sexually transmitted infection. It causes skin tumors called **papillomas** (L. *papilla* = pimple + *oma* = tumor, i.e., epithelial tumor), which are classified as:

- **Common or seed warts:** Painless, elevated, rough growth on the fingers, face or trunk, common in young children.
- **Plantar warts:** Deep, painful, flat, benign tumors on feet and trunk, elbows and knees.
- **Genital warts:** Genital warts, a special form of verruca, that start as tiny bumps on membrane or skin of genitals, a very common STD and is linked to some kind of cancer.

Warts are spread by close contact with infected skin or fomites. The incubation period ranges from 2 weeks to more than a year.

CONDYLOMATA ACUMINATA (CERVICAL CANCER)

The genital warts, especially the external and internal membranes of the vagina and head of the penis may progress to large branched, cauliflower-like masses, called **condylomata acuminata** that may extend into labial perineal, and periunal regions. The chronic infection especially with two HPV types (16 and 18) may lead to **cervical cancer**. It takes 15 to 20 years (in women with normal immune system) and only 5 to 10 years in women with weakened immune system. It mainly spreads through sexual contact. Cervical cancer is the second most common cancer worldwide. WHO in 2018 reported death of 3,11,000 women of the 5,70,000 new cases in one year.

DIAGNOSIS

WHO recommeds three types of screening tests. Visual infection with acetic acid (VIA); conventional (PaP) test and liquid-based cytology, and HPV testing by DNA probes.

Treatment for all types of warts includes: direct chemical application of podophyllin and physical removal of the skin or membrane by cauterization, freezing or laser surgery, and immunotherapy with interferon.

POLYOMAVIRUSES

Polyomaviruses (L. *poly* = many + *oma* = tumor) are small non-enveloped dsDNA viruses that exist in symbiosis with humans and animals. 14 human PyVs have been identified, most of which cause infections with little or no symptomes. The diseases caused among immunocompromised people are:

- **BK virus** – **nephropathy** in renal transplant patients
- **JC virus** – progressive multifocal leukoencephalopathy characterized by a slow destruction of the brain.
- **Merkel cell viruses** – MCV, discovered in 2008 in Pennsylvania, is an oncovirus. It causes Merkel cell corcinoma an aggressive form of skin cancer.
- **SV 40** – Cancer in rodents; may be involved in brain and bone tumors (cancer)

PARVOVIRUSES – ssDNA VIRUSES

Parvoviruses (PVS) are the tiniest viruses (18–26 nm) and unique among the viruses having single-stranded DNA genome. Important diseases include.

Canine parvovirus (**CPV** or **parvo**) causes a highly infectious disease in dogs that can be fatal.

Parvovirus B 19 (human parvovirus) infects only humans and causes **fifth disease** a mild rash illness that usually affects children and rarely adults. It spreads through respiratory route and may cause erythematous maculopapular rash called **erythema infectiosum (slapped check disease)**, painful swollan joints (polyarthropathy syndrome) and severe sickle-cell anaemia in children with immunodeficiency.

KEY POINTS

- The viruses having DNA as their genetic material are called **DNA viruses**.
- DNA viruses of humans exist in the enveloped or naked state and can carry double-stranded or single-stranded DNA.
- **Smallpox**, a skin disease caued by variola virus, has been eradication as a result of vaccination.
- **Herpesviruses** are enveloped DNA viruses that are known for being latent in host cells after initial infection.
- Cold sores, gential herpes, chickenpox, shingles, mononucleosis and roseola (common diseases) and Kaposi's sarcoma and lymphoma (rare cancers) are caused by the **herpesviruses**.
- **Hepatitis B virus,** an enveloped DNA virus, is one cause of hepatitis that damages the liver and may cause cancer.
- **Papovaviruses**, dsDNA naked viruses, include papillioma, polyoma or vacuolating viruses, are the causative agents of various kinds of warts and cancer.
- **Parvoviruses,** the ssDNA, non-enveloped viruses, are the tiniest viruses.

IMPORTANT QUESTIONS

1. Write short notes:
   (a) Kinds of DNA viruses.
   (b) Name the types of herpesviruses.
   (c) Chickenpox and shingles.
   (d) Epstein-Barr virus.

MULTIPLE-CHOICE QUESTIONS

1. All of the following are double-stranded DNA viruses EXCEPT:

(a) Poxviruses (b) Parvoviuses

(c) Herpesviruses (d) Adenoviruses.

2. Which of the following viral infections is not caused by a poxvirus?

(a) Cowpox (b) Smallpox

(c) Chickenpox (d) Molluscum contagiosum.

3. Which virus was used in smallpox vaccination?

(a) Cowpox virus (b) Variola virus

(c) Varicella virus (d) Vaccinia virus.

4. Varicella and zoster are caused by:

(a) Herpes simplex and herpes zoster

(b) Cytomegalovirus and varicella-zoster virus

(c) Two different strains of varicella-zoster virus

(d) The same (or a single) virus.

5. Parvoviruses are unique because they contain ....

(a) Reverse tanscriptase

(b) An envelope without spikes

(c) A single-stranded DNA genome

(d) A double-stranded DAN genome.

6. Which of the following causes genital warts and cervical cancer?

(a) Papillomavirus (b) Polyomavirus

(c) Parvovirus (d) Adenovirus.

7. Burkitt's lymphoma, that swells cheek or abdomen, and prevalent in African children is caused by:

(a) Cytomegalovirus

(b) Herpesvirus-6

(c) Papillomavirus

(d) Epstein-Barr virus.

ANSWERS TO MCQs

1. (b)	2. (c)	3. (d)	4. (d)
5. (c)	6. (a)	7. (d).	

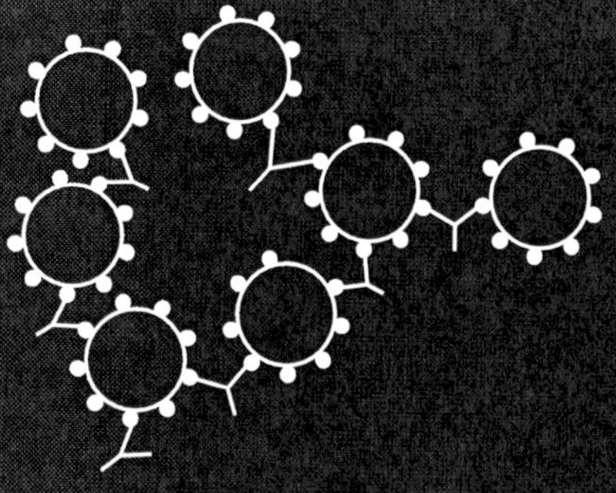

Unit IV C

FUNGI-MEDICAL MYCOLOGY

- Characteristics and Classification of Fungi and Laboratory Diagnosis of Mycotic Infections
- Superficial, Cutaneous and Subcutaneous Mycoses
- Systemic (Deep) Mycoses by True Pathogens
- Opportunistic Mycoses

64

Characteristics and Classification of Fungi and Laboratory Diagnosis of Mycotic Infections

WHAT ARE FUNGI?

The **fungi** (sing. **fungus**) are achlorophyllous, heterotropic, **eukaryotic** microscopic and macroscopic, spore-producing unicellular and multicellular mycelial organisms having a cell wall composed of chitin and β-glucans. **Fungus** is the Latin word for mushroom that, in turn, is derived from the Greek word *sphongos* for **sponge** which refers to the macroscopic structures and morphology of mushrooms and molds. Fungi include mushrooms, yeasts, molds and related organisms, which occur either free-living in soil or parasitic or symbiotic relationships with plants or animals. These organisms are classified as a Kingdom–*Fungi* (or *Myceteae*), which is separate from the other eukaryotic life kingdoms of plants and animals.

The study of fungi is known as **mycology** (from the Greek word *mykes*, mushroom and *logos*, study).

Fungal biodiversity is enormous–estimated at 2.2 million to 38 million species and of these only 1,48,000 species have been described so far, with over 8000 species pathogenic to plants and more than 600 species are associated with humans, either as commensals and members of our microbiota or as pathogens that cause some of the lethal infectious diseases. Fungi are beneficial to us as food/products of food, bread, alcoholic beverages (beer, wine), antibiotics (penicillin, griseofulvin, cephalosporin), human hormones, citric acid, organic matter decomposers, biopesticides, and as versatile tools in medical research.

The applied branch of mycology/microbiology that deals with the study of human mycotic infections (mycoses) is termed **medical mycology.**

CHARACTERISTICS OF FUNGI

- They are **eukaryotic** (i.e., have organelles with true nucleus).
- They lack chlorophyll and are nonphotosynthetic.
- Cell wall is made up of **chitin** instead of cellulose like that of a plant.
- Reproduce **asexually** (budding spores, conidia) and **sexually** (ascospores, basidiospores, zygospores).
- **Heterotrophic** with absorptive mode of nutrition.
- Plant body is a **thallus** (thallophyte) may be nonmycelial (yeasts) or mycelial made up of tubular filaments called **hyphae.**
- **Decomposers** – the best recycles around.
- More related to animals than plants.

MORPHOLOGICAL TYPES OF FUNGI

Based on their morphology, they are classified into five groups, each of which has some human pathogenic species.

1. **Yeasts:** Single-celled, microscopic fungi which reproduce asexually by budding (blastoconidia formation) or fission.

   Examples: *Cryptococcus neoformans*, *Saccharomyces*.

2. **Molds or filamentous fungi: Mold** is a fungus that grows in the form of filaments called hyphae, and the network of branching hyphae is termed **mycelium** which have incomplete cross-walls called septa, each compartment (cell) containing one (uninucleate), or multiple, genetically identical nuclei (multinucleate). Mold growth results in discoloration and a fuzzy appearance, especially on food (e.g., bread, orange or citrus fruits).

   Examples: *Aspergillus, Penicillium, Mucor, Trichophyton, Microsporum* and *Epidermophyton*.

3. **Yeast-like fungi:** Some fungi exist as a yeast (single budding cells) for part of their life cycle and are hyphal (filamentous) for a significant portion of it, such organisms are called yeast-like fungi (e.g., *Candida albicans*).

4. **Dimorphic fungi:** The fungi that can switch between two morphologies: yeast and mold are called **dimorphic fungi,** depending upon the environmental conditions and the phenomenon is termed as **fungal dimorphism** (Gr. *di* = two +

morphe = form). They are also **thermally dimorphic**–occuring as hyphae in natural habitat (such as soil) and converting to yeast form while growing as parasites at body temperature, or when grown at 37°C and enriched media.

Examples: *Histoplasma capsulatum, Blastomyces dermatitids, Coccidioides* and *Paracoccidiodes.*

5. **Mushrooms:** A mushroom is a **macrofungus**, a reproductive structure which is fleshy, spore-bearing typically produced above the ground, on soil, or on its substrate from the dikaryotic septate mycelium.

   Examples: *Agaricus bisporus* (edible mushroom) and *Amanita muscaria* (poisonous mushroom that causes death of a person on consumption).

SYSTEMATIC CLASSIFICATION OF FUNGI

C.J. Alexopoulos and **C.W. Mims,** American mycologists, in 1979 proposed a **fungal classification system** and put the fungi including **slime molds** in the kingdom ***Myceteae*** of the superkingdom ***Eukaryota***, which in addition includes four other kingdoms.

Formerly fungi were classified in four classes:
Phycomycetes, Ascomycetes. Basidiomycetes and *Deuteromycetes* (Fungi imperfecti).
Currently *Myceteae* is classified into six divisons/phyla, based on sexual spores/sexual reproduction, morphology (spore colour, microscopic features, nature of hyphae) and DNA analysis:

- *Chytridromycota* (**chytrids,** aquatic molds) – Reproduce asexually by zoospores.
- *Zygomycota* (**conjugate fungi,** bread molds) – Aseptate hyphae, sporangiospores (asexual spores in sporangia) and zygospores (sexual spores in zygosporangia). Examples: *Mucor, Rhizopus.*
- *Ascomycota* (**sac fungi**) – **Ascospores** produced in sac-like structures **asci** and fruiting bodies called **ascocarps.** Examples: *Saccharomyces* (yeast), and *Aspergillus, Penicillium* (molds).
- *Basidiomycota* (**club fungi**) – **Basidiospores**, the sexual spores produced externally on club-like structures called **basidia** and **basidiocarps**. Examples: *Cryptococcus neoformans, Amanita.*
- *Glomeromycota* (**arbuscular mycorrihrzal fungi**) – Growing in symbiotic association with plant roots. Example:

- *Amastigomycota* (***Deuteromycota***) – The imperfect fungi – fungi producing asexual spores only, i.e., lacking a sexual state hence called **imperfect fungi** and were placed in the *Fungi imperfecti* or *Deuteromyetes*. Most fungi of medical importance belong to this division.

MYCOSES (HUMAN FUNGAL INFECTIONS)

Human diseases resulting from fungal infections, primarily by yeasts and molds, are called **mycoses** (sing. **mycosis**) (the term derived from Greek *mykes* – fungi and *osis* – disease process). Mycotic infections occur on the skin, mucous membranes, and internal organs or systems. Fungi also cause **respiratory allergies, mycotoxicoses** (intoxications due to ingesting fungal toxins e.g., aflatoxins) and **mycetism (or mycetismus)** (due to consuming poisonous mushrooms, e.g., *Amanita* spp).

The human mycotic agents are classified into two types:

- **True fungal pathogens** – cause diseases in healthy, noncompromised individuals.
- **Opportunistic fungal pathogens** – These fungi invade only when host defenses are weakened (*Candida, Cryptococcus*).

Mycoses are categorized based on the type and level of infection and their degree of pathogenicity into four types:

- **Superficial mycoses**
- **Cutaneous mycoses**
- **Subcutaneous mycoses**
- **Systemic mycoses**

LABORATORY DIAGNOSIS OF MYCOTIC INFECTIONS

Early diagnosis of fungal infections is critical for effective treatment. Common approaches for the laboratory diagnosis of fungal infections are:

- **Direct microscopic examination** of clinical samples, (e.g., sputum, biopsy, CSF and/or skin scrapings) including histopathology and identification.
- **Culturing of the fungus** (especially on Sabouraud dextrose agar, SDA). Based on colour of colonies, hyphae (septate or aseptate), asexual spores (sporangiospores, conidia-colour, septation, shape), sexual spores (ascospores basidiospores, zygospores) and fruiting bodies.

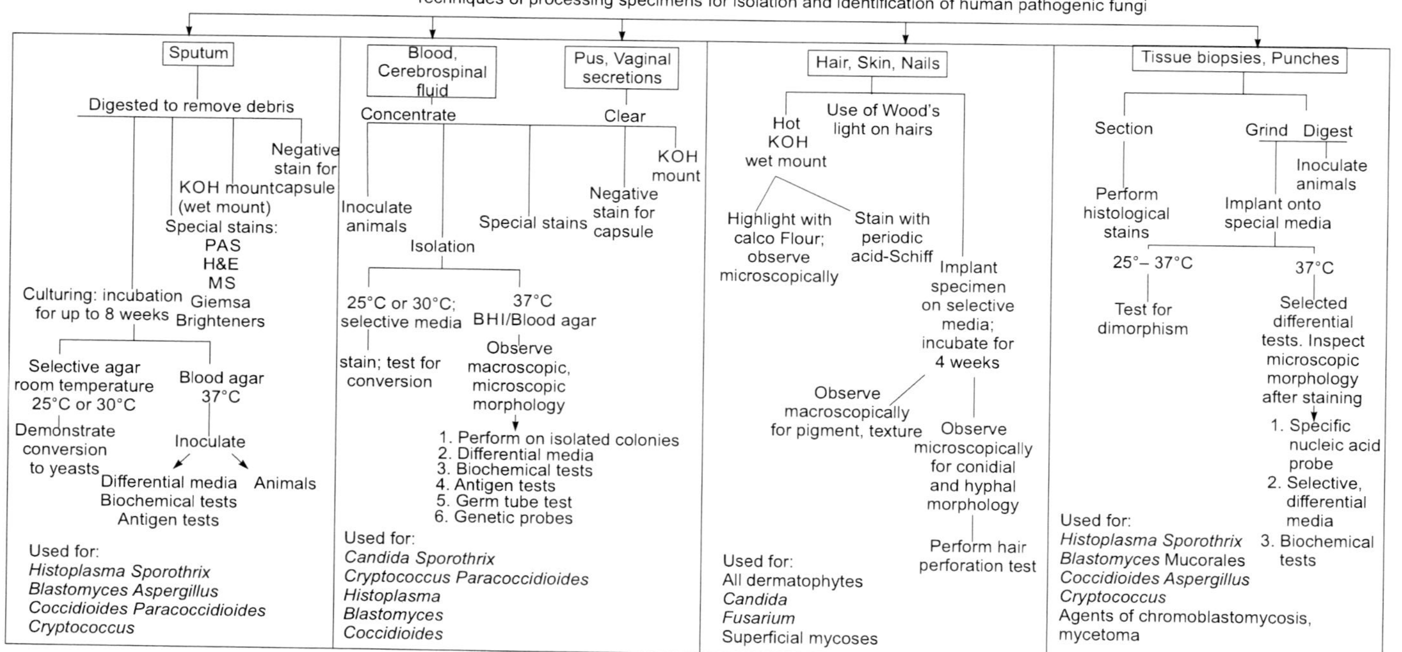

Fig. 64.1 Diagnosis of mycotic infections. Laboratory procedures used for processing specimens applicable to specific fungal pathogens.

- **Antigen detection tests** — tests to detect fungal polysaccharides or proteins in the body fluids using specific antibodies.
- **Serologic tests** — tests to detect antibodies in the patient's semen or spinial fluid by immunodiffusion, complement fixation (CF) and enzyme immunoassay (EIA).
- **Molecular diagnostics** (DNA probe tests): Polymerase chain reaction (PCR) and proteomics profiling/finger printing.

Animal inoculations: Test performed only to help diagnose systemic mycoses when other methods are indeterminant.

A suitable specimen for laboratory diagnosis can be obtained from skin scrapings, hair , nails, skin biopsies, sputum, blood, cerebrospinal fluid, tissue exudates, urine or vaginal samples, based on the patient's symptoms. Methods of processing different specimens to diagnose mycotic agents are outlined in Fig. 64.1.

KEY POINTS

- **Fungi** are eukaryotic, achlorophyllous, heterotrophic, spore producing microorganisms having cell wall composed of chitin and glucans.
- They are classified in the kingdom *Myceteae* (*Fungi*).
- Study of human pathogenic fungi-**mycoses** is called **medical mycology.**
- Fungi include microscopic organisms—molds and yeasts and macroscopic organisms mushrooms.
- Human pathogenic fungi show the phenomenon of **dimorphism,** exist in two forms, yeasts and molds when grown at two different temperatures: 25°C and 37°C.
- **Mycoses** are classified as superficial, cutaneous, subcutaneous, systemic and opportunistic mycoses.
- **Diagnosis** and identification of mycotic infections is made by direct microscopic examination and stained specimens, culturing of pathogen on selective and enriched media, serology and molecular methods (DNA).

IMPORTANT QUESTIONS

1. Describe the diagnosis of mycotic infections from different kinds of samples.
2. Write short notes on:
   (a) Based on morphology how fungi are classified?
   (b) How mycoses are classified?
   (c) Systematic classification of fungi.

MULTIPLE-CHOICE QUESTIONS

1. All are true for fungi EXCEPT:
   (a) Eukaryotic
   (b) Heterotrophic
   (c) Chitin in cell wall
   (d) Do not produce spores.

2. Most fungi of medical significance belong to:
   (a) *Deuteromycota* (*Deuteromycetes*)
   (b) *Ascomycota* (*Ascomycetes*)
   (c) *Basidiomycota* (*Basidiomycetes*)
   (d) *Zygomycota* (*Zygomycetes*).

3. The ability of a fungus to alternate between hyphae and yeast phases in response to temperature is known as:
   (a) Binary fission
   (b) Dimorphism
   (c) Sporulation
   (d) All of the above.

4. All of the following fungi are molds EXCEPT:
   (a) *Cryptococcus*
   (b) *Epidermophyton*
   (c) *Aspergillus*
   (d) *Penicillium*.

ANSWERS TO MCQs

1. (d) **2.** (a) **3.** (b) **4.** (a).

65

Superficial, Cutaneous and Subcutaneous Mycoses

Pityriasis versicolor; Piedras; Dermatophytoses; Sporotrichosis; Mycetoma; Chromoblastomycosis

Superficial mycoses are fungal infections localized on hair shafts and superficial skin cells, i.e., outer layer of epidermis. These include:

- **Pityriasis versicolor** and **tinea nigra** (causing skin infections)
- **Black piedra** and **white piedra** (causing hair infections)

PITYRIASIS VERSICOLOR (DANDRUFF)

Dandruff (also called **scurf, tinea versicolor** or **pityrasis capitata**) noncontagious superficial mycosis, is caused by *Malassezia furfur* (*Pityrosporum orbiculare* = *P. ovale*) a lipophilic basidiomycetous yeast. It is one of the most common superficial mycoses. Discolored skin pigmentation is the characteristic symptom, hence called **tinea versicolor.**

M. furfur is a budding yeast resembling phialides bearing phialoconidia and short angular hyphae requiring fats to grow, hence common in areas with many sebaceous glands, on the scalp, face and upper part of the body where it grows too rapidly. On Sabouraud's agar supplemented with olive oil at 37°C produces budding cells (8 μm) showing phialidic ontogeny (Fig. 65.1).

M. furfur is characterized by the short curved hyphal elements along with round yeast cells that are round at one end and flattened at the point of conidiation.

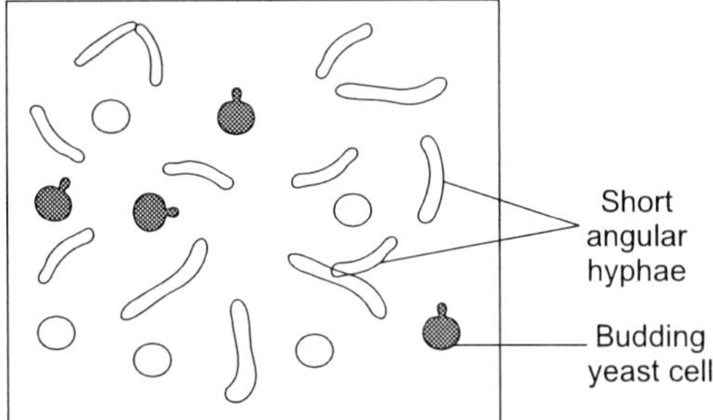

Fig. 65.1 ***Malassezia furfur*, a lipophilic basidiomycetous yeast.**

SYMPTOMS

The disease manifests as hyper- or hypo-pigmented macules of the skin alongwith flaking of dead skin that forms on the human's scalp, redness and irritation. Aggravated by exposure to dust, UV light, hair dyes and harsh shampoos.

DIAGNOSIS

- Skin lesions will fluoresce under Wood's lamp.
- Scrapings treated with KOH will reveal both the hyphae and yeast forms microscopically.

TREATMENT

- Apple cider vinegar, and salt and lemon juice, are the common household remedies.
- Selenium sulfide found in dandruff shampoo can be spread over lesions, in most cases.

PIEDRAS — WHITE AND BLACK

Piedra (a Spanish word for **stone**) is a fungal disease of the hair that appears as white or black small stony nodules (masses) on individual hair shafts. It is of two types: white piedra and black piedra.

WHITE PIEDRA

White piedra (or **tinea blanca**) is a superficial mycosis of the terminal hair shaft caused by *Trichosporon beigelii* (= *T. cutaneum*) a basidiomycetous pleomorphic yeast.

SYMPTOMS

It is characterized by the presence of numerous light coloured – white, light brown or yellow soft nodules (stones) loosely attached to the hair shafts. The disease may develop on scalp hair, eyebrows and eyelashes, beard, mustaches, underarm hair and pubic hair.

TRICHOSPORON BEIGELII

It is a urease-positive, soil-borne yeast, having cells with a diameter of 3–8 μm septate hyaline hyphae, each cell acts as an arthroconidium, either of which can predominate in the tissue.

On cornmeal–tween agar at 25°C after 72 hr of incubation, colonies white to creamish, waxy, wrinkled producing abundant, pseudohyphae, hyphae, blastoconidia with barrel or elongate arthroconidia. Production of urease-enzyme is a significant feature.

TRANSMISSION

The disease can spread to people when they come in contact with contaminated soil, water, plants and animals. Person-to-person spread is uncommon.

DIAGNOSIS

Microscopic examination of the affected hair for the presence of yeast-like cells and septate hyphae.

TREATMENT

- Shaving the affected area is the preferred treatment
- Topical application of antifungal lotions or creams (e.g., clotrimazole 1% or ketaconozole 2%).

BLACK PIEDRA

It is a superficial mycosis of the scalp hair shaft caused by an ascomycetous, soil-borne fungus *Piedraia hortae* (*Ascomycota*), usually seen in the tropics worldwide where it is hot and humid. *P. hortae* in some societies is used for cosmetic purposes to darken hair.

SYMPTOMS

Characteristic dark brown to black oval nodules (1–2 mm) firmly adherent on hair shafts causing disintegration and breakage of the hair fiber, predominantly produce on the hair of the scalp and beard.

PIEDRA HORTAE

P. hortae, on agar media at 25°C, grows very slowly producing red pigmented greenish-black colonies. It is keratinolytic producing characteristic arthroconidia (asexual spores), tightly packed darkly pigmented hyphae and asci, each ascus containing 2–8 crescent-shaped ascospores within black nodules that are actually fruiting bodies of the fungus called **ascostromata.**

LABORATORY DIAGNOSIS

- Characteristic red pigmented greenish colonies on agar media.
- Microscopically it shows thick-walled resting cells (**chlamydoconidia**) on short dark hyphae.
- KOH treated infected hair fluoresce under UV light.
- Microscopic examination of hair nodules (ascostromata) for asci and ascospores.
- Sequence analysis of the nuclear ribosomal internal transcribed spacer region.

TREATMENT

The infection is usually treated with cutting or shaving of the hair followed by the application of antifungal topical agents.

CUTANEOUS MYCOSES (DERMATOPHYTOSES)

Fungal infections that affect keratin-containing tissues such as hair and nails and skin are called **cutaneous mycoses.** These are caused by three genera of **dermatophytes** (***Trichophyton, Epidermophyton*** and ***Microsporum***), molds that require **keratin,** a protein, found in skin and nails for their growth hence are termed **dermatophytoses** (Gr. *dermato* = skin, fungal, *phyton* = plant, osis). Fungal infections of the skin was the 4th most common skin disease in 2010 affecting 984 million and an estimated 1.6 million people dying each year of fungal infections.

Common terms used for these diseases are **ringworm** because of the dramatic ringed appearance that results from the gradual spread of inflammation from the center to the newest area of invasion in a circumferential pattern, and **tinea** infections (from Latin a larva or worm) because early observers thought they were caused by worms.

Based on the body region infected, dermatophytoses (tineas) are, clinically classified into seven types:

• Tinea corporis (ringworm)	Body smooth parts
• Tinea capitis (ringworm)	Scalp
• Tinea pedis (athlete's foot)	Feet
• Tinea barbae (barber's itch)	Beard
• Tinea cruris (jock itch)	Groin
• Tinea unguium (onychomycosis)	Toes and finger nails
• Tinea mannum (two feet one hand)	Hands

CHARACTERISTICS OF DERMATOPHYTIC GENERA

Dermatophytes are differentiated based on: macroconidia, microconidia and unusual type of hyphae (Fig. 65.2).

These **anamorphic** (imperfect or deuteromycetous) mold genera (*Trichophyton, Microsporum* and *Epidermophyton*) with over 40 known species belong to *Arthroderma*, a teleomorphic genus of *Ascomycota*.

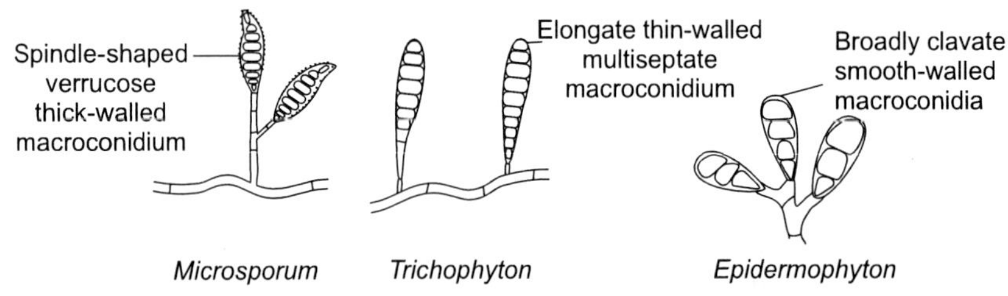

Fig. 65.2 Dermatophyte macroconidia forms. Two types of asexual spore: macroconidia and microconidia are produced by many dermatophyte species and their classification is based on the morphology.

Trichophyton: **Macroconidia** are clavate to fusiform, thin-walled smooth, borne laterally directly on the hyphae or short pedicels, 8–50 µm and 4–8 µm, and **microconidia** are numerous, spherical, pyriform to clavate, 2-3 µm × 2-4 µm.

The members cause athlete's foot, ringworms and jock itch.

Microsporum: **Macroconidia** are multiseptate, fusiform, spindle-shaped to ovate, echinulate to verrucose cell walls, 30–160 µm × 7–20 µm. **Microconidia** are unicellular, pyriform to clavate, smooth walled 4–7 µm × 2.5–3.5 µm. Both are borne on short conidiophores (conidiogenous cells).

Species cause tinea capitis and tinea corporis.

Epidermophyton: **Microconidia** are not produced in this fungus. **Macroconidia** are thin-walled, 1-9 septate, Beaver tail shaped, borne singly or in clusters of 2 to 3, 20-40 μm × 7-12 μm. Arthroconidia are also produced in culture. *E. floccosum* causes athlete's foot, tinea cruris, tinea corporis and onychomycosis.

TRANSMISSION

The natural reservoirs of dermatophytes are other humans, animals and the soil. They are transmitted by direct contact with an infected host (human or animal), or by direct or indirect contact with infected shed skin or hair in fomites such as clothing, towels, combs, hair brushes, caps, theatre seats, furniture, bed linens, shoes, shocks, hotel rugs, sauna, bathhouse, locker room floors, coolers and air conditioners. Transmission may also occur from soil-to-skin contact. Depending upon the fungal species, the organism may survive in the environment for up to 15 months.

SYMPTOMS

Symtoms begin 4–14 days after exposure resulting in a red, itchy, scaly and raised red rings of ringworm on the skin. Multiple areas can be affected at a given time, nails may thicken, discolor or begin to crack (onychomycosis).

DIAGNOSIS

- By their physical appearance on the body.
- Direct microscopic examination of KOH treated samples of hair, skin scarpings and nail debris.
- Wood's lamp (UV) examination of infected hairs for specific dermatophytes (e.g., *microsporum*) that fluoresce.
- Culturing on Sabourand's agar medium at 25°C for 3-4 weeks and identification based on colony, morphology, hyphae and sporulating structures.
- Culturing of specimen on a special agar medium (e.g., *dermatophyte test medium, DTm* based on a simple colour test) at room temperature and observed for bright red colour within 14 days of incubation, identifies a dermatophyte.

TREATMENT

Ringworms are treated with the application of antifungal topical agents (e.g., micronazole, terbinatine, clotrimazole, ketoconazole and tolnaftate) twice daily until symptoms resolve. To prevent recurrence, topical treatments are to be continued for a further 7 days after resolution of visible symptoms, the total duration lasting for 2-3 week.

In more severe cases for scalp ringworm, systemic antifungal treatment with oral medications is recommended.

PREVENTION

Preventive measures include:

- Avoid sharing clothing, towels, sheets and sport equipment.
- Avoid walking barefoot.
- Avoid touching pets with bald spots.
- Wash clothes in hot water with fungicidal soap after suspected exposure to ringworm.
- To prevent spreading the infection, lesions should not be touched, and good hygiene to be maintained with washing hands and the body.

SUBCUTANEOUS MYCOSES

Subcutaneous mycoses are localized fungal infections beneath the skin. These are caused by soil saprophytes.

Sporotrichosis, mycetoma (mycotic) and chromoblastomycosis are the well known examples.

SPOROTRICHOSIS

Sporotrichosis, also called **rose thorn** or **rose-gardener's disease,** (because roses can spread it) is a skin infection caused by a saprophytic fungus *Sporothrix schenkii,* associated with soiled plant matter (e.g., rose thorns, sphagnum moss). It usually affects gardeners, farmers and agricultural workers.

SYMPTOMS

The first symptom of sporotrichosis is usually a small bump or nodule on the arm, finger or hand that appears 1–12 weeks after exposure which eventually becomes larger and resembles a sore or ulcer. Immunocompromised individuals develop disseminated infections/ or pneumonia, called *pulmonary sporotrichosis* that can cause shortness of breath, cough and fever.

CHARACTERISTICS OF *SPOROTHRIX SCHENKII*

S. schenckii is a deuteromycetous **dimorphic fungus**, with hyphal and conidial growth in the environment and at 25°C on Sabouraud's agar and yeast phase at body temperature (i.e., 37°C) and in host's tissues.

It is characterized by cream to dark brown moist mycelial colony commonly with wrinkled or folded surfaces at 25°C on SDA producing hyaline (glass-like) or dark coloured single-celled conidia developing as floral clusters on sympodially growing conidiophores (Fig. 65.3).

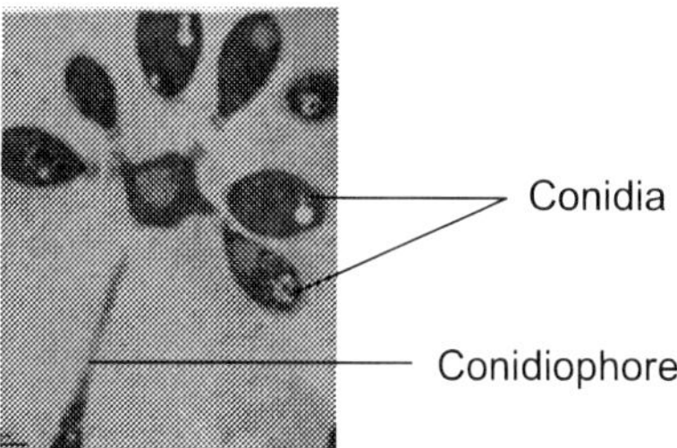

Fig. 65.3 ***Sporothrix schenckii.*** A conidiophore with conidia arranged as a floral cluster at its tip.

Yeast phase is characterized by elongated cigar-shaped budding cells (2–6 μm long), white or off-white colonies at 37°C.

DIAGNOSIS

- Swabbing or taking a biopsy of an infected site by culturing the fungus on SDA at 25°C and 37°C.
- **Sporothrichin skin test** that uses the antigen produced from the fungus.
- Molecular methods – PCR (amplification of the gene) and ELISA (serum antibody).

TREATMENT

Treated by antifungal drugs that include:

- Itraconazole (or terbinafine) taken orally for 3–6 months
- Amphotericin B is the drug of choice for disseminated infection
- Oral administration of saturated **potassium iodide** solution, the first effective treatment, is still the drug of choice.

MYCETOMA (MADURA FOOT)

Mycetoma (**Madura foot, mycetoma pedis** and **maduromycosis**) is a localized chronic subcutanous tumor-like inflammation of the foot or leg caused by fungi and filamentous aerobic bacteria (actinomycetes). The disease was initially named **Madura foot** and **Maduromycosis,** after the place Madurai, in South India, where it was first identified in 1842 by Gill. It is characterized by nodules that discharge an oily, pus, and looks superficially like a tumor, hence named **mycetoma** meaning fungal tumor. When it is caused by fungi, it is termed **mycotic mycetoma** (or **eumycetoma**), and when caused by bacteria, it is called **actinomycotic mycetoma** (or **actinomycetoma**).

The disease is endemic to Sudan, Venezuela, Mexico and South India (TN state) frequently in rural people, particularly, farmers and shepherds.

It is caused by common fungal and bacterial saprotrophs found in soil such as:

- *Madurella mycetomatis* – Deuteromycetous fungus producing pigmented colonies (due to pyomelanin) with black grains (sclerotia) (1–2 mm) on potato carrot agar. Two types of conidia — oval to pyriform (3–5 µm) on simple or branded conidiophores, and small spherical conidia (3 µm) on phialides and collarettes.
- *Nocardia brasiliensis**
- *Streptomyces somaliensis**
- *Actiomadura madurae**
- *Actinomadura pelletieri**

  * Filamentous bacteria called actinomycetes are Gram-positive, aerobic bacteria producing spores in chains from the aerial branches.

TRANSMISSION

The causative agents (fungi and aerobic bacteria) are saprophytes of soil or vegetable matter always that gain entry through traumatic inoculation, such as stepping on a needle or weed splinter, or through a pre-existing wound.

DIAGNOSIS

- Primary diagnosis is made by the presence of grains in pus collected from draining sinuses or in biopsy material.

- Microscopic examination of granules (sclerotia).
- Culturing of the fungus on Sabouraud's dextrose agar (supplemented with chloramphenicol, an antibacterial antibiotic, and cycloheximide, an antifungal antibiotic, to inhibit the growth of fungal contaminants) at 25°C for 7 days.

TREATMENT

Combined surgical and antifungal treatment is used to treat eumycetomas. Drugs like ketoconazole, itraconazole or voriconazole (200–400 mg) are used daily for 6 months or until complete cure.

CHROMOBLASTOMYCOSIS

Chromoblastomycosis (also called **chromomycosis, phaeosporotrichosis, cladosporiosis, Foriseca' disease,** and **pedroso's disease)** is a long-term mycosis of the skin and subcutaneous tissue (a chronic subcutaneous mycosis) caused by dematiaceous (pigmented or melanized) fungi that produce sclerotic bodies in tissue. The term is derived from Greek: *Chroma* = color + *blasto* = germ + *mycosis* due to the presence of pigmented yeasts resembling copper pennies in infected tissue. The disease is worldwide in distribution, however, Madagascar and Japan have the highest incidence. Males between the ages of 30 and 50 are affected more.

SYMPTOMS

It is characterized by warty dry nodule or plaque crusted lesions usually involving the limb which can enlarge abnormally (elephantiasis).

CHARACTERISTICS OF MYCOTIC AGENTS

The fungi causing chromoblastomycosis are:

- *Fonsecacea predosoi*
- *Phialophoa verrucosa*
- *Cladophiarophora carrionii*
- *Fonsecacae compacta*

These organisms, members of the family *Dematiaceae* belonging to *Deuteromycetes* (currently classified in the *Ascomycota*), are identified on the basis of conidial pigmentation, morphology, septation and mode of production from the conidiogenus cell/conidiphore.

DIAGNOSIS

- Microscopic examination of KOH treated lesion scrapings for the presence of *medlar bodies* (also called *muriform bodies* or *sclerotic cells*) and pigmented yeasts after staining with lactophenol or periodic acid shiff.
- Culturing the mold from the lesion scrapings on SDA at 25°C for 1 to 3 weeks resulting in dark brown/black velvetty colonies.

TREATMENT

Although it is very difficult to cure the disease, the primary treatment of choice consists of:

- Oral use of itraconazole alone or in combination with flucytosine.
- Alternatively, it is treated with *cryosurgery* with liquid nitrogen.

KEY POINTS

- **Superficial mycoses** are localized on hair shafts and superficial skin cells which include **tinea versicolor** and **white** and **black piedras.**
- **Cutaneous mycoses** or **dermatophytoses** caused by dermatophytes (*Trichophyton*, *Microsporum* and *Epidermophyton*), are infections of epidermis, hair and nails and include **ringworm** of the body, scalp, foot and hand.
- **Mycetoma**, or **Madura foot,** that looks superficially like a tumor, is caused by *Madurella* that invades traumatized skin, is an example subcutaneous mycosis.
- **Chromoblastomycosis,** characterized by tough, warty (verrucous) lessions, is caused by dematiaceous (pigmented), soil-borne saprophytic fungi.
- **Sporotrichosis (rose-gardener's disease)** is caused by *Sporothrix schenckii,* a dimorphic fungus, that is characterized by conidia arranged as floral clusters on conidiophores.

IMPORTANT QUESTIONS

1. Write short notes on:
   (a) Tinea versicolor (dandruff).
   (b) Dermatophytes.
   (c) Madura foot.
   (d) Chromoblastomycosis.
   (e) Sporotrichosis.

MULTIPLE-CHOICE QUESTIONS

1. All of the followings are examples of superficial mycoses, EXCEPT?
   (a) Black piedra
   (b) Tinea versicolor
   (c) Tinea pedis
   (d) Tinea nigra.

2. All of the following are examples of subcutaneous mycoses EXCEPT?
   (a) Mycetoma
   (b) Pityriasis versicolor
   (c) Sporotrichosis
   (d) Chromoblastomycosis.

3. Which of the following is a dimorphic fungus?
   (a) *Sporothrix schenckii*
   (b) *Madurella*
   (c) *Trichophyton*
   (d) *Phialophora verrucosa.*

4. Which of the following dermatophytes does not produce microconidia?
   (a) *Microsporum*
   (b) *Trichophyton*
   (c) *Epidermophyton*
   (d) None of the above.

5. Which of the following is the most common and effective method used for treatment of localized infection caused by dermatophytes that does not involve hair and nails?
   (a) Surgery
   (b) Oral antifungal therapy
   (c) Use of topical antifungal ointments
   (d) All of the above.

ANSWERS TO MCQs

1. (c) **2.** (b) **3.** (a) **4.** (c)
5. (a).

66

Systemic (Deep) Mycoses by True Pathogens

Histoplasmosis; Coccidioidomycosis; Paracoccidiodomycosis, Blastomycosis

Systemic mycoses, also called **deep mycoses,** are fungal infections deep within the body that affect internal organs. These are usually causd by soil-borne fungi and belong to any one of the two categories: primary (or true) pathogens and opportunisitic pathogens.

Systemic mycoses caused by true pathogens include:

Histoplasmosis, coccidioidomycosis, paracoccidiodomycosis and blastomycosis. These mycoses do not spread from human-to-human (i.e., non-contagious). These fungi are usually **dimorphic**.

Amphotericin B, an antifungal cidal antibiotic, first isolated in 1955 from *Streptomyces nodosum,* is the standard treatment for life-threatening, serious systemic mycoses. WHO in 2019 has considered it as the safest or most effective medicine needed in a health system.

HISTOPLASMOSIS: DARLING'S DISEASE

Histoplasmosis is a disease of the lung caused by inhaling conidia of *Histoplasma capsulatum,* a dimorphic ascomycetous, fungus, which is abundantly found is soil supplemented by bird and bat droppings called **guano** (from the Spanish *huanu* for dung). The disease is not **contagious** i.e., does not spread from person-to-person.

The disease is often called **Darling's disease,** named after **Dr. Samuel Darling** who first described the causative agent in 1905. Other synonyms used are **Ohio Valley fever** and **reticuloendotheliosis.** The disease is worldwide in distribution, but it is particularly common in North Central America especially Ohio and Mississippi River Valleys. Around 2,50,000 people are infected each year in the U.S.

CHARACTERISTICS OF *HISTOPLASMA CAPSULATUM*

H. capsulatum is typically dimorphic, producing mycelial growth on agar medium at 25°C (or below 35°C) and at 37°C on blood agar dense and waxy yeast colony (Fig. 66.1).

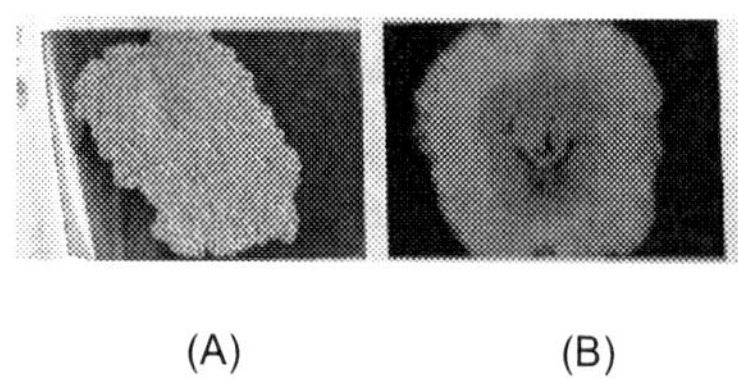

(A) (B)

Fig. 66.1 Cultural characteristics of *Histoplasma capsulatum*. (A) A colony at 25°C produces a fuzzy mycelium. (B) A yeast colony (37°C) is dense and waxy.

Mycelial stage is characterized by two types of conidia:

Macroconidia–thick-walled, globose (8–15 μm) tuberculate with finger-like projections produced terminally on conidiogenous cells and **microconidia**–thin-walled, small (2–4 μm) produced in natural habitat (or at 25°C) (Fig. 66.2)

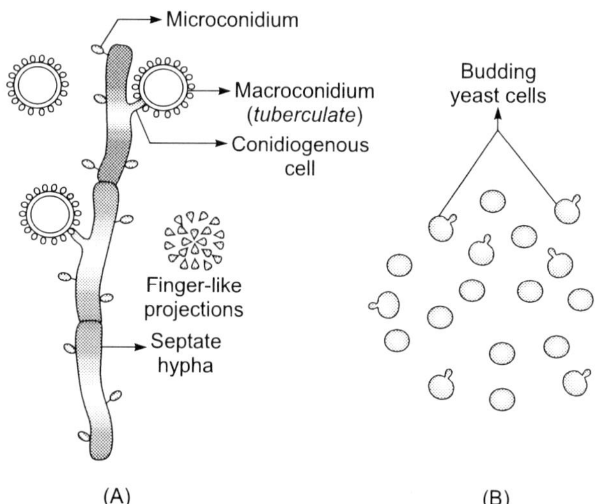

Fig. 66.2 ***Histoplasma capsulatum:*** (A) Mycelial phase at 25°C and in soil. (B) Yeast phase in tissues and at 37°C in culture medium.

Budding stage is characterized by clusters of budding yeast cells (2-4 μm) within phagocytes (in human's tissue) and at 37°C.

Teleomorphic state (or perfect state or ascomycetous state) is called *Ajellomyces capsulatus* (syn. *Emmonsiella capsulata*) which is characterized by **cleistothecia** (ascocarps) having 8-spored evanescent asci.

MODE OF INFECTION/TRANSMISSION

The disease is acquired by inhaling airborne conidia in demolition projects that contain bat and bird droppings. The airborne spores can travel hundreds of feet. Infants, young children and elderly are more likely to be infected. People with suppressed immune system are at higher risk.

CLINICAL TYPES AND SYMPTOMS

Symptoms appear between 3 and 17 days after exposure. Clinically it is of two types:

Pulmonary histoplasmosis: Symptoms are similar to those of pneumonia, similar to flu such as fever, chills, sweats, a dry cough, malaise and chest pain. Joint pain is also experienced by some people.

Disseminated histoplasmosis: Infection spreads and multiple organs are involved, such as *central nervous system* involvement leads to severe symptoms including seizures, headaches and confusion may develop. Eye involvement can cause loss of vision.

LABORATORY DIAGNOSIS

The diagnosis of histoplasmosis rests upon demonstrating the fungus or an immune response to the fungus. The lab tests used are:

- **Direct microscopy:** KOH treated samples of infected tissues are examined microscopically to detect oval yeast cells within macrophages and free tissue.
- Culture of body fluids or tissues on Sabouraud's agar at 25°C and at 37°C in glucose cystein blood agar to identify the fungus.
- Detection of surface markers of *Histoplasma* antigens in a urine test.
- Blood tests to measure antibody response to *Histoplasma* by ELISA or PCR.
- **CT scans** are useful to identify areas of spread in disseminated histoplasmosis.

TREATMENT

Severe infections or disseminated histoplasmosis is treated with amphotericin B (IV) followed by oral itraconazole for a period ranging from 6–12 weeks to several months or one year.

Mild symptoms do not require any treatment.

COCCIDIOIDOMYCOSIS: VALLEY FEVER

Coccidioidomycosis is a pulmonary fungal disease caused by *Coccidiodes immitis,* a dimorphic fungus. It is also called **Valley fever** or **San Joaquin Valley fever** because of its frequent occurrence in the San Joaquin Valley of California (USA). An estimated one lakh infections occur every year in the United States.

CHARACTERISTICS OF *COCCIDIOIDES IMMITIS*

C. immitis (Fig. 66.3) is a dimorphic saprophytic ascomycetous fungus and belongs to the family *Onygenaceae*. Its family grows as a mycelium that fragments into thick-walled, block-like (or barrel-shaped) arthroconidia (arthrospores), the infection stage occurring in dry alkaline soils and forms a moist, white, cottony colony on Sabouraud's agar medium at 25°C.

In tissues, the fungus forms a thick-walled body called a **spherule** (30 μm in diameter) filled with endospores which are formed by cleavage, each spherule resembling a giant sporangium. Each endospore after its release, spreads in tissue developing into a new spherule.

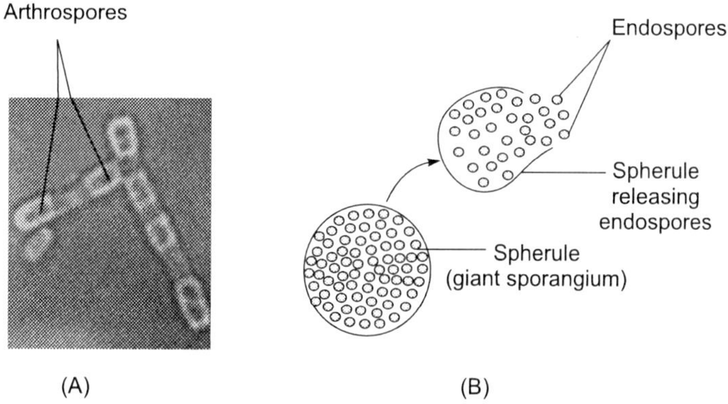

Fig. 66.3 ***Coccidioides immitis.*** (A) Arthrospores (conidia) produced by fragmentation of hyphae. (B) Formation of endospores from a spherule.

MODE OF INFECTION

The infection occurs when arthroconidia (asexual spores) are inhaled from dust after disruption of soil, especially during a dust storm, and reach the lungs. Wind storms may also cause epidemics in far from endemic areas. Signs and symptoms appear 1–3 weeks after exposure.

CLINICAL TYPES

The initial form of coccidiomycosis is the **Valley fever** (or acute coccidioidomycosis) with few or no symptoms, which can develop into a more serious disease: **chronic coccidioidomycosis** and **disseminated coccidioidomycosis.** The major symptoms are: fever, coughing, chest pain, headache, tiredness, rash, muscle or joint pain, and loss of smell or taste. In a few cases, the symptoms resembling tuberculosis spread throughout the body.

LABORATORY DIAGNOSIS

- By identifying distinctive spherules in sputum, spinal fluid and biopsies by Grocott's methenamine silver staining.
- Culturing of the fungus from fluids or lesions on Sabourauds's agar and induction of spherules.
- By DNA probes (PCR using specific nucleotide primers).
- By detecting fungal antigen (tube precipitin (TP) assay and ELISA).
- A tuberculin-like skin test is used in screening.

TREATMENT

Amphotericin B (intravenous) is the drug of choice to treat serious infections.

PARACOCCIDIOIDOMYCOSIS: SOUTH AMERICAN BLASTOMYCOSIS

Paracoccidioidomycosis (PCM), also called *South American blastomycosis*, is a mycosis of the lungs, skin, mucous membranes, lymph nodes and other internal organs caused by ***Paracoccidioides brasiliensis***. It is a chronic, often fatal, respiratory in origin, however, not transmitted directly from person-to-person. PCM has the highest prevalence of all systemic mycoses. It is endemic to South America with over 10 million people infected with the asymptomatic form with 2% developing clinically significant form.

CHARACTERISTICS OF *PARACOCCIDIOIDES BRASILIENSIS*

P. brasiliensis (= *Blastomyces brasiliensis*) named for its superficial resemblance to *Coccidioides* and its prevalence in Brazil, is **thermally dimorphic deuteromycetous**, soil-borne fungus. It produces thick-walled **chlamydoconidia**, the infection spores, on Sabouraud's dextrose agar supplemented with cycloheximide at 30°C (room temperature) for 4 weeks. They convert to invasive yeasts characterized by globose yeast cells, each mother cell with a series of narrow-necked buds that look like the spokes of a wheel (Fig. 66.4).

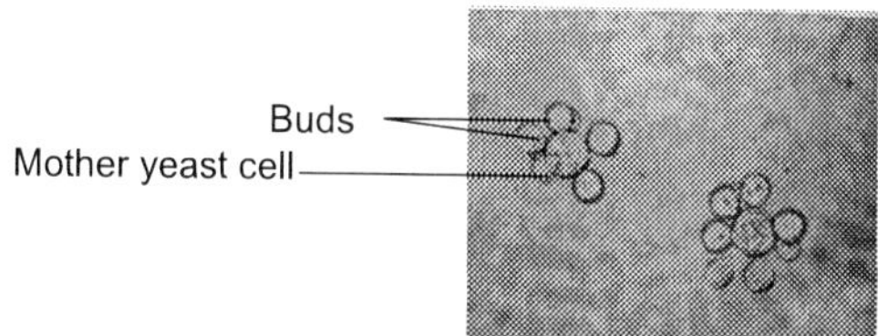

Fig. 66.4 ***Paracoccidioides brasiliensis* yeast phase.** Budding yeast cell looks like the spokes of a wheel, as observed in infected tissue (*in vivo*) and at 37°C on agar medium (*in vitro*).

CLINICAL TYPES

Chlamydoconidia (spores) produced from the mycelia are inhaled that convert to invasive yeasts in the lungs and from there spread to other sites via blood and lymphatics resulting in three clinical types:

- **Mucocutaneous:** Involve face, especially the nasal and oral mucocutaneous borders revealing enlarged lymph nodes discharging necrotic material through the skin.
- **Lymphatic:** Enlarged, but painless, cervical, supraclavicular or axillary nodes.
- **Visceral (multi-organ):** Enlargement of the liver, spleen and abdominal lymph nodes, sometimes causing abdominal pain.

An acute/subacute form usually manifests as *disseminated paracoccidioidomycosis* involving the lymph nodes, liver, spleen and bone marrow.

DIAGNOSIS

Specimens used for diagnosis include: blood, sputum and skin.

- **Direct microscopic examination** of fresh or stained clinical specimens for the distinctive large yeast mother cells with characteristic multiple buds (spokes of a wheel).
- **Culturing of the fungus** at 25–30°C and at 37°C.
- **Serological tests**

TREATMENT

- Oral itraconazole is generally considered the drug of choice.
- Intravenous amphotericin B is often used in severe cases.
- Sulfonamides (sulfa drug) such as trimethoprim/sulfa-methoxazole are also used in some countries due to their low cost.

BLASTOMYCOSIS: NORTH AMERICAN BLASTOMYCOSIS

Blastomycosis (also called **North American blastomycosis, Gilchrist's disease**) is a systemic fungal infection caused by inhaling conidia of *Blastomyces dermatitidis,* dimorphic fungus occurring in soil wood near lakes and rivers. It is a chronic infection of lungs (called **pulmonary blastomycosis**) which may spread to other tissues, particularly skin, bones and central nervous system.

The disease was first reported by **Thomas Casper Gilchrist** in 1894, hence also called **Gilchrist's disease.** It is endemic to some parts of United States and Canada.

CHARACTERISTICS OF *BLASTOMYCES DERMATITIDIS*

Blastomyces dermatitidis (Gr. *blastos* = germ + *myces* = fungus + *dermato* = skin + *itis* = inflammation) is a dimorphic fungus showing hyphal growth at 25°C, septate mycelium bearing ovoid conidia resembling tiny lollipops (Fig. 66.5) and budding yeast cells with thick walls with buds as large as the mother cell at 37°C/human body (Fig. 66.5). Sexual state of the fungus is ***Ajellomyces dermatitidis,*** a member of the phylum ***Ascomycota*** (family **Ajellomycetaceae**).

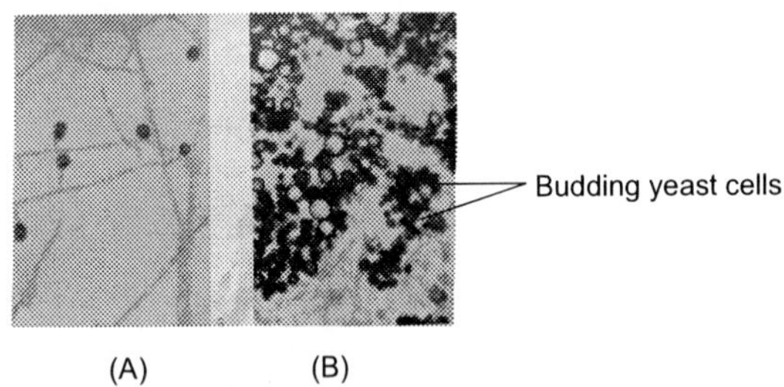

Fig. 66.5 ***Blastomysis dematitidis*, a dimorphic mycotic fungus.** (A) Mycelial phase at 25°C : septate hyphal filaments bearing conidia that resemble tiny lollipops. (B) Yeast phase in a sputum sample: Budding thick-walled yeast cells.

CLINICAL FEATURES

Respiratory tract infection occurs through inhalation of conidia, inhaling only 10 to 100 conidia is enough to initiate infection, and symptoms develop between 3 weeks and 3 months after exposure.

Mild disease is accompanied by non-productive cough, chest pain, hoarseness (dysphonia), fever, night sweats and muscle pain. More severe chronic blastomycosis to progress to lungs, skin (causing lesions–wart-like or ulcerated with smell particles at the margins) or bones (causing bone and joint pain).

LABORATORY DIAGNOSIS

- **Direct microscopy:** Demonstration of the characteristic broad-based thick walled buds in smears of sputum or tissues by KOH preparation is the most reliable diagnostic test.
- **Culturing of the fungus:** Dimorphic characteristics is the definitive diagnostic method, its slow growing nature can lead to delays in treatment of up to several weeks.
- **Antibodies test:** By complement fixation and ELISA tests.
- **Antigen testing:** Commercially available urine, antigen testing kit is used. It is quite sensitive and quick.

TREATMENT

- Oral use of itraconazole is the treatment of choice.
- Ketaconazole may also be used.
- For severe cases, amphotericin B, though toxic, is required.

KEY POINTS

- **Systemic mycoses** are fungal diseases of the internal organs and tissues.
- **Histoplasmosis** (**Darling's disease**), a disease of the lungs, is caused by dimorphic ascomycetous soil-borne (guano rich) fungus *Histoplasma capsulatum* (perfect state *Ajellomyces capsulatus*).
- **Coccidioidomycosis** (**Valley fever**), a pulmonary systemic disease, caused by *Coccidioides immitis* characterized by the production of arthroconidia in nature and *spherule* in tissues.
- **Paracoccidioidomycosis** (South American blastomycosis), a mycosis of lungs, is caused by *Paracoccidioides brasiliensis*, a thermally dimorphic deuteromycetous fungus.

- **Blastomycosis** (North American blastomycosis), a chronic infection of lungs, is caused by *Blastomyces dermatitidis,* that produces sexual, an ascomycetous perfect state *Ajellomyces dermatitidis.*
- Amphotericin B, an antifungal antibiotic, is the **drug of choice** to treat histoplasmosis and coccidioidomycosis.

IMPORTANT QUESTIONS

1. Write short notes on:
   (a) Thermally dimorphic fungi with their significance.
   (b) Histoplasmosis.
   (c) Systemic mycoses.

MULTIPLE-CHOICE QUESTIONS

1. The ability of a fungus to alternate between hyphae and yeast phases in response to temperature is termed:
   (a) Conversion
   (b) Binary fission
   (c) Sporulation
   (d) Dimorphism (thermally dimorphic).
2. Skin testing with antigen is a useful diagnostic procedure for:
   (a) Blastomycosis
   (b) Histoplasmosis
   (c) Coccidioidomycosis
   (d) Candidiasis.
3. Which fungus *does not* commonly cause systemic infection?
   (a) *Histoplasma*
   (b) *Malassezia*
   (c) *Coccidioides*
   (d) *Blastomyces.*
4. Which of the following fungal infections primarily involve the lungs?
   (a) Blastomycosis
   (b) Paracoccidioidomycosis
   (c) Histoplasmosis
   (d) All of the above.
5. Which of the following mycoses is acquired by inhalation of conidia from bird droppings?

(a) Blastomycosis
(b) Histoplasmosis
(c) Coccidioidomycosis
(d) Paracoccidioidomycosis.

6. Which of the following fungal agents of systemic mycoses are diagnosed by the presence of spherules in the infected organ?
(a) *Blastomyces dermatitidis*
(b) *Histoplasma capsulatum*
(c) *Coccidioides immitis*
(d) None of the above.

7. Which of the following drugs/antibiotics is the drug of choice to treat most of the systemic mycoses?
(a) Griseofulvin
(b) Thiabendazine
(c) Amphotericin B
(d) Fluconazole.

ANSWERS TO MCQs

1. (d)	**2.** (c)	**3.** (b)	**4.** (d)
5. (b)	**6.** (c)	**7.** (c).	

67

Opportunistic Mycoses

Candidiasis; Cryptococcosis; Aspergillosis; Pneumocystosis; Mucormycosis

Opportunisitic mycoses are infections of a compromised host caused by fungi which are not usually pathogenic; and are called **opportunisitic fungal pathogens**.
These mycoses are usually systemic, hence called **opportunisitic systemic mycoses**.

Common examples of opportunisitic pathogens are: The yeasts (*Candida, Cryptococcus, Pneumocystis*) and filamentous fungi (*Aspergillus, Mucor, Rhizopus, Cladosporium, Geotrichum*); and opportunisitic mycoses caused by these are candidiasis, cryptococcosis, aspergillosis, mucormycosis (zygomycosis) and pneumocystosis.

CANDIDIASIS: CANDIDIOSIS OR MONILIASIS

Candidiasis, also called **candidosis, moniliasis,** and **oidiomycosis,** is an opportunisitic fungal infection typically on the skin or mucous membranes caused by *Candida albicans,* a yeast that normally affects the skin, mouth, and vagina. Infection predominates in cases of lowered resistance (babies, pregnancy, AIDS and drug therapy) and arises from normal flora, or is transmissible through intimate contact.

CHARACTERISTICS OF *CANDIDA ALBICANS*

Candida, a genus of yeasts with over 61 species, is a member of the family *Saccharomycetaceae* (divison *Ascomycota*), formerly classified in the class *Deuteromycetes.* Many species are harmless commensals, including *C. albicans* found in the gut flora. *C. albicans* is the common cause of candidiasis (or thrush) in humans worldwide.

Its species name, *albicans*, comes from the Latin word *albus* for white. The yeast colony appears white when cultured on an agar plate at 25–30°C. And in case of certain infections, like thrush, it can create "white patches". *C. albicans* is a unique asexual (anamorphic) diploid and polymorphic fungus. It has budding yeast cells of varying size that may form elongate pseudohyphae, septate true hyphae and chlamydospores (encapsulated thick-walled cells) in host tissues (Fig. 67.1).

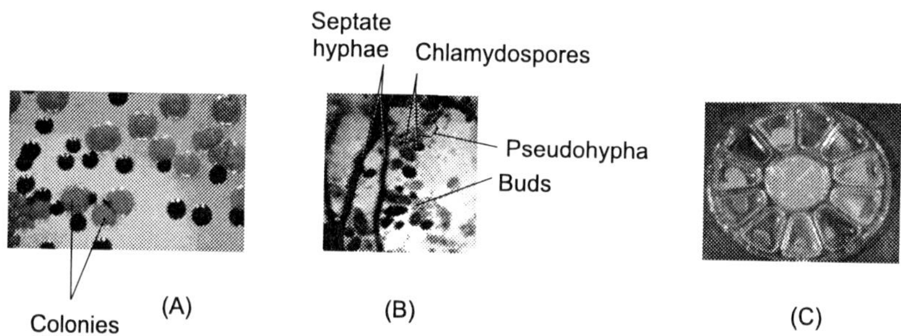

Fig. 67.1 ***Candida albicans***. (A) Pale blue colonies on trypan medium. (B) Septate hyphae, pseudohyphae, buds and chlamydospores in a vaginal smear. (C) Rapid yeast identification system using biochemical reactions to 12 test substances.

CLINICAL TYPES OF CANDIDIASIS

Infections caused by *C. albicans* range from human skin mycoses to fatal systemic diseases which are classified into five types based on the part of the body infected:

- **Urinary yeast infection:** Infection in the lower part of GT accompanied by a painful or burning sensation, abdominal or pelvic pain and blood in urine.
- **Genital yeast infection (genital candidiasis or VVC):** An itchy or painful swelling and redding and tissues at the opening of the vagina (ulva) with abnormal white discharge.
- **Penile candidiasis:** Men also have yeast infection *itchy rash* on his penis.
- **Oral thrush (or oropharyngeal candidiasis):** As a thick, white (appearance of cottage cheese), adherent growth on the mucous membranes of the mouth and throat.
- **Cutaneous (mucocutaneous) candidiasis:** An infection of the sweaty or moist areas of the skin (e.g. armpits, groin, skin between fingers and toes, under breasts) shining red rash.

- **Napkin (diaper) candidiasis** — Characterized by a scald-like rash on the skin in infants especially where diapers are not changed frequently.
- **Invasive candidiasis:** Bloodstream infection that travels to heart, brain, blood and eyes, a serious life-threating infection showing fever and chills.

LABORATORY DIAGNOSIS

- **Direct microscopy** of KOH treated clinical specimens (swab or scraping of the affected area) for visualization of budding yeast cells and pseudohyphae of *Candida*.
- **Culturing** of the yeast at 37°C (98.6°F) on agar plate (SDA, corn meal, trypan media), streaking the skin rubbed swab on agar media for characteristic yeast colonies that appear pale blue on **trypan media**.
- **Germ tube test.**
- **Rapid-multiple panel system** — It uses biochemical reactions to 12 test substances.
- **Molecular method** — DNA amplification technique (PCR) is used to identify the yeast directly from clinical samples.

TREATMENT

- Candidiasis is usually treated with topical antifungal agents, such as nystatin (mycostatin), miconazole (Monistat, Vagistat), clotrimazole (Lotrimin) and tioconazole used as creams, and are generally curative.
- One-time oral therapy (i.e., a single oral use) with **fluconazole** (150 mg) and **itraconazole** (600 mg) is effective and may be a more attractive alternative to some patients.

  Mild yeast infections are cured within 3 days while moderate to severe infections may take one to two weeks.

CRYPTOCOCCOSIS

Cryptococcosis (formerly known as **European blastomycosis, torulosis**), a life-threatening opportunisitic systemic infection involving the lungs and CNS, is caused by *Cryptococcus neoformans.* Globally one million cases of cryptococcosis are reported each year resulting in 6,25,000, deaths. It is most common in AIDS patients and infects respiratory, mucocutaneous and nervous system.

CHARACTERISTICS OF *CRYPTOCOCCUS NEOFORMANS*

C. neoformans occurs in soil, especially in bird droppings. It is a basidiomycetous encapsulated yeast with a perfect state (teleomorph) *Filobasidiella neoformans* (class *Tremellomycetes* divison *Basidiomycota*). In tissues, the yeast cells are large, spherical to ovoid with large constricted buds surrounded by a nonstaining large capsule (Fig. 67.2). In culture, they produce whitish mucoid colonies producing encapsulated spherical budding cells (5–10 µm in diameter). It is a melanin forming, urease producing yeast.

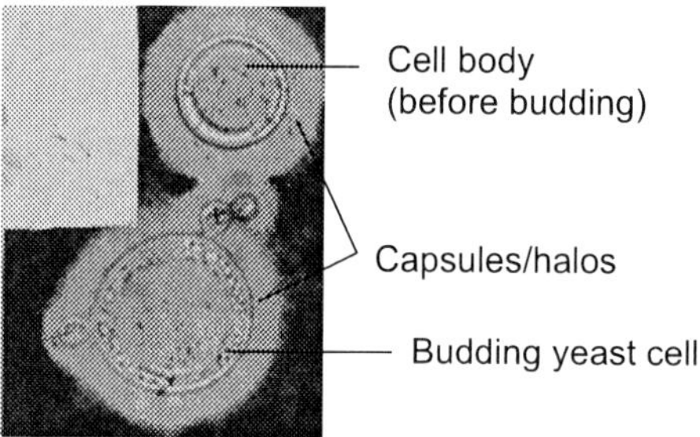

Fig. 67.2 ***Cryptococcus neoformans*** **from infected spinal fluid stained negatively with India ink.** Halos around the large spherical yeast cells are thick capsules. Also note the buds forming on one cell. Encapsulation is a useful diagnostic sign for cryptococcosis, although the capsule is fragile and may not show up in some preparations.

CLINICAL TYPES OF CRYPTOCOCCOSIS

Cryptococcosis is acquired by inhalation of airborne yeast cells, most likely biasidospores, from the enviornment which causes three types of infections in immunocompromised patients:

- *Pulmonary cryptococcosis*
- *Wound or cutaneous cryptococcosis*
- *Cryptococcal meningitis*

SYMPTOMS

These include fever, dry cough, headache, fatigue, blurred vision and confusion. Onset of symptoms is often subacute, progressively worsened over several weeks leading to pulmonary (lung) infection and meningitis (an infection in and around brain).

DIAGNOSIS

- **Direct microscpy** — Negative staining with media ink of the CSF to detect encapsulated (halos) budding cells, is the most useful diagnostic method.

- **Detection of cryptococcal antigen** (capsular material) in a specimen by serological tests. Latex agglutination test to detect antigen is a rapid diagnostic method.
- **Polymerase chain reaction** (PCR), a genetic identification method, is used on tissue specimens.
- **Culturing of the pathogen**.

TREATMENT

Intravenous amphotericin B with flucytosine (or fluconazole) by mouth is the best therapy over a period of weeks or months to treat systemic cryptococcosis.

ASPERGILLOSIS

Aspergillosis is an opportunisitic infection, allergic reaction or fungal growth caused by the *Aspergillus* fungus, especially *Apergillus fumigatus* commonly found indoors and outdoors. The illness is a result of a combination of exposure to the *Aspergillus* mold and a weak immune system. Aspergillosis is not contagious.

CHARACTERISTICS OF *ASPERGILLUS FUMIGATUS*

A. fumigatus, a thermophilic anamorphic (deuteromycetous) (can grow at as high as 55°C), is a fast-growing fungus. On Sabouraud's dextrose agar at 35°C, the colonies are dark blue green to slate gray. The **foot cell** produces long conidiophore bearing dome-shaped vesicles having phialides in one series on upper half only; head strongly columnar; conidia are smooth to echinulate (2–3.5 μm) (Fig. 67.3).

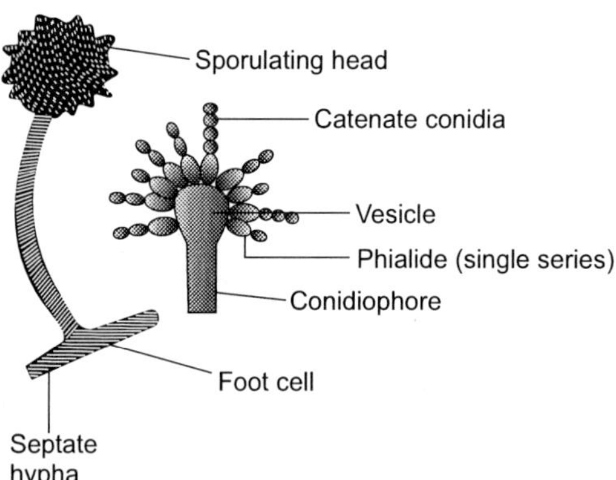

Fig. 67.3 ***Aspergillus fumigatus*** **sporulating structures:** Conidiophore arises from a foot cell and single series of phialides (sterigmata) bearing conidia in chains (catenate) arranged in basipetal manner (i.e., youngest conidium at the base and oldest at the top in the chain).

MODE OF INFECTION

Aspergillosis occurs by inhaling airborne conidia of ***Aspergillus*** (e.g., *A. fumigatus, A. terreus, A. niger*). *A. fumigatus* being the common cause responsible for mild to serious infections in persons with chronic infection and weak immune system (not in healthy individuals).

CLINICAL TYPES OF ASPERGILLOSIS

- **Allergic bronchopulmonary aspergillosis (ABPA)**. An allergy to *Aspergillus* showing coughing or sneezing without causing infection.
- **Allergic aspergillus sinusitis** — Inflammation of the sinuses showing drainage, stuffiness with headache.
- **Aspergilloma (fungus ball)** — Localized ball of the mold in the lungs called fungal ball or aspergillosis which is made up of fungus growth (mycelial mass), clots and white blood cells, often linked to CPA.
- **Chronic pulmonary aspergillosis (CPA)** — A long-term lung infection causing cavities with one or more balls.
- **Invasive pulmonary aspergillosis (IPA)** — A life threatening infection in lungs that produces a necrotic pneumonia with symptoms of a cough with or without blood, fever, chest pain and shortness of breath and disseminates to the brain, heart and other parts of the body (i.e., disseminated mycosis).
- **Cutaneous (skin) aspergillosis** — The fungus causes skin infection when it enters the body through a break on the skin (e.g., after surgery or a burn wound).

SYMPTOMS OF ASPERGILLOSIS

A repeated coughing up of blood, chest pain, with fever (38°C or above), wheezing (a whistling sound when breathing), shortness of breath, weight loss, shock, chills and blood clots.

DIAGNOSIS

- **Direct microscopy of specimens (lungs):** For the molds hyphae.
- **Fungus culture:** On Sabouraud's dextrose agar at 37°C (or higher temperature) since it is a thermophile. It produces abundant growth with conidia, a diagnostic feature of *A. fumigatus.*
- **Blood tests:** To check for antibodies and allergens.

- **Skin test:** Development of a hard, red bump on injecting a small amount of *Aspergillus* antigen into the skin of forearm, indicates the presence of antibodies to the mold in your blood.
- **Rapid antigen detection test:** By radioimmunoassay.

TREATMENT

The current medical treatment consists of combined antifungal therapy of voriconazole and amphotericin B in combination with surgical removal of the fungus tumor (ball) from the lung.

PNEUMOCYSTOSIS (PCP)

Pneumocystosis or **Pneumocystis jirovecii pneumonia**, PJP (previously known as PCP or **Pneumocystis carinii pneumonia**) is an infection of lungs caused by *Pneumocystis jirovecii,* an opportunisitic fungus. Originally classified as a protozoan, it is now known to be related to the yeast *Saccharomyces* and classified in the family *Pneumocystidaceae* (divison *Ascomycota*). PCP is seen in people with HIV/AIDS or among immunocompromised hosts.

CHARACTERISITICS OF *PNEUMOCYSTIS JIROVECII*

P. jirovecii is an ascomycetous, obligate **biotrophic** yeast, obtaining essential nutrition from living host cells, and has not been cultured *in vitro* (i.e., on agar media) It has a high tropism for the lung, hence its life cycle/morphology has been studied in lungs.

Three morphologically distinct stages observed in the lung are:

- **Ascus** with eight ascospores (= **spore case,** formerly known as **cyst**) (Fig. 67.4).
- **Diploid young ascus** before meiosis (= **pre-cyst**)
- **Ascospores** (= trophic form stage) that reproduce asexually by binary fission.

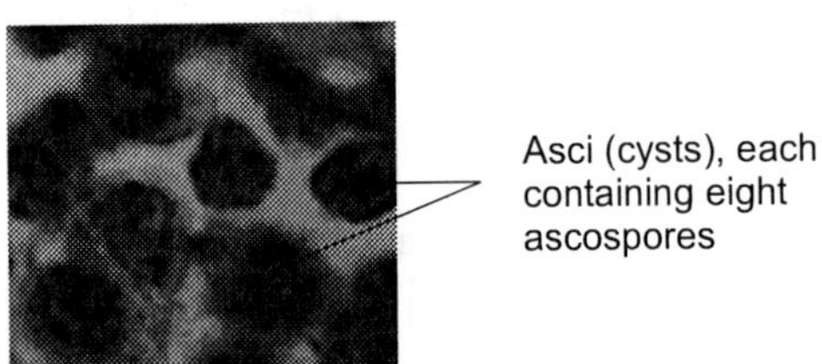

Fig. 67.4 ***Pneumocystis jirovecii*** **asci in the lung tissue of an AIDS patient.**

SOURCES AND SPREAD

PCP spreads from person-to-person through the air in droplets after being exposed to a person who has PCP or who is carrying the fungus in their lungs without having symptoms. The primary site of *Pneumocystis* infection is the lung alveoli.

SYMPTOMS

The symptoms of PCP can develop over several days to weeks and include: fever, cough, difficulty in breathing, chest pain, chills and tiredness.

DIAGNOSIS

- Microscopic examination of lung secretions (sputum or bronchoalveolar lavage) or lung tissue sample (a biopsy) stained with methenamine silver stain for asci (or cysts) each containing 8 ascospores (Fig. 67.4).
- PCR to *Pneumocystis* DNA
- A blood test to detect B-D glucan (a cell wall constituent of a fungus).

TREATMENT

Trimethoprim/sulfa methoxazole (TMP/SMX), which is also called co-trimoxazole, taken orally or given through a vein for 3 weeks, is the treatment of choice.

MUCORMYCOSIS (ZYGOMYCOSIS)

Mucormycosis also called **zygomycosis** and **phycomycosis**, is an opportunisitic mycosis caused by saprobic mucoraceous fungi, belonging to the class *Zygomycetes* (earlier called *Phycomycetes*) hence named. People with acidotic (diabetes and malnutritious) are severely affected by mucormycosis. The species in the genera most often involved are *Rhizopus, Mucor, Absidia* (now termed *Lichtheimia*) and *Cunninghamella* which are abundantly found in soil, organic debris and food.

CHARACTERISITICS OF MUCORACEOUS FUNGI

Mucor Exhibits rapid growth producing greyish-brown colonies–coenocytic hyphae producing hyaline erect unbranched to sympodially branched sporangiophores.

The sporangia are spherical, non-apophysate with pronounced columellate and conspicuous collarette at the base following sporangiospore dispersal and producing mucus bound sporangiospores (Fig. 67.5). *Mucor circinelloides* is the most infectious species.

Rhizopus: Characterized by horizontal aerial hyphae, called **stolons,** producing unbranched sporangiophores in clusters (umbels) just opposite the dark colored (pigmented) rhizoids, (named *Rhizopus,* from Gr. *rhiza* = root and *pous* = foot), columellate sporangia which produce, dry easily, wind-borne sporangiospores. *R. stolonifer* (syn *R. nigricans*) is commonly called **"bread mold"** (Fig. 67.6). *R. arrhizus* and *R. microsporus* are clinically significant.

Lichtheimia (Absidia): In *L. corymbifera* (*A. corymbifera*) sporangiophores arise from stolons in groups of 3–7 but never opposite the rhizoids as in *Rhizopus*. Spores are single celled, ellipsoidal, hyaline produced inside pyriform sporangia having a conical-shaped columella with a short projection (called apophysis) on the top (Fig. 67.5). It is a thermophilic mold.

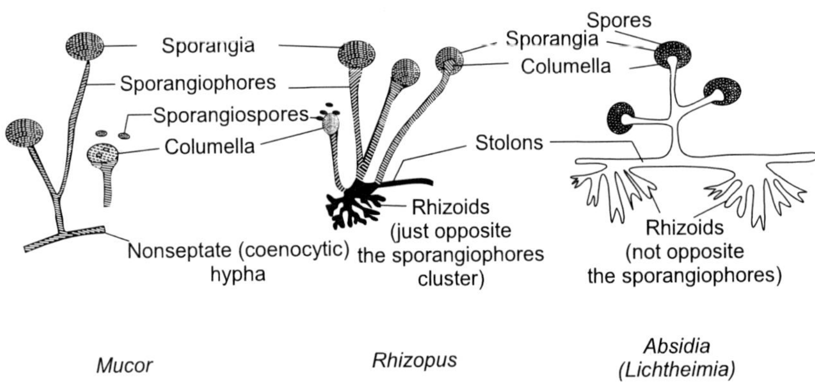

Fig. 67.5 Sporulating structures of three mucoraceous genera, the causative agents of mucormycosis.

CLINICAL TYPES

- **Rhinocerebral (sinus and brain) mucormycosis:** One side facial swelling, headache, sinus congestion, fever, black lesions on nasal bridge.
- **Pulmonary (lung) mucormycosis:** Fever, cough, chest pain and shortness of breath.
- **Cutaneous (skin) mucormycosis:** Blisters and ulcers surrounded with black skin.
- **Gastrointestinal mucormycosis:** Abdominal pain, nausea, vomiting and gastrointestinal bleeding.

- **Disseminated mucormycosis:** Infection in brain can develop mental status changes, coma and sometimes death.

MODE OF INFECTION

There are several portals of entry for a fungus such as nose, lungs, skin and oral cavity and progresses rapidly to a systemic infection.

LABORATORY DIAGNOSIS

- **Direct microscopic examination:** KOH treated tissue samples (biopsies/phlegm or nasal discharge) are examined for thick-walled, aseptate (nonseptate) hyphae scattered throughout the tissue for the mold.
- **Isolation and identification of molds on agar media** at 25° on Sabouraud's agar media for 4 days and identification by the colonial morphology, nature of hyphae and rhizoids, and sporangia.
- **Use of PCR**-based techniques on histologic specimens.

TREATMENT

Treatment consists of surgical removal of infected areas (called debridement) accompanied by antifungal drugs such as: amphotericin B (IV), posaconazole (IV or oral) and isavuconazole (IV or oral).

KEY POINTS

- **Candidiasis,** an opportunisitic mycosis, is caused by ***Candida albicans***, common yeast that normally resides in the mouth, vagina, intestine and skin of humans.
- **Cryptococcosis,** an opportunisitic mycosis, is caused by ***Cryptococcus neoformans***, an encapsulated basidiomycetous yeast that inhabits soils around pigeon roosts.
- **Aspergillosis,** an opportunisitic deep mycosis, is caused by ***Aspergillus fumigatus***, a themophilic common airborne mold.
- **Pneumocystosis** (called PCP), an infection of lungs in AIDS patients, is caused by an opportunisitic fungus, ***Pneumocystis jirovecii*** (previously considered to be a protozoan).
- **Mucormycosis** (or **zygomycosis**) is caused by mucoraceous fungi, such as ***Mucor circinelloides*, *Rhizopus arrhizus*, *R. microsporus* and *Lichtheimia* (= *Absidia*) *corymbifera*.**

IMPORTANT QUESTIONS

1. Write brief notes on:
   (a) Opportunisitic systemic mycoses.
   (b) Candidiasis.
   (c) Aspergillosis.

MULTIPLE-CHOICE QUESTIONS

1. Which of the following diseases is an opportunisitic mycosis?
   (a) Ringworm (b) Candidiasis
   (c) Histoplasmosis (d) Paracoccidioidomycosis.
2. Aspergillosis is recognized in the tissue by the presence of:
   (a) Budding cells (b) Pseudohyphae
   (c) Metachnomatic granules (d) Septate hyphae.
3. Which of the following is the least frequently responsible for causing infections in immunocompromised persons?
   (a) *Aspergillus fumigatus* (b) *Cryptococcus neoformans*
   (c) *Mucor* spp. (d) *Malassezia furfur*.
4. Each of the following statements concerning *Candida albicans* is true *EXCEPT:*
   (a) It causes thrush.
   (b) It is transmitted primarily by respiratory aerosol.
   (c) It is a budding yeast and forms both psudohyphae and hyphae.
   (d) Impaired cell mediated immunity is an important predisposing factor to disease.
5. Which of the following fungi can cause mucormycosis (zygomycosis)?
   (a) *Mucor* (b) *Rhizopus*
   (c) *Absidia* (d) All of the above.
6. Cryptococcosis, an opportunisitic mycosis, is associated with
   (a) Pigeon droppings
   (b) Plant debris
   (c) Blowing wounds
   (d) Sacaration of ancient swellings.

ANSWERS TO MCQs

1. (b) 2. (d) 3. (d) 4. (b)
5. (d) 6. (a).

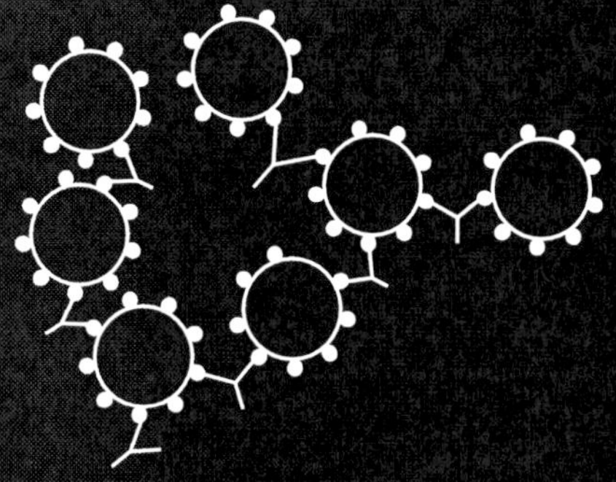

Unit IV D

PARASITES AND ARTHROPODS OF MEDICAL SIGNIFICANCE

- Protozoans and Human Diseases
- Helminths: Nematodes, Cestodes, Trematodes and Human Diseases
- Rodents and Arthropods: Vectors of Medical Importance

68

Protozoans and Human Diseases

Malaria; Amebic dysentery; Primary amebic meningoencephalitis; Giardiasis; Tricohomoniasis; Periodontitis; African sleeping sickness; Chagas' disease; Leishmaniasis; Balandiasis

WHAT IS A PARASITE, HOST, MEDICAL PARASITOLOGY AND PROTOZOOLOGY?

A **parasite** is a living organism that acquires its basic nutritional requirements through its intimate contact with another living organism. The word parasite hold its origin from Gr. *parasitos* (*para* = beside and *sitos* = food) means "one who eats at the table of another". There are three main classes of parasites that can cause disease in humans: protozoa, helminths and ectoparasites (arthropods).

Parasitology: It is the branch of microbiology that is concerned with the study of parasites.

Medical parasitology: It is a branch of medical science/medical microbiology that deals with the study of human infections caused by parasites (protozoa and helminths). Notable diseases caused by these are malaria, amebiasis, giardiasis (protozoans), ascariasis, river blindness and schistosomiasis (helminths).

Host: An organism that harbours a parasite is called its *host*. Hosts are classified as:

- **Definitive host:** The host that harbours the adult stage of the parasite or where the parasite replicates/reproduces sexually is called the *definitive host.*
- **Intermediate host:** The host where the parasite replicates asexually or that harbours the larval stage of the parasite is called the *intermediate host.*

- **Reservoir host:** The host that harbours the parasite and acts as an important source of infection is known as the *reservoir host.*

Medical Protozoology

Medical protozoology is a branch of medical parasitology that is largely concerned with the study of parasitic protozoa that infect or cause diseases in humans. The term *protozoan* means the first animal which has been derived from two Greek words (*protos*–first and zoon–animals) which describes its animal-like nutrition.

Protozoa are one-celled, eukaryotic and heterotrophic microorganisms that either exist as parasites or free-living organisms. They have the ability to multiply in humans and are transmitted by fecal-oral route (contaminated food and water), person-to-person contact or by arthropod vectors (through the bite of a mosquito or sand fly), resulting in serious infections from just a single organism.

Clinically important protozoans are *Plasmodium, Entamoeba* and *Giardia*.

CLASSIFICATION OF PARASITIC PROTOZOANS

The protozoa consists of 65,000 species classified as a phylum in the kingdom *Protista* (or *Animalia*). Based on the mode of locomotion important protozoa are classified into four groups:

• **Apicomplexa (sporozoa)**	– non-motile in their natural forms (spores)	*Plasmodium vivax* *P. falciparum* *P. malariae* *Toxoplasma gondii* *Cryptosporidium*
• **Sarcodina**	– the **amoebae** (pseudopodia)	*Entamoeba histolytica* *Entamoeba coli* *E. gingivalis*
• **Mastigophora**	– the **flagellates** (flagella)	*Giardia lamblia* *Trichomonas vaginalis* *Leishmania* *L. tropica donovani* *L. brasiliensis*
• **Ciliophora**	– the **ciliates** (cilia)	*Balantidium coli*

Current schemes of classifying protozoan species into phyla are based on DNA data and morphology of the organism.

PLASMODIUM AND MALARIA

Plasmodium (commonly called ***malaria parasite***) is an obligate intracellular unicellular eukaryotic sporozoan that causes malaria in humans. **Charles Laveran** first identified it in the blood of malaria patients in 1880 and was named as *Oscillaria malariae*. Malaria is the dominant protozoan disease which affects 10% of the world's population, with 228 to 300 million new cases and 0.4 to one million deaths annually worldwide; about two-thirds of them in Africa alone, killing an African child every 30 seconds.

The origin of the name is from the Italian words = *mal* = bad, *aria* = air due to the superstition of the Middle Ages that are spirits or mists and vapours arising from swamps that caused malaria.

Currently, the genus contains over 200 species classified in the phylum *Apicomplexa*. (*Sporozoa*). Four species of *Plasmodium* cause malaria in humans which are spread by female *Anopheles* mosquito.

P. falciparum causes life-threatening malaria, invades erythrocytes, of all ages.

P. vivax and *P. ovale* cause *benign tertian malaria*: febrile episodes typically occur every 48 hours or every third day.

P. malariae causes *quartan malaria*: febrile episodes typically occurring at an interval of 3 to 4 days.

LIFECYCLE OF *PLASMODIUM*

The lifecycle of *Plasmodium* involves two hosts (Fig. 68.1):

- Female *Anopheles* mosquito which carries the infective stage (sporozoite) in its saliva, the **vector host**, also called the **definitive host** because it harbours the sexually reproducing stage **(sporogamy)** of the parasite.
- Humans, the **intermediate host**, because the parasite undergoes asexual reproduction in liver.

Cycle in Humans (Asexual Cycle)

Infection in humans is initiated by the bite of a mosquito that inoculates *the infective stage*, called **sporozoite** (Gr. *sporo* = seed and *zoon* = animal), into the human's blood, followed by invasion of the liver cells and multiplication asexually resulting in large number of **merozoites**, the process called *schizogony* (Gr *schizo* = to divide and *gonia* = seed).

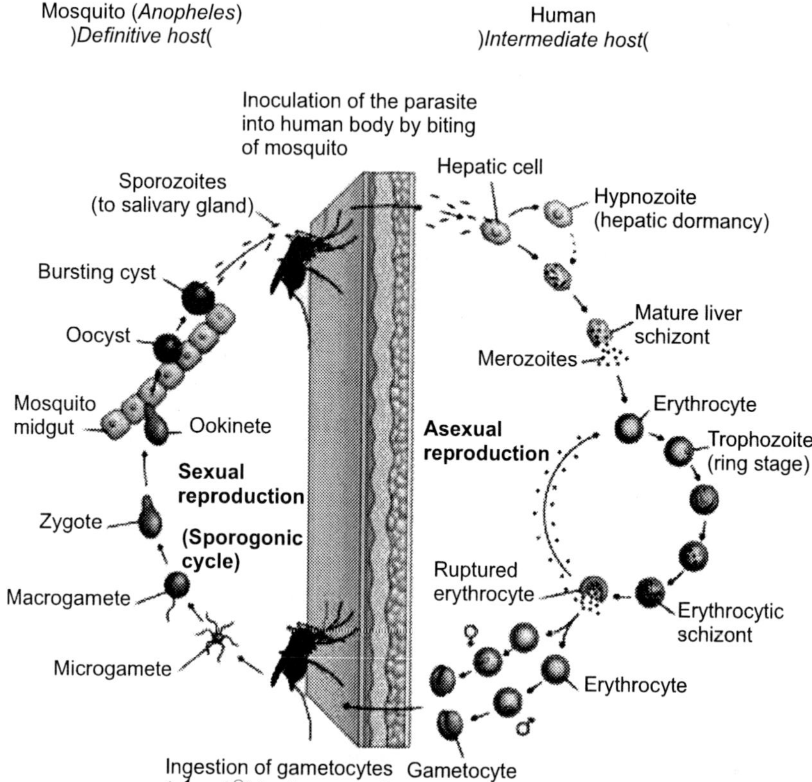

Fig. 68.1 Lifecycle of *Plasmodium*, the cause of malaria. The protozoan parasite involves two hosts: human, the intermediate most, in which asexual reproduction occurs in the liver (*exo-erythrocytic cycle*) and blood (*erythrocytic cycle*); and sexual reproduction takes place in the female *Anopheles* mosquito (the definitive host).

This phase of development in liver is called ***exo-erythrocytic (or liver) phase or development),*** which lasts for 5 to 16 days, depending upon the *Plasmodium* species.

The merozoites, after their release, from the liver, enter the blood circulatory system, infect red blood cells transforming in a short time to circular trophozoites, looking like a ring in which the nucleus and cytoplasm are visible under a microscope, this is called the **ring stage** (Fig. 68.2), an important diagnostic characteristic for malaria. **Schizogony** of the ringed form trophozoites produces additional merozoites that burst out and is responsible for the clinical manifestations of malaria. This phase of development is called

erythrocytic schizogony. Eventually, certain merozoites differentiate into **sexual erythrocytic stages,** i.e. differentiation into two types of gametes: *macrogametocytes* (female) and *microgametocytes* (male), called the *gametocyte phase* with the end of the cycle in humans.

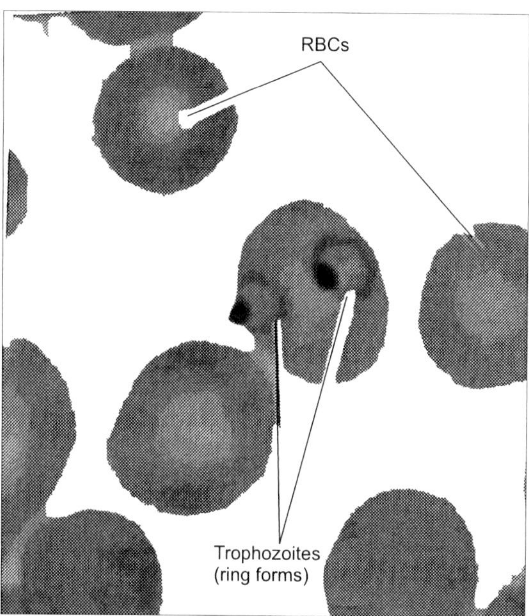

Fig. 68.2 The ring trophozoite stage in *Plasmodium falciparum* infection. A smear of peripheral blood shows the feeding protozoan (trophozite) resembling a ring within the RBC, a characteristic feature used to diagnose malaria.

Cycle in Mosquito (Sporogony)

Sporogonic cycle in mosquito involves fertilization and formation of sporozoites. During a human bite, male or female gamocytes are ingested by an *Anopheles* mosquito and in the digestive tracts they unite to form zygotes, which in turn, become motile and elongated, called **ookinetes** which involve the mosquito's midgut walls where they develop into **oocysts**. Each **oocyst** undergoes multiple meiotic divisions, releasing haploid sporozoites that migrate to the saliary glands and lodge there, for infecting the next victim (Fig. 68.1).

The malaria parasite is transmitted by female *Anopheles* mosquitoes, which bite mainly between dusk and dawn.

Blood products (e.g., uncleaned needles and unscreened blood) are also involved in its spread.

PATHOGENESIS AND CLINICAL TYPES OF MALARIA

Mosquito-borne infection with malarial parasite causes intermittent high fever 105° F (40.6°C) or higher which is called **malaria**. It is characterized by chills and high fever, vomiting, severe headache, sweating with tiredness.

In severe cases, it can cause yellow skin, seizure, coma and death. Symptoms usually begin after weeks (7 days after) after being bitten by an infected mosquito and typically appear at intervals of 2 to 3 days, alternating with asymptomatic periods.

There are four major forms of malaria:

- **Benign malaria** caused by *P. vivax*, most prevailed in temperate countries, the cycle of paroxyms occurs every 2 days; the parasite can remain dormant in the liver for months to years.
- **Relatively benign malaria** caused by *P. ovale* and *P. malariae*; lower in incidence and restricted geographically.
- **Malignant malaria** caused by *P. falciparum*. Most dangerous causing maximum deaths especially of young children, spleen, kidney and liver are damaged.
- **Cerebral malaria** caused by *P. falciparum* affecting the brain with neurological symptoms, including coma.

DIAGNOSIS

- **Microscopic examination** of blood smear to detect ring forms and gametocytes of *Plasmodium* in RBCs of infected persons is the 'gold standard' for diagnosis of malaria.
- **Antigen** based rapid diagnostic tests (RDT).

  In addition, other lab tests used to diagnose include:

  - Low number of platelets in the blood
  - Higher-than-normal levels of bilirubin in blood

PREVENTION

Methods used to prevent malaria include:

- **Mosquito elimination and prevention of bites** by using mosquito nets, insect repellent and mosquito control by spraying insecticides and draining standing water, an effective way of reducing its incidence.

- **Prophylaxis drugs**
- **Vaccination:** As of 2020, there is one vaccine for malaria (known as **RTS, S**) which is licensed for use.

Treatment

Antimalarial drugs include:

- WHO recommends **artemisinin** based combination therapies (ACTs) such as **coartem** (artemether and lumefantarin) for treatment of malaria worldwide. Alternative drugs used are:

  Mefloquine, lumefantarine, sulfadoxine + pyrimethamine or quinine + doxycycline.

  Chloroquine, a cost effective treatment is the preferred treatment for malaria.

SARCODINIAN (AMOEBOID) PROTOZOA

The **Sarcodinian protozoans** or **amebae** (also spelled **amoebae**) are unicellular organisms that move by extending blunt, lobe-like projections of the cytoplasm termed **pseudopods** and have the ability to alter their shape (basis of naming for Greek *amoibe* meaning 'to change'). Disease causing amebas include:

- *Entamoeba histolytica* – **Amebic** or **amoebic dysentery**
- *Naegleria fowleri* – **Naegleriasis (or primary amoebic meningoencepalitis)**
- *Acanthamoeba keratitis* – **Blindness** (or visual impairment)
- *Balamuthia mandrillaris* – **Granulomatous amoebic encephalitis**

ENTAMOEBA HISTOLYTICA AND AMEBIC DYSENTERY

Entamoeba histolytica is an anaerobic parasitic amebozoan that causes amebic dysentery. The name of the protozoan parasite is derived from Greek words: *ento* = within + *histos* = tissue + lysis = dissolution) means disintegration and dissolution of tissues in the intestine.

Amebic dysentery or **amebiasis** (also spelled **amoebic dysentery** and **amoebiasis**) is an intestinal protozoan infection characterized by blood stools, fever with cramping. It is present all over the world, though more prevalent in the developing world, especially in the tropical and subtropical climate, 480 million people are currently infected globally, with about 40 million new cases reported every year, and killing between 40,000 and 1,10,000 people a year. Infection is common in homosexuals means having anal sex.

Morphology and Lifecycle

The parasite produces two stages – **motile trophozoite** and **nonmotile cyst**–with an intermediate **precyst** in its lifecycle (Fig. 68.3). The trophozoites move by pseudopods, each 20–30 μm in diameter, and contain a large single nucleus with a prominent nucleolus called **karyosome,** peripheral chromatin and radial chromatic fibrils imparting a cart-wheel appearance. These cannot survive in the environment.

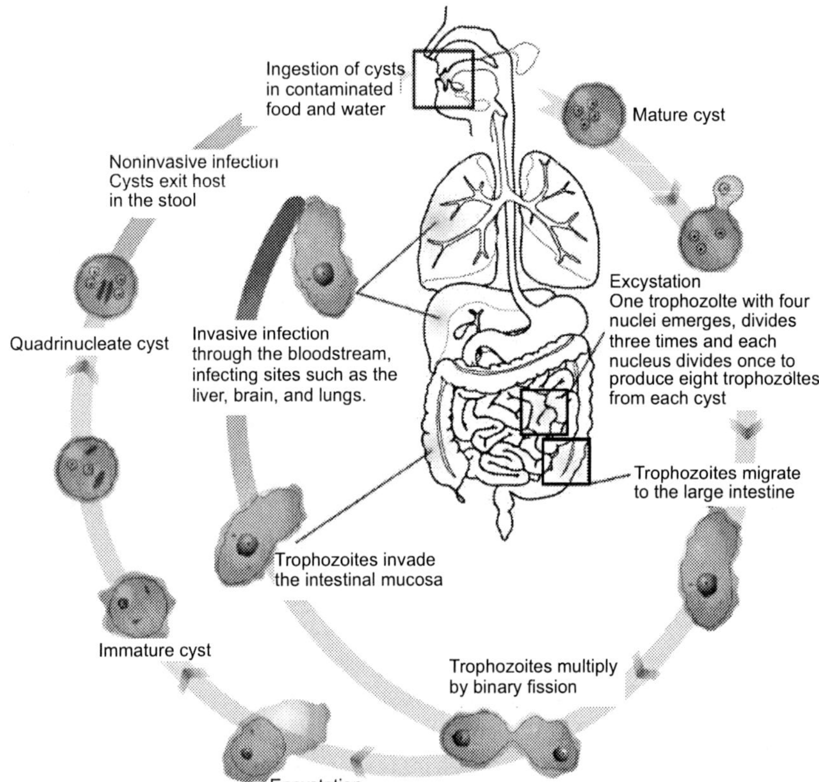

Fig. 68.3 Life cycle of *Entamoeba histolytica,* the cause of amebic dysentery. Cysts and trophozoites are passed in feces. Infection of humans occurs via ingestion of mature cysts (typically found in formed stool).

The cysts are spherical, nonmotile 10–15 μm in diameter (i.e., smaller than trophozoites) and having 4 nuclei each with distinctive bodies called **chromatoidals** (which are actually dense clusters of ribosomes) and surrounded by a double tough wall.

Transmission: Amoebasis is usually transmitted by the fecal-oral route through the ingestion of the cysts of the parasite, a semi-dormant and hardy structure found in the faeces.

Lifecycle and Pathogenesis

Humans are the primary hosts of *E. histolytica* and the infection is spread mostly by food and water contaminated with cysts released by the asymptomatic carrier. When cysts are swallowed they reach the small intestine where the cyst wall is digested and the trophozoites are released (4 trophozoites/cyst), the process called **excystment** (Fig. 68.4). The trophozoites are swept into the **cecum,** the pouch-like anterior portion of large intestine near the appendix and large intestine where they multiply on the epithelial cells and feed on the tissue in the gastrointestinal tract resulting in severe symptoms of dysentery (the feces containing blood and mucus).

Both the cysts and trophozoites are passed in the feces; cysts are typically found in the formed stool, whereas trophozoites are typically found in diarrheal stool. Infection only occurs via ingestion of mature cysts since these can survive for up to a month in soil due to the protection conferred by their walls. Trophozoites passed in the stool are unable to cause infection because they are rapidly destroyed once outside the body and if ingested would not survive exposure to the gastric environment in the body.

Clinical Features

E. histolytica causes two types of infections:

- Intestinal infection (luminal amebiasis)
- Extraintestinal infection.

Intestinal Infection

Majority of the infections restricted to the lumen of the intestine are asymptomatic. **Amebic colitis** or **amoebic dysentery** occurs when the wall of the intestine (mucosa) is invaded by the amoebas. These amoebas may pass to the bloodstream and travel to the liver or, infrequently, to the brain, where they form pockets of infection (called **abscesses**).

Symptoms usually begin within months after amoebas first enter the body. Various initial symptoms include:

- In over 90% of cases, no symptoms (**asymptomatic**)
- **Mild symptoms** include mild pain and gurgling sounds in the lower abdomen, alongwith 2 or 3 loose stools daily.
- **Full-blown symptoms** include high fever, severe abdominal pain, 10 or more episodes of diarrhea (watery or mixed with blood and mucus) daily, and intestinal ulcers with perforation resulting in *peritenitis*.
- **Liver abscess symptoms** include fever, nausea, vomiting and pain in abdomen, weight loss and an enlarged liver.

Laboratory Diagnosis

- **Direct microscopy** – Microscopic identification of cysts and trophozoites in the stool (fresh stool/concentrated from fresh stool) in wet mounts and iodine stained smears.
- **Immunodiagnosis** – Enzyme immunoassay (EIA) kits for antibody detection as well as EIA kits for antigen detection are commercially available. Most accurate test is finding specific antibodies in the blood.
- **Molecular diagnosis:**
    - **Use of conventional PCR-based assays.**
    - **A Real-time PCR** – The assay targets the 18SrRNA gene with species-specific TaqMan probes in a duplex format, making it possible to detect both *E. histolytica* and *E. dispar* in the same reaction vessel.
- **Biochemical test** – An increased white blood level.

Treatment

- Amebiasis is treated with nitroimidazole drugs such as metronidazole and timidazole followed by luminal agents such as paromomycin or diloxanide furate to prevent relapse.

  Metronidazole (Flagyl) is the drug of choice for treating adult and children. Usually it is given for 10 days either by mouth or directly into veins (intravenously). To avoid recurrence, a combination of metronidazole plus iodoguinol/paromomycin/ diloxanide furoate (which will kill both amoebas and cysts) is used.

ENTAMOEBA COLI

Entamoeba coli is a **nonpathogenic intestinal amoeba** that frequently exists as a commensal parasite with the human gastrointestinal tract, however, is very important in medicine because it can be confused during microscopic examination of stained stool specimens with the pathogenic *Entamoeba histolytica*, the cause of amebic dysentery in humans. Its distinguishing diagnostic features are:

- Trophozoites (10.5–20.0 μm in diameter) provided with wide and tapered pseudopodia.
- The amoeba is immobile and keeps its round shape and creates a *sur place* (nonprogressive) *movement* inside the large intestine.
- Mature cysts of *E. coli* are characteristic each having 8 nuclei (but may have as many as 16 or more).
- It does not have an invasive stage or does not ingest red blood cells.

NAEGLERIA FOWLERI AND PRIMARY AMEBIC MENINGOENCEPHALITIS

Naegleria fowleri is a thermophilic flagellated protozoan, commonly referred to as the **brain-eating** amoeba, the causal agent of **primary amebic meningoencephalitis** (**PAM**) (also known as **naegleriasis**), a fatal infection of the brain that causes sudden tragic deaths usually of heathy people. The disease was first documented in Australia in 1965. The genus was named after **M. Naegler**, (a French) and species after **M. Fowler** (an Australian) who first discovered this protozoan in 1899 and described the disease process in 1965, respectively. The disease is lethal but rare in occurrence but the problem is getting worse every year in the USA since these amoebas are surviving the US rivers and lakes.

Only four of the 145 Americans infected by *N. fowleri* have survived. On Sept. 28, 2020, death of a 6-year-old boy occurred due to this parasite present in the hose at the boy's house in Lake Jackson, Texas.

Morphology and Lifecycle

N. fowleri is a thermophilic (heat-loving) free-living amoeba which is typically found in warm bodies of fresh waters (e.g., ponds, lakes, rivers, hot springs) and unchlorinated swimming pools and water-heaters and is able to grow at temperatures up to 45°C (115°F).

This amaeboflagellate goes through three stages in its lifecycle: cyst, flagellate and trophozoite (amoeboid), the cysts do not occur in human tissue.

The **trophozoite** is a feeding, dividing by binary fission and infective stage for humans. It is a flask-shaped amoeba having a nucleus surrounded by halo that moves by means of a single broad pseuodopod. It has a prominent feeding structure or **amebostomes** that look-like 'eyes' and 'mouth' face-like appearance in scanning electron micrographs. It forms a spherical (7–15 µm diameter), thick-walled, uninucleate **cyst** that is resistant to temperature extremes and mild chlorination. The **biflagellate** form occurs when trophozoites are exposed to a change in ionic concentration and can be inhaled into the nasal cavity during swimming or diving.

Pathogenesis and Clinical Features

The infection occurs through the nasal route during swimming, diving and water skiing and enters the CNS after inhalation of the contaminated water. The parasite furrows in nasal mucosa, multiplies and subsequently migrating along the olfactory nerve, through the cribriform plate into the brain causing a rapid, massive destruction of the brain and spinal tissues that cause haemorrage or coma eventually leading to death.

Symptoms are similar to meningitits which progress rapidly over around five days and include headache, fever, nausea, vomiting, stiff neck, confusion, hallucination and seizures. Death usually results within one to two weeks after the onset of symptoms.

Laboratory Diagnosis

DM is diagnosed from specimens (CSF, biopsy, tissue) or using the culture by

- **Direct microscopy** – Detection of mobile trophozoites in a fresh sample of CSF.
- **Antigen detection** by indirect immunofluorescence.
- **Detection of DNA by PCR.**
- **Culturing of amoeba** – Inoculation of a bacterial growth plate and incubating at 108°F (42°C).

Treatment

The treatment of choice is a combination of oral miltefosine (impavidol) and intravenous amphotericin B.

FLAGELLATED PROTOZOA (MASTIGOPHORANS)

The **flagellates,** commonly called **mastigophorans,** are uninucleate organisms that possess one to many flagella for locomotion and sensation. The major flagellate genera of clinical, significance include: *Giardia, Trichomonas, Leismania* and *Trypanosoma*. The notable human diseases caused by the flagellates are:

DISEASE	HUMAN PATHOGEN/S
• **Giardiasis (Giardial enteritis)**	*Giardia duodenalis*
• **Trichomonasis**	
Urethritis, vaginitis	*Trichomonas vaginalis*
Gingivitis	*T. tenax*
• **Leishmaniasis**	
Kala-azar	*Leishmania donovani*
Oriental sore	*L. tropica*
• **Trypanosomiasis**	
African sleeping sickness	*Trypanosoma brucei gambiense, T.B. rhodesiense*
Chagas' disease	*T. cruzi*

GIARDIA DUODENALIS AND GIARDIASIS

Giardia duodenalis (also called *G. lamblia* and *G. intestinalis*), a flagellated parasitic protozoan, colonizes and reproduces in the small intestine, causes a diarrheal disease called **giardiasis.** Giardiasis is popularly known as **beaver fever.** It is one of the most common parasitic human diseases globally. Over 280 million people are found to have giardiasis, rates of infection being over 4.5 times higher in the developing countries as compared to developed countries. About 1 million persons are infected with this disease every year in India. **Antonie van Leeuwenhoek** was the first to observe this protozoan in his own stool in 1681 and described the trophozoites an "**animalcules**". This protozoan was initially named *Cercomonas intestinalis* by a Czech physician **Lambl** in 1859. It was renamed *Giardia lamblia* by **Charles Stiles** in 1915 in honour of Professor **A. Giard** of Paris and Dr. **V. D. Lambl** of Prague. In fact, it is the most common flagellate isolated in clinical specimens.

Morphology

The **trophozoites** are 10–20 μm long and 7–10 μ wide, each having two nuclei with a unique symmetrical heart-shape with organelles positioned in such a way that it resembles a human's face or simply face symbol (Fig. 68.4). They are motile by way of four pairs of flagella that emerge from the vertical surface, which is concave. Trophozoites adhere to host epithelial cells via a specialized disk-shaped organelle named the **ventral adhesive disc** or **sucker**.

The cysts are oval-shaped, slightly smaller than trophozoites, covered by a smooth, clear cyst wall. Each cyst contains the organelles for two trophozoites that includes four nuclei and two vertical disks.

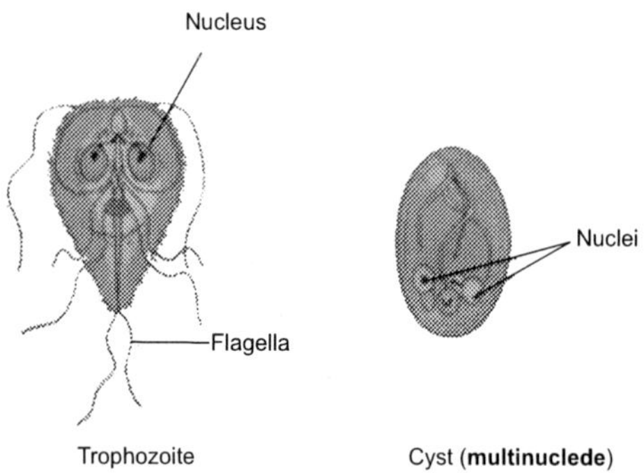

Fig. 68.4 Trophozoite and cyst of *Giardia*, the causative agent of giardiasis. Flagelleted trophozoites, a characteristic heart-shaped morphology resembling human face.

Life and Disease Cycle

Giardia cysts, the resistant forms that can survive for 2 months (in the environment) to 3 months (in cold water), are responsible for transmission of giardiasis. Infection occurs by the ingestion of cysts in contaiminated water, food and by the fecal-oral-route (hands or fomites) and contaminated objects; as few as 10 cysts can cause infection.

Lifecycle consists of two stages: cysts and trophozoites. Excystation of cysts occurs in the duodenum (small intestine), each cyst producing two trophozoites which either float free or are attached to the mucosa of the lumen, and reproduce by binary fission. Some trophozoites, encyst in the small intestine. Giardiasis is transmitted via **fecal-oral route** with the ingestion of cysts.

Symptoms

Symptoms usually start 1 to 3 weeks after ingestion of cysts and usually lasts for up to 6 weeks without treatment. These include diarrhea (greasy stool that floats), abdominal pain, nausea, flatulence (intestinal gas) and weakness. The distinctive odour of H_2S can often be detected in the breath and stools.

Laboratory Diagnosis

- Detection of antigens on the surface of stool specimen is the current test of choice for diagnosis of giardiasis.
- A trichome stain of preserved stool is another method used to detect *Giardia.*
- Microscopic examination for the presence of cysts or trophozoites of the parasite in the stool.
- The **string test** (or **Entero test**) that uses a gelatin capsule with an attached fine string (or thread). One end is attached to the inner aspect of the host's cheek and the capsule is swallowed to the patient. After a few hours, the thread is withdrawn and shaken in saline to release trophozoites which can be detected microscopically.
- ELISA tests are used to detect both ova and parasites in stool specimens.
- Hydrogen peroxide breath tests are also useful in diagnosis.

Treatment

Metronidazole (Flagyl) is the drug to choice to treat giardiasis. Tinidazole, nitazoxanide are the other effective drugs which are to be administered for 5 to days (a complete course).

TRICHOMONAS VAGINALIS AND TRICHOMONIASIS (OR TRICH)

Trichomonas vaginalis, an anaerobic flagellated protozoan, causes a very common sexually transmitted disease (STD) called **trichomoniasis** in both males and females. WHO has estimated that 160 million cases of infection are acquired annually worldwide, with over 10 million cases per year in India. The parasite is mainly found in the vagina of females and urethra of males.

Morphology

T. vaginalis exists in only one **morphological** stage, trophozoites and does not produce cysts. **Trophozoites** are pear shaped, measuring 9 × 7 μm, with four anterior flagella and an undulating membrane (whip-like tail) which together produces a characteristic **twitching motility** in live preparations.

Lifecycle

The parasite resides in female lower genital tract and male urethra and prostate, where it replicates by binary fission. It does not survive well in the external enviornment due to the absence of cysts. The trophozoites can survive for up to 24 hours in urine, semen or even in water samples.

Clinical Features

In women, trich can cause a foul-smelling vaginal discharge, genital itching and painful urination. Men typically have no symptoms. Premature delivery may occur in pregnant women. It is a sexually transmitted disease and spreads from person-to-person during sex. Symptoms appear within 5 to 28 days after being infected.

Diagnosis

- **Microscopic examination** of samples of vaginal fluid (for women) and urethral discharge (men) for the motile protozoa.
- **Rapid antigen test** (antibodies bind, if the *Trichomonas* is present diagnosing infection).
- **Culturing** of the parasite on CPLM.
- **Trichomans DNA** by nuclei acid amplification test.

Treatment

- Metronidazole or tinidazole are used orally for five days.
- Vaginal douching with lactic acid and vinegar to promote acid pH is also useful to treat the infection.

TRICHOMONAS TENAX AND PERIODONTITIS

Trichomonas **tenax** (or **oral trichomonas**) is a flagellated aerotolerant protozoan, commonly found in the oral cavity of humans. Routine hygiene is generally not sufficient to eliminate the parasite, hence its Latin name, meaning 'tenacious' (*L. tencre* = keep, hold fast). It causes ulcerative gingivitis and necrotizing ulcerative periodontitis.

Morphology

It occurs as a flagellated vegetative stage measuring 5–14 µm long and 6–9 µm wide with four free flagella at the anterior pole and a lateral recurrent one, reproducing by repeated longitudinal binary fission. They feed on bacteria by phagocytosis.

Transmission

It is found in human oral cavity and spreads through saliva, droplet spray and kissing, use of contaiminated dishes and drinking water.

Clinical Features

T. tenax alone is not known to cause any symptoms. In diseased persons, the parasite worsens the preexisting periodontal disease.

Diagnosis

- **Microscopic examination** of tonsillar crypts and pyorrhea pockets for trophozoites.
- **Phase-contrast microscopy** of biofilm harvested from the infested areas of the periodontal pockets mounted on a slide, especially by using the patient's saliva as the medium, is used for easy detection of the trophozoites.
- By **culturing** of the parasite on the appropriate media.

Treatment

Oral hygiene instructions in combination with **scaling** and **root planning** are used to treat the patients.

TRYPANOSOMA BRUCEI AND AFRICAN TRYPANOSOMIASIS

Trypanosoma is a unicellular parasitic hemoflagellate protozoan that is characterized by its infective stage, the **trypomastigote,** an elongate, spindle-shaped cell with tapered ends and an eel-like corkscrew like motion. The name is derived from the Greek *trypano* (borer) and *soma* (body). It is a **hemoflagellate,** i.e., it lives in the blood and tissues of the human host. It is a **heteroxenous** organism, i.e., requiring more than one obligatory host to complete its lifecycle and is transmitted by a blood-sucking vector.

Trypanosoma was discovered in 1894 by **Sir David Bruce**, after whom the scientific name was given in 1899. Two sub-species of *T. brucei* are parasites of humans and cause African trypanosomasis.

African trypanosomiasis (also called **African sleeping sickness** or simply **sleeping sickness**), a disease of the nervous system, is caused by two sub-species of *T. brucei* (*T. brucei gambiense, TbG* and *T. brucei rhodesiense,* TbR). It is a vector-borne disease transmitted by **tsetse fly bites. Winston Churchill** in 1907 described Uganda during an epidemic of sleeping sickness as *beautiful garden of death*. Even today, estimates are that as many as half a million Africans are infected, and there are about one lakh new cases.

Morphoglogy of *T. brucei*

T. brucei forms trypomastigotes in human hosts and epimastigotes in insect vector (tsetse fly). The **trypomastigotes** have basal body and kinetoplast posterior to the nucleus, with a single flagellum that arises from the posterior end of the body. The **kinetoplast** (an unusual organelle made up of numerous circular DNA that functions as a single large mitochondrion) is spindle-shaped with tapering ends measuring 18–50 µm × 1–3 µm. The flagellum is attached to the cell membrane (pellicle) forming an undulating membrane with its tip free at the anterior end.

In **epimastigote**, the kinetoplast and the basal body lie anterior to the nucleus and the flagellum starts from the centre of the body.

The flagellar function is twofold: locomotion via oscillations and attachment to the fly gut during the procyclic phase.

The two subspeices *TbG* and *TbR* are morphologically indistinguishable but differ significantly in their epidemiology, that is, in their ability to infect nonhuman hosts:

- *TbG* is parasitic on humans only.
- *TbR* is parasitic on domestic livestock and many wild animals.

Lifecycle

T. brucei completes its lifecycle (Fig. 68.5) between tsetse fly (*Glossina* spp.) and mammalian host. The saliva of a fly infected with *T. brucei* inoculates the human skin from where it enters the lymphatic system and pass into the bloodstream and carried to other body fluids (as lymph, spinal cord) and continue replication by binary fission without entering the cells (i.e., extracellular). Its cumulative effects cause central nervous system damage. The trypanosome is spread to other hosts through another fly in whose alimentary tract the parasite completes a series of developmental stages:

tryptomastigotes → procyclic tryptomastigotes → epimastigote. Thereby reaching to salivary's gland in 3 weeks.

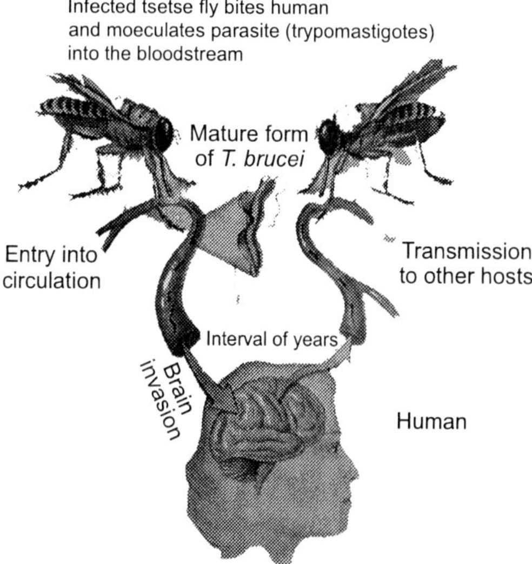

Fig. 68.5 Lifecycle of *Trypanosoma brucei*, the causative agent of African sleeping sickness between humans and the vector (tsetse fly).

Clinical Features

African trypanosomiasis symptoms appear 1 to 3 weeks after the bite and occurs in two stages. In both forms, the CNS is affected.

Early symptoms (stage 1) include: Fever, headache of joint pain and itchiness.

Later symptoms (stage 2) include: Confusion, poor coordination numbness and trouble in sleeping. Death results from coma, secondary infections or heart damage.

The disease is commonly called **sleeping sickness**, but in fact, uncontrollable sleepiness occurs primarily in the day and is followed by sleeplessness at night.

Diagnosis

The gold standard for diagnosis is identification of trypanosomes by microscopic examination by two ways:

Wet preparation is used for examining live trypanosomes, or fixed (dried) stained (Giemsa's) smear of blood can be used. Characteristics trypomastigote with a posterior kinetoplast, a centrally located nucleus, and an anterior flagellum are observed.

Serological tests: Three serological tests to detect specific antibodies from the blood samples are available for the diagnosis. These include: The **micro-CATT** (card agglutination test) that uses dried blood sample; **Wb-CATT** and **Wb-LATEX** these two use whole blood samples.

Treatment

First stage due to TbG is treated with flexinidazole (mouth) orpentamidine (injection); or due to TbR by suramin (injection).

Second stage (severe infection) is treated with eflornithine alone or a combination of two drugs: nifurimox eflornithine, or nifurtimox-eflornithine.

TRYPANOSOMA CRUZI AND CHAGAS' DISEASE

Trypanosoma cruzi, the caustive agent of Chagas' disease (also called **American trypanosomiasis**) is a flagellate protozoan parasite that is transmitted by **triatomine bug**, commonly called the **kissing bug** because it often bites people near the lips.

Chagas' disease, named after the Brazilian physician **Carlos Chagas** who discovered the disease in 1909. It is a life-threating illness common in South and Central America or Mexico where it chronically infects 6–7 million people.

Morphology

T. cruzi has three morphological forms: the **trypomastigote** (in feces of bug and transformed in human), the **epimastigote** (in gut of bug); and **amastigote** (intracellular in human macrophages, liver, heart, or spleen)

Trypanosomes are single-celled, slender 20 mm long with a thin, irregularly shaped membrane, a centrally positioned nucleus and a posterior kinetoplast. The trypansome has an undulating membrane, the flagellum that follows the outer margin of the membrane and then projects beyond the body of the trypansome as a free flagellum (Fig. 68.6).

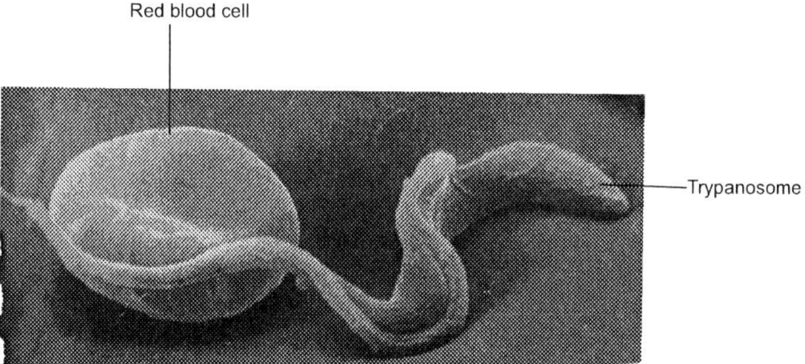

Fig. 68.6 ***Trypanosoma cruzi*, a flagellated protozoan, the cause of Chagas' disease (American trypanosomiasis).** The trypansome has an undulating membrane; the flagellum follows the outer margin of the membrane and then projects beyond the body of the trypansome as a free flagellum.

Lifecycle

The kissing bug infects humans through its feces deposited at the bite region. Infection occurs if the infected bug defecates while biting a human, it can release trypanosomes that can contaminate the bite wound. Human also inoculates the wound by accidentally rubbing the bug feces into it. Infection can also occur when bug feces fall onto the mucous membrane or conjunctiva or through contact with blood. Infection progresses in stages: Inside the host, the trypomastigotes invade cells near the site of inoculation, where they differentiate into intracellular amastigotes which multiply by binary fission and differentiate into trypomastigotes, and then burst out of the cell, and enter the blood stream, and clinical manifestation can occur during the infective cycle of the parasite.

The trypomastigotes are ingested by the kissing bug while feeding on infected humans and rapidly multiply schizogamy in the midgut.

Clinical Manifestations

The acute (or early) stage of the disease is characterized by fever, swollen lymph nodes, headaches or swelling at the site of the bite, lasting for a few weeks only and not cause alarm.

After 4 to 8 weeks, up to 45% of people infected develop a chronic form of the disease — affecting heart leading to heart failure after 10 to 30 years of illness, and in some cases enlarged esophagus or an enlarged colon causing digestive complications, and in some people damaging the nerves.

Diagnosis

- In microscopic examination of Giemsa stained blood smear, search for the presence of the characteristic S or C-shapted trypomastigotes of the parasite having more pronounced kinetoplast compared to other species.
- Detecting DNA by PCR.
- Serology: finding antibodies for the parasite in the blood by ELISA.
- Rapid diagnostic tests are available for searching purpose.
- Isolation of the parasite by inoculating blood into a guinea pig, mouse or rat.

Treatment

Benznidazole and nifurtimox are the drugs of choice for treating Chagas' disease. Two to three oral doses/day for 60–90 days are required for complete cure.

LEISHMANIA AND LEISHMANIASIS

Leishmania, a genus of trypanosomes, is a protozoan dimorphic parasite, that causes a vector-borne disease **leishmaniasis** dating back to the 7th century BC. However, the causative agent for the disease *Leishmania donovani* was only discovered in 1901 independently by **William Boog Leishman** and **Charles Donovan**. Between 4 and 12 million people are currently infected worldwide. Two million new cases and 20,000 to 50,000 deaths occur each year. The infectious disease is transmitted by sandflies.

Morphology

Leishmania species exist in two structural forms:

Amastigote (ovoid form) in humans and **promastigote** (flagellated form) in sandfly.

The **amastigote** are oval, 3-6 μm in length and 1–3 μm in breadth with the kinetoplast and basal body present at the anterior end and occur in the mononuclear phagocytes.

The **promastigote** are larger, spindle shaped, tapering at both ends, 15–30 μm in length and, 5 μm in width with the central nucleus provided with a long flagellum (about the body length) at the anterior end.

Lifecycle

The *promastigote*, the infective form of the parasite is present in the saliva of sandfly, which loses its flagellum when it penetrates the human skin, transforming to an *amastigote* that proliferates in phagocytic cells which are ingested by feeding sandflies, renewing the lifecycle (Figure 68.7).

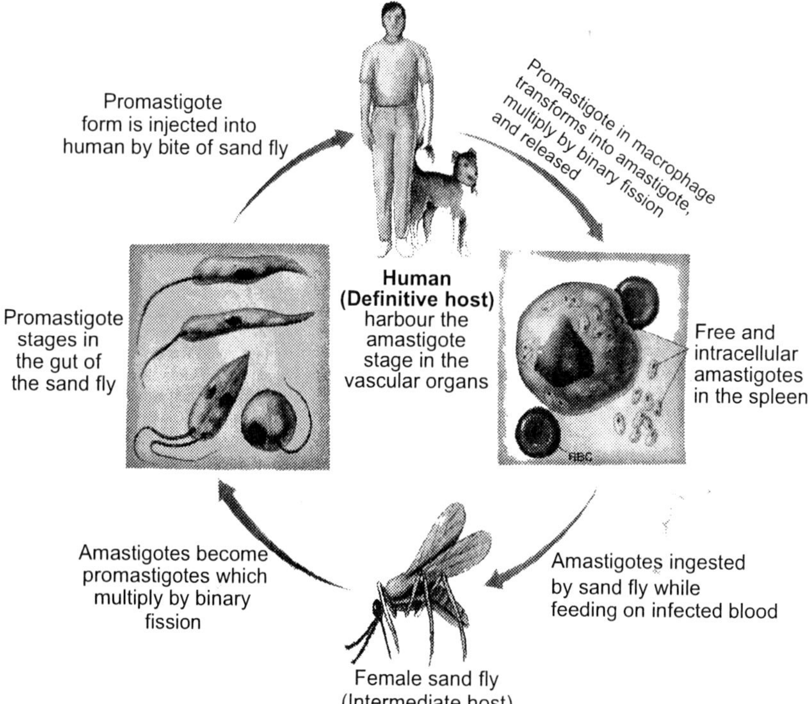

Fig. 68.7 Lifecycle of *Leishmania*, the cause of leishmaniasis, where the vector sandfly acts as the intermediate host and the human as the definitive host.

Infection can also occur through contact with contaminated blood from transfusions or shared needles.

Clinical Manifestations

There are three main clinical forms of leishmaniasis which are caused by different species of *Leishmania*.

- **Visceral leishmaniasis (VL)**, also known as ***Kal-azar***. The most serious form of the disease is caused by *Leishmania donovani*. It is characterized by irregular bouts of fever, weight loss, enlargement of the spleen and liver, and anaemia. In 95% of the cases, the disease is fatal.

It is a disease of the tropical world recorded mainly from 10 countries (WHO, 2018): Brazil, India, Bangladesh, Sudan, Kenya, Iraq, Nepal, China, Ethiopia, Somalia and South Sudan.

- **Cutaneous leishmaniasis (CL),** sometimes called **oriental sore,** is caused by *Leishmania tropica* and *L. major*. It is the most common form of leishmania and causes skin lesions, mainly ulcers on exposed part of the body, leaving life-long scars and serious disability or stigma. It mainly occurs in the Americas, the Mediterranean basin, the Middle East and Central Asia.
- **Mucocutaneous leishmaniasis** often called **American leishmaniasis** is caused by *Leishmania braziliensis*. It affects mucous membranes of nose, mouth and throat (the name). It mainly occurs in Bolvia, Brazil, Ethiopia and Peru.

Laboratory Diagnosis

- **Direct light microscopic examination** for the visualization of the **amastigotes** (**Leishman-Donovan bodies**) in the Leisnman stain or Giemsa stain smears prepared of the peripheral blood or aspirates from bone marrow, spleen, lymph nodes or skin lesions (bone marrow smear is preferred).
- **Culturing the parasite** – Culture of bone marrow or blood in Novy-McNeal-Nicolle (NMN) medium at 24°C for one week and observed for the growth of **promastigote** form of the parasite. The specimen is declared negative only 5 to 6 weeks of incubation.
- **Immunological assays:** ELISA (that uses monoclonal antibody dipsticks) and direct agglutination test are available.

- **PCR** tests are used to detect the DNA of ***Leishmania***. The most sensitive PCR tests use minicircle kinetoplast DNA found in the parasite.

Treatment

- Amphotericin B, single dose, is the treatment of choice for VL in India, South America and Mediterranean.
- A combination of pentavalent antimonials (sodium stibogluconate and meglumine antimoniate) and paromomycin is used to treat VL in Africa
- Miltefosine (Impavido), an oral drug, is used to treat both VL and CL.
- Paromomycin and fluconazole are effective against CL.

CILIATED PROTOZOAN PARASITE – *BALANTIDIUM* AND BALANTIDIASIS

Balantidium coli, the cause of **balandial dysentery,** is the largest protozoan pathogen and the only parasitic ciliate of humans. The name *Balantidium* is derived from the Greek *balantidium* means a "bag" small sac, pouch purse). The parasite inhabits large intestine of man and pigs where it is asympatomatic. The disease is common in Philippines, however, occurs worldwide affecting less than 1% of the human population.

Morphology

Balantidium coli exists in two developmental stages: the trophozoites and cysts (Fig. 68.8).

The ***trophozoites*** are oblong, giant (30–150 μm × 25–120 μm), two-nucleated (sausage-shaped macronucleus and globose micronucleus) ciliates. Surface is covered with cilia. These replicate by binary fission.

The **cysts** are spherical, 40-60 μm in diameter with one or more layered tough wall.

Lifecycle

The cysts are passed in stool which are ingested with contaminated water and food resulting in infection. Excystation occurs in the intestinal wall, trophozoites develop which live and subsequently multiply by transverse binary fission to the mucosa of large intestine. Mucosal damage results causing small superficial ulcer.

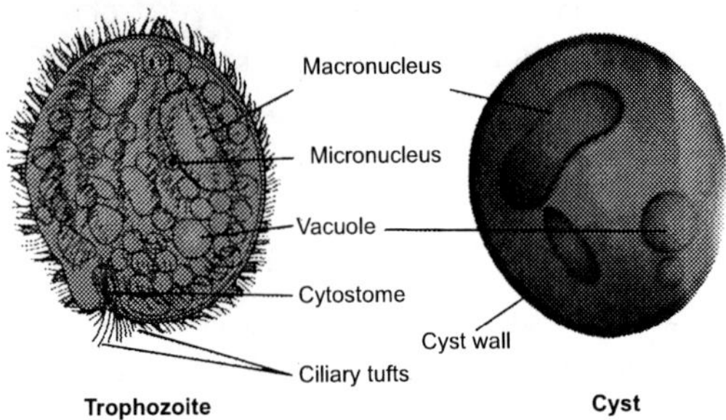

Fig. 68.8 ***Balantidium coli,*** **the causative agent of balantidial dysentery.** Morphology of ciliated trophozoite and a mature cyst.

Symptoms

The most common symptoms are intermittent diarrhea that may occur as often as every 20 minutes and constipation or inflammation of the colon combined with abdominal cramps and bloody stools.

In acute infection, perforation of the colon may occur which can lead to life-threatening conditions.

Laboratory Diagnosis

Microscopic examination of stools for the visualization of living large sized trophozoites and cysts which are yellowish or greenish in color.

Treatment

Tetracycline, carbarsone, metronidazole or di-iodohydroxyquin are used to treat balantidiasis.

KEY POINTS

- **Protozoans** are heterotrophic, wall-less, single-celled animal-like, eukaryotic parasitic microoganisms.
- The four commonly recognized protozoan groups are: **sarcodinians** (amoeboid protozoa), **flagellates, ciliates** and **apicomplexans**.
- All protozoans propagate sexually via their trophozoite, or active feeding stage.
- *Entamoeba histolytica*, an amoebae, the causative agent of amebic dysentery, infects humans via quadrinucleate cysts.

- *Giardia duodenalis* (*Giardia lamblia*), a flagellate protozoan, causes **giardiasis** (diarrhea and malabsorption), and exists in two morphological forms: trophozoite and cyst.
- *Trichomonas vaginalis,* a urogenital protozoan, contains only the trophozoite stage.
- **Malaria** is caused by four species of *Plasmodium,* through the bite of female *Anopheles* mosquito having the sporozoites (infective stage).
- *Leishmania donovoni,* a haemoflagellate causes **Kala-azar** (viceral leishmaniasis) through the sandfly (*Phlebotomus argentipes*).
- *Trypanosoma cruzi,* the causative agent of Chagas', disease, is spread by the kissing bug (*Triatoma*) through its feces deposited at the bite site.
- **African sleeping sickness** is caused through the bite of tsetse fly infected with *Trypanosoma brucei* (*TbG* or *TbR*).
- *Balantidium coli,* the cause of **balantidial dysentery**, is the largest and the only ciliate known to be pathogenic to humans.

IMPORTANT QUESTIONS

1. Write short notes on:
   (a) Characteristics of parasitic protozoans.
   (b) Amoebic dysentery.
   (c) Malaria.
   (d) Giardiasis.
   (e) Kala-azar.
   (f) Chagas' disease.
2. Describe in brief the laboratory diagnosis of malaria, Kala-azar and amoebic dysentery.

MULTIPLE-CHOICE QUESTIONS

1. All protozoan pathogens have a ____________ phase.
   (a) Cyst (b) Trophozoite
   (c) Sexual (d) Blood.
2. *Entamoeba histolytica* primarily invades the ____________.
   (a) Lungs (b) Liver
   (c) Large intestine (d) Small intestine.
3. Mosquito (*Anopheles*) is the definitive host for *Plasmodium,* the malaria parasite
   (a) True (b) False.

4. *Plasmodium ovale* and *Plasmodium malariae* most commonly causes malaria in humans.
   (a) True (b) False.
5. Laboratory diagnosis of *Entamoeba histolytica*, the causative agent of entamoebic dysentery in humans, depends on identification in ____________.
   (a) Saliva (b) Blood
   (c) Stool (d) Urine.
6. Which of the following protozoans causes African sleeping sickness in humans?
   (a) *Plasmodium vivax* (b) *Leishmania donovani*
   (c) *Trypanosoma bruci* (d) *Entamoeba dispar.*
7. In malaria, the schizonts enter which body part of humans?
   (a) Spleen (b) Liver
   (c) Bloodstream (d) Mouth.
8. After how many days of infection by mosquitoes do the symptoms for malaria occur?
   (a) 1–2 (b) 3–5
   (c) 10–16 (d) 20–30.
9. *Leishmania*, the causative agent of leishmaniasis, is transmitted to humans by:
   (a) Tsetse flies (b) Sandflies
   (c) Mosquitoes (d) Bugs.
10. Which of the following protozoans causes Chagas' disease?
    (a) *Trypanosoma cruzi* (b) *Leishmania donovani*
    (c) *Acanthamoeba* (d) *Balantidium coli.*
11. Where are the protozoa present during the acute stage of Chagas' disease?
    (a) Stool (b) Blood
    (c) Spleen (d) Liver.
12. In *Plasmodium* lifecycle, the merozoites develop into ring stage in:
    (a) Liver (b) Spleen
    (c) Red blood cell (d) Salivary gland.
13. Which one of the following is a ciliated parasitic protozoan?
    (a) *Balantidium coli* (b) *Leishmania donovani*
    (c) *Trypanosoma cruzi* (d) *Entamoela histolytica*.

ANSWERS TO MCQs

1. (b)	**2.** (c)	**3.** (a)	**4.** (b)	**5.** (c)
6. (c)	**7.** (b)	**8.** (c)	**9.** (b)	**10.** (a)
11. (b)	**12.** (c)	**13.** (a).		

69

Helminths: Nematodes, Cestodes, Trematodes and Human Diseases

Intestinal worm infections; Elephantiasis; River blindness, loa loa filariasis; Schistosomiasis; Taeniasis; Cysticercosis; Hydatid disease;

WHAT ARE HELMINTHS?

Helminths or parasitic worms are large multicellular worms that are generally visible to the naked eye in their adult stages and have microscopic infective forms. They are chemoheterotropic macroparasites which obtain their nutrient through a mouth. Most parasitic helminths have two hosts: the **definitive host** (where sexual reproduction occurs) and the **intermediate host** (which supports immature or larvae forms). They can be monoecious or dioecious and have elaborate lifecycles involving egg, larva and adult. The word **helminth** is derived from the Greek word ***helmins*** for "worms". The disease caused by a helminth is known as **helminthiasis** or **worm infection**. The study of parasitic worms is called **medical helminthology**.

Helminths of medical significance are classified into two phyla *Nematoda* (round body) and *Platyhelminthes* (flattened body), and consists of three groups.

1. **Roundworms (nematodes):** Elongated, cylindrical, round and unsegmented with a body cavity.
2. **Flatworms (platyhelminths)**
    - **Trematodes (flukes and blood flukes)** – Flat or leaf-like unsegmented worms.
    - **Cestodes (tape worms)** – Tape-like segmented worms.

NEMATODES OR ROUNDWORMS

Nematodes or **roundworms** constitute the phylum *Nematoda* which is the second largest phylum in the animal kingdom – *Animalia*. Members are elongated with bilaterally symmetric bodies that contain an intestinal system and a large body cavity.

Over 60 species of roundworms parasitaze humans which are classified according to the site location on the body: intestine, blood and tissue, as shown in Fig. 69.1. **Intestinal roundworm infections** constitute the largest group of helminthic diseases of humans.

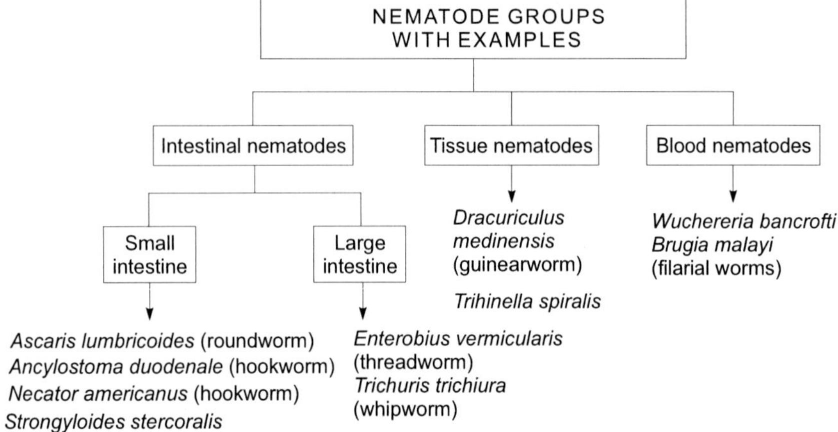

Fig. 69.1 Three types of parasitic nematodes, classified on the basis of their site of infection/location on the body.

ASCARIS LUMBRICOIDES AND ASCARIASIS

Ascaris lumbricoides, a member of the *Nematoda*, is the giant intestinal most common roundworm of humans. It infects between 807 million and 1.2 billion people worldwide, especially in tropical and subtropical countries.

Carolus Linneaus, the Swedish botanist, in 1758 named it based on its presence in the intestine and resembling to an earthworm (Gr *askaris*, an intestinal worm, L. *lumbrian*, earthworm, and Gr *eidos*, resembalance). The male and female exist as separate worms.

Morphology

The adults are large and fleshy 25–40 mm in length and 5 mm in diameter. The female is larger than the male, the latter can be recognized by his characteristically cooked tail (Fig. 69.2). The adult female worm produces eggs (ova) in huge numbers: 2 lakh – 2.5 lakh every day which may be fertilized or unfertilized. The eggs are thick-walled, bile-stained and typically exhibit a corrugated albuminous coat. The fertilized eggs are oval (45.7 μm × 35.50 μm), each containing a single unsegmented ovum with clear crescenteric areas on either side. The unfertilized eggs are irregular and more elongated measuring 88–94 μm long and 44 μm wide.

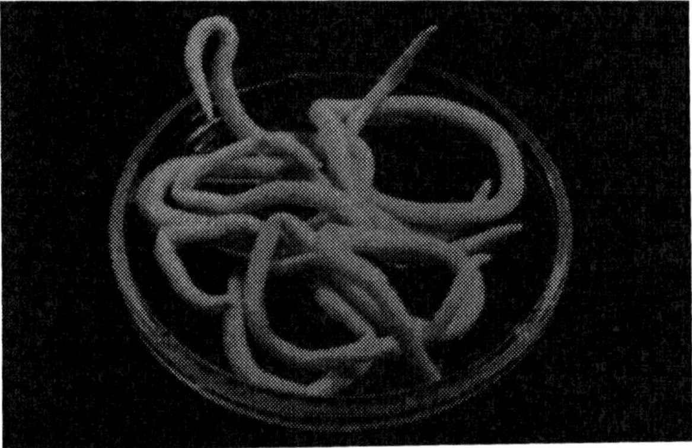

Fig. 69.2 ***Ascaris lumbricoides*, a large roundworm.** The female roundworm may reach a length of 30 cm and can produce several hundred eggs each day.

Lifecycle

Humans are the only definitive hosts in which this worm completes its lifecycle. It infects humans via fecal-oral-route. Eggs are ingested through food, drink or soiled objects, hatch into larvae and burrow through the intestine into circulation. From there, they travel to the lungs and pharynx and are swallowed. The adult worms complete the reproductive cycle in the intestine. The embryonated eggs are released with feces onto the soil (Fig. 69.3).

Clinical Features

Abdominal pain, nausea and vomiting are the major symptoms. Diarrhea or bloody stools may also occur. Intestinal obstruction can occur, if there are large number of adult worms which cause severe pain and vomiting.

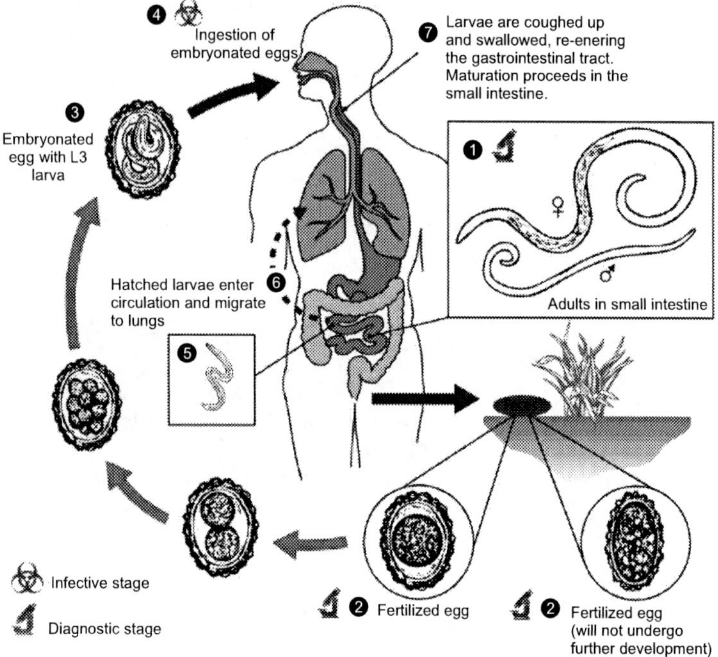

Fig. 69.3 Lifecycle of *Ascaris lumbricoides*, the cause of ascariasis.

Laboratory Diagnosis

- **Microscopic examination of stool:** For visualization of worm eggs in a saline preparation of stool is a gold standard method. (However, eggs will not be present, if the infection is caused by male worms).
- Detection of larval worms in sputum by naked eye.
- **Imaging tests:** X-ray, MRI scan, ultrasound and endoscopy for visualization of worm numbers in the body.

Treatment

Albendazole and mebendazole, are the drugs of choice for treatment. Infections are generally treated for 1–3 days.

ANCYLOSTOMA DUODENALE AND *NECATOR AMERICANUS*: HOOKWORM INFECTIONS

Two species of hookworm (*Ancylostoma duodenale* and N*ecator americanus*) cause **hookworm infection (ancylostomiasis and**

necatoriasis collectively termed helminthiasis) of humans. These cause infection of the intestine that can cause an itchy rash, respiratory and gastrointestinal problems, and eventually iron deficiency anemia due to ongoing loss of blood. Worldwide, between 576 and 740 million people are infected with hookworms, especially in the tropical areas where sanitation is poor. Hookworms thrive best in warm, moist places.

A. duodenale is endemic to the Old World (Middle East, North Africa and Southern Europe) and *N. americanus* is endemic to the New World (mainly Americas and Australia). In hookworms, the *hook* refers to the adult's oral cutting plates by which it anchors to the intestinal walls and its curved anterior end.

Morphology

The two hookworms that infect humans share a similar morphology. The head is bent a little in relation to the rest of body, forming a *hook* shape, hence the name. The two species produce indistinguishable thin-walled eggs which hatch on soil. *N. americanus* is generally smaller (males 5-9 mm long and females 1 cm long) than *A. duodenale* (males 1 cm long and females longer than males) and has a pair cutting plates in the buccal capsule in place of two pairs of teeth in *A. duodenale.*

Lifecycle

The host is infected by larvae, not by eggs, and the usual route is through the skin. The larvae migrate from the blood to the lungs to the intestine where they mature and reproduce. Eggs are released with feces and hatch in the soil after 1–2 days and develop in the environment producing more larvae (Fig. 69.4). A person can become infected by walking barefoot and sitting in contaminated soil. Worms need 5–7 weeks to reach maturity and symptoms of infection can therefore appear before eggs are to be found in the feces, making a diagnosis of hookworm infection difficult.

Clinical Features

At first, people may have an itchy rash at the site of skin penetration, followed by fever, coughing and sneezing or abdominal pain, loss of appetite and diarrhea. Chronic infections can cause loss of blood and anemia leading to heart failure and swelling.

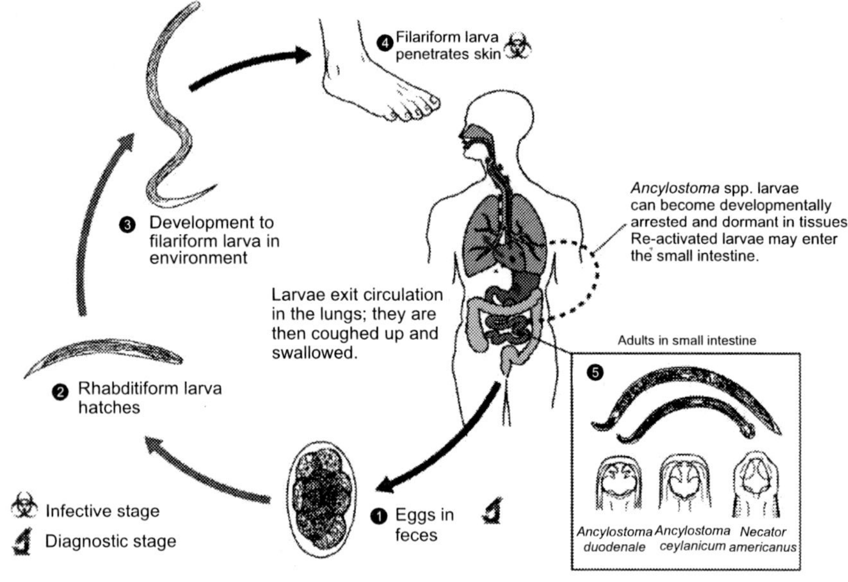

Fig. 69.4 Lifecycle of *Ancylostoma duodenale*, the cause of ancylostomiasis.

Laboratory Diagnosis

- **Microscopic examination of stool:** For visualization of hookworm eggs in a sample of stool.
- **Blood smear for eosinophilia:** The peripheral blood smear is used to count eosinophils, a type of WBCs. Higher eosinophilia than normal number of eosinophils, is indicative of hookworms infection.
- **Blood tests** for anemia and iron deficiency are also used for diagnosis.

Treatment

Hookworms infection is treated with anthelminthic drugs: *Albendazole* (400 mg orally as a single dose), *mebendazole* (100 mg orally twice a day for 3 days or 500 mg as a single dose) or *pyrantel pamoate* (11 mg/kg, maximum dose or 1 g orally once a day for 3 days). Iron supplements are given to cure iron deficiency anemia.

STRONGYLOIDES STERCORALIS AND STRONGYLOIDIASIS

Strongyloides stercoralis, commonly called **threadworm**, the cause of **strongyloidiasis**, is a tiny nematode that completes its lifecycle in humans or in moist soil (from Greek words: *strongylos*, round and *stercoral*, pertaining to feces). **Strongyloidiasis**, a soil-transmitted helminthiasis, affects 30 to 100 million people worldwide, mainly in tropical and subtropical countries.

Morphology

S. stercoralis is one of the smallest parasites known to infect humans. Females are 2.0 to 2.5 mm in length and males are 0.9 mm in length, ♂ and ♀ can be distinguished by the spicules and gubernaculum.

Lifecycle

It is a soil-transmitted disease acquired through direct penetration of the skin by infective larvae through direct contaminated soil during agricultural, domestic and recreational activities. The worm then enters the circulation, is carried to the respiratory tract and swallowed and reacts the small intestine where it matures into adult and produces eggs, the eggs hatch in the gut lumen and yield larvae that are evacuated in feces (Fig. 69.5).

The interesting thing about this worm is that some larvae are not excreted but reinvade the intestine or perianal skin to perpetuate the infection ("**autoinfection cycle**").

Clinical Features

A red, intensely itchy skin rash at the site of entry is the first sign of threadworm infections. The infection is mild that may cause intermittent symptoms that mostly affect the intestine (intestinal pain and intermittent or persistent diarrhea), the lungs (cough, wheezing, chronic bronchitis) or skin (pruritus, urticaria). It is severe and life-threatening through **hyperinfection,** especially in immunodeficient patients.

Laboratory Diagnosis

- Microscopic identification of larvae in the stool (wet normal) or duodenal fluid.

- Detection of larvae in sputum from patients.
- Serology – Detection of antibodies by ELISA.
- By elevated eosinophils count in blood.

Treatment

- Ivermectin (stromectol) in a single oral dose, 200 µg/kg is the drug of choice for the treatment.
- Thiabendazole and albendazole (25 mg/kg twice daily for 5 days – 400 mg maximum) are the other effective drugs.

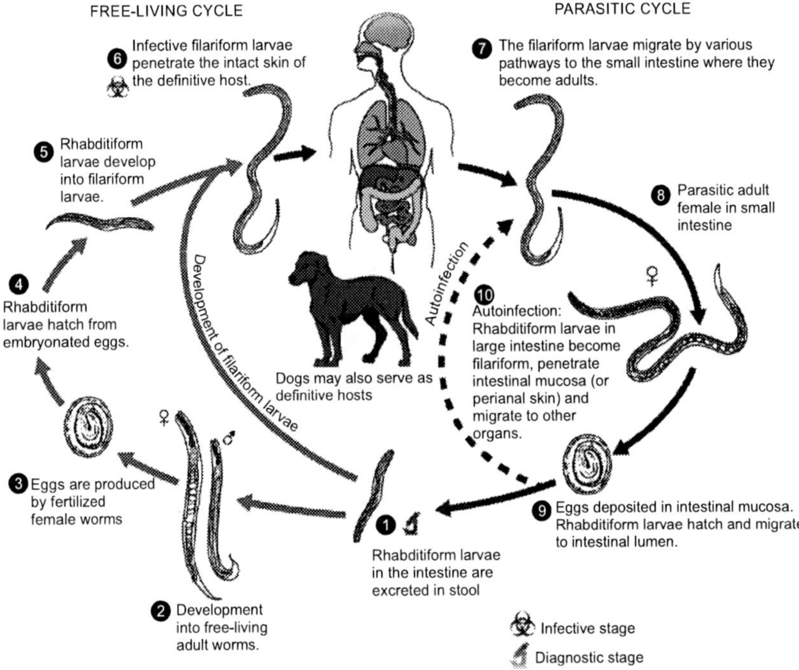

Fig. 69.5 Life cycle of *Strongyloides stercoralis*, the cause of strongyloidiasis.

ENTEROBIUS VERMICULARIS AND ENTEROBIASIS

Enterobius vermicularis, commonly known as the **human pinworm** (due to the female's long pointed tail), is one of the most common nematode infections – **pinworm infection** (or **enterobiasis**), especially among children, worldwide. The disease is more prevalent in the United States and Western Europe.

Morphology

The adult females are 8–13 mm long and 0.5 mm thick with a shortly pointed posterior end. The males are smaller than the females measuring 2–5 mm long and 0–2 mm thick. The eggs are translucent, small sized (50-60 μm × 20-30 μm), thick-shell and have a surface that adheres to object. The larvae are 140–150 μm in length.

Lifecycle

The lifecycle begins with ingestion of the pinworm embryonated eggs through contaminated hands, food and nail biting. The entire lifecycle from egg to adult takes place in the human gastrointestinal tract of a single host from about 2 to 8 weeks (Fig. 69.6).

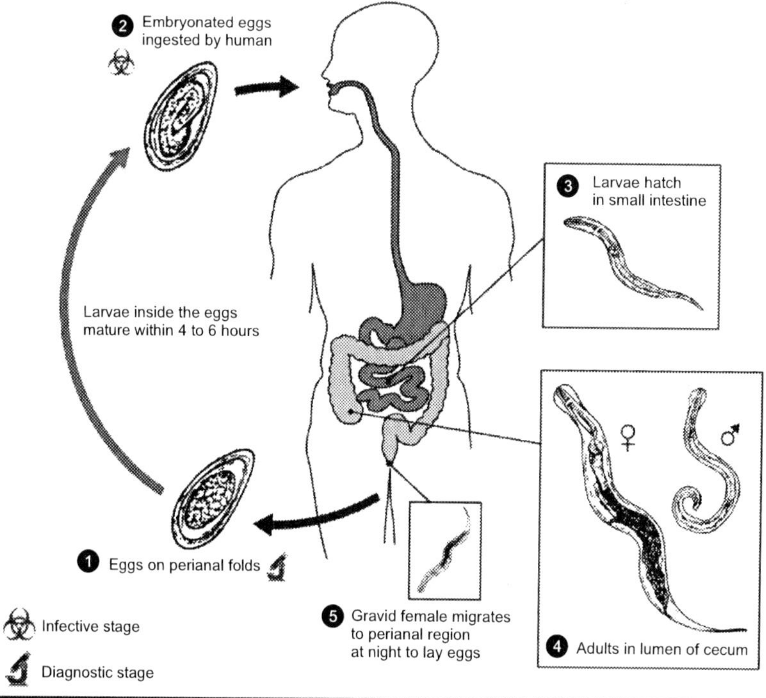

Fig. 69.6 Lifecycle of *Enterobius vermicularis*, the cause of enterobiasis.

Symptoms

Severe rectal itching (anal area) is the major symptom. It may be associated with restlessness and difficulty in sleeping.

Laboratory Diagnosis

- By visualization of eggs and pinworms (1 cm long).
- Microscopic examination of fecal matter for the presence of eggs.
- Presence of light-yellowish, thread-like adult pinworms (1 cm long) by microscopic examination of anal area applied scotch tape (transparent) for the eggs and pinworms that have a characteristic (i.e., protruding ridges) running the length of the worm.

Treatment

Two doses of mebendazole, pyrantel parmoate or albendazole at two weeks interval are given for treatment.

FILARIAL NEMATODES AND FILARIASIS

Filarial worms (or **nematodes**) are long, thread-like tissue nematodes that produce characteristic–tiny larvae, called **microfilariae,** and cause **filariasis** of different types in humans. These worms can live in host tissues for several years. They have a biphasing lifecycle that alternates between humans (the **definitive host**) and blood-sucking mosquito or fly vectors (the **intermediate host)**. Eight filarial worms are known to cause infections in humans, 3 species that cause serious filariasis are:

- *Wuchereria bancrofti,* the cause of **lymphatic filariasis**
- *Onchocerca volvulus,* the cause of **river blindness**
- *Loa loa,* the cause of ***Loa loa* filariasis.**

WUCHERERIA BANCROFTI AND LYMPHATIC FILARIASIS (ELEPHANTIASIS)

Lymphatic filariasis, commonly called **elephantiasis**, is a human disease caused by filarial worms that affects the lymph nodes and lymph vessels. It is marked by severe swelling due to collection of fluids in the legs, arms, breasts and genitals with pain in which the skin takes on the appearance of an elephant's hide, hence called **elephantiasis** (Gr. *elephas* = elephant). The disease is most common in tropical Africa and Asia. An estimated 15 million people currently live with lymphedema worldwide, the condition developing years after first becoming infected with the parasite.

Three species of filarial worms cause the disease: *Wuchereria bancrofti, Brugia malayi* and *Brugia timori*, with *W. bancrofti* being the most common causing over 90% of the infections. The male worms are 3-4 centimeters in length and female worms 8–10 cm.

Transmission and Lifecycle

The disease spreads from person-to-person by mosquitoes (female *Culex Anopheles* and *Aedes*). When a mosquito bites an infected person, microscopic worms (called microfilariae) circulating in the patient's blood enter and infect the mosquito. When the infected mosquito bites another person the larvae pass from the mosquito through the skin, and travel to the lymph vessels where they grow into adult worms. An adult worm lives for about 5 to 7 years. Mating of adult worms releases millions of microfilariae into the blood. People with worms in their blood give the infection to others through mosquitoes (Fig. 69.7).

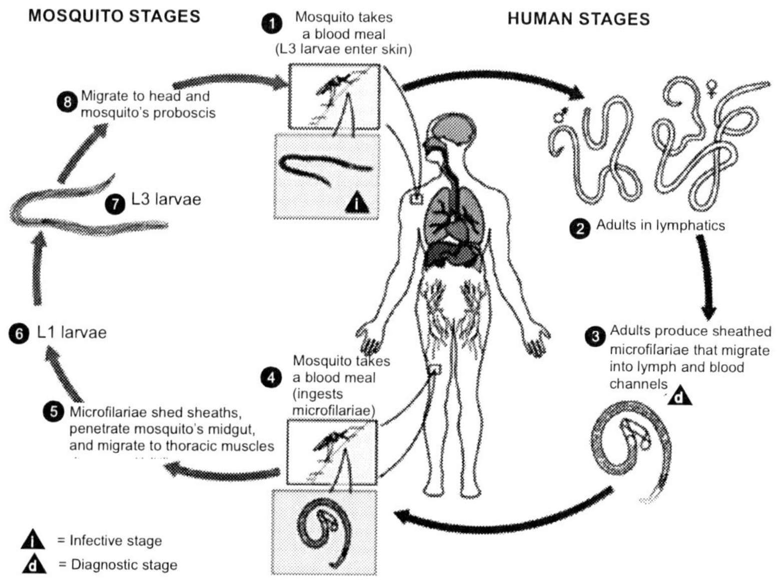

Fig. 69.7 Lifecycle of *Wuchereria bancrofti*, the cause of lymphatic filariasis (elephantiasis) showing infective and diagnostic stages.

Symptoms

The disease shows abnormal enlargement (swelling) called **lymphedema** mostly of legs but sometimes of arms, breasts and genitalia causing pain, and severe disability. **Hydrocele**, (i.e., swelling of the scrotum) develops in some men. In affected persons, hardening and thickening of the skin, called elephantiasis, develops. Most people develop these clinical manifestations years after being infected by the parasite.

Laboratory Diagnosis

- **Microscopic examination** of Giemsa stained peripheral blood collected during night for demonstration of microfilarial (larval stage of parasite). The worms are only active at night (called nocturnal periodicity), so the sample should be collected in the night between 10 pm and 2 am.
- **Serological testing**. Testing the blood serum for antibodies. (elevated levels of antifilarial Ig G4) against the disease may also be used for diagnosis.

Treatment

Antiparasitic drugs used for the treatment are albendazole with diethylcarbamine, or albendazole with ivermectin.

ONCHOCERCA VOLVULUS AND RIVER BLINDNESS

River blindness or **onchocerciasis** is a parasitic disease caused by the filarial worm ***Onchocerca volvulus*** that affects the eyes and skin. It is the second-most common cause of blindness due to infection, after trachoma. The disease is spread by the repeated bites of a black fly (*Simulium*) which lives near rivers, hence the name of the disease.

River blindness is a serious problem in Sub-Saharan Africa. The Global Burden of Disease study estimated in 2017 that there were 20.9 million prevalent infections worldwide and 14.6 million had skin disease and 1.15 million had vision loss.

Morphology

O. volvulus is a dioecious worm in which males are much smaller (23 mm in length) than females (230–700 mm) and the macrofilariae, the first larval stage, are 300 µm in length. Male and female worms form nodules under the skin in humans. The mature females, with an average lifespan of 15 years, can produce from 500 to 1500 microfilariae per day.

Lifecycle

It is spread from person-to-person via female biting blackflies. In infected humans, the microfilariae of the parasite are found in the dermis layer which are ingested by a female blackfly during a feed (i.e., blood meal) only during the daytime. The larvae are deposited into the bite wound and develop into adults in the immediate subcutaneous tissues, where disfiguring nodules form within 1-2 years after initial contact between the host and parasite. Microfiliariae given off by the adult females migrate via the blood to many locations, but especially eyes. It is the blood phase that infects other feeding black flies (Fig. 69.8).

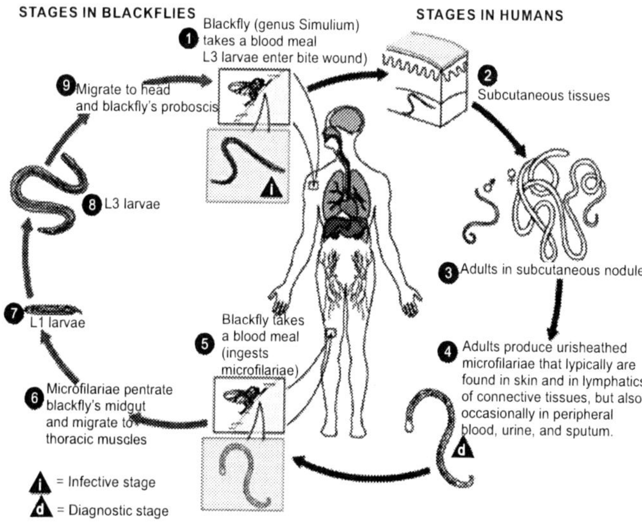

Fig. 69.8 Lifecycle of *Onchocerca volvulus*, the cause of river blindness (onchocerciasis), showing both the infective and diagnostic stages.

Clinical Features

Onchocerciasis is an eye and skin disease, characterized by severe itching and bumps under the skin, vision changes and permanent blindness. In most cases, nodules under the skin form around the adult worms.

Laboratory Diagnosis

- It is diagnosed via skin biopsies called **snips.** Skin snips are put into saline, and if larvae (parasitic eggs) exist they will emerge from the skin.
- Examination of eyes for the presence of larvae.
- Looking within the bumps under the skin for the presence of adult worms.
- **Serology blood testing** for antibodies of the parasite.

Prevention

There is no vaccine or medication to prevent infection with *O. volvulus.*

Treatment

- Ivermectin, every six to twelve months, is the drug of choice used for the treatment. It kills the larvae but not the adult worms.
- In addition, doxycycline is also recommended to control *Wolbachia* an associated bacterium, with the worms.

LOA LOA AND FILARIASIS

Loa loa, a filarial nematode, commonly known as the "**African eye worm**", causes a skin and eye disease—the ***Loa loa* filariasis**. *Loa loa* actually means "worm worm" but is commonly referred to as the "eye worm", as it localizes to the conjunctiva of the eye. This worm is commonly found in Africa. It mainly inhabits rain forest in West Africa and has native origins in Ethiopia. Currently over 10 million humans are infected with *L. loa* larvae.

Morphology

Loa worms have a simple structure consisting of a head (that lacks lips), a body, and a blunt tail. It is sexually dimorphic, the male adults are smaller and range from 30–34 mm long and 350–420 µm wide, and the female adults are between 40 and 70 mm long and 500 µm (0.5 mm) wide and vary in colour. Microfilariae are 250–300 µm long and 6–8 µm wide, sheathed and contain body nuclei that extend to the tip of the tail.

Lifecycle

The human is the *definitive host*, in which the parasitic worms attain activity, mate and produce microfilariae. Two species of deer flies (*Chrysops*), the vectors serve as the *intermediate host* in which the microfilarae undergo part of their morphological development, and they are borne to the next definitive host. The larvae mature into adult worms in 5 months after entry into the human's body and can live up to 17 years in the human host. These parasitic worms have a **diurnal periodicity**—they circulate in the peripheral blood during day time and migrate into the vascular parts of the lungs during the night, where they are considered non-circulatory.

Symptoms

The major symptoms include localized angioedema, called **Calabar swellilngs**, in skin which is itchy but non-painful, more common near joints in the arms and legs. Migration of an adult worm to the eyes can also occur frequently, and this is the reason *Loa loa* is often called the "African eye worm" Eosinophilia is often prominent in filarial infections.

Laboratory Diagnosis

- Microscopic examination of Giemsa stained thick blood smear for the presence of microfilariae, in the blood sample collected between 10 am and 2 pm.
- Antigen detection using an immunoassay.

Treatment

- Diethylcarbamazine (DEC) (8-10 mg/kg/day taken 3 times daily for 21 days) is the drug of choice for treatment. Surgical removal of adult worms from the conjunctiva is also employed for early recovery.

TREMATODES OR FLUKES

Trematodes, also called **flukes**, are parasitic flat worms (leaf-shaped) that have flattened, bilaterally symmetrical body. The name **trematode** (Gr. *trema*, a hole) comes from the muscular sucker containing a mouth (hole) at the fluke's anterior end. They have an oral and ventral sucker with which they attach to the host tissue. Based on the system of the vertebrate host they infect, they are classified into:

- **Blood flukes**

  Schistosoma spp. the cause of **schistosomiasis** in humans:

  S. haematobium, S. mansoni and *S. japonicum*
- **Lung flukes**

  Paragonimus westermani seen in Manipur
- **Hepatid (liver) flukes**
- *Clonorchis* (*Opisthorchis*) *sinensis*–seen in Assam and Manipur
- *Fascicola hepatica*–seen in Assam and Uttar Pradesh.

Trematodes are relatively uncommon in India. The common trematodes seen in India are *Paragonimus westermani* (lung fluke), and *Schistosoma hematobium* (blood fluke).

SCHISTOSOMIASIS

Schistosomiasis, also known as **bieharziasis** and **snail fever** is a systemic infestation of bladder and intestine caused by parasitic flatworms (blood flukes) called **schistosomes** (Gr. *schisto,* split and *some,* body). The disease has been considered the second-most socio-economically devastating parasitic disease (after malaria), with 200 to 250 million people infected worldwide. It is most commonly found in Africa, Asia and South America. Three main *Schistosoma* species causing the disease are *S. haematobium, S. japonicum* and *S. mansoni.*

Morphology

The adult human schistosomes are dioecious, male and female worms having different morphologies. They are white-greyish worms with a basic bilateral symmetry, 10-20 mm long, and have both digestive system and oral and ventral suckers for attachment and stabilization.

Lifecycle

Unlike most flatworms, the schistosomes are **gonochristic**, the male surrounds the female and encloses her within his gynecophoral canal for the entire adult lives of the worms.

Human infection occurs through the larval forms of the parasite released by freshwater snails penetrate the skin during contact with infested water.

Transmission occurs when people suffering from schistomoiasis contaminate freshwater sources with their excreta containing parasite eggs, which hatch in water.

In the body, the larvae develop into adult schistosomes. Adult worms live in the blood vessels where the female releases eggs. Some of the eggs are passed out of the body in the feces or urine to continue the parasites lifecycle (Fig. 69.9). Others become trapped in body tissues, causing immune reactions and progressive damage to organs.

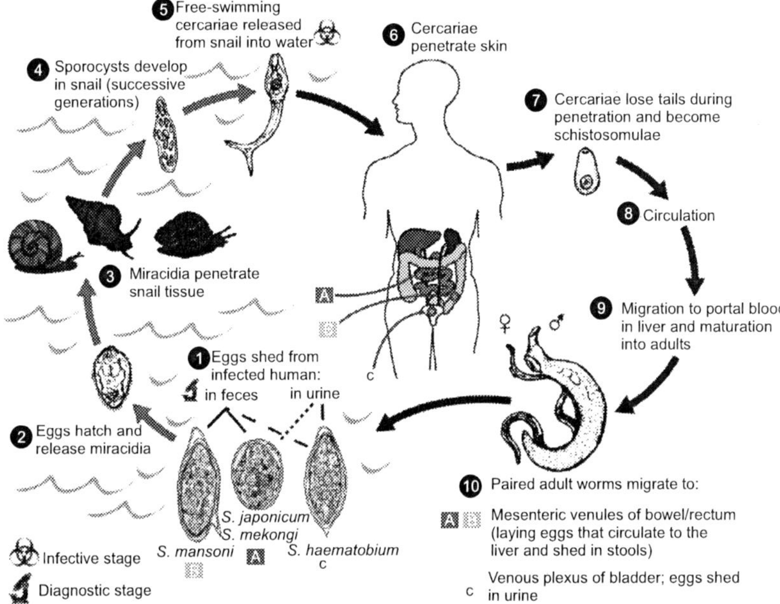

Fig. 69.9 Lifecycle of *Schistosoma* spp., the cause of schistosomiasis.

Clinical Features

Clinically schistosomiasis is of two types: **Intestinal schistosomiasis** and **urogenital schistosomiasis.**

Symptoms usually appear between 4 and 6 weeks of infection. These initiate with light rash, commonly called "**swimmer's itch**" at the point of entrance of the parasite. These are followed by abdominal pain, diarrhea, bloody stool or blood in the urine (haematuria). Long time infection may lead to liver damage, kidney failure, infertility or bladder cancer. In children, it may cause anaemia, poor growth and learning difficulty.

Laboratory Diagnosis

- **Microscopic examination** of urine or stool for detection of eggs of the parasite. Eggs of *S. mansoni* are 140 × 60 μm with a prominent lateral spine near the posterior end.
- **Tissue biopsy** (rectal/bladder) for demonstration of eggs is also used.
- **Urine reagent strips** for identification of microhematuria in urine is a reliable method.
- **Detection of antibodies in blood**–Serum specimen are tested by FAST-ELISA using *S. mansoni* adult microsomal antigen (79 units/ml serum indicates a positive reaction, i.e., infection with *Schistosoma* spp).
- **Molecular method**–PCR based testing is accurate and rapid.

Treatment

Praziquantel is the drug of choice to prevent and treat *Schistosoma* infections as per WHO. A single oral dose of the drug is taken annually.

Other possible treatments include a combination of praziquantel with metrifonate, artesunate, and mefloquine.

CESTODES (TAPEWORMS)

The **cestodes** (L. *cestus*, girdle, belt) commonly called **tapeworms,** are long tape- or ribbion-like multisegmented parasitic worms that can be found in the gastrointestinal tract of humans. Their bodies consist of many similar units, called **proglottids** as they lack a digestive tract and absorb nutrients directly from the host's small bowel. Interestingly, whale tapeworm (*Polygonoporus giganticus*) is 40-m long, known to be the longest parasite in the world.

Some of the most common cestodes include:

- ***Taenia saginata*** (beef tapeworm) → the cause of **taeniasis.**
- ***Taenia solium*** (pork tapeworm) → the cause of **cysticercosis.**
- ***Taenia asiatica*** (Asian tapeworm) → the cause of **taeniasis.**
- ***Echinococcus granulosus*** (dog tapeworms) → the cause of **hydatid.**
- ***Diphyllobothrium latum*** (fish or broad tapeworm) → the cause of **diphyllobothriasis.**
- ***Hymenolepis diminuta*** (rat tapeworm) → the cause of **hymenolepiasis**.
- ***Hymenolepis nana*** (dwarf tapeworm) → the cause of **hymenolepiasis.**

TAENIASIS AND CYSTICERCOSIS

Taeniasis is an intestinal tapeworm. Infection is caused by eating undercooked beef or pork containing eggs of three *Taenia* species *Taenia saginata* (beef tapeworm), *Taenia solium* (pork tapeworm) or *Taenia asiatica* (Asian tapeworm).

The larvae of *T. solium* called **cysticerci**, when enter brain, liver and other organs cause **cysticercosis** (**neurocysticercosis**).

The disease (taeniasis or cysticercosis) is worldwide in distribution affecting 50 million people globally. It is most common in the developing world. In India, it is a very common parasitic infection with over 10 million cases reported each year.

T. solium and *T. saginata* are worldwide in distribution, *T. solium* being more prevalent in poorer communities and *T. asiatica* is limited to Asia.

Morphpology

These flatworms have long, very thin, ribbon-like bodies (**strobilia**) composed of sacs (**proglottids**) and a **scolex** that grips the host intestine. Each proglottid is an independent unit adapted to absorbing food and making and releasing eggs.

Taenia saginata (*L. taenia* = a flat band or ribbon, *sagi* = a pouch and *natore* = to swim) is flat, white, or semi-transparent, the adults measure 5 metres, however, it may reach up to 25 metres. It can produce up to 1 lakh eggs per proglottid. An adult usually has 1000 to 2000 proglottids.

Taenia solium is also called **armed tapeworm** due to the presence of rostellum and hooklets. The adults are somewhat smaller than the *T. saginata*, measuring 2 to 7 m usually have 1000 proglottids and produce 50,000 eggs per proglottid.

Taenia asiatica body is yellowish-white, about 350 cm long and 1 cm broad (i.e., shorter body than both the taenids) with 700 to less than 1000 proglottids in the strobilia and produce 44,180 to 1,32,500 (average 90051) eggs per proglottid and infection is acquired by eating pork, not beef.

Lifecycle

Humans (the definitive host) are infected through cysticerci (larvae) of the pork tapeworm or by ingesting eggs in pork or drink. After ingestion, the larvae mature into adults and attach to the intestine where they produce **proglottids** (segments bearing eggs), which become gravid; detach from the tapeworm and migrate to the anus or pasted on the feces (stool) (Fig. 69.10). Autoinfection may occur in humans if proglottids pass from the intestine to the stomach via reverse peristalsis.

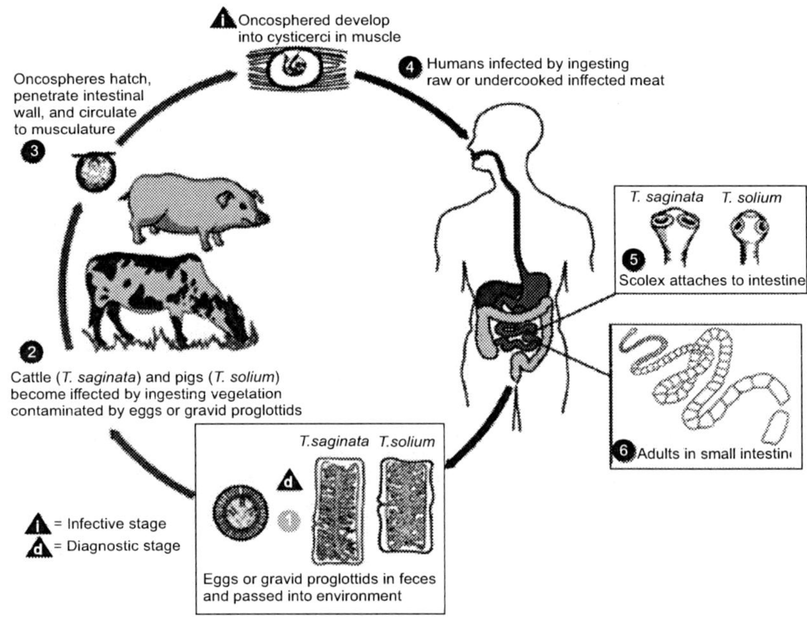

Fig. 69.10 Lifecycle of *Taenia* spp., the cause of taeniasis.

After eggs of the worm are ingested, they hatch in the intestine and release **onchospheres** which penetrate the intestine wall and through the bloodstream travel to the straited muscles and to the brain; liver and other organs, where they develop into **cysticerci** and cause damage resulting to **cysticercosis. Neurocysticercosis**, a common manifestation of the disease, occurs when several larvae settle in the brain, which gives rise to seizers in affected humans.

T. saginata lifecycle begins with the ingestion of raw undercooked beef containing the encysted larvae form (cysticercus), which gets digested out of the beef in the human intestinal system and the worm then attaches on the intestine of mucosa of the upper small intestine and becomes an adult tapeworm. Animals are infected by grazing on land, contaminated with human feces containing gravid detached from the adult tapeworms.

Clinical Features

Taeniasis generally has few or no obvious symptoms (i.e., asymptomatic). It takes about 8 weeks from infection for adult worms and can last a few years without treatment. Heavy infection can result in abdominal pain, indigestion and weight loss.

Cysticercosis of brain called neurocysticercosis is characterized by epileptic seizures, dizziness, dementia and low eosinophil levels, sometimes leading to death.

Laboratory Diagnosis

Intestinal infection with adult *T. solium* worms can be diagnosed by examination of stool samples for segments of worms (proglottids) and microscopic examination of saline preparation for characteristic eggs.

Neurocysticercosis is diagnosed by CT scan or MRI to reveal solid nodules, ring-enhancing lesion or hydrocephalus.

Immunoblot assay, using a serum specimen is a reliable method. Peripheral blood smear reveals eosinophilia in case of cysticercosis.

Treatment

- *Praziqunatel tablets* 5 to 10 mg/kg orally as a single dose is used to treat intestinal infection (without neurocystecercosis).
- Niclosamide, a single dose of the 2 gm tablet (that is to be chewed) is the alternative drug.

Neurocysticercosis is treated with corticosteroids (prednisone up to 60 mg orally once/day or dexamethasone 12-24 mg orally once/day). Sometims albendazole or praziquantel and/or surgery are used to treat the serious patients.

ECHINOCOCCUS GRANULOSUS AND HYDATID DISEASE

Hydatid disease (also known as **hydatidosis** or **cystic echinococcosis**) is sometimes a fatal disease of the liver, lungs and brain caused by dog tapeworm *Echinococcus granulosus*. **Hydatid** is the larval stage of a tapeworm occurring in a fluid-filled sac contaning daughter cysts in which scolices develop. The disease occurs worldwide and currently affects about 1.4 million people globally.

Morphology

E. granulosus, also called the **hydatid worm**, **hyper tapeworm** and **dog tapeworm** is 3 to 6 mm in length, provided with three proglottids (segments) when intact: an immature proglottid, mature proglottid and a grand proglottid with 823 eggs. It has four suckers on its scolex (head) and a rostellum with hooks.

It is a cyclophyllid cestode that dwells in the small intestine of canids as an adult. The lifecycle involves dogs as a definitive host were parasites reach maturity and reproduce. The wild ungulates, such as sheep and humans serve as **intermediate hosts** where larval stage results in the formation of echinococcal cysts, the cause of cystic echinococcosis in humans that affects the liver, lungs, brain and other organs (Fig. 69.11).

Lifecycle

It is a *zoonotic disease,* i.e., transmitted to humans from animals. Infection results by ingestion and contact of dog feces containing eggs of the tapeworm (fecal-oral route, swallowing of feces by children and eating salads) and attaches to the mucosa of the intestines in the definitive host and there the parasite will grow into the adult stages. Adult *E.granulosus* releases eggs within the intestine which will be transported out of the body via feces. When contaminated waste is excreted into the environment, intermediate host has the potential to contract the parasite by grazing in contaminated pasture, perpetuating the lifecycle (Fig. 69.11).

Pathogenesis

Hydatid disease is characterized by the presence of a cyst called **hydatid cyst** that contains tapeworm larvae. The cyst wall is provided with three layers: the pericyst, ectocyst and endocyst. The formation of a cyst takes several years. The infection may be acquired in childhood and may manifest only in adulthood.

Echinococcosis occurs in two main forms: **cystic echinococcosis (hydatidosis)** and **alveolar echinococcosis**.

Symptoms

Symptoms of the disease depend on size and location of the cysts in the body.

- Abdominal pain, weight loss, along with yellowish skin (due to jaundice during liver infection).

- Pain in chest, coughing and shortness of breath occur in lung infection.

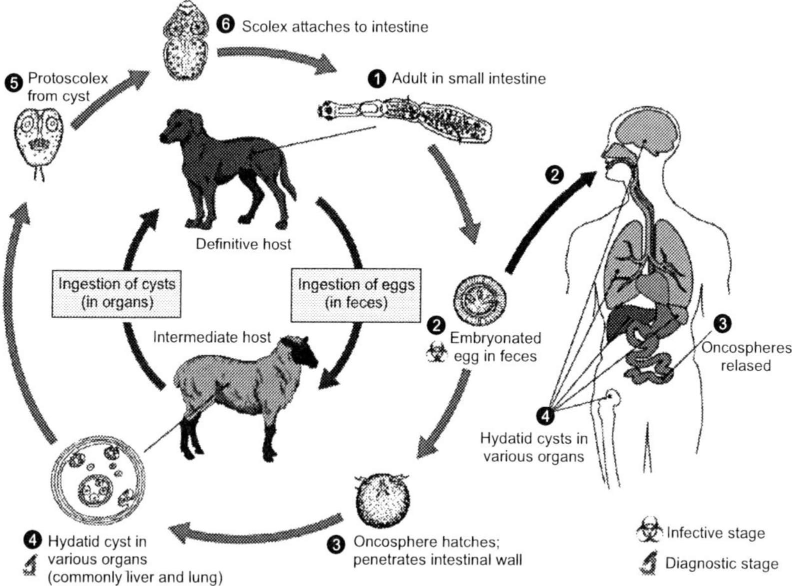

Fig. 69.11 Lifecycle of *Echinococcus granulosus*, the cause of hydatid (cystic echinococcosis).

Diagnosis

- **Examination of cyst fluid** to visualize the presence of scolices and blood capsules in surgically removed cysts.
- **Casoni test** or **immediate hypersensitivity skin test** in which the antigen, (0.25 mL fluid from hydatid cysts/human cyst and sterilized by seitz filtration) is injected intradermally in the patients arm and equal volume of saline injected on the other forearm and observed for large wheel (> 5 cm diameter) within 20 minutes at the injection site a positive reaction.
- **Radiological examination:** Ultrasound through CT or MRI to visualize hydatid cysts in the lungs, liver and other tissues.
- **Blood tests:** To look for antibodies against the parasite.

Treatment

Human echinococcosis is treated with:

- Surgical removal of cysts (without rupturing to prevent acute anaphylactic shock).
- Surgical removal of fluid from the cysts. Surgery is followed by administering the drug praziquantel (oral or injection).

KEY POINTS

- **Helminths**, commonly called **worms**, are characterized by the attachment organs which include suckers, hooks, lips, teeth and dentary plates.
- The diseases caused by the parasitic helminths (worms) are called **helminthiasis** (**worm infections**).
- **Helminthic parasites** are classified into **roundworms** (**nematodes**), **flukes** (**trematodes**) and **tapeworms** (**cestodes**).
- Helminthic infections are more common in children.
- Soil-transmitted helminthiasis (e.g., ascariasis) and schistosomiasis are the most important helminthiasis.
- Helminthic parasites are spread by eggs and larvae that are eaten or exposed to skin surfaces (walking bare foot)
- Human tapeworms are acquired from eating poorly cooked beef and pork.
- Six intestinal nematodes infect more than 25% of the humans causing **ascariasis**, **hookworm infection**, **strongyloidiasis**, **enterobiasis**, and **trichuriasis**.
- Eggs are classified as bile-stained and non-bile stained eggs or ova based on the saline and iodine preparations.
- Praziquantel and albendazole are used to treat helminth infections that kill or paralyze the worms by interrupting their lifecycles.

IMPORTANT REVIEW QUESTIONS

1. What are helminths? How clinically significant helminths are classified? Name the intestinal roundworm diseases, their mode of spread, diagnosis and treatment.
2. Write short notes on:
   (a) Ascariasis.
   (b) Microfilaria.
   (c) Enterobiasis.

(d) Hydatid disease.
(e) Elephantiasis.
(f) River blindness.
(g) Schistosomiasis.
(h) Cysticercosis.

MULTIPLE-CHOICE QUESTIONS

1. Which of the following is the most common worldwide nematode infestation?
(a) Ascariasis (b) Trichinosis
(c) Hookworm infection (d) Enterobiasis.

2. All of the following are intestinal nematodes (roundworms) EXCEPT:
(a) *Ascaris lumbricoides*
(b) *Necator americanus*
(c) *Trichinella spiralis*
(d) *Enterobius vermicularis.*

3. Which of the following is a cestode?
(a) *Taenia solium*
(b) *Ascaris lumbricoides*
(c) *Enterobius vermicularis*
(d) *Strogyloides stercoralis.*

4. Which of the following causes enterobiasis disease?
(a) Hookworm (b) Pinworm
(c) Roundworm (d) Filarialworm.

5. Which of the following disease is caused by a nematode?
(a) Poliomyelitis (b) Leprosy
(c) Covid-19 (d) Filariasis.

6. All are true for lymphatic filariasis EXCEPT:
(a) Mainly affects the lower limb
(b) Caused by the parasitic worms *Wuchereria bancrofti* and *Brugia malayi*
(c) Intermediate vector is the mollusc
(d) Also known as elephantiasis.

7. Which of the following is a whipworm?
   (a) *Ascaris lumbricoides*
   (b) *Trichuris trichura*
   (c) *Ancylostoma duodenale*
   (d) *Enterobius urmicularis.*
8. Which of the following are segmented flatworms (tapeworms)?
   (a) Cestodes
   (b) Trematodes
   (c) Nematodes
   (d) None of these.
9. Which of the following helminths causes river blindness in humans?
   (a) *Loa loa*
   (b) *Onchocerca volvulus*
   (c) *Schistosoma gaponium*
   (d) *Trichinella spiralis.*
10. Which of the following helminths causes iron deficiency anemia?
   (a) *Enterobius vermicularis*
   (b) *Loa loa*
   (c) *Ancylostoma duodenale*
   (d) *Trichinella spiralis.*
11. Which of the following helminths is classified as a blood fluke?
   (a) *Paragonimus westermani*
   (b) *Schistosoma haematobium*
   (c) *Clonorchis sinensis*
   (d) *Fasciola hepatica.*
12. Smallest parasite known to infect humans is:
   (a) *Strongloides stercoralis*
   (b) *Ascaris lumbricoides*
   (c) *Ancylostoma duodenale*
   (d) *Necator americanus.*

ANSWERS TO MCQs

1. (a) **2.** (c) **3.** (a) **4.** (b) **5.** (d)
6. (c) **7.** (b) **8.** (a) **9.** (b) **10.** (c)
11. (b) **12.** (a).

70
Rodents and Arthropods: Vectors of Medical Importance

WHAT ARE ARTHOROPODS?

Arthropods are invertebrate animals characterized by the presence of a jointed skeletal hard covering composed of chitin (exosekleton), segmented bodies bearing paired jointed appendages (legs), from which the name *arthropod* (jointed feet) is derived.

The members are classified in the phylum ***Arthropoda***, the largest phylum in the animal kingdom—***Animalia*** consisting of over 1 million species, which include, such familiar forms as crabs, lobsters, spiders, mites, insects, centipedes, and millipedes.

Arthropods though are not microbes themselves, but they are still studied in microbiology because a variety of arthropods–insects, spiders and crustaceans–cause human diseases directly and serving as vectors of pathogenic organisms. Arthropods that transmit the infectious diseases are called **disease vectors** and the diseases are termed **vector-borne diseases**.

The first major discovery of a disease vector—*mosquito transmission of malaria* came from **Sir Ronald Ross** on 20th August 1897. Since then several arthropods have been reported as vectors of disease causing organisms belonging to different groups such as bacteria, viruses, protozoa and helminths (parasitic worms). The stings and bites of arthropods may be irritating or painful but very few inject dangerous toxins. Medically arthropods are more significant as carriers of diseases such as malaria, yellow fever, dengue and elephantiasis (via mosquitos), African sleeping sickness (via tsetse flies), typhus fever (via lice), bubonic plague (via fleas) and Rocky Mountain spotted fever, Lyme disease (via ticks). Many diseases of domesticated animals are also transmitted by arthropods. Figure 70.1 illustrates some of the arthropods of clinical/medical significance.

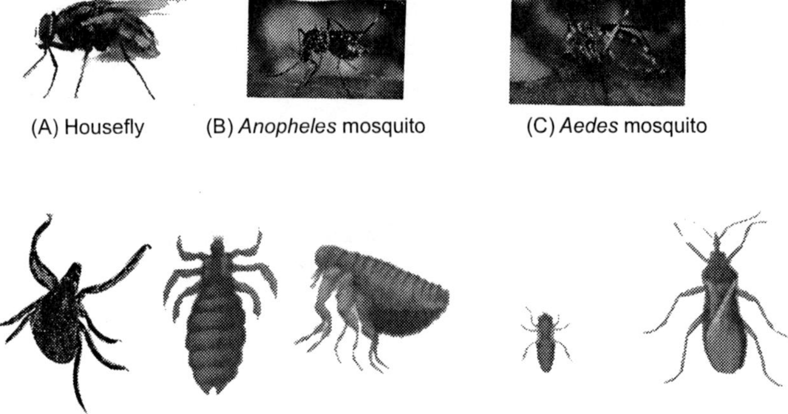

(D) Tick (E) Human louse (F) Rat flea (G) Deer fly (H) Kissing bug

Fig. 70.1 Representative arthropods that are parasitic or can serve as disease vectors. (A) The house fly (*Musca domestica*), spreads diseases by carrying microbes on its body; (B) *Anopheles* mosquito transmits malaria (*Plasmodium*) from humans to humans; (C) *Aedes* mosquito transmits chikungunya virus and dengue virus. (D) Tick (*Ixodes*), vector for Lyme disease and babesiosis; (E) Human louse (*Pediculus*), a vector of epidemic typhus;

(F) Rat flea (*Xenopsylla cheopis*), a vector for endemic murine typhus and bubonic plague;

(G) Deer fly (*Chrysops*), a vector for tularemia;

(H) Kissing bug (*Triatoma*) a vector for (Chagas' disease).

The study of insects and related arthropods is called **entomology** (*entomon* = insect + *logia* = study) and the discipline involved with the study of insects of medical importance is called **medical entomology** (or **public health entomology**).

CLASSIFICATION OF ARTHROPODS

Based on the number of legs/appendages, the phylum *Arthropoda* includes three classes:

- *Arachnida* (8 legs): Ticks, mites, spiders, scorpions.
- *Insecta* (**hexpods**) (6 legs): Mosquitoes, flies, lice, flees, bees, true bugs.
- *Crustacea* (one pair of appendages on each body segment): crabs, crayfish, copepods.

ECTOPARASITIC INFESTATION

A parasitic disease in which an organism lives primarily on the skin of its host without killing it, is called the **actoparasitic infestation**. Lice, flies, bed bugs and ticks are examples of ectoparasitic. arthropods responsible for tick paralysis, chigger dermatitis, scabies, pediculosis and myiasis in humans. Pains, itching, fever, allergic reactions and anaphylactic shock are the results of bites and toxins production by arthropods, respectively. A summary of these diseases is given in Table 70.1.

Table 70.1 A summary of ectoparasitic human diseases caused by arthropods bites

Disease	Agent	Characteristics
• **Tick paralysis**	Various ticks	Toxins introduced with tick bite cause fever and ascending motor paralysis.
• **Chigger dermatitis**	*Trombicula* mites	Larvae burrow into skin and cause itching and inflammation: can cause violent allergic reactions.
• **Scabies**	*Sarcoptes scabiei*	Widespread lesions with intense itching; other mites cause house dust allergy when their feces are inhaled by allergic individuals.
• **Flea bites**	*Tunga penetrans*	Itching and inflammation from adult females in skin.
• **Pediculosis**	*Pediculus humanus* (human louse)	Inflammation at louse bite sites and itching; *Phthirus pubis* (pubic louse) found in public areas.
• **Blackfly fever**	Blackfly	Bites cause severe inflammatory reaction in sensitive individuals.
• **Myiasis**	Fly larvae	Maggots infect wounds in animals: Congo floor maggot sucks human blood: screwworms injure cattle.
• **Mosquito and other bites**	Mosquitoes, some flies, bedbugs	Painful, itchy bites, several insects serve as disease vectors.

MODES OF TRANSMISSION IN ARTHROPOD VECTORS

Arthropods transmit pathogenic organisms mechanically or biologically (Fig. 70.2) and the vectors are appropriately called mechanical and biological vectors.

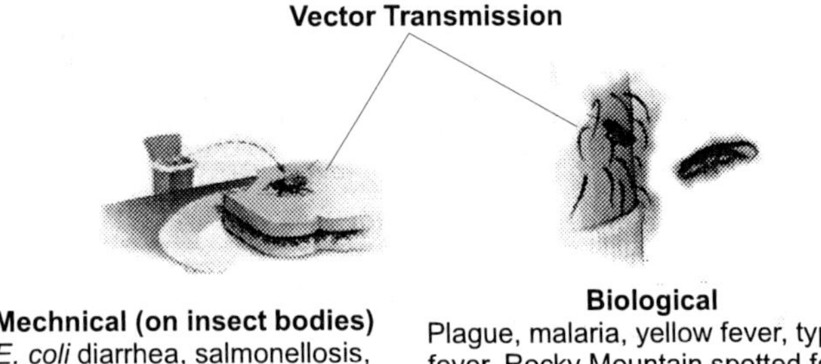

Fig. 70.2 Two modes of disease transmission in arthropod vectors.

Mechanical vectors: Mechanical transporters transmit diseases passively by picking up infections from feces and then contaminating human food and the diseases are contracted orally (flies, cockroaches). A vector in which the parasite does not go through any part of its life-cycle during transit on or in it, is termed a **mechanical vector**. The housefly is a very common and cosmopolitan species which carries over 100 pathogens and parasitic worms and transmits these through their feet and body parts from feces to human food mechanically. These include:

- *Amoebic and bacillary dysenteries*: From feces to food
- *Typhoid bacteria*: From feces to food
- *Yaw germs*: From a yaw ulcer to ordinary sore
- *Poliomycelitis*: Viruses from infected feces to food or drink.

Other diseases transmitted by houseflies are salmonellosis, tuberculosis, anthrax, cholera, hepatitis and some forms of opthalmia.

Biological vectors: Actively transmit parasitic disease causing organisms. The pathogen develops and multiplies in the vectors, and is transmitted to humans via arthropods bite or excreta (mosquitoes, tsetse flies, body lice, fleas) compared with direct transmission through animal bites, the transmission of zoonoses through arthropod vectors is more common.

Arthropods form a major group of vectors transmitting a huge number of pathogenic organisms that affect human health. Many such vectors are *haematophagus*, which feed on blood at some or all stages of their lives. According to a recent study of May 2018 by CDCA, USA, diseases caused by insect bites have tripled from 2004 to 2016 resulting in millions of deaths of the over billions infections caused every year globally.

Examples of important arthropod vectors of human diseases belonging to insects and arachnids are:

Vectors		Diseases
Common name	**Scientific name**	
• **Mosquitoes**	*Anopheles*	Malaria
	Aedes	Dengue fever, yellow fever
	Culex	Arboviral encephalis
• **Kissing bug**	*Triatoma*	Chagas' disease
• **Rat flea**	*Xenopsylla*	Bubonic plague, endemic murine typhus
• **Human louse**	*Pediculus*	Relapsing fever, epidemic typhus
• **Tsetse fly**	*Glossina*	African trypanosomiasis
• **Deerfly**	*Chrysops*	Tularemia
• **Sand fly**		Kala-azar
• **Bed bug**		Typhus fever
• **Mango fly**	*Chrysops*	Loaiasis, eye worm *Loa loa*
	ARACHNIDA (mites and ticks)	
• **Ticks**	*Diermacentor*	Rocky Mountain spotted fever, Colorado tick fever
	Ixodes	Lyme disease, babesiosis, Ehrlichiosis
	Ornithodorus	Endemic relapsing fever
• **Mite**	*Leptotrombidium*	Scrub typhus fever

TREATMENT AND PREVENTION OF ARTHROPOD-BORNE DISEASES

Treatment

The recommended treatment of an arthopod-borne disease depends upon the specific disease. Treatment often involves a course of drugs and in some cases, through a vaccine available for the specific disease.

Prevention

Arthropod-borne diseases transmitted by biological vectors can be prevented by:

- Avoiding being bitten by the arthropod vectors, by wearing clothing that covers bare skin, using repellants to deter insects, avoiding outdoor activities at times when arthropods are most active, and sleeping under mosquito net.
- Avoiding visiting countries/places where certain arthropod-borne diseases are common.
- Vaccination, where vaccines are available, to prevent development of the disease if transmission occurs.

For mechanically transmitted arthropod infections, the preventive methods employed are:

- By excluding insects from areas where food is prepared and served.
- Washing or thoroughly cooking any food that may have come into contact with an arthropod.
- Avoiding aquatic bodies inhabited by arthropods.

WHAT ARE RODENTS?

Rodents (from Latin *redere*, "to grow, eat away") are small mammals with continuously growing sharp front teeth (incisors) and lacking canine teeth. They are included in *Rodenta*, one of the largest order of mammals. Well-known examples include mice, rats, squirrels, praire dogs, guinea pigs, beavers, lamsters and gerbils. Rabbits, hare and pikas, were once included with them, but are now considered to be in a separate order the *Lagomorpha*. Figure 70.3, illustrates some of the rodents of medical significance.

Rodents are almost everywhere and are well-known reservoirs and carriers for a number of infectious diseases caused by bacteria, viruses, protozoa and helminths and play an important role in their transmission and spreading. Rodents can act as both intermediate infected hosts or as hosts for arthropod vectors such as fleas and ticks. A well known example is: Plague popularly known as "black death" in the 14th century, the most notorious bacterial disease killing 25 million people over a 50-year period is linked to rats in the human environment. It is a zoonosis caused by the bacterium *Yersinia pestis* that is transmitted to humans by fleas (vector) feeding on black rats (*Rattus rattus*). Since then rodents have been linked to hanta virus, lymphocytic choriomeningitis, leishmaniasis, salmonellosis, relapsing fever, pulmonary infection and viral hemorrhagic fevers and are thought to be responsible for more deaths than all wars over the last 1000 years.

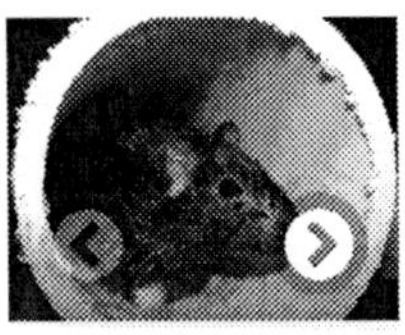

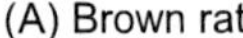

(A) Brown rat

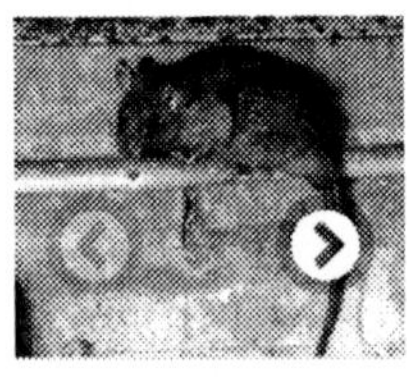

(B) Black rat

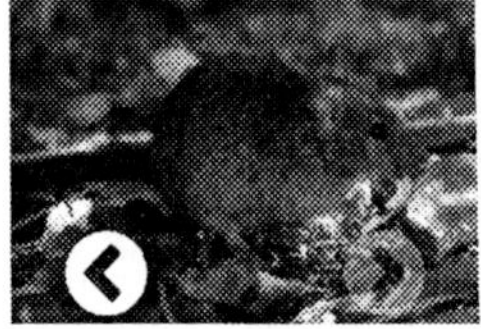

(C) House mouse

Fig. 70.3 Some of the common rodents. (A) Brown rat (common rat, or street rat, and Norway rat) (*Rattus norvegicus*), pathogen carrier of Weil's diseases, rat-bite fever, Q-fever, cryptosporidiosis, viral hemorrhagic fever, hantavirus pulmonary syndrome). (B) Black rat (house rat, roof rat, ship rat) (*Rattus rattus*), a serious pest to farmers. (C) House mouse (*Mus musculus*), a carrier of lymptocytic choriomeningitis (LCMV).

Rodent-Borne Diseases

Rodents carry a wide range of disease causing organisms belonging to bacteria, viruses, protozoa and worms (helminths). Worldwide, rats and mice, two common rodents, spread over 30 human diseases. Rodent diseases can be spread to humans directly and indirectly (Fig. 70.4).

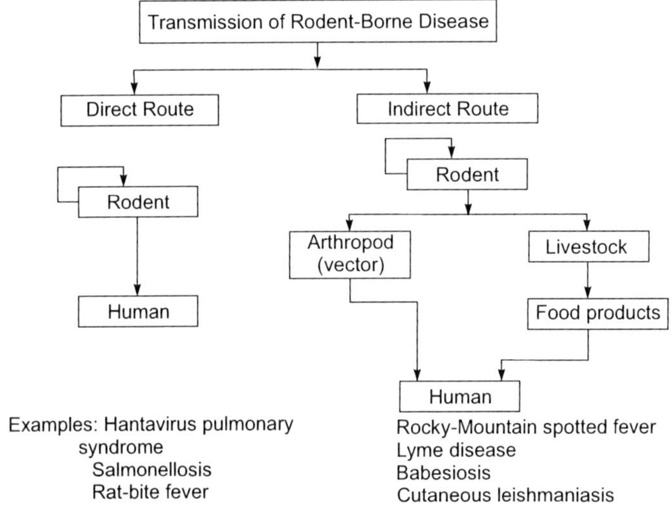

Fig. 70.4 Two different transmission pathways of rodent-borne infections, direct and indirect routes.

Direct Route of Transmission: The rodent harbours the disease causing agent (no or limited symptoms of the disease), i.e., a **carrier** and passes it directly onto humans via:

- Handling of live or dead rodents.
- Direct contact with rodent urine, feces (droppings) or saliva.
- Breathing in dust that is contaminated with rodent urine or feces.

Rodent-borne diseases are directly transmitted to humans with the causative agent, rodent involved and mode of infection are summarized in Table 70.2.

Table 70.2 A summary of directly transmitted rodent diseases

Disease	Causative agent(s)	Rodents as vectors	Mode of infection(s)
• **Hantavirus pulmonary syndrome (HPS)** and **Hantavirus**	Virus	Deer mouse, cotton rat, rice rat, white footed mouse	Inhalation of aerosolized virus shed in infected rodents droppings, urine or saliva; direct contact with rodents or their droppings.

Contd.

Table 70.2 Contd.

• **Leptospirosis**	Bacteria (*Leptospira*)	Rodents	Eating food or drinking water contaminated with urine from infected rodents; contact with urine contaminated water and soil.
• **Lymphocytic choriomeningitis (LCM)**	Virus	House mouse (*Mus musculus*)	Breathing in dust that is contaminated with rodent urine or droppings; direct contact with diseased rodents and their urine or droppings.
• **Plague (Black death)**	Bacteria	Wild rodents especially rats	As a zoonosis, the disease is spread by infected rats, humans are infected by contact with carcasses of plague infected rats.
• **Rat-bite fever**	Bacteria	Rats and mice	Bite or scratch wound human infected rodents, contact with a dead rodent. Rat feces contaminated food or water.
• **Salmonellosis**	Bacteria	Rats and mice	Rat feces contaminated food or water.
• **Tularemia**	Bacteria	Wild rodents, including musk rats, ground squirrels, beavers	Handling infected common carcasses, eating or drinking contaminated food or water.
• **South American arenaviruses**	Virus	Cane rat, drylands vesper mouse, large vesper mouse	Breathing in dust contaminated with rodent urine or droppings. Direct contact with rodents and their urine and droppings.

Indirect Mode of Transmission: In this mode, the rodents harbour disease causing organisms (reservoir) and spread the pathogen to humans via a vector such as ticks, mites, fleas or sandfly that have fed on an infected rodent or spread through livestock (Fig. 70.4). The major rodent-borne diseases transmitted through indirect mode of transmission with their reservoirs and vectors are summarized in Table 70.3.

Table 70.3 A summary of rodent-borne diseases transmitted through indirect mode of transmission

Disease	Causative agents	Rodents microbes (reservoir)	Vectors	Mode of infection
• **Babesiosis**	Parasite	Deer mice, voles	Tick	Bite
• **Colorado tick fever**	Virus	Deer mouse, bushy-tailod woodrat, ground squirrel, chipovink	Tick	Bite
• **Cutaneous leishmaniasis**	Parasite	Wild wood rat	Sandfly	Bite
• **Lyme disease**	Bacteria	White-footed mouse (*Peromyscus*), tree squarrel	Tick	Bite
• **Murine typhus**	Bacteria	Rats	Fleas	Bite
• **Omsk hemorrhagic fever**	Virus	Muskrat	Tick	Bite
• **Scrub typhus**	Bacteria	Rats	Mite	Bite
• **Rickettsialpox**	Bacteria	Mice	Mite	Bite
• **Relapsing fever**	Bacteria	Wild rodents	Tick	Bite
• **Rocky Mountain spotted fever**	Bacteria	Wild rodents	Tick	Bite
• **Sylvatic typhus**	Bacteria	Flying squirrel	Flea, louse	Bite from an infected flea, contact of brokan skin or wound with infected flea, louse or their droppings or inhaling thier aerosolized fever

Contd.

Table 70.3 Contd.

• **West nile virus**	Virus	Ground squirrel, snowsphoe hare		Bite
• **Plague** * **(Bubonic)**	Bacteria		Oriented rat flea (*Xenophylla chcopsis*)	Bite

* It also spreads by handling an infected animal (i.e., direct mode).

A few rodent-borne diseases are transmitted through both routes of transmission, i.e., directly and indirectly. Plague (bubonic and septicemic plague) generally spreads to people by the bite of an infected flea (oriental rat flea (*Xenopsylla cheopsis*), (the primary vector). It can also spread through direct contact with an infected animal or person or by eating an infected animal.

PREVENTION OF RODENT-BORNE DISEASES

The primary strategy for preventing humans exposure to rodent associated diseases is effective rodent control in and around home which can be achieved by adopting the following means: by eliminating the food sources by keeping foods in thick plastic or metal containers with light lids and cleaning spilled food right away and washing dishes and cooking utensils soon after use; by sealing even the smallest entries such as holes inside and outside the homes to prevent their entry; to trap rodents in and around the home to reduce their population; preventing contact with rodents by cleaning your homework place and camp site at regular intervals; and avoid illness by taking precautions before and while cleaning rodent-infested areas such as nesting sites.

KEY POINTS

- **Arthropods** are animals with jointed legs that include licks, flies, fleas, lice and mosquitoes.
- The arthropod that transmit infectious diseases are called **vectors** and the diseases are called **vector-borne diseases**.
- Mechanism of vector transmission can be **mechanical** or **biological**.
- Typhoid, polio, amoebic and bacillary dysenteries are mechanically transmitted by arthropod vectors.

- Dengue fever, malaria, kala azar, plague and yellow fever are transmitted by arthropod vectors biologically.
- Strategies for prevention of illness due to arthropod-borne diseases include avoidance, vector reduction programs, repellents and chemoprophylaxis.
- **Rodents** are small animals characterized by continuously growing sharp front teeth (incisors).
- Rats, mice, squirrels, gunea pigs, hamsters and gerbils are rodents of medical significance.
- **Rodent-borne diseases** are transmitted by direct and indirect routes.
- In **direct mode of transmission**, the rodent passes the pathogenic organism directly to humans (e.g. hantavirus, salmonellosis, rat bite fever).
- In **indirect mode of transmission**, rodent acts as a reservoir of pathogen and transmits it via arthropod vector (e.g., Rocky Mountain spotted fever, Lyme disease, Cutaneous leishmaniasis).
- Human exposure to rodent diseases can be prevented by effective rodent control by eliminating any food sources, sealing entries in homes and successfully traping rodents in and around home.

IMPORTANT QUESTIONS

1. Write brief notes on:
   (a) Define arthropod vector. Name 5 arthropod vectors and name a disease transmitted by each.
   (b) Medical significance of arthropods.
   (c) Modes of disease transmission in arthropods.
   (d) How can arthropod-borne diseases be prevented?
   (e) How rodent-borne diseases are transmitted?
   (f) Give examples of directly and indirectly transmitted diseases by rodents, three each with the rodent involved.
   (g) Rat and mice-borne human diseases.

MULTIPLE-CHOICE QUESTIONS

1. Parasites that have a jointed, chitinous exoskeleton with segmented bodies and jointed appendages (legs) would be classified as:
   (a) Protista (b) Flukes
   (c) Arthropods (d) Nematode.

2. Which of the following arthropod has six legs?
   (a) Arachnid (b) Insect
   (c) Crustacean (d) None of these.
3. The organisms that transmit diseases are called vectors. True or false?
4. All of the following diseases are transmitted by biological arthropod vector EXCEPT:
   (a) Malaria (b) Chagas' disease
   (c) Kala-azar (d) Amoebic dysentery.
5. All of the following are ectoparasitic diseases caused by arthropod-bites EXCEPT:
   (a) Scabies (b) Chigger dermatitis
   (c) Poliomycelitis (d) Tick paralysis.
6. Which of the following is *not* the mosquito-borne viral disease?
   (a) Yellow fever (b) Lassa fever
   (c) Dengue (d) Japanese B encephalitis.
7. Name the vector via which viruses causing yellow fever and encephalitis is transmitted to humans?
   (a) Rodents (b) Mosquitoes
   (c) Ticks (d) Sandflies.
8. All are rodent-borne diseases transmitted by indirect mode of transmission or by vectors EXCEPT:
   (a) Lyme desease
   (b) Babesiosis
   (c) Lymphocytic choriomeningitis (LCM)
   (d) Rocky Mountain spotted fever.
9. All of the following are directly transmitted diseases by rats EXCEPT:
   (a) Salmonellosis (b) Rat-bite fever
   (c) Plague (d) Lyme disease.
10. Plague (also called Black death) caused by *Yarsinia pestis* is a rodent-borne disease transmitted through direct and indirect mode of transmission. True or False?

ANSWERS TO MCQs

1. (c)	2. (b)	3. True	4. (d)	5. (c)
6. (b)	7. (b)	8. (c)	9. (d)	10. True.

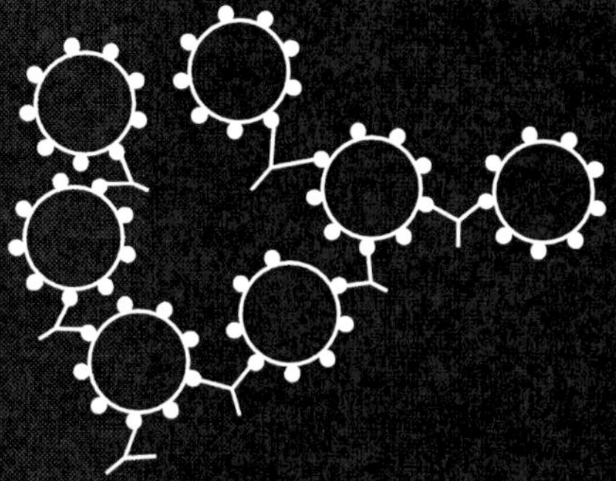

Unit IV E

DIAGNOSTIC-CLINICAL MICROBIOLOGY

- Diagnosis of Pathogenic Microorganisms in Clinical Microbiology Laboratory
- Collection, Handling and Transportation of Various Laboratory Specimens

71

Diagnosis of Pathogenic Microorganisms in Clinical Microbiology Laboratory

Bacterial, Viral, Fungal and Parasitic Diseases

WHAT IS DIAGNOSTIC OR CLINICAL MICROBIOLOGY?

The infectious agents (such as bacteria, viruses, fungi and parasites: protozoa and helminths) that cause the infectious diseases are diagnosed/identified in a clinical laboratory by microbiologists.

The branch of microbiology that makes it possible to identify the exact pathogens of infectious diseases and the most optimal therapy at the level of individual patients is called **diagnostic microbiology, clinical microbiology** and **diagnostic medical microbiology**.

A diagnostic test for an infectious agent is used to demonstrate the presence or absence of infection to detect evidence of a previous infection (for example, the presence of antibodies). A medical professional presents a test to diagnose or to exclude possible illness. Diagnostic testing has become indispensable for diagnosing and monitoring diseases for providing prognoses and for predicting treatment responses.

PROTOCOL FOR PROCESSING A SPECIMEN IN THE LABORATORY

Diagnosis of a disease and isolation of pathogens from samples of infected tissues or fluids (e.g., blood, urine, stool, mucus, serum, vaginal fluids, CFS) require a wide array of procedures which are described here.

- Direct specimen examination and testing
- Cultivation on different media, pure culture isolation and identification
- Examination of biochemistry, antigenicity and genetics of microbes
- Examination of patient for symptoms and serological tests

Scheme of examination to be followed for presumptive evidence or confirmatory evidence of a pathogen is given in Fig. 71.1. Some tests are performed on the specimen immediately and yield 'same day' results (**preliminary report**). Cultures of specimen involve a minimum of 18 hours incubation before colonies are visible and can be identified (**interim report**) after 2nd day. Antibiotic susceptibility tests and complete identification involve a further incubation period of 18–20 hours (**final report** after 3rd day).

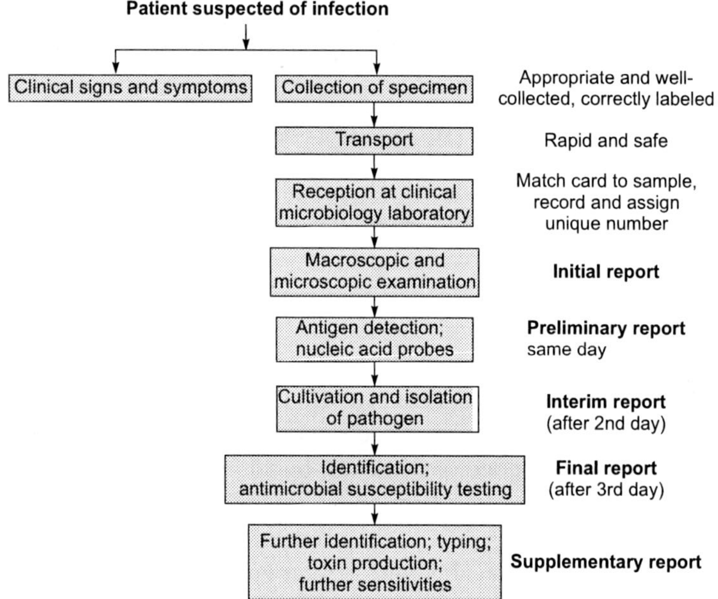

Fig. 71.1 A protocol for diagnosis of an infectious disease from a clinical (biological) specimen in a microbiology laboratory.

Direct Tests and Cultural Tests

Samples are analysed by two routes: direct tests and cultural tests.

- **Direct tests (noncultural techniques)** include microscopic examination of stained specimens (Gram stain, acid-fast stain), direct antibody fluorescent test and macroscopic antigen tests, all of which provide immediate clues to the identity of the microbe and microbes in the sample.
- **Cultural tests** isolate and identify the pathogen by performing various tests on the isolates (biochemical, slide serum typing, antimicrobic sensitivity, gene probes, phage typing), and animal inoculation.

MICROSCOPIC EXAMINATION OF MICROBIAL SPECIMENS

Direct specimen tests (or **noncultural techniques)** include microscopic examination of stained specimen, direct fluorescent antibody tests, and macroscopic antigen tests, all of which provide rapid clinical data. **Microscopy** (i.e., use of microscope) is an important first step in the examination of all specimens. The different uses of two basic types of microscopy (light and electron microscopy) are given in Fig. 71.2. Many test specimens can be examined in their native state. Examination of stained material, either direct test specimens or samples of growth from cultures, is the most useful method for presumptive identification of several microorganisms. Bright-field microscopy is commonly used in diagnostic microbiology, stained smears from lesions are examined with the oil immersion objective (100×) using the 10× eyepiece, yielding a magnification of 1000×.

Wet films are examined with a dry objective (40×) (for example, to demonstrate the motility of bacteria). Examination can be enhanced with either phase-contrast or dark-field microscopy. Dark-field microscopy is generally used for the detection of spirochetes in skin lesions associated with early syphilis or in blood specimens of people with early leptospirosis. Fluorescence microscopy can be used to identify acid-fast microorganisms such as *Mycobacterium tuberculosis* after they are stained with fluorochromes such as auramine-rhodamine.

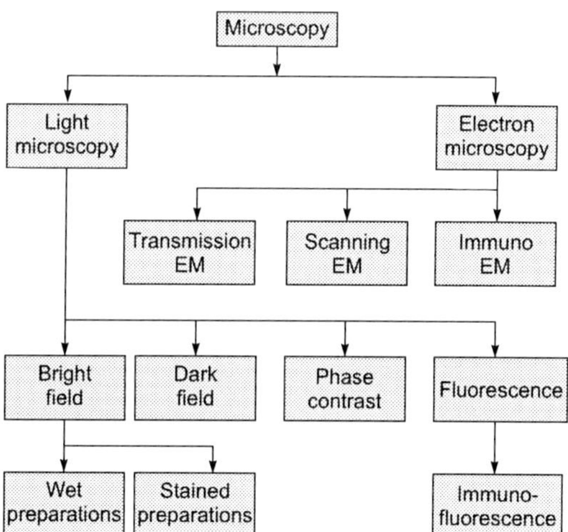

Fig. 71.2 Various types of microscopy used in clinical microbiology laboratory.

DIAGNOSIS OF BACTERIAL DISEASES

Bacterial infections can be diagnoted by microscopic culture based and non-culture based (serology and PCR) tests.

MICROSCOPIC METHODS

Microscopy is a simple and rapid method for the detection of microorganisms and can be performed quickly. Most specimens are treated with stains that colour the pathogens, although **wet mounts** of unstained samples can be used to detect certain pathogens. Gram stain and acid-fast stain are often used for bacterial identification.

Because microscopic detection usually requires a bacterial concentration of at least $1 \times 10^{4\text{-}5}/m^2$, host body fluid specimens (e.g. cerebrospinal fluid) are concentrated by centrifugation before examination.

• Gram Stain

In **Gram staining**, (Fig. 71.3), specimen material is heat-fixed to a slide and stained by sequential exposure to Gram crystal violet (20–60 sec),

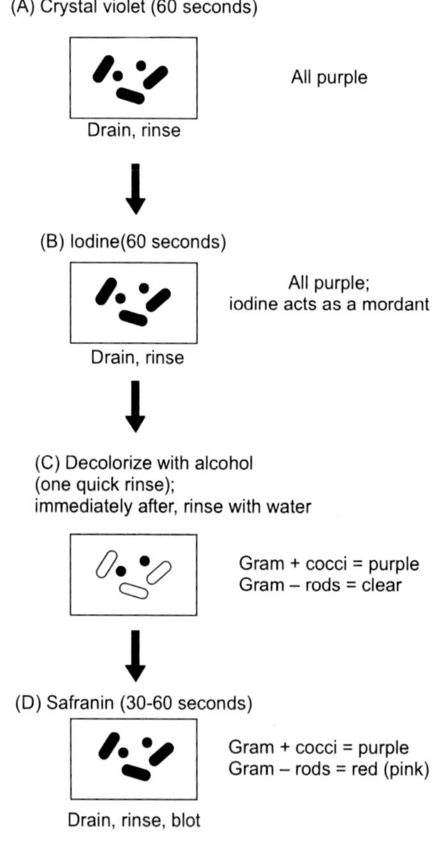

Fig. 71.3 The Grain stain (A – D). Steps in Gram staining: Gram-positive cells retain the purple colour of crystal violet, whereas Gram-negative cells are decolorized with alcohol and subsequently pick up the red colour of the safranin counter-stain.

iodine (60 sec) decolorized with C_2H_5OH 95% or acetone (10–20 sec) and counterstained with safranin (20 sec). Microscopic examination of the stained smear would **classify**: **purple-blue or blue** (Gram-positive bacteria) and **red** (Gram-negative reaction), thus classifying bacteria;

- **High lights cell morphology** (e.g. bacilli, cocci) and **cell arrangement** (e.g., diplo, chains, clumps).
- **Identifies polymorphonuclear leukocytes** indicating bacterial infection rather than colonization.

Based on these characteristics and on the presumptive identification of the organism, the antibiotic-therapy can be initiated pending definitive identification.

• Acid-Fast Stain (Ziehl-Neelson)

In **Ziehl–Neelson acid-fast stain,** the bacterial smear is heat-fixed (over the flame 2–3 times), covered (flooded) with carbolfuchsin and heated over the flame for 5 minutes, water rinsed and decolorized with acid-alcohol mixture (3% HCl-95% C_2H_5OH) for 15–20 seconds, rinsed again and then stained with Loeffler's methylene blue, washed with water, and blot dry. This stain produces bright red colours in ***acid-fast*** organisms (e.g., *Mycobacterium*) due to the presence of lipid components in their cell wall. Non-acid fast bacteria appear blue.

Acid-fast stain is used to diagnose tuberculosis and leprosy caused by *Mycobacterium* species.

• Fluorescent Stains

Fluorescent stains (e.g., auramine D, acridine orange) are used to detect mycobacteria (e.g., *M. tuberculosis*) by using a fluorscence microscope. The advantage is that these stains allow detection of microbes at lower concentrations ($<1 \times 10^4$ cells/mL).

Coupling a fluorescent dye to an antibody directed at a pathogen (direct or indirect immunofluorescence) increases sensitivity and specificity. Direct fluorescent antibody tests are commercially available and commonly used in diagnostic kits (e.g., *Pnenmocystis* and *Legionella*).

Wet Mounts

Wet mounts of unstained samples can be used via dark field microscopy to detect the following:

- Vaginal clue cells (present in bacterial vaginosis)
- Motile organisms (e.g., *Trichomonas*)
- *Treponema* spirochetes (present in syphilis).

Special Stains

- **Fontana's stain** for *Treponema pallidum*
- **Polychrome methylene blue** for *Bacillus anthracis*
- **Warthin-Starry stain** for *Helicobacter pylori* and spirochetes
- **Albert's and Ponder's stain** for *Corynebacterium diphtheriae.*

CULTURE-BASED METHODS

Culture is a microbial growth on or in a nutritional solid or liquid medium (broth) as increased number of organisms simplify identification. Culture also facilitates testing of antimicrobial susceptibility.

In **culture-based methods**, the isolation and identification of bacteria from various specimens is achieved by plating on general purpose media (e.g. blood or chocolate agar), some pathogens require inclusion of specific nutrients and inhibitors called selective media or other special conditions for incubation (e.g., a specific temperature, oxygen or CO_2 concentration, and duration).

• Blood Culture

Blood samples are inoculated into bottles containing enriched nutrient broth (brain-heart infusion agar, biphasic Mac-Conkey medium) and incubated at 37°C for 5 to 7 days or until growth occurs.

Used commonly for Gram-positive bacteria (*Staphylococcus aureus, Enterococcus* spp), Gram-negative bacteria (e.g. *Escherichia coli. Enterobacter* spp. and *Klebsiella* spp.).

• CFS Culture

Blood agar is used for isolation of *S. pneumoniae* and chocolate agar for *H. influenzae* and *N. meningtidis* from CFS and examined using Gram stain and methylene blue for studying the morphology of these bacteria.

• Feces Culture

Salmonella and *Shigella* from feces are cultured on blood agar, Mac-Conkey agar and desoxycholate agar (DCA) and xylose lysine desoxycholate (XLD). TCBS (thiosulphate citrate bile salt sucrose) is used for *Vibrio cholerae.*

• Urine Culture

Blood agar, MacConkey agar and CLED (cystine lactose electrolyte deficient) are used for urine specimens to diagnose urinary tract infections caused by Gram-positive (e.g. *S. aureus, Enterococcus.* spp.)

and Gram-negative bacteria (e.g., *E. coli, P. aeruginosa*, species of *Klebsiella, Enterobacter* and *Proteus*).

A quantitative culture, based on the presence of CFUs per ml of clean-catch mid-stream urine sample, is used to diagnose UTI (presence of $>10^5$ CFUs/ml is indicative of significant bacteiuria).

• Pus (Wound Exudates) Culture

Blood agar and MacConkey agar are used for the presence of *S. aureus, Enterococcus* (Gram+ive), *E. coli, P. aeruginosa, Klebsiella, Enterobacter* (gram +ve) and *Staphylococcus* (coagulase-negative) bacteria.

• Throat Swab Culture

Blood agar and Loeffler's serum slope are used to detect group A β-hemolytic *S. aureus* and *C. diphtheriae.*

• Sputum Culture

Blood agar, MCA and CA are used for sputum culture for diagnosing longer respiratory tract infectious especially *S. aureus* and *S. pneumoniae* (Gram +ive) and *Klebsiella, Enterobacter, E. coli* and *H. influenzae*.

NON-CULTURE BASED METHODS

These methods include: immunological tests and serological methods, nucleic acid-based methods, and non-nucleic acid-based methods.

Immunological Tests–To detect antigens and antibodies in the patients specimen:

Antigen detection Latex agglutination test to diagnose infections caused by *S. pneumoniae, H. influenzae* and *N. gonorrhoeae*.

Antibody detection–Tube agglutination test for typhoid fever and slide agglutination test for *T. pallidum.*

• Nucleic Acid-Based (Molecular) Identification Method

These methods detect organism-specific DNA and RNA sequences extracted from the microorganism, by nucleic acid amplification techniques (e.g. polymerase chain reaction, especially that are difficult to culture), *Mycobacterium tuberculosis* and several others are detected by PCR.

• Non-Nucleic Acid Based Identification Methods

These identification methods use phenotypic (functional and morphologic) characteristics of organism rather than genetic identification.

Characteristics of an organism's growth on culture media (e.g., colony size and shape) provide clues to species identification and combined with Gram stain, direct further testing of the organism by biochemical tests (eg. coagulase test, catalase test and several others).

Non-nucleic acid based identification tests may involve:

- Manual methods
- Automated methods
- Chromatographic methods
- Mass spectroscopy

Currently, commercial kits are available in the markets that contain battery individual tests that may be done simultaneously using a single inoculation of a microbe and are useful for a wide range of microorganisms.

DIAGNOSIS OF VIRAL DISEASES

Due to emerging viruses and growing number of viral infections, a few serious and causing pandemic (e.g., COVID-19), there is explosion in clinical testing. Three approaches are used to diagnose viral infections: direct detection of virions, viral antigens or viral nucleic acids (RNA, DNA) in clinical sample; isolation of virus in cultured cells (indirect detection); and detection and measurement of virus, specific antibodies in a patient's serum (serology), a majority of the common viral infections can be diagnosed in the laboratory. Various methods employed to diagnose viral infections are described.

DIRECT EXAMINATION OF SPECIMEN

- **Light microscopy**–histological appearance (e.g., inclusion bodies–negri bodies (rabies) and cytomegalic inclusion bodies (CMV infection).
- **Electron microscopy**–Electron micrographs of feces for virus particles morphology (X 50000) – gastroenteritis caused by rotavirus, adenovirus, astrovirus, calcivirus and norwalk-like virus; detection in vesicles and skin lesions for herpeviruses and papillomaviruses.
- **Demonstration of viral antigens**

  Immunoflorescence testing–for respiratory viruses (e.g., RSV, flu A, flu B and adnoviruses), detection of rotavirus antigen in feces.
  - *Counter immune electrophoresis* (CIE): Hepatitis B.
  - *ELISA*: Hepatitis B virus, rotavirus.

- **Molecular techniques for direct detection of viral genome (DNA/RNA)**

  Polymerase chain reaction (PCR), an extremely sensitive and rapid diagnostic reliable method being commonly used to identify several viruses, epidemiological investigation and drug susceptibilily testing

INDIRECT DIAGNOSIS BY ISOLATING THE VIRUS

Cell culture embryonated eggs and animals are used for virus isolation and the presence of growing viruses is usually detected by:

- *Cytopathic effect (CPE)* which may be specific, e.g., HSV and CMV) or nonspecific (e.g. enterovirus)
- *Hemadsorption:* For influenza and parainfluenza viruses.

SEROLOGICAL DIAGNOSIS

Serological diagnosis is based on either the demonstration of the presence of virus-specific IgM antibodies or a significant increase in the events of specific IgG bodies. The presence of IgM in the blood is indicative of acute infection and IgG indicates an infection sometime in the past.

Antibody testing is the main method used for the diagnosis of the large majority of viral infections. Commonly used serological tests are neutralizing antibody assay, hemagglutination inhibition test (HAI), complement fixation test (CFT), enzyme-linked immunosorbent assays (ELISA) and immunoblot assays (e.g. western blot). Automated panels that can screen for many viruses at once are currently being used.

DIAGNOSIS OF FUNGAL DISEASES

Laboratory diagnosis of fungal infections is done by direct microscopic examination of clinical samples, including histopathology, culturing of the fungus, by exposing the sample to UV, antigen detection, serology and DNA probe tests (molecular diagnostics).

- **Direct Microscopic Examination** of clinical specimens (e.g., sputum CSF, biopsy) and/or skin scrapings provide rapid and accurate diagnosis of some fungal infections. It can be performed by the following methods:
  - *KOH preparation* The specimen is treated with 20% KOH to dissolve the tissue material, leaving alkali-resistant fungi intact, making fungi readily visible.

- *Calcifluor white* when CW is mixed with KOH detects fungi rapidly because of bright fluorescence.
- *India ink preparation* is used to detect *Cryptococcus neoformans* in CSF for cryptococcal meningitis.
- *Wright stain* Examination of bone marrow and peripheral blood sample to detect *Histoplasma capsulatum* and *C. neoformans*.

- **Scotch tape Lactophenol Cotton Blue Wet mount Preparation**

A transparent scotch tape with its adhesive side is touched on the surface of a fungus colony, the sprorulating structure adheres to it as they are produced, thus making possible the arrangment of conidia, an important feature for identification in deuteromycetous fungi (dermaotophytes).

- **Histopathology of Skin Biopsy** With special stains, such as Periodic acid-Schiff (PAS) and examinated for dermatophytes.

- **Wood Lamp** Exposing the infected site to long-wavelength UV radiation (Wood Lamp) used to, identify fungal infections of hair (tinea capitis) because the infected hair fluoresces green.
- **Culturing the fungus** Culture of the fungus from a clinical sample is the gold standard for the diagnosis of fungal infections. Sabouraud dextrose agar (SDA) is the standard medium used for culturing human pathogenic fungi as it facilitates the growth of slow-growing fungi by inhibiting bacterial growth due to low PH by the medium. Common fungal pathogens can be identified on the basis of the colony characteristics, nature of the mycelium, sporulating structures (spores/conidia, their mode of production and arrangement).

ANTIGEN DETECTION TEST

Latex agglutination test, a rapid test used to diagnose:

- **Cryptococcal meningitis** is caused by *C. neoformans* due to the presence of polysaccharide capsular antigen in the spinal fluid.
- **Invasive aspergillosis** caused by various aspergilli due to the presence of galactomannan (polysaccharide antigen) in the cell wall.
- **Histoplasmosis** caused by *Histoplasma capsulatum* due to polysaccharide antigen in the body fluids, especially urine.

  Immunoassays used to detect galactomannan from *Blastomyces dermatitidis* and *Coccidioides immitis* in urine and other body fluids.

SEROLOGICAL TESTS

Several serological tests (presence of antibodies in the patient's serum or spinal fluid) are used to diagnose systemic (endemic) mycoses (e.g. cocccidioidomycosis, histoplasmosis, blastomycosis). These include immunodiffusion (ID), complement fixation (CF) and enzyme immunoassay (EIA)

MOLECULAR DIAGNOSTICS

- PCR performed on positive blood culture and detects species of *Candida*.
- DNA probe tests are available to identify growing fungal colonies of *Coccidioides*, *Histoplasma*, *Blastomyces* and *Cryptococcus*.

DIAGNOSIS OF PARASITIC DISEASES

Parasitic diseases (those caused by protozoa and helminths) are diagnosed by examining stool and blood by the following tests.

STOOL TEST

Fecal Stool Examination Test (O and P Test)

Fecal (stool) exams, (also called an **ova and parasite test** or **O and P**) is used to find parasites that cause diarrhea, loose or watery stools, cramping flatulance (gas) and other abdominal illnesses. In this test three or more stool samples, collected on separate days, are examined for the presence of ova, eggs and the parasite by two ways: macroscopic and microscopic examination.

1 Macroscopic examination The fecal specimens are examined for their consistency, presence of blood and mucus, and whole worms (e.g. *Ascaris lumbricoides* and *Enterobius vermicularis*), larvae (e.g. *Strongloides stercoralis*), and segments of tapeworms.

2 Microscopic examination of unstained and stained samples

- **Wet mounts in saline (unstained preparation)** – This is used to examine diarrhea specimens for the presence of trophozoites in the freshly passed stool.
- **Iodine stained preparation** – This preparation is used to observe the nuclear characteristics of a cyst.

BLOOD TESTS

Two kinds of blood tests are used: smear and serology.

- **Blood smear**– Stained blood smear is used to look for parasites that are found in the blood such as malaria, filariasis and babesiosis. Ramanowsky's stain and Leishman's stain are used for staining the blood smear.
- **Serology** This test is used to look for antibodies and for parasite antigens produced in the blood.

KEY POINTS

- Laboratory diagnosis of infectious diseases is done using microscopy, culture, serology and genomic analysis of the agent involved.
- **Diagnostic methods for bacterial disease** include microscopy (Gram stained, acid-fast stain, fluorescent stains, wet mounts), culturing, antibody, antigen detection, molecular and biochemical tests.
- **Diagnosis of viral diseases** is based on the direct detection of virions, viral antigens or viral nucleic acids (DNA or RNA) in the specimen; isolation and identification of the virus in cultured cells; detection and measurement of antibodies in the patient's serum.
- **Fungal infections are commonly diagnosed** by microscopic examination of clinical samples, culture of the fungus, antigen and antibody detection and DNA probes.
- **Parasitic diseases** are diagnosed by examining stool (macroscopic and microscopic) and blood smear.

IMPORTANT QUESTIONS

1. Write short notes on:
   (a) Diagnosis of bacterial diseases by microscopy.
   (b) Diagnosis of viral infections.
   (c) How fungal infections are diagnosed in a clinical laboratory?

MULTIPLE-CHOICE QUESTIONS

1. Acid-fast stain is used to identify:
   (a) Tuberculosis (b) Malaria
   (c) Cryptococcosis (d) Typhoid.

2. Immunological methods are used to detect antigens in patient's body fluids. True or False?
3. Following Gram's staining method, Gram-positive bacteria take up which colour?
   (a) Purple (b) Pink
   (c) Yellow (d) Green.
4. Which of the following methods can be used to diagnose fungal diseases?
   (a) Lactophenol cotton blue mount
   (b) KOH preparation
   (c) Wood lamp
   (d) All of these.
5. Calcoflour white, which has the ability to bind to the cell wall, is used to detect:
   (a) Protozoa (b) Helminths
   (c) Fungi (d) None of these.
6. Which of the following techniques can be used to diagnose malaria?
   (a) Stool examination
   (b) Blood smear preparation
   (c) KOH preparation
   (d) Culture of the organism from tissue.
7. Which of the following methods is/are used to diagnose a viral infection?
   (a) Demonstration of the virus by EM
   (b) Demonstration of the antibodies in the sample
   (c) Isolation of the virus on cells/tissues.
   (d) All of these.
8. Haemagglutination can be used to detect antibodies against any antigen that can be linked to surface of red blood cells.
   True or False?

ANSWERS TO MCQs

1. (a) **2.** False **3.** (a) **4.** (d) **5.** (c)
6. (b) **7.** (d) **8.** True.

72

Collection, Handling and Transportation of Various Laboratory Specimens

WHAT IS A SPECIMEN?

Laboratory diagnosis of diseases begins with the collection of a clinical specimen for examination or processing into laboratories. **Specimen** is defined as 'any' substance which is taken from the body of a person for testing in the laboratory. The terms '**sample**' or 'specimen' are considered interchangeable in a chemical, diagnostic or microbiology laboratory. The word specimen comes from the Latin word *specere*, meaning 'to look'.

Specimen collection requires withdrawing blood, cerebrospinal fluid (CSF), collecting urine, feces or swabs from mucosal surfaces. A fundamental step to diagnose an infectious disease is the choice of appropriate specimen (also called biological specimen, chemical specimen or laboratory specimen). The types of biological samples accepted in most clinical laboratories are: serum samples, virology swab samples, urine samples, cerebrospinal fluid, blood for PCR, biopsy (tissue from a living body) or necropsy (pathological dissection of a corpse tissue). Serum is the preferred specimen source for serological testing. Appropriate selection, collection, storage and transportation of specimens is necessary for a meaningful microbiological laboratory report.

SELECTION OF THE SITE FOR SPECIMEN SAMPLING

The specimen selected should adequately represent the diseased area in order to isolate and identify potential agents of the particular disease process. Hence always select the correct/proper anatomical site and the specimen must be representative of the active site of infection. Clinical specimens such as swabs (nasopharynx, throat or tonsils, skin, vaginal), blood, saliva, CSF, sputum, urine and feces, collected from various sampling sites is shown in Fig. 72.1.

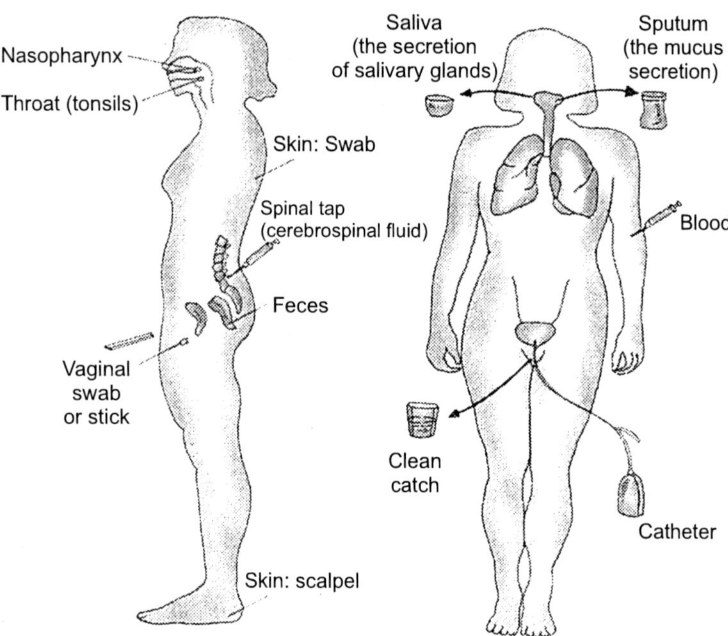

Fig. 72.1 Common sampling sites of human body for clinical specimens and their mode of sampling.

Some sites in the body of a healthy individual are free from microorganisms (i.e., sterile) (Table 72.1) so growth of any organism from these sites is indicative of infection provided that the specimen has been properly collected, transported, and examined in the laboratory without delay. The significance of isolates from sites that have a commensal flora (Table 72.2) depends upon the identity of the isolate and the quantity, as well as the immune status of the patient.

Table 72.1 Sampling sites and the normal flora associated with these sites

Body sites free from microorganisms (i.e., normally sterile)	Body sites that have a normal commensal flora
• Tissues	• Skin
• Bladder	• Mouth
• Lower respiratory tract	• Nose
• Blood	• Upper respiratory tract
• Bone marrow	• Gastrointestinal tract
• Cerebrospinal fluid (CSF)	• Female genital tract
• Serous fluids	• Urethra

GENERAL PRINCIPLES/GUIDELINES FOR COLLECTION OF SPECIMENS

- Always use universal precautions for collecting and handling specimens.
- Appropriate specimen should be collected from the correct anatomical site of the body.
- Specimen should be collected at the appropriate time during the active phase of the disease (as in the preparation of malarial films, virus isolation, virus genome and IgM detection).
- Whenever possible, collect all culture specimens prior to administration of any antimicrobial agents.
- All specimens must be properly labelled with the patient's name, location, date and the desired test.
- Adequate amount of the specimen and number of samples should be collected to allow for all the tests (for instance enough blood/serum for more than one set of blood cultures).
- Avoid contamination of the specimen with indigenous biota, for instance oral flora sputum, skin flora in wound swabs, normal flora or in case of midstream urine, no sterile equipment, as the undesirable microbes can over grow the causative agent and interfere with transportation of results.
- Specimens should be collected in appropriate in leak proof, well labelled (e.g., patient name, identification number and desired test) containers.
- Specimens for an anaerobic bacterial culture should be collected in proper anaerobic collection containers.
- Proper instructions should be given for patient when they have to collect the sample himself/herself, e.g., feces, urine or sputum.

COLLECTION OF BLOOD AND CSF

Blood

Blood specimens are obtained aseptically using approved **veripuncture techniques** by qualified personnel. Specimens are allowed to clot at room temperature and then are centrifuged. Serum, the preferred specimen for serological testing, is transferred to tightly-closing plastic tubes and stored at 28°C before shipment. Acute serum should be collected at the inset of symptoms. Convalescent specimens should follow 2-4 weeks later. Paired sera are tested together.

Cerebrospinal Fluid (CSF)

A **lumbar puncture** (or LP, or colloquially called a **spinal tap**) (Fig. 72.1) is performed to collect CSF. LP consists of the insertion of a hollow needle beneath the arachnoids membrane of the spinal cord in the lumber region to withdraw CSF which should be clear of any visible contamination or blood. This should be transported in tightly-closing plastic tubes.

Refrigerated CSF is acceptable for a limited number of serological tests, however, if PCR is to be performed for viral panels, the specimen must be frozen and shipped on dry ice.

SPECIFIC SAMPLING PROCEDURES FOR MICROBIAL CULTURE

Stool

For **bacteriological examination**, only a small sample is needed. This may be obtained by inserting a sterile swab into the rectum or feces. The swab is then placed in a tube of sterile enrichment broth for **transport to the laboratory**.

For examination of parasites, a small sample may be taken from a morning stool. The sample is placed in a preservative (polyvinyl alcohol, buffered glycerol, saline, or formalin) for microscopic examination for eggs and adult parasites.

Sputum

1. A morning sample is best because microorganisms would have accumulated while the patient is sleeping.
2. The patient should rinse his or her mouth thoroughly to remove food and normal microbiota.
3. The patient should coughed up far from down the bronchial free of expectorate immediately into a steroid glass wide-mouth jar/containers, keeping in view that it should not be mixed with saliva or orpharangial secretion and delivered to the laboratory as soon as possible.
4. Care should be taken to avoid contaminating healthcare workers.
5. In some cases, such as tuberculosis in which there is little sputum, stomach aspiration may be necessary.
6. Infants and children tend to swallon sputum. A fecal sample may be of some value in these cases.

Urine

1. Clean-catch technique is used to collect urine for Gram-negative bacillus involved in UTI.

2. Provide the patient with a sterile container.
3. Instruct the patient to first void a small volume from the urinary bladder before collection (to wash away extraneous bacteria of the skin microbiota) then to collect a midstream sample.
4. A urine sample may be stored under refrigeration (4–6°C) for up to 24 hours.

Blood

1. Close the windows to avoid contamination.
2. Clean the skin around the selected vein with 2% tincture of iodine on a cotton swab.
3. Remove the dried iodine with gauze moistened with 80% isopropyl alcohol.
4. Draw a few milliliters of venous blood.
5. Aseptically bandage the puncture.

Wound or Abscess

1. Cleanse the area with a sterile swab moistened in sterile saline.
2. Disinfect the area with 70% ethanol or iodine solution.
3. If the abscess has not ruptured spontaneously, the physician will open it with a sterile scalpel.
4. Wipe the first pus away.
5. Touch a sterile swab to the pus, taking care not to contaminate the surrounding tissue.
6. Replace the swab in its container, and properly label the container.

Ear

1. Clean the skin and auditory canal with 1% tincture of iodine.
2. Touch the infected area with a sterile cotton swab.
3. Replace the swab in its container.

Eye

1. Anesthetize the eye with topical application of a sterile anesthetic solution.
2. Wash the eye with sterile saline solution.
3. Collect material from the infected area with a sterile cotton swab. Return the swab to its container.

A summary of specimen collection method with the clinical significance of each from skin and soft tissue, eye, respiratory secretions, gastrointestinal tract, urine, CNS, genital tract and blood is given in Table 72.2.

Table 72.2 Summary of specimen collection methods from different tissues/sites for detection of pathogens

Specimen collection method	Applications
Skin and soft tissue	
Skin scrapping/nail clipping	For isolation of dermatophytic fungi
Skin swab	For pus examination
Vesicle fluid	For electron microscopy of viruses
Wound swab	For pus examination
Pus, tissues, aspirates	For describing site of infection and other operative details
Eye	
Conjunctival swab	For virus and chlamydia detection
Aspirates	For detection of pathogen
Respiratory secretions	
Anterior nasal swab	For detection of staphylococci and streptococci
Nasopharygeal swab	For detection of COVID-19, pertusis and meningococci
External ear swab	For examination of wide range of microbes including fungi
Throat swab	For examining the presence of streptococci and diphtheria
Saliva	Used to detect antibodies
Laryngeal swab	Used to detect mycobacteria
Sputum	For detection of mycobacteria, legionellae, pneumocystis
Transtracheal aspirate, bronchoscopy specimens, lung biopsy	For diagnosis of the disease by carrying out specific tests
Pleural fluid	Used to examine mycobacteria
Gastrointestinal tract	
Gastric washings	For mycobacteria (in children)
Gastric biopsy	For detection of *Helicobacter pylori*
Duodenal/jejunal aspirates	Protozoa (*Giardia lamblia*, microsporidia etc.)
Liver aspirate	For detection of anaerobes in pus
Spleen puncture	For detection of *Leishmania* spp.
Rectal biopsy	For diagnosis of schistosomiasis

Contd.

Rectal swab	For detection of gonococci and chlamydia
Colonic biopsy	Histopathological diagnosis of amoebiasis and pseudomembranous colitis
Feces	For detection of clostridial toxins and presence of parasites
Perianal swab	For presence of eggs of threadworm
Urine	
Suprapubic aspirate	Used in infants and neonates for detection of microbial contaminants
Ureteric/bladder washout	For localizing infection
Prostatic massage	Sample collection before, during and at the end of micturition
Terminal urine	For detection of *Schistosoma* ova and for chlamydia DNA amplification
Complete early morning or 24-hour urine	For detection of mycobacteria
Central nervous system	
Cerebrospinal fluid by spinal tap	For detection of meningitis, and also for detection of virus, fungi or syphilis serology
Brain ascess	For detection of anaerobes
Genital tract	
Urethral swab	Detection of pus for gonococci, scrape for chlamydia
Adult vaginal swab	For diagnosis of *Candida, Trichomonas,* bacterial vaginosis
Cervical swab	For detection of *Chlamydia*
Ulcer scrape	For detection of viruses
Blood	
Culture media	Strict aseptic technique, usually large sample is taken in special sterile vials before adding antibiotics
Bone marrow	Valuable for diagnosis of *Leishmania,* mycobacteria, *Brucella*
Film	For diagnosis of malaria, filarial, borrelia, trypanosomes
Whole blood	For detection of filaria
Serum antigen	Rapid diagnosis of many microbial diseases
Serum antibody	Retrospective diagnosis of common viral diseases and syphilis

TRANSPORTATION OF SPECIMENS

- Deliver all specimens to the clinical laboratory as soon as possible after collection.
- Appropriately label specimens with the patient's name, medical record number, location, date and time of specimen collected.

- A requisition needs to accompany each different specimen type.
- Specimens should be in tightly sealed, leak-proof containers and transported in sealable, leak-proof plastic bags. Specimens for TB should be double bagged.
- Specimens for bacterial culture should be transported at room temperature. The following specimens should be refrigerated, if transport is delayed: urine (within 30 min), stool (within 60 min), and respiratory specimens.
- Specimens for viral culture must be transported immediately in ice.

PROCESSING OF CLINICAL SPECIMENS

Sample processing is a process done to a sample to prepare it for testing/culturing in the laboratory as quickly as possible within 24 hours to ensure that the causative agents do not die before being transported to the culture media and the accuracy of the microbiological results. Generally, the processing of a specimen is initiated by placing a portion of the specimen on glass slides, stained appropriately and examined microscopically (direct mount). Simultaneously, the material is processed for inoculating by inoculating appropriate broth/culture media aerobically/aerobically or cell lines for main trial growth.

KEY POINTS

- **Clinical specimens** (samples of blood, urine, feces, CSF, swabs, skin, tissues) are to be detected aseptically from the appropriate site in the right containers.
- CSF samples of blood culture bottles are not to be refrigerated.
- Urine culture samples are to be stored at low temperature before their transportation.
- Specimens should be transported/processed rapidly within 2 hours in the laboratory.
- Specimens must be collected aseptically and before the initiation of antimicrobial therapy.

IMPORTANT QUESTIONS

1. Write short notes on:
   (a) Common sites on the human's body for collection of specimens.
   (b) General principles for specimen collection.
   (c) Collection of urine and sputum for bacterial culture.

MULTIPLE-CHOICE QUESTIONS

1. Which specimen is ideal for COVID-19 (Coronavirus disease 2019)?
(a) Sputum (b) ESF
(c) Nasopharygeal swab (d) Stool.

2. Ideally, specimens for cultures should be collected:
(a) At any shape of the desease
(b) After completion of antimicrobial therapy
(c) Before the start of the antibodies therapy
(d) It is irrelevant.

3. Which of the following specimen should not be refrigerated, in case of delay in the transportation of the specimen?
(a) Feces (b) Urine
(c) Sputum (d) CSF.

4. Which of the following is the ideal specimen to diagnose TB?
(a) Feces (b) Blood
(c) Sputum (d) CSF.

5. For which microbe culture, the specimens are to the transported on ice?
(a) Bacteria (b) Fungi
(c) Virus (d) Mycoplasma.

ANSWERS TO MCQs

1. (c) **2.** (c) **3.** (d) **4.** (c) **5.** (c).

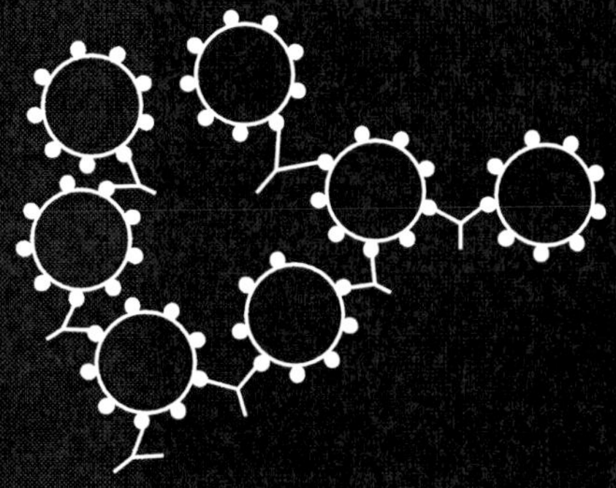

Unit V

FUNDAMENTALS OF IMMUNOLOGY

- Immunology and Immunity: Introduction and Types
- Antigens: The Antibody Generators
- Antibodies: The Immunoglobulins
- Antigen-Antibody Interactions and Serological Diagnostic Tests
- Hypersensitivity Reactions (Immune Hypersensitivity)
- Autoimmunity and Autoimmune Diseases
- Vaccines, Sera-Types and Cold Chain Management
- Immunoprophylaxis (Immunization/Vaccination) and Immunization Schedule

73

Immunology and Immunity: Introduction and Types

WHAT IS IMMUNITY?

Immunity is defined as the ability of an organism to ward off disease through body defenses. It is derived from Latin word *immunes* means free of burden.

Lack of immunity or vulnerability of the host to harm by infectious agents is termed **susceptibility** (derived from Latin word *susceptibly* means especially sensitive, or likely to be affected). The term immunity was coined by **Elie Metchnikoff** in 1882 who first observed the phenomenon of **phagocytosis,** and received the Noble Prize for his work in 1908. **von Behring** recognized antibodies in serum against diphtheria toxin. **Karl Landsteiner** in 1900 described ABO blood groups and natural isohemagglutinin. **Edward Jenner** pioneered the smallpox vaccines in the 18th century.

WHY IS IMMUNITY IMPORTANT?

Our immune system does a lot of amazing things and is essential for our survival. It helps keep us healthy by figuring out when something harmful enters our body, and then fighting it, so you don't get sick. The stronger your immune system is, the more likely you are to stay healthy. We can boost our immunity with vaccination against serious diseases.

WHAT IS IMMUNOLOGY?

Immunology is a branch of biology/medical science that deals with the study of human immune system, functions and how our body protects itself against infectious diseases caused by microorganisms and infectious agents, and the use of antibody-based laboratory techniques or immunoassays.

WHY IS IMMUNOLOGY IMPORTANT?

Immunology is important in varied ways:

- It interacts with multiple areas of biomedical science from infectious diseases and vaccination to the management and treatment of chronic diseases such as diabetes, cancer, asthma, allergies, rheumatic fever and acute glomerulonephritis.
- It is also fundamental to life sciences industry: the discipline is core to the development of modern antibodies therapies, vaccines, small molecule drugs and biologics (therapeutic molecules).
- It helps to diagnose several diseases using ELISA.

TYPES OF IMMUNITY

There are two major types of immunity:

1. Innate immunity (or natural immunity)
2. Acquired immunity (or adaptive immunity).

Innate Immunity: Nonspecific Defenses of the Host

Innate Immunity, also called **inborn** or **natural** or **genetic immunity**, refers to the defenses (physical, chemical and genetic) that are present at birth and protect the body against any kind of pathogen, regardless of species, and without prior **exposure**, hence this immunity is **nonspecific** (Fig. 73.1). This is the basic immunity that is passed on from one generation to other generation, hence referred to as the **genetic immunity**.

Types of innate Immunity: It is of three types:

- **Species immunity** is the total immunity shown by all members of a species against pathogen, e.g., birds immune to **tetanus**; polio, measles, syphilis, gonorrhea occur only in humans.
- **Racial immunity** is in which various races show marked differences in their resistance to certain infectious diseases, e.g., Negros are resistant to yellow fever and malaria.
- **Individual immunity** is very specific for each and every individual, despite having racial background and opportunity for explosure, e.g., homozygous twins exhibit similar degree of resistance or susceptibility to TB and lepromatous leprosy.

Mechanism of Innate Immunity

Innate defenses act by four ways: **first line of defense** (skin and mucous membranes) and the **second line of defense** (natural killer cells and

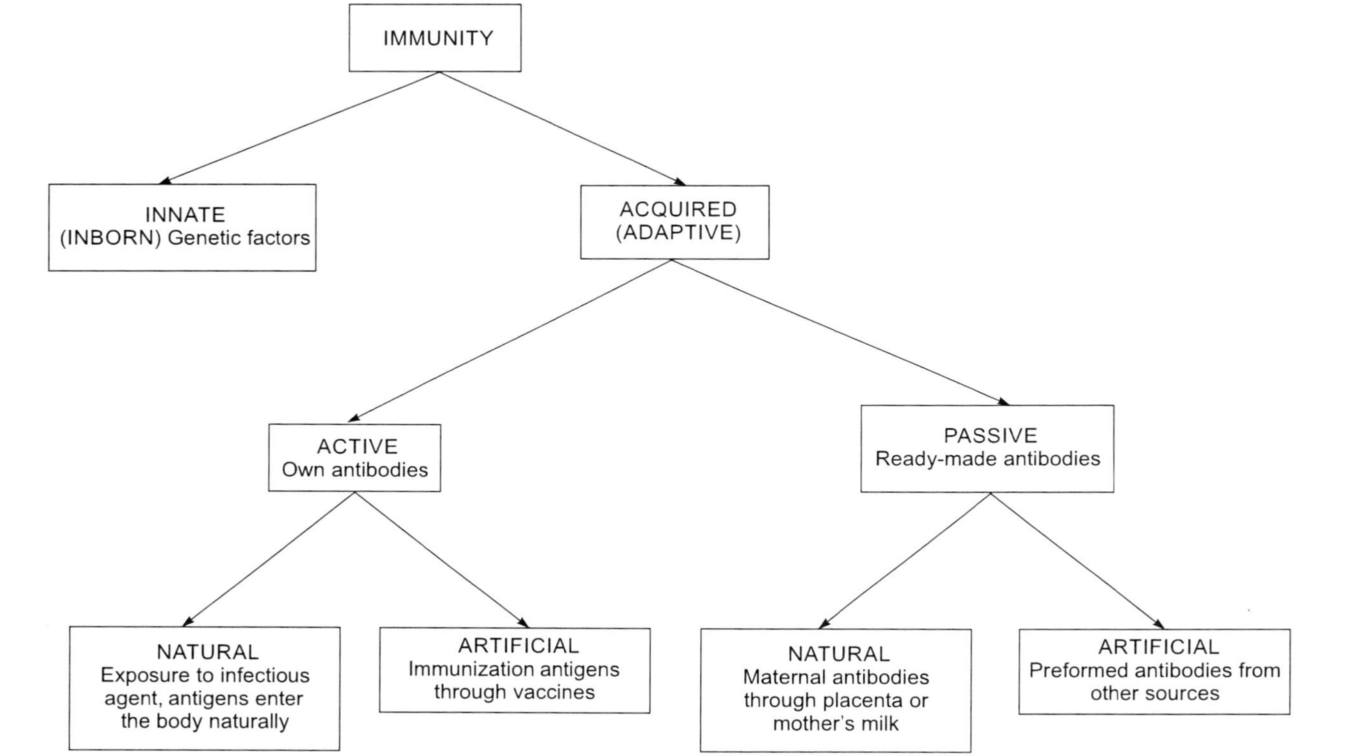

Fig. 73.1 The various types of immunity. Nonspecific immunity is largely innate or inborn, whereas specific immunity is acquired.

phagocytes, inflammation, fever and antimicrobial substances). Their mode of action includes the following:

1. **Physical barriers:** In fact, skin and mucous membranes and the chemicals secreted by these stop the entrance of the microbes in the body.
2. **Chemical barriers:** Including antimicrobial substances in body fluids (e.g., saliva, mucus, gastric juices) and the iron limitation mechanisms.
3. **Cellular defensive cells:** Phagocytes (neutrophils, easinophils, dendrite cells at macrophages) are specialized cells that engulf (phagocytize) and clear invading microbes, foreign molecules or particles.
4. **Inflammation:** A sequential protective response to injury that results in reddening, swelling and increase in temperature in tissues at infection sites, providing protection against infection and further damage at that site and initiates tissue repair.
5. **Fever:** The elevation of body temperature to kill invading microbes and/or inactivate their toxic product and speeds up body reactions that aid repair.
6. **Molecular defenses (antimicrobial substances):** Such as interferons, complement system, iron-binding proteins of antimicrobial peptides that kill or impede invading microbes.

ADAPTIVE (ACQUIRED) IMMUNITY: SPECIFIC DEFENSES OF THE HOST

Adaptive (**acquired** or **specific**) immunity refers to the protection (resistance) that an individual acquires against certain specific pathogens or foreign substances during his lifetime. Adaptive immunity is **induced,** that is, it adapts to a specific microbial invader or a foreign substance. It can be acquired either actively or passively and can be obtained by natural or artificial ways, and forms the basis of naming of different types of adaptive immunity.

Adaptive immunity differs from innate immunity in the following respects:

- It is specific for a single type of microbe.
- It is not inherent in the body.
- The pathogen specific receptors are acquired during the lifetime of the organism.

The major functions of the acquired immune system are:

- Generation of responses that are tailored to maximally eliminate specific pathogens or pathogen infected cells.

- Recognition of specific 'non-self' antigens in the presence of 'self' during the process of antigen presentation.
- Development of immunological memory, in which pathogens are remembered by memory B cells and memory C cells.

In humans, it takes 4–7 days for the adaptive immune system to mount a significant response.

Types of Adaptive Immunity

Adaptive immunity is of two types: active immunity and passive immunity and each is further subdivided into artificial immunity and natural immunity (Fig. 73.2).

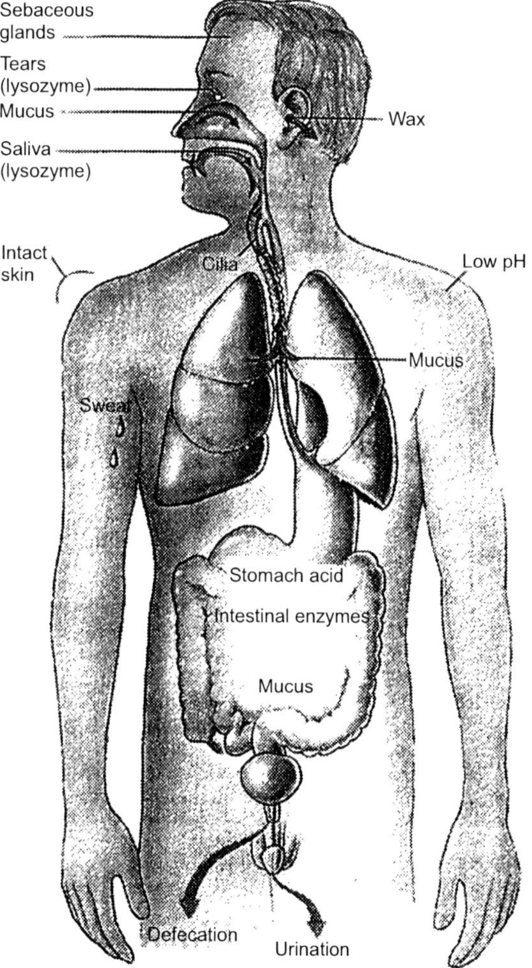

Fig. 73.2 The primary physical and chemical defense barriers: nonspecific defenses of the host due to innate immunity.

Active immunity: Immunity that develops actively after exposure to a microbe or other foreign substance (antigen), such as following infection or vaccination is called **active immunity**. It is long lasting. If an immune person who has been immunized against one antigen, experiences the same antigen in the future. The immune system will recognize it and immediately produce the antibodies needed to fight it.

- **Naturally acquired active immunity:** Immunity resulting from infection is called naturally acquired active immunity. Once acquired, this immunity is life-long for some diseases, such as measles and chickenpox.
- **Artificially acquired active immunity:** Immunity resulting from vaccination (also called immunization) is called artificially acquired active immunity which can be long lasting. Resistance is induced by vaccines in the body. Vaccines are antigens such as killed or living microbes (bacteria or viruses) or inactivated bacterial toxins.

Passive Immunity: The immunity is acquired passively when antibodies (readymade immunity) are transferred from one person to another. This immunity lasts for a few weeks, as long as antibodies are present in the system.

Two types of passive immunities are:

- **Naturally acquired passive immunity** involves the natural transfer of antibodies from a mother to her foetus (transplacental transfer) or to a newborn (nursing infant) in *colostrums* (first secretions of breast milk) results in naturally acquired passive immunity in the newborn (e.g., diphtheria, rubella, polio). This type of immunity can last up to a few months.
- **Artificially acquired passive immunity** involves the injection of antibodies into the body. These antibodies come from a person or animal who is already immune to the disease (e.g., pooled human gamma globulin, hyper immune sera of human or animal (origin). Serum containing antibodies is often termed **antiserum**. This type of immunity can last for a few weeks.

LOCAL IMMUNITY

Local immunity refers to natural or acquired immunity to an infectious agent manifested by a particular organ or tissue. It acts at the entry site and prevents the entry of certain infectious agents. It is conferred by secretory **immunoglobulins,** namely, IgA (secretory IgA) produced locally by plasma cells present on mucosal surfaces or in secretory glands. Examples include:

- Live oral vaccines in poliomyelitis immunization augment the resistance at the level of the gut mucosa, the site of entry of polio virus.
- Provides protection against intestinal infections medicated by intestinal immunoglobulins which are different from those found in the bloodstream.

HERD IMMUNITY

The term h**erd immunity** (also called **community immunity, herd organ protection**) was coined by **W.W. Topley** and **G.S. Wilson**, an American scientist in 1923, who studied how an entire herd of laboratory mice) could become immune to a disease even though not every member of the herd had been immunized.

Herd immunity happens when large proportion of the population in a community (or herd) becomes immune to an infectious disease, that is, it stops the disease from spreading. This can happen in two ways:

- Many people contact the disease and in time build up an immune response to it (natural immunity).
- Many people are vaccinated against the disease to achieve immunity.

The goal of herd immunity is to prevent others from catching or spreading an infectious disease. Many viral and bacterial infections spread from person-to-person. This chain is broken when most people don't get or transmit infection. This helps protect people who aren't vaccinated who have weak immune system and may develop an infection more easily (e.g., older, adult, babies, young children, pregnant women, people with certain health conditions).

The percentage of people that have immunity to safely slow or stop an infectious disease is called the **herd immunity threshold (HIT)**. HIT varies with every disease, for example, for measles and polio, it is 95% and 80 to 85% respectively. Experts estimate that herd immunity would require around 80-90% of their population to have COVID-19 immunity, either through prior infection or vaccination.

KEY POINTS

- **Immunity** is defined as the ability of an organism to ward off disease through body defenses.
- Lack of immunity is known as **susceptibility**.
- **Innate (or natural or genetic) immunity** refers to the resistance to infection an individual possesses against any kind of pathogen (i.e., nonspecific).
- **Adaptive (acquired) immunity** refers to the resistance against specific microorganisms that an individual acquires during his lifetime.
- Adaptive immunity is **induced**: that is, it adapts to a specific microbial invader or a foreign substance.
- In **active immunity,** an individual's own immune system makes antibodies.
- In **passive immunity** ready-made antibodies are introduced into the body.
- **Artificial active immunity** is the resistance induced by vaccines through vaccination/immunization.
- **Herd immunity** (also known as **community or population immunity**) refers to the level of resistance or immunity of a community to a specific disease.
- Herd immunity can be achieved through prior illness and/or vaccination thereby reducing the likelihood of infection and spread of a disease.

IMPORTANT QUESTIONS

1. Describe in brief:
   (a) Distinguish between innate and acquired immunity, with examples of each type.
   (b) Distinguish between active and passive immunity, with examples of each type.
   (c) What is herd immunity, what is its significance in the current scenario?

MULTIPLE-CHOICE QUESTIONS

1. The branch of biology involved in the study of immune system in all organisms is called:
   (a) Manifold science
   (b) Biotechnology

(c) Molecular biology
(d) Immunology.

2. Immunity refers to:
(a) The number of a disease fighting RBCs in the body
(b) An organism's ability to fight off disease
(c) A measure of overall health in an organism
(d) The amount of antibodies in a person's system.

3. Which of the following immunity is present from our birth?
(a) Active immunity
(b) Passive immunity
(c) Innate immunity
(d) Acquired immunity

4. Which of the following conveys the longest lasting immunity for an infectious agent?
(a) Naturally acquired active immunity
(b) Naturally acquired passive immunity
(c) Artificially acquired passive immunity
(d) Both (a) and (c).

5. All of the following act as a protective barrier for the body surface EXCEPT:
(a) Mucus
(b) Skin
(c) Salivary amylase
(d) Gastric acid.

6. Which of the following immunity is obtained during a lifetime?
(a) Active immunity
(b) Passive immunity
(c) Innate immunity
(d) Both (a) and (b).

7. Which of the following immunity is called the first line of defense in the body?
(a) Innate immunity
(b) Active immunity
(c) Passive immunity
(d) Acquired immunity.

8. Naturally acquired active immunity would be most likely acquired through which of the following processes?
(a) Natural growth
(b) Vaccination

(c) Drinking colostrum
(d) Infection of the host with disease causing organism followed by recovery.

9. All are true for herd immunity EXCEPT:
(a) Immunity in a herd of cows
(b) The number of people that opt out of getting vaccination
(c) The protection the whole population has against an infectious disease because a threshold number of individuals are immune to the disease
(d) The number of disease-fighting white blood cells in a person.

10. Herd immunity threshold–for the population need to be vaccinated for polio is:
(a) 100% (b) 95%
(c) 80% (d) 70%

11. Which of the following immunity lasts longer?
(a) Active immunity
(b) Passive immunity
(c) Both (a) and (b)
(d) None of the two.

ANSWERS TO MCQs

1. (a)	2. (b)	3. (c)	4. (a)	5. (c)
6. (d)	7. (a)	8. (d)	9. (c)	10. (c)
11. (a).				

74

Antigens: The Antibody Generators

WHAT IS AN ANTIGEN?

An **antigen (Ag)** is a foreign molecule (substance) that stimulates the immune system to produce an antibody against it. **Ag** abbreviation stands for an **antibody generator**. The word antigen comes from French antigene from Gr. *anti*, against and *gen*, thing that produces or causes. It was coined by a French scientist **Ladislas Deutsch** in 1899 for substances halfway between bacterial constituents and antibodies. **Immunogen** is another term for an antigen (i.e., the substance that can elicit an immune response). The property of behaving as an antigen is called **antigenicity**. Antigens are large molecules of proteins, present on the surface of pathogens such as bacteria, fungi, viruses, other foreign particles, human cells and pollens. Vaccines are the common examples of antigens.

PROPERTIES OF ANTIGENS

- The antigen is a foreign substance (i.e., not a normal constituent of the body) to induce an immune response.
- Entire molecule reacts not fragments.
- The antigens have a molecular mass of 14,000 to 6,00,000 Da.
- Antigens are species specific.
- They are mainly proteins and polysaccharides.
- The more chemically complex they are, the more immunogenic they will be.
- Each antigen has many antigenic determinants (**epitopes**).
- Combination occurs as surface antigens to surface of antibodies.

SOURCES OF ANTIGENS

Based on the sources, antigens are categorized as:

- **Microbial antigens:** components of the involving micro-organisms:

  - Capsules, cell walls, flagella, fimbria, bacterial toxins, coats of viruses.
  - Surface of other microbes.
- **Nonmicrobial antigens:** Pollens, egg white, blood cell surface molecules; serum proteins from other individuals and species, and surface molecules of transplanted tissues and organs.

CHEMICAL NATURE OF ANTIGENS

Based on the chemical nature, antigens fall into five categories:

- **Proteins and polypeptides** — enzymes, albumins, antibodies, hormones and exotoxins.
- **Lipoproteins:** cell membranes
- **Glycoproteins:** blood cell markers
- **Nucleoproteins:** DNA combined to proteins, but not DNA.
- **Polysaccharides:** 'Certain bacterial capsules' and lipopolysaccharides.

CLASSIFICATION/TYPES OF ANTIGENS

Antigens have been classified differently on the basis of origin and immune response, such as:

A. On the Basis of Origin

1. **Exogenous antigens:** These are external antigens that enter the body from outside, e.g., inhalation, injection, etc. These include food allergens, pollen, aerosols, and are the most common type of antigens.
2. **Endogenous antigens:** These are generated inside the body due to viral or bacterial infections or cellular metabolism.
3. **Autoantigens:** There are the 'self' proteins or nucleic acids that due to some genetic and environmental alterations get attacked by their own immune system causing autoimmune diseases (e.g., rheumatoid arthiritis)
4. **Tumor antigens:** An antigenic substance present on the surface of tumor cells that induces an immune response in the host, e.g., MHC-1 or MHC-II. Many tumors develop a mechanism to avoid the immune system of the body.
5. **Alloantigens:** Cell surface markers of one individual that are antigens to another of the same species that form the basis for an individual blood groups and are responsible for incompatibility that can occur in blood transfusion or organ grafting.

6. **Heterophilic antigens:** Molecules from unrelated species that bear similar antigenic determinants. Examples include carbohydrate residues on the surface of bacteria. These antigens are involved in rheumatic fever.
7. **Allergens:** The antigens that evoke allergic reactions.

B. On the Basis of Immune Response

These are classified into two types:

1. **Immunogens:** The antigens that can generate an immune response on their own. Proteins and polysacarharides are the examples of immunogens. These molecules are complex with several antigenic determinants.
2. **Haptens** (also called **incomplete immunogen**) (Fig. 74.1) are non-protein foreign substances that require a carrier molecule to induce an immune response since they are unable to stimulate antibody formation by itself (i.e. they are not antigenic). When a hapten attaches to a carrier molecule usually a serum protein, forms a **conjugate** (hapten-carrier conjugate) and becomes antigenic, stimulating an immune response. Penicillin is a good example of a hapten.

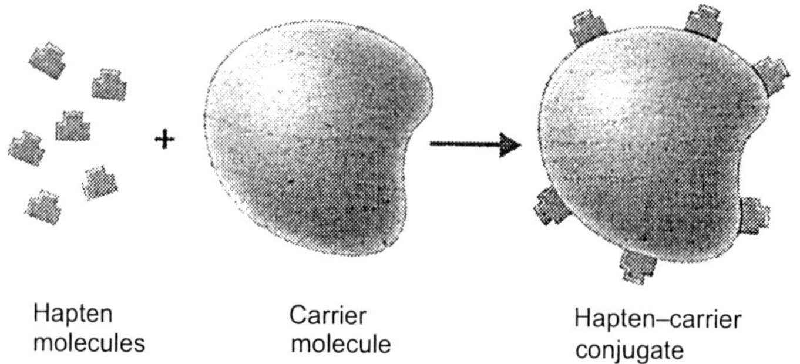

Fig. 74.1 Hapten. A hapten is a molecule too small to stimulate antibody formation by itself. However, when it is combined with a larger carrier molecule, usually a serum protein, the hapten and its carrier together form a conjugate that can stimulate the immune response.

Allergic reaction, a type of immune response, occurs in some people when penicillin, not antigenic by itself, combines with host proteins forming a combined molecule that causes an immune response.

EPITOPES

The **epitopes** also called **antigenic determinants** (Fig. 74.2) are the components of an antigen. An **epitope** is defined as the specific small region of an antigen to which an antibody binds. The part of the antibody that binds to the epitope is called a **paratope**.

Each epitope is usually 1–6 monosaccharides or 5-8 amino acid residues on the surface of the antigen. Each antigen carries more than one epitope.

Epitopes are used to develop vaccines–**epitope-based vaccines** where multiple epitopes can be used to increase the vaccine's efficiency.

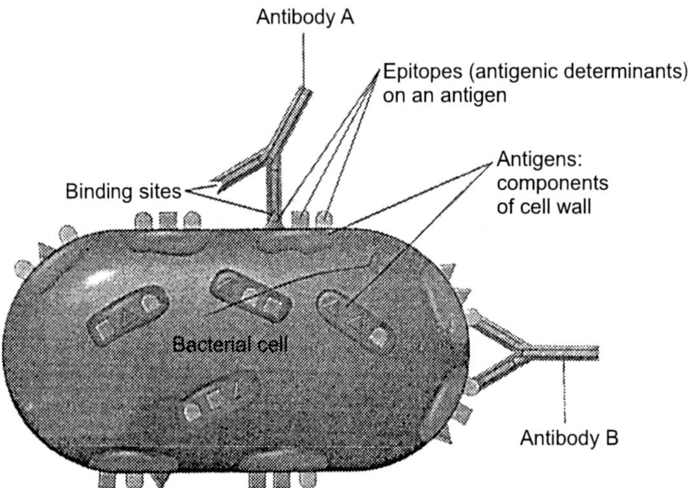

Fig. 74.2 Epitopes (antigenic determinants). In this illustration, the epitopes are components of the antigen–the bacterial cell wall. Each antigen carries more than one epitope. Each Y-shaped antibody molecule has two binding sites that can attach to a specific epitope on an antigen. An antibody can also bind to identical epitopes on two different cells at the same time which can cause neighboring cells to aggregate.

KEY POINTS

- Any substance that stimulates an immune response in the body is called an **antigen (Ag)**.
- The specific regions of an antigen to which an antibody binds is called an **epitope** or **antigenic determinant**.
- **Haptens** (molecules less than 1000 MW) are not antigenic unless attached to a larger molecule.
- Each antigen has several epitopes or antigenic determinants.
- Cells, viruses and large molecules have numerous epitopes.
- Foreign cells or large complex molecules (over 1000 MW) are most antigenic.

IMPORTANT QUESTIONS

1. Write brief notes on:
   (a) How antigens are classified?
   (b) Differentiate between antigen, epitope and hapten.

MULTIPLE-CHOICE QUESTIONS

1. Which of the following substances will not stimulate an immune response unless they are bound to a larger molecule?
   (a) Virus (b) Antibody
   (c) Antigen (d) Hapten.
2. As a rule, antigens are proteins or large polysaccharides. True or False?
3. Which of the following is true for epitope or antigenic determinant?
   (a) Substance that causes the body to produce specific antibodies
   (b) It is a low-molecular weight substance that cannot itself form antibodies
   (c) Antibodies are formed against specific regions on antigens
   (d) Protein is produced in response to an antigen.
4. Each antigen carries one epitope. True or False?

ANSWERS TO MCQs

1. (d) **2.** True **3.** (c) **4.** False.

75
Antibodies: The Immunoglobulins

WHAT IS AN ANTIBODY OR IMMUNOGLOBULIN?

An **antibody (Ab)**, also called **immunoglobulin (Ig)** is a protective protein produced by the immune system, specialized NBCs called B-lymphocytes or B-cells, in response to the presence of a foreign substance, called an antigen. Antibodies recognize bonds and neutralize the antigen. Antibodies are produced by the specialized white blood cells, and **B lymphocytes** (or **B cells**), or **plasma cells** and secreted into the bloodstream and lymphatic system. The term antibody (in German called *Antikorper* means anti-toxic body) was coined in 1891 by **Paul Ehrlich**.

Immunoglobulins (Ig), (another name used for antibodies), was coined by WHO in 1964, because antibodies are chemically **globular proteins (**a protein family with a compact globular form) belonging to the immunoglobulin (immune + globulin) super family. These are classified into five classes (or types): IgG, IgM, IgA, IgD and IgE. All antibodies are immunoglobulins, but all immunoglobulins are not antibodies.

B cells and antibodies together provide one of the most important functions of immunity, which is to recognize an invading antigen and to produce a tremendous number of protective proteins that scour the body to remove all traces of that antigen. Sera having high antibody levels following infection or immunization is called **immune sera**.

Preformed antibodies, which are derived from the **blood serum** of previously infected people or animals, are often administered in an **antiserum** to another person in order to provide immediate **passive immunization** (**plasma therapy**) against fast-acting toxins or microbes (as in COVID-19), such as snakebites or tetnus infections.

Major properties of antibodies are:

- Globular proteins
- Formed by B lymphocytes or B cells.

- Millions of antibodies are secreted into the bloodstream and lymphatic system by **plasma cells** (i.e., mature B cells).
- Antibodies attack antigens by binding and inactivate them.
- Antibody produced by one B cell can bind to only one type of antigen.
- Each antibody has two identical antigen binding sites.

STRUCTURE OF AN ANTIBODY

The basic unit of antibody or immunoglobulin (Ig), called a **monomer,** is a Y-shaped protein molecule. It is composed of four polypeptide chains (lengths of amino acids linked by peptide bonds): two identical **light (L) chains** and two identical **heavy (H) chains** ('Light' and 'heavy' refer to the relative molecular weights) linked by disulfide bonds (S–S) that form a flexible Y shape. Each chain is composed of a **variable (V) region** and a **constant C region** (Fig. 75.1).

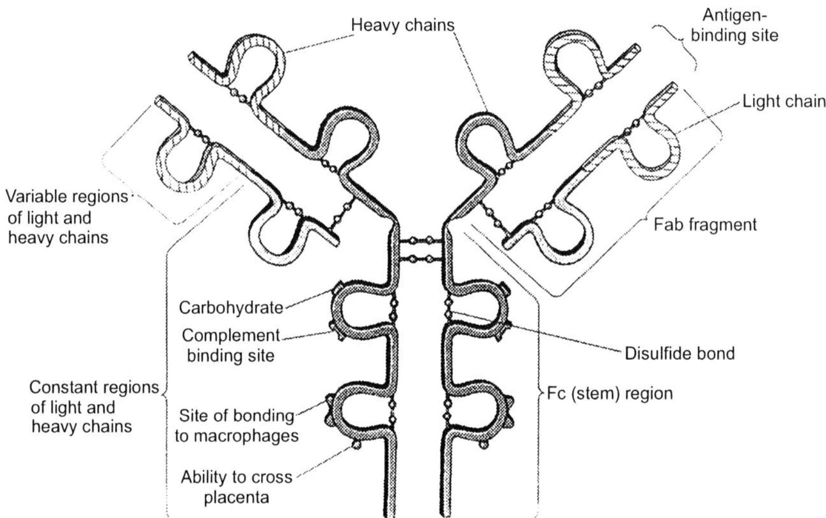

Fig. 75.1 Structure of an antibody molecule.

Most of the molecule is made up of C regions, which are the same for all antibodies of the same class. The amino acid sequences of the V regions, present at the upper ends of the Y, which form the two antigen antibody sites (part of the Fab segment), differ from molecule to molecule, and are responsible for the specificity of the antibody.

The stem of the Y-shaped antibody monomers, called the **Fe region** (so named because when antibody structure was first being identified, it was a fragment (F) that crystallized (C) in cold storage (Fig. 75.1), determine the role antibody plays in the body's immune responses, that is, immunological reactions.

Classes of H Chains: There are 5 classes of heavy chains, therefore 5 classes of antibodies, and are designated by the Greek letters: gamma (γ), alpha (α), mu (μ), delta (Δ) and epsilon (ε) corresponding to the immunoglobulin class.

Classes of L Chains: The L chains are similar in all 5 classes of immunoglobulin. They occur in two varieties kappa (κ) and lambda (λ).

IMMUNOGLOBULIN CLASSES

Five classes of immunoglobulin have been identified. The antibody molecules: IgG, IgM, IgA, IgD, IgG distinguished by the type of heavy chain found in the molecule (Fig. 75.2). These constitute 20–25% of total serum constituents, each class has a different role in the immune response.

1. Immunoglobulin G (IgG)

IgG (the name derived from the blood fraction gamma globulin) is present in the largest amounts, constituting 80% of total antibodies in the serum. It has a molecular weight of **1,50,000**, sedimentation coefficient of **7S** of normal serum concentration of 8-16 ml/ml, half-life in serum of **23 days**, and distributed equally between extra and intravascular spaces. IgG is the only immunoglobulin that can cross the placenta from mother to fetus. It can also be found in milk.

Functions of IgG include: Enhances phagocytosis; neutralizes bacterial toxins and viruses; provides passive immunity to a fetus and newborn.

2. Immunoglobulin M (IgM)

IgM (from *macro,* reflecting their large size)–MW of 9,70,000 daltons, 19S) hence called **millionaire molecule**) has a pentamer structure consisting of five monomers held together by a polypeptide called a J **(Joining) chain** (Fig. 75.2). IgM constitutes 5–10% of the total antibodies in the serum and generally remains in the blood vessels. The normal serum level of IgM is 1.2 mg/mL. It is the first antibody formed in life, being synthesized by the fetus.

IgM is the predominant type of antibody involved in response to the ABO blood group antigens on the surface of RBCs. It is the first antibody produced in response to initial (primary) infection and is relatively short lived (5 days half life in serum) hence their demonstration in serum indicates recent infection and is a valuable tool in disease diagnosis.

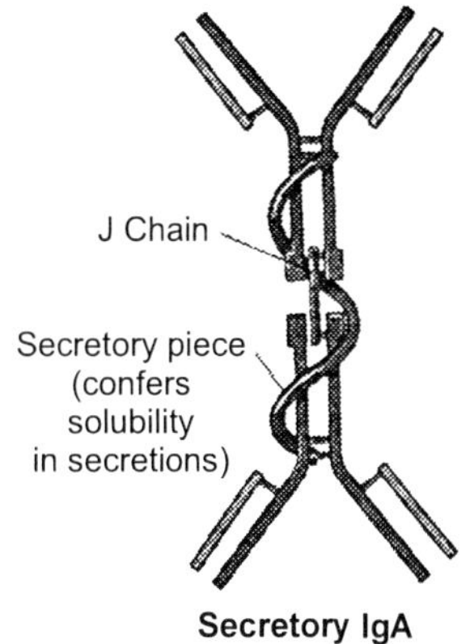

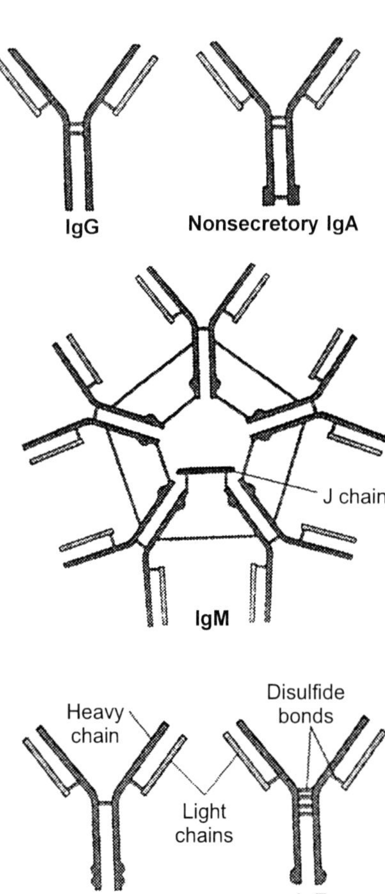

Fig. 75.2 The structure of the five classes of antibodies (immunoglobulins).

IgM is especially effective against microorganisms and agglutinating antigens.

3. Immunoglobulin A (IgA)

IgA (Fig. 75.2) (the molecule having alpha chains) is the main class of antibody found in body secretions such as tears, saliva, gastric fluid, sweat and colostrum (the first milk produced by lactating mothers). It is produced by B cells located in the mucous membranes of the body and secreted into the blood. It is the second most abundant antibody constituting 10-15% of serum immunoglobulins with a MW of 405,000 daltons, and 6 day's half life in serum. The normal serum level is 0.6-4.2 mg/ml.

IgA occurs in two forms distinguished by subtle amino acid differences.

- **Serum IgA** is a *monomer* and circulates in serum.
- **Secretory IgA:** It is a *dimer* and produced by plasma cells in the mucous membranes. Each day, humans secrete 5-15 grams of secretory IgA into their mucous secretions. IgA provides localized protection on mucosal surfaces by preventing the attachment of microbial surfaces. IgA's presence in a mother's milk, especially the colostrum provides protection to infants from gastrointestinal infections.

4. Immunoglobulin D (IgD)

IgD (Fig. 75.2) is found mainly on B cell membranes and is found in trace amounts in blood (0.2%). Its MW is 1,75,000 daltons of a half-life of 3 days in serum. It functions in initiation of immune response.

5. Immunoglobulin E (IgE)

IgE (Fig 75.2) (also called reagin) characterized by epsilon-chains, constitutes only 0.0002% of the total serum antibodies. IgE has the special property of binding to receptor, on basophils or mast cells, specialized cells that participitate in allergic reactions (e.g., hay fever) by releasing histamines. Allergy medicated by IgE is called a **type 1 hypersensitivity response**. IgE antibody provides protection against parasitic worms.

Levels of IgE are elevated in patients with allergies (e.g., asthma and hay fever) and in those harbouring helminthic parasites.

KEY POINTS

- An **antibody** or **immunoglobulin** is a globulin protein (glycoprotein) formed by the immune system in response to an antigenic stimulus.
- Antibodies bind to epitopes (or antigenic determinants) on the antigen.
- Maximum concentration of antibody in the human serum is IgG (80%) followed by IgM (5-10%), IgA (10-15%), IgD (0-2%) and IgE is minimum (0.002%).
- IgG crosses the placental barrier and enters the fetus from the mother.
- IgA is secretory antibody and provides mucosal or local immunity.
- IgG antibody has the maximum half life of 23 days in serum.

IMPORTANT QUESTIONS

1. Write short notes on:
   (a) Definition and structure of an immunoglobulin (antibody).
   (b) List the five types of immunoglobulins with functions of each.

MULTIPLE-CHOICE QUESTIONS

1. Another term for antibody is:
   (a) Antigen (b) Protein
   (c) Immunoglobulin (d) Hapten.
2. The specificity of an antibody is due to:
   (a) The light chain
   (b) The heavy chain
   (c) The variable region of the heavy and light chain
   (d) The Fe portion of the protein.
3. Antibodies are:
   (a) Proteins
   (b) Globulin proteins
   (c) Polypeptides
   (d) Nucleic acids.
4. Light chains and heavy chains in antibodies are joined by
   (a) Covalent bond (b) Hydrogen bond
   (c) Disulphide bond (d) Ionic bond.

5. The antigen binding site of an antibody is called:
   (a) Epitope (b) Antitope
   (c) Paratope (d) None of these.
6. Which of the following antibody can cross placental barrier and enters the fetus from mother?
   (a) IgG (b) IgA
   (c) IgM (d) IgE.
7. Which of the following is the earliest (first) antibody formed in life or synthesized by fetus?
   (a) IgG (b) IgM
   (c) IgA (d) IgE.
8. All antibodies are immunoglobulins, but all immunoglobulins are not antibodies. True or False?

ANSWERS TO MCQs

1. (c)	**2.** (c)	**3.** (b)	**4.** (c)	**5.** (a)
6. (a)	**7.** (b)	**8.** True.		

76

Antigen-Antibody Interactions and Serological Diagnostic Tests

WHAT IS AN ANTIGEN-ANTIBODY INTERACTION?

Antigen-antibody interaction, or **antigen-antibody reaction** (abbreviated as **Ag – Ab Interaction**), is a specific chemical interaction between antibodies produced by B cells of the WBCs and antigens to form an antigen-antibody (**AgAb**) complex. It is the fundamental reaction in the body by which we are protected from foreign molecules. **Richard J. Goldberg**, an American scientist, in 1952 gave the first complex description of the Ag-Ab reaction, hence this reaction, is called the **Goldberg's theory**.

Ab-Ag reactions *in vitro* are termed **serological reactions**, and their study is called **serology**, so named because these tests are performed in serum samples. These tests, called immunologic (or serologic)-based diagnostic tests, form the basis for detection of infectious diseases, identification of the causative agents and determination of ABO blood group.

FEATURES OF ANTIGEN-ANTIBODY REACTIONS

- The reaction is highly **specific**, that is, an antigen combines only with its homology antibody and vice versa.
- The molecules are held together in **lock and key arrangement.**
- All molecules react (not the fragment).
- Neither the antigen nor the antibody is denatured during the reaction.
- During combination only **surface antigens** participate, therefore, surface antigens are immunologically relevant.
- Antigens and antibodies can be combined in varying proportions.
- The combination between Ab and Ag is **firm** but **reversible**.
- **Affinity** (intensity of attraction between Ab and Ag) and **avidity** (strength of the bonds after the formation of AgAb complex) influence the firmness of the serum in combination.

TYPES OF ANTIGEN AND ANTIBODY REACTIONS: SEROLOGICAL REACTIONS

Antigen-antibody (Ab-Ag) reactions (or interactions) *in vitro* are called **serological reactions**. Various types of these are:

1. **Precipitation reactions**
    - **Sample precipitation**
    - **Immune diffusion (precipitation in gel)**
        - Single diffusion in one direction
        - Double diffusion in one direction
        - Single diffusion in two directions (radial immune diffusion)
        - Double diffusion in two dimensions (Ouchterlony method)
        - Immunoelectrophoresis
        - Electroimmunodiffusion
            - Counter immunoelectrophoresis
            - One-dimensional single electroimmunodiffusion
2. **Agglutination reactions**
    - Direct (active) agglutination tests
        - Slide tile agglutination
        - Tube agglutination
        - Coomb's (antiglobulin) test
        - Indirect (passive) agglutination tests
        - Coagglutination
        - Hemagglutination
3. **Neutralization reactions**
4. **Complement fixation reactions**
5. **Labelled (tagged) immunoassays**
    - Immunofluorescence (fluorescent-antibody technique)
    - Radioimmunoassays (RIA)
    - Enzyme-linked immunosorbent assay (ELISA)
    - Western blotting

PRECIPITATION REACTIONS

Precipitation reactions involve the reaction of soluble antigens with antibodies (IgG or IgM) called *precipitins* to form an insoluble visible precipitate, called **precipitation**. It was **Marrack** who in 1934 proposed *lattice hypothesis* for the mechanism of precipitation reaction which occurs in two stages: first, antigens and antibodies diffuse towards each other and quickly form small complexes (i.e. within seconds). Ab-Ag complexes form lattice-like network (cross-linking), which may take minutes to hours (second is a slower reaction) and precipitation takes place which is visible is a line or hazy "**precipitin ring**" (Fig. 76.1). The maximum amount of precipitate forms (i.e., largest precipitation reaction) where the ratio of Ab and Ag is similar or roughly equivalent, (i.e. the **zone of equivalence**) and the test is called the *precipitin ring test* for antibodies. Precipitation is greatly influenced by the relative amount of Ab or Ag in the mixture; precipitation is initiated by excess amount of antibody called the **frozen effect** as well as by the excess amount of antigen in the mixture — known as the **postzone effect,** in other words, a weak reaction due to nonproduction of lattice on either site of the zone of equivalence (Fig. 76.1). This is called the **zone phenomenon**.

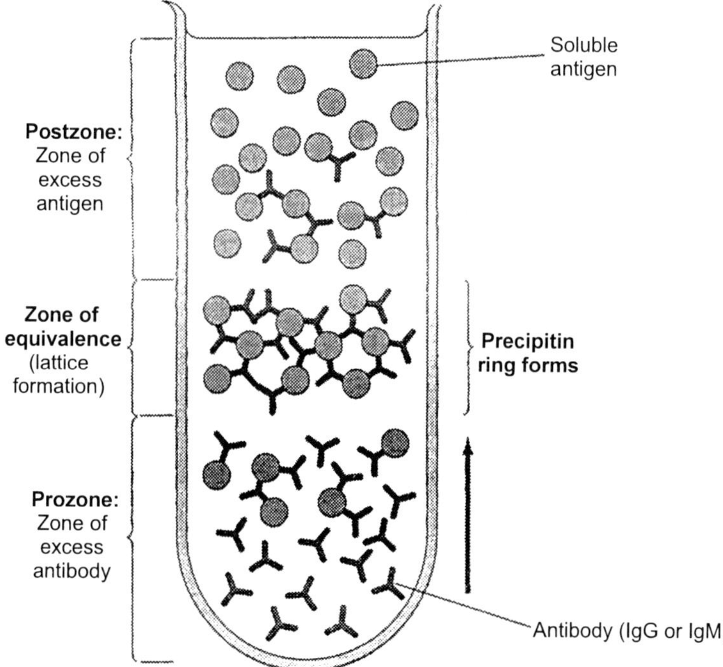

Fig. 76.1 Mechanism of precipitation reaction by lattice formation and zone phenomenon - the precipitin test for antibodies. Weak reaction occurs in: prozone (no precipitation) of largest reactioned lattice formation occurs in zone of equivalence (i.e., procipitation occurs as a hozy precipitin ring).

Applications of Precipitation Reactions

- To identify microbes (bacteria)
- To detect antibody in serum or other samples
- To detect toxin or anti-toxin
- To measure concentration (quantitative estimation) of antigen or antibody
- To detect food adulteration
- Forensic application in the identification of blood and seminal stains

Types of Precipitation Tests

1. **Simple precipitation tests:** These are of three types:

- **Slide precipitation/flocculation test**: In this test, one drop of an antigen is placed on a glass slide followed by addition of one drop of antiserum, and mixed by rotating the slide. Appearance of floccules/precipitates, indicates a positive test. VDRL (veneral disease research laboratory), a most widely used test to diagnose syphilis, is an example of slide flocculation test.
- **Tube flocculation test:** Flocculation test can be carried out in tubes also. Kohn test for syphilis and standardization of toxins and toxoids are examples of tube flocculation.
- **Ring test:** This test consists of layering a clear solution of sample containing antigen over a column of antiserum (antibody) in a capillary tube (narrow test tube). After a short period, a white ring of precipitate appears at the junctions of the liquids. The clinical applications of the ring test are: grouping of streptococci and detection of adulterants in food stuffs.

2. Immunodiffusion tests (precipitation reactions in gels): Immune diffusion refers to a precipitation reaction that occurs between an antibody and antigen in a thin layer of soft agar (1%) gel (or agarose gel) that results in an opaque band of precipitation at the junction of their diffusion front.

The main advantages of gel diffusion methods are:

- The reaction appears as a distinct band of precipitation that can be stained for better visibility and preservation.
- Several antigens can be reacted with one kind of antibody or several kinds of antibodies with one antigen on a single test medium.

Types of Immunodiffusion Tests

1. **Single immunodiffusion in one dimension (Qudin method):** The antibody is incorporated in agar gel in a test tube followed by layering of sample containing antigen over it. The antigen diffuses downwards through the agar gel forming a line of precipitation where it meets the antibody (Fig. 76.2).

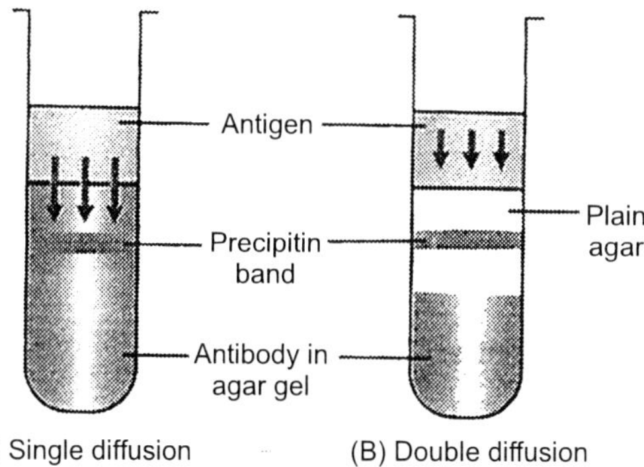

Fig. 76.2 Immunodiffusion tests: Single and double immunodiffusion in one dimention.

2. **Double immunodiffusion one dimension (Oakley-Fulthorpe method):** The antibody is incorporated on to gel in a test tube followed by placing a column of plain agar. The sample containing antigens is placed above the solidified plain agar. Both the Ag-Ab diffuse (double diffusion), i.e., move towards each other (in one direction) forming a band of precipitation where they meet in optimum concentration in the column of plain agar (Fig. 76.2B).
3. **Single immunodiffusion in two dimensions (radial immunodiffusion):** This method is used to determine the quantity or concentration of antigen or antibody in a serum sample.

   Antiserum solution containing antibody is added to molten agar and allowed to solidify on a glass slide. Number of wells are cut into the gel followed by addition of antigen samples of different dilutions/concentrations into various wells. The antigen diffuses outwards, complexing with antibody precipitate as a ring around the wells when the ratio of Ab to Ag is optimal (Fig. 76.3). The diameter of the precipitation ring formed is directly proportional to the concentration of the antigen.

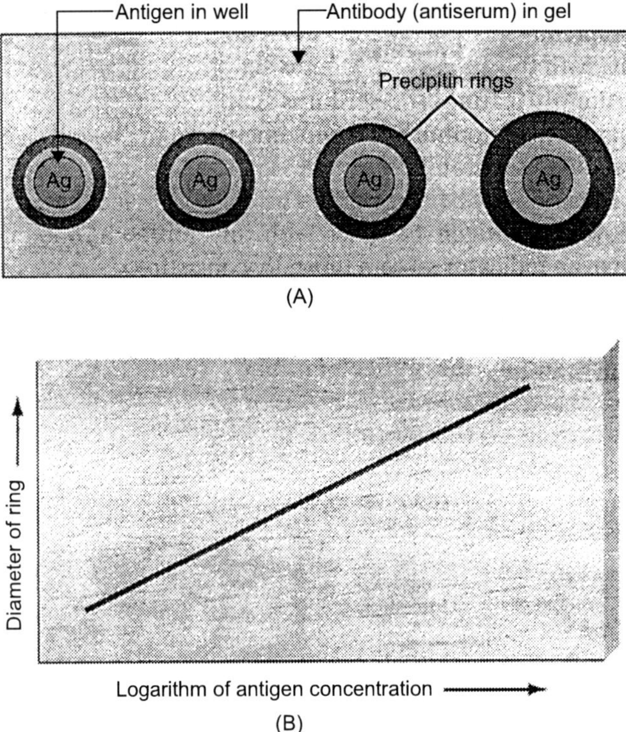

Fig. 76.3 Radial immunodiffusion: Single immunodiffusin in two dimensions. (A) Method: Wells cut into antibody-containing agar sheets are filled with antigen. The antigen diffuses outwards complexing with antibody as it goes. When the ratio of antigen to antibody is optimal, the complexes precipitate in a ring. (B) The diameter of the ring is proportional to the logarithm of the antigen concentration, which can be determined by reference to a standard curve. The concentration of an antibody can also be determined by reference to standard curve. The concentration of an antibody can also be determined by placing it in a well cut into an antigen-containing agar sheet and comparing the size of the resulting ring with a standard curve for that antibody.

4. **Double immunodiffusion in two dimensions (Ouchterlony immunodiffusion method):** This technique named after **Ouchterlony,** a Swedish physicians who invented it in 1948, is the most widely employed immunodiffusion method in serology. Both Ab and Ag diffuse independently through agar gel in two dimensions, horizontally and vertically (Fig. 76.4).

   In this method, agar gel is poured on a slide and wells are cut. The known antiserum (i.e., antibody) is placed in the central well and different antigens are placed in the surrounding wells. Ab and Ag diffuse and precipitation bonds are formed where they meet in optimal conditions. If two adjacent antigens are identical, the precipitate lines formed by them will fuse; and the precipitate lines will cross each other, if they are unrelated.

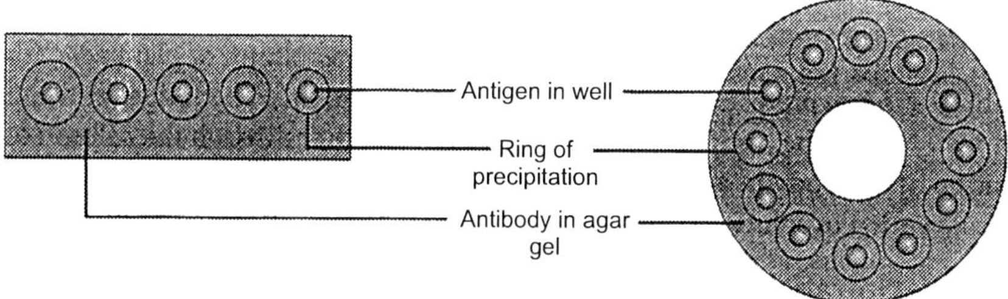

Fig. 76.4 Double immunodiffusion in two dimensions (Ouchterlony method), also known as passive double immunodiffusion).

5. **Immunoelectrophoresis:** It refers to precipitation in agar under an electric field. As the name implies, this process is a combination of immunodiffusion and electrophoresis. An antigen mixture is first separated into its component parts by electrophoresis and then tested by double immunodiffusion. It can be used to detect separate antigen-antibody complexes, and to test normal and abnormal protiens in serum and urine.

   In this test (Fig. 76.5), the antigens are placed in a well on an agar coated slide and are separated by passing an electric current (electrophoresis). The positively charged molecules are drawn towards the negative pole and negatively charged ones move towards the positive pole. A trough is cut into the agar gel between the wells and filled with antibody and precipitin bands result wherever matching antigen and antibody diffuse to meet, react and precipitate.

6. **Electroimmunodiffusion (EID):** It is an immune precipitation method in which antigen diffuses under the influence of an electric field, into a layer of agar containing specific antiserum. It is a sample rapid method for quantitation of immunoglobulins. Two common methods in use in a clinical laboratory are:

   - **Countercurrent immunoelectrophoresis** (One-dimensional double electroimmunodiffusion) (Fig. 76.6). The precipitation line apposed in 30 minutes as opposed to 24 hours in diffusion and is 10 times more sensitive than diffusion. It is used to detect meningococcal, cryptococcal and hemophilic antigens in CSF and Hepatitis B surface antigen in serum.

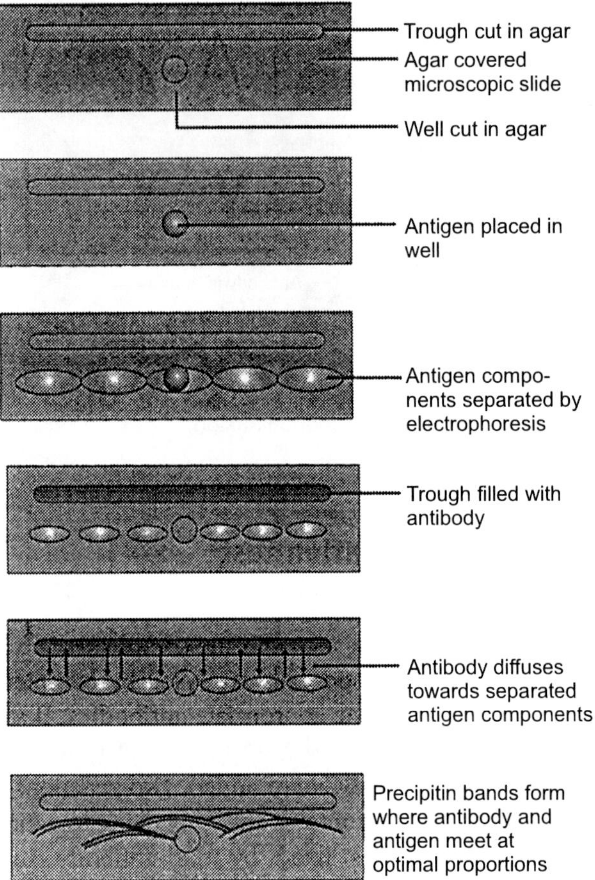

Fig. 76.5 Immunoelectrophoresis.

Lauren's rocket electrophorsies (one-dimensional single electroimmunodiffusion) (Fig. 76.6): The sensitivity of this technique is 0.5 mg/ml. It is used to detect antigens of *Cryptococcus,* Maningococcus and Hemophilus in CSF.

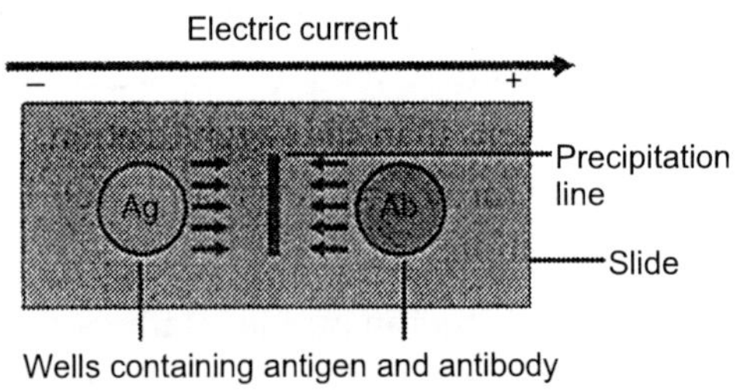

(A) Counterimmunoelectrophoresis

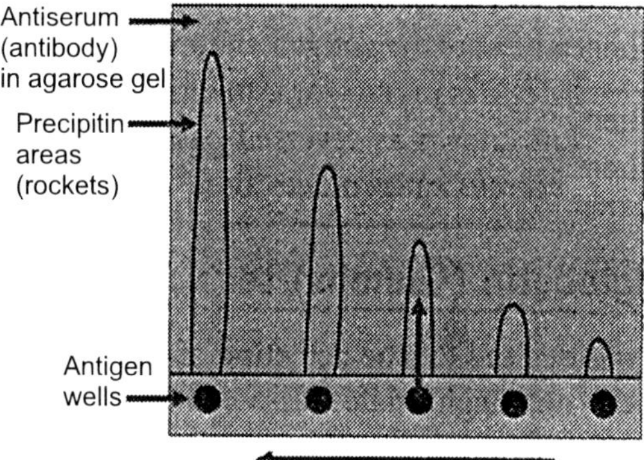

(B) Rocket electrophoresis

Fig. 76.6 Electroimmunodiffusion-an immunoprecipitation method, (A) Counter current electrophoresis, (B) Lauren's rocket electrophoresis.

AGGLUTINATION REACTIONS

Visible expression of clumping together of antigen-antibody complexes during reaction of a particulate antigen with specific antibody is called **agglutination**. The word agglutination comes from the Latin *agglutinare* means 'glueing to' antibodies that produce such reactions are called **agglutinins**. Agglutination occurs optimally when Ab and Ag are in equivalent proportion agglutination reaction is analogous to the precipitin reaction, in that antibody acts as a bridge to form a lattice network of antibody and cells. The quantity of the antibodies is called the **antibody titer**. It is reported as the reciprocal of the highest serum dilution in which agglutination (or clumping) occurs. The condition of excess antibody, however, is called a **prozone phenomenon**. Because the clumping reaction occurs quickly and is early to produce, agglutination is an important technique in clinical diagnosis.

Applications of agglutination reactions

- Cross-matching and grouping of blood.
- Identification (serotyping) of *Vibrio cholerae*, *Salmonella* Typhi and Paratyphi.
- Serological diagnosis of diseases that are difficult to detect or grow in clinical laboratory (e.g., syphilis (by RPR test), rheumatic fever (ASO test).
- Detection of unknown antigens in clinical specimens (e.g., detection of Vi antigen of *Salmonella* Typhi in urine).

Types of agglutination reactions

1. **Active/direct agglutination**
   (a) Slide/tile agglutination test
   (b) Tube agglutination test
   (c) Coombs/antiglobin test
2. **Passive agglutination**
3. **Coagglutination**

1. Active/direct agglutination

(a) **Slide/tile agglutination test:** Basic type of agglutination reaction performed on a slide/tile. Suspension of unknown antigen/ bacterial culture made in saline is placed on a glass slide or tile followed by the addition of a drop of standardized appropriate antiserum. Formation of visible clumps within 60 seconds is a positive reaction.

(b) **Tube agglutination test:** A fixed volume of a particulate antigen suspension is added to an equal volume of serial dilutions of a patient's serum in a series of test tubes and incubated at 37°C overnight. Positive Ab-Ag reaction is indictated by visible clamps of agglutination.

The last tube showing positive test will reflect the serum antibody **titer** of the patient. The reciprocal of the highest serum dilution that causes clamping is called the **agglutinin titer**. Thus, the serum that agglutinates at 1:216 dilution is reported to have a titre of 216 and if the test has been carried out in 1 mL volumes, the titer of the serum is 256 units/mL of serum.

Tube agglutination is a quantitative test which is routinely employed for diagnosis of enteric fever (**Widal test**), typhus fever (**Weil-Felix reaction**).

(c) **Antiglobulin test (Coomb's antiglobulin test):** The test was devised by **Coombs, Mourant** and **Race** for detection of incomplete anti-RH antibodies that do not agglutinate Rh^+ erythrocytes in saline. The erythrocytes are treated with antiglobulin or Coombs serum (rabbit antiserum against human gamma globulin) and the agglutination of the cells (i.e., hemagglutination) occurs (Fig. 76.7) revealing that the person with these RBCs would be Rh-positive. It is of two types:

- **Direct Coombs test (Direct antiglobulin test, DAT):** The sensitization of the RBCs (erythrocytes) with incomplete antibodies takes place *in vivo*. DAT is usually used to diagnose hemolytic anaemia (in which blood does not contain enough RBCs, because they are destroyed prematurely), a disease of the newborns due to Rh incompatibly (i.e. anti-Rh antibodies)

- **Indirect Coomb's test (Indirect antiglobulin test, IAT):** The sensitization of the RBCs with the antibody globulin is performed *in vitro*. It looks for antibodies floating in serum.

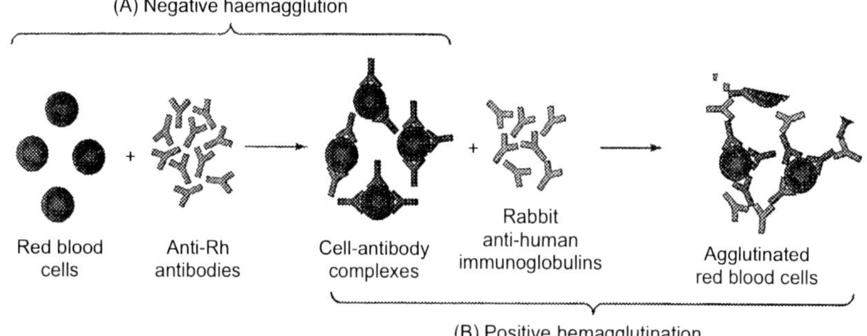

Fig. 76.7 The Coomb's antiglobulin test. (A) Anti-Rh antibodies are allowed to react with RBCs. If Rh antigens are present on the blood cells, there are not enough of them to produce a hemagglutination. (B) Therefore, anti-human antibodies prepared in rabbits are reacted with the red blood cell-antibody complexes. If Rh antigens are present on the red blood cells, hemagglutination will occur.

In IAT, the patient's serum (i.e., recipient) is mixed with normal RBCs and antiserum to human immunoglobulin. Agglutination occurs if antibodies are present in the serum. It is used for testing blood prior to blood transfusion. A negative IAT indicates, serum lacking antibodies, hence blood transfusion is safe from the donor.

2. Indirect agglutination/Passive agglutination: This test employs the use of carrier particles (e.g., RBCs, latex, bentonite, gelatin) that are coated with soluble antigens (i.e., converting soluble antigen to insoluble antigen). When corresponding antibody reacts, the particles or cells get agglutinated. In this a precipitation reaction is converted into agglutination reaction, hence it is called **indirect agglutination**. For example, antigens coated in latex particles are used in ASO test.

When the antibody instead of antigen is absorbed on the carrier particles in tests for detection of antigens, it is called **reverse passive agglutination**. For example, cryptococcus antigen detection.

3. Coagglutination test: Coagglutination is a type of agglutination reaction in which Cowan I strain of *Staphylococcus aureus* is used as a carrier particle to coat antibodies. Fc portion of any antibody gets attached to protein A of the Cowan strain leaving the Fab region free to react with the antigen present in the specimens.

In a positive test, protein A bearing *S. aureus* water with antibodies will be agglutinated if mixed with specific antigen. This test is used for

- Detection of cryptococcal antigen in the CSF for diagnosis of cryptococcal meningitis.
- Detection of amoebic and hydatid antigens for diagnosis of amoebiosis and cystic echinococcsis.
- Grouping of streptococci and mycobacteria and for typing of *Neisseria gonorrhoeae*.

4. Hemagglutination Test: Hemagglutination or **agglutination of red blood cells** is a specific form of agglutination that involves RBCs that carry antigens on their surface. Two common uses are:

- **Blood typing (grouping):** It is determined by using antibodies that tend to A or B blood group antigens in a sample of blood.
- **Viral hemagglutination:** many viruses bind to and cross-link RBCs causing **viral hemagglutination**. This test is used to detect viruses that cause measles and influenza.

This assay may be modified to include the addition of an antiserum (antibodies to the viruses), thereby inhibiting the agglutination of RBCs by the virus, the test called **hemagglutination inhibition test**, which can be used to diagnose measles, influenza and other viral diseases.

COMPLEMENT-FIXATION REACTIONS

A group of normal serum proteins is collectively called a **complement**. Complement can only link to **ground antibody** (i.e., Ab attached to Ag) at Fc portion and is used up, or fixed. The process in which complement combines with an Ag-Ab complex is called **complement fixation**, thereby making complement unavailable for hemolysis of indicator RBCs. This test is used to detect the presence of antibodies to a known antigen (even in very small amount). Complement-fixation test (CFT) was once used for the diagnosis of syphilis (caused by *Treponema*) and is still used to diagnose certain fungal, rickettisial and virus antibodies in patient sera or CSF during an acute infection. This test mainly measures IgG antibodies.

In the CFT (Fig. 76.8), the complement in the patient's serum is first destroyed by heating (complement is heat-labile protein); the serum is then mixed with appropriate antigen and after incubation, when Ab-Ag complex is formed, exogenous complement (usually from fresh guinea pig serum) is added. This complement then binds to the complexes and having been fixed, no hemolysis results of added indicator red cells – so the CFT is positive for the presence of antibodies. Lysis of RBCs (i.e., hemolysis) indicates a **negative CFT** (due to no Ab-Ag reaction and availability of uncombined complement in the reaction).

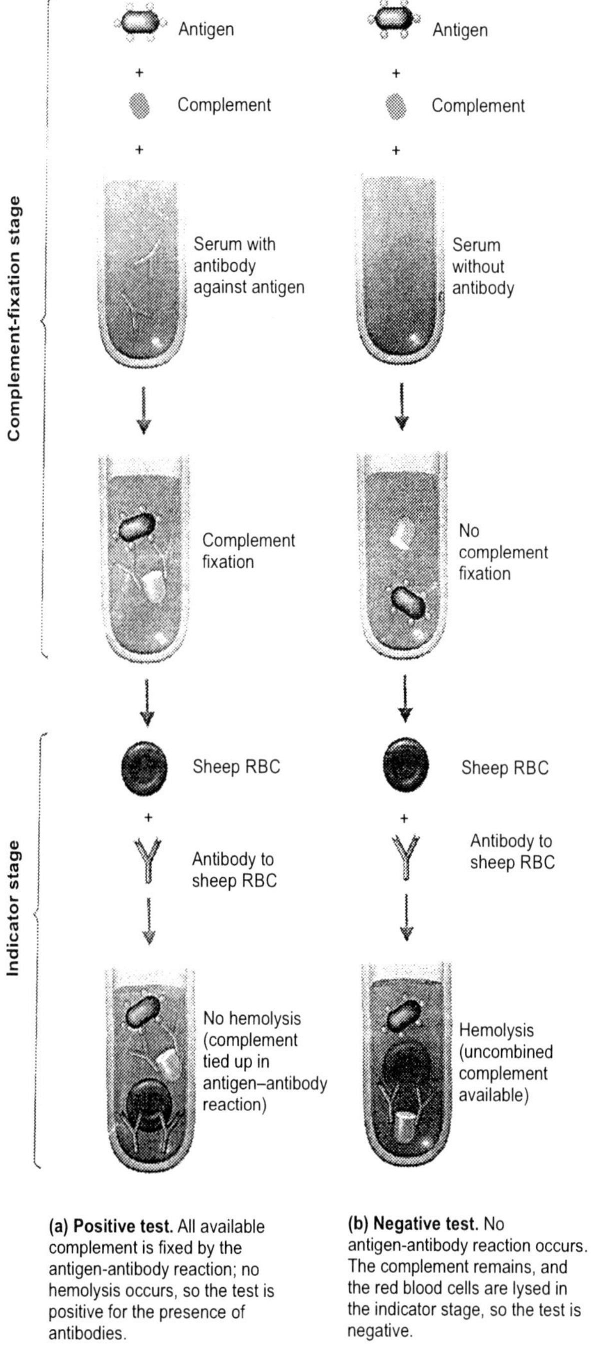

(a) Positive test. All available complement is fixed by the antigen-antibody reaction; no hemolysis occurs, so the test is positive for the presence of antibodies.

(b) Negative test. No antigen-antibody reaction occurs. The complement remains, and the red blood cells are lysed in the indicator stage, so the test is negative.

Fig. 76.8 The complement-fixation test. Complement will combine (be fixed) with an antibody that is reaction with an antigen. If all the complement is fixed in the complement-fixation stage, then none will remain to cause hemolysis of the red blood cells in the indicator stage.

NEUTRALIZATION REACTIONS

Neutralization is an antigen-antibody reaction in which the harmful effects of a bacterial exotoxin or a virus are blocked by specific antibodies called **neutralizing antibodies (NAb)**. Neutralization tests are of three types:

(a) **Virus neutralization test:** The patient's serum is mixed with a suspension of infectious virus particles of the same type as those suspected of causing the disease in the patient. A control suspension of the virus is mixed with normal serum and inoculated into an appropriate cell culture. If the patient's serum contains antibody of the virus, the antibody will bind to the virus particles, thereby neutralizing the infection of the virus (e.g., vaccinia, influenza and poliomyelitis).

(b) **Toxin neutralization tests:** Toxin neutralization tests (Fig. 76.9) are based on the principle that biological action of toxin is neutralized on reacting with specific neutralizing antibodies called antitoxins. Examples of neutralization tests includes:

- **Schick test** – to demonstrate immunity against diphtheria toxin.
- **Anti-streptolycin 'O' test** – in which antitoxin present in the patient's serum neutralizes the hemolytic activity.
- **Nagler's reaction** – used for rapid detection of *Clostridium welchii*.

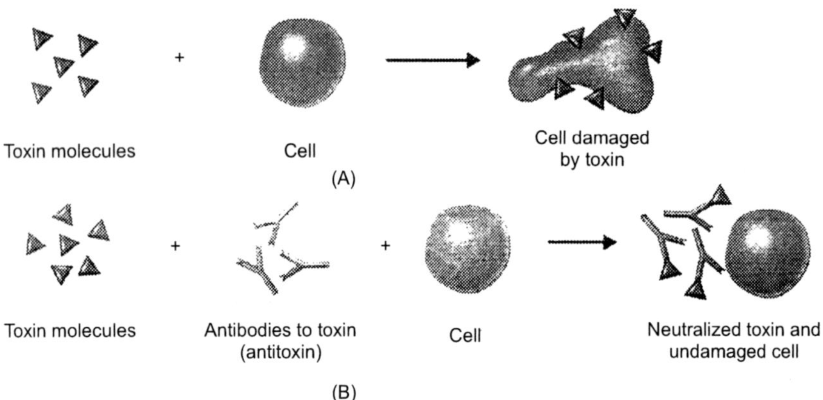

Fig. 76.9 Neutralization reaction. The effects of a toxin on a susceptible (A) and neutralization of the toxin by antitoxin (B).

(c) **Viral hemagglutination inhibition test:**

This test is used to detect antibodies to a virus. It is an example of **virus neutralization test** (Fig. 76.10) frequently used in the diagnosis of viral infections, such as influenza, mumps and measles. These viruses have surface proteins that cause the agglutination of red blood cells (i.e., hemagglutination). If the person's serum contains antibodies against these viruses, these antibodies will react with the viruses, neutralize them and inhibit hemagglutination (hence the test named hemagglutination inhibition test).

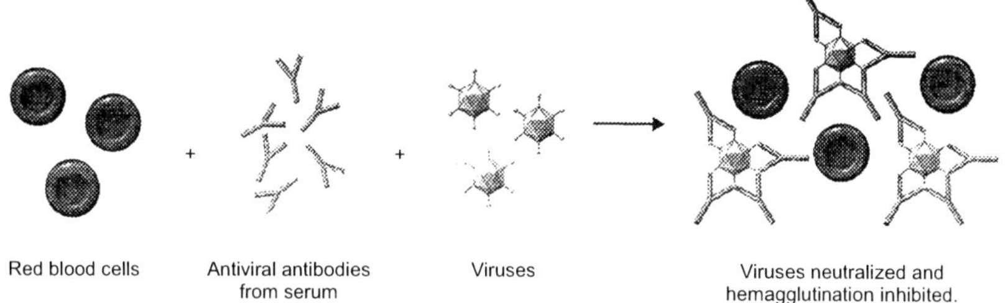

Fig. 76.10 Neutralization reaction. Viral hemagglutionation test to detect anibodies to a virus. These viruses will normally cause hemagglutination when mixed with red blood cells. If antibodies to the virus are present, as shown here, they neutralize and inhibit hemagglutination.

OPSONIZATION

Opsonins are freely circulating serum proteins that facilitate phagocytosis and cell lysis by making antigen. The process of the enhancement of phagocytosis by creating microorganisms with certain opsonins is called **opsonization**. The ratio of phagocytic activity of patiens blood having bacterium to the phagocytic activity of blood from a healthy individual is called **opsonic index**. This is measured by incubating the fresh citrated blood with bacterial suspensions for 15 minutes at 34°C and number of phagocytized bacteria per leukocyte from stained blood is calculated.

LABELLED OR TAGGED IMMUNOASSAYS

Labelled immunoassays (or **tagged antibody tests**), the most sensitive with better visualization of the antibody-antigen reaction, are used to detect/isolate/purify antibodies or antigens even at very low concentrations. In these assays, antibodies like other proteins, are attached to a specific tag (e.g., fluorescent dyes, radioisotopes, enzymes, biotin) called **antibody labelling**. Examples of labelled immunoassays include:

1. **Immunofluorescence** (**Fluorescent – antibody techniques**)
2. **Radioimmunoassay**
3. **Enzyme-linked immunosorbent assay** (**ELISA**)
4. **Western blot**

1. Immunofluorescence: Immunofluorescence (also called **fluorescent-antibody (FA) techniques**) uses antibodies labelled with fluorescent dyes (e.g., fluorescein isothiocyanate). When viewed with UV light under a fluorescence microscope, it will **fluoresce** (or emitting an intense yellow-green light), revealing the presence of the tagged molecule. These assays are extensively used for:

- To identify microorganisms in clinical specimens.
- To detect the presence of a specific antibody in serum.
- To detect tissue antigens.
- To detect antigen-antibody complexes.

FA techniques are of two types:

Direct IF (Direct FA tests): Only one labelled antibody is used in this test. A solution of fluorescein tagged antibody to that antigen is prepared, added to cells or clinical specimen, incubated and washed and examined with fluorescence microscopy for fluorescing-tagged antibody-antigen complex (Fig. 76.11A). It is used to identify specific microorganisms (e.g., Group A streptococci from patients throat).

Indirect IF (Indirect FA tests): Two labelled antibodies are used to demonstrate the presence of antibody in serum, and the antibody to the antigen being sought is not itself tagged. Syphilis is diagnosed by this test: The fluorescent dye is attached to anti-human immune serum globulin, which reacts with any human immunoglobulin (e.g., *Treponema pallidum*-unspecific antibody) that has previously reacted with the antigen and fluorosed spirochaete (Ab- dye tagged Ag) glows (fluoresces) on examination with fluorescence microscope (Fig. 76.11 B).

A **fluorescence-activated cell-sorter (FACS),** a modified form of flow cytometer, can be used to detect and count cells labelled with fluorescent antibodies. It is used to assess the progression of disease in AIDS patients.

2. Radioimmunoassay (RIA)

Radioimmunoassay (RIA): Refers to the immunoassay of a substance that has been radiolabelled. It is an extremely sensitive technique for measuring minute quantities (nanograms) of antigens or antibodies using gamma spectrometer.

In this procedure, a known antigen is overlayed on a plastic plate to which antigen molecules adhere. A solution of antibody (to be tested) is applied to the same plate and allowed to react and if the Ab is specific to the Ag it will combine with it. It is followed by the addition of radioactively labelled second antibody (anti-antibody) (Fig. 7.12) which is allowed to react or then washed off. The radioactivity that remains on the plate is a measure of the amount of antibody that combined with the known fixed antigen.

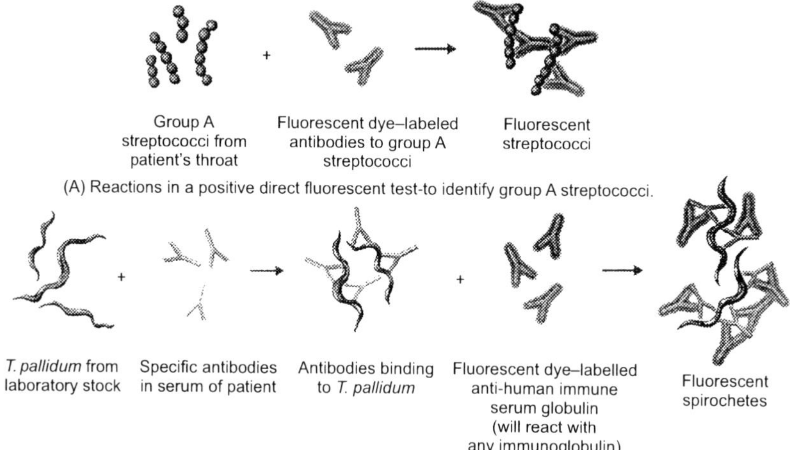

Fig. 76.11 Fluorescent-antibody (FA) techniques: (A) A direct FA test to identify group A streptococci. (B) In an indirect FA test such as that used in the diagnosis of syphilis, the fluorescent dye is attached to anti-human immune serum globulin, which reacts with any human immunoglobulin (such as the *Treponema pallidum*-specific antibody) that has previously reacted with the antigen. The reaction is viewed through a fluorescence microscope, and the antigen with which the dye-tagged antibody has reacted fluoresces (glows) in the ultravioiet illumination.

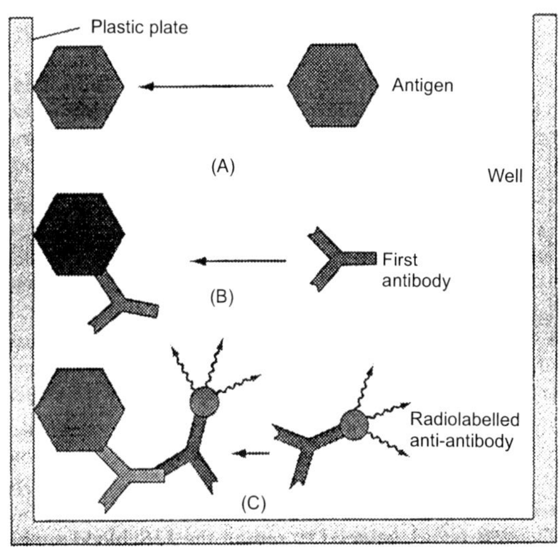

Fig. 76.12 Radioimmunoassay (RIA) is used to detect very small quantities of antibody. (A) Antigen first is bound to a well of a plastic plate. After excess unbound antigen is washed out, the solution being tested for antibody is added and allowed to react. (B) If antibody is present, it reacts with the antigen. (C) After any unbound antibody is washed out, a radioactively labelled second antibody (anti-antibody) specific to the first antibody is added. The amount of bound radioactive anti-antibody present is measured. It is proportional to the concentration of the antibody in the original solution.

3. Enzyme-linked Immunosorbent Assay (ELISA)

ELISA, as the name implies, uses an enzyme system, as an indicator of an antigen-antibodies combination. It is a plate-based assay technique usually run in 96-well microplates in which the targetted antibody or antigen is linked to a specific enzyme, and if the target substance is present in the sample, the test solution turns a different colour which is detected and read using a colorimeter spectrophotometer linked to a computer.

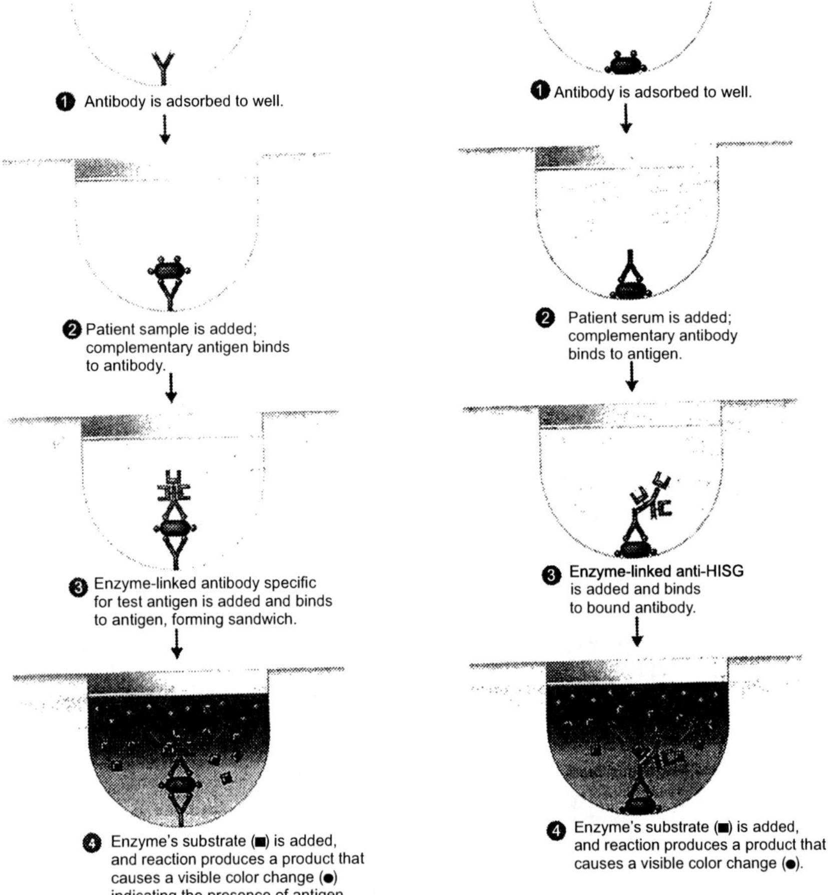

Fig. 76.13 Enzyme-linked immunosorbent assay (ELISA). This method is a modification of radioimmunoassay (**RIA**), the ELISA, uses enzymes instead of radioisotopes to detect antigen-antibody complexes. The components are usually contained in small wells of a microtiter plate and the resultant-colored product (end product of the reaction) are read by the ue of a computer. ELISA tests are done rountinely as an initial test to detect HIV and Covid-19 virus in blood samples. Antigens are detected by direct ELISA and antibodies by indirect ELISA test.

ELISAs, a type of immunoassay, that are commonly used to quantify levels of a specific target (antibody, antigen) within a sample. Clinical samples routinely used in ELISAs include blood (serum and plasma), cell culture supernates, saliva, urine, cell lysates and tissue lysates.

It is a very useful tool to diagnose diseases caused by viruses (e.g., AIDS, hepatitis, rubella, respiratory syncytial infections), bacterial (syphilis, salmonellosis, brucellosis), fungi (histoplasmosis, aspergillosis) and parasites (amoebiasis, leishmaniasis cysticercosis lymphatic filariasis). For clinical use, several ELISAs test kits are available in the market. Automated version of ELISA is used to detect antigens and antibodies simultaneously for *Clostridium*, *Chlamydia*, *Toxoplasma gondii* and several viruses-mumps, measles, rubella, cytomegalovirus, respiratory syncytial virus in the sophisticated diagnostic labs.

ELISA TYPES

The four main types of ELISA are direct, indirect, sandwich and competitive.

- **Direct ELISA:** Only single, an enzyme-labelled antibody, is used in the assay. It is a very fast and simple test used to detect antigens against a specific antibody bound in a test well (Fig. 76.13).
- **Indirect ELISA :** It uses two antibodies (primary and secondary) and the enzyme is linked to the secondary antibody that reacts with the substrate to produce a visible signal proportional to the amount of antigen bound in the well (Fig. 76.13). It is used for measuring endogenous antibodies.
- **Sandwich ELISA:** The most common types of ELISA. It uses two specific antibodies to sandwich the antigen, commonly referred to as **matched antibody pairs**. This assay is highly straight and is used for determining analytic concentration in biological sample.
- **Competitive ELISA:** It is also called **antibody capture ELISA**. It uses conjugated antigen used to compete for bonding with the antigen present in the sample. Since the assay involves the use of initiator antigen, hence also called **inhibition ELISA**. It is highly sensitive at best for detection of small molecules of antigen, even when they are present in low concentration in a sample.

Western Blot

The **Western blot**, or **Western blotting** or **protein immunoblot** (simply called **immunoblotting**) is an enzyme-linked antibody technique widely used to identify a specific portion in a sample (a mixture tissue homogenate extract). In this proteins are first separated by gel electrophoresis, then transferred (blotted) to a protein binding sheet (blotter) such as cellulose filter paper. Now the protein/antigen is flooded with the enzyme-linked antibody. Location of the antigen of the enzyme-linked antibody react and can be visualized, usually with a colour-reading label similar to an ELISA test reaction.

The term 'Western blot' was given by **W. Neal Burnette** in 1981 in honour of **Edwin Southern** and of the West coast location of its invention.

The diagnostic uses of this technique are:

- Confirmatory test for HIV infection by determining the exact viral antigens to which the HIV antibodies are specific in a human serum sample.
- Confirmatory test for **Hepatitis B-infection** or HSV-2 (Herpes Type 2) infection.
- Definite test for **variant Creutzfeldt disease**, a prion disease.
- To diagnose **tularemia** (caused by *Francisella. tularensis*).

KEY POINTS

- **Serology** is the study of blood serum used to detect antibody, and the antigen-antibody reactions.
- **Immunology based diagnostic tests** to identify infectious diseases are categorized into: precipitation reactions, agglutination reactions, neutralization reactions, complement fixation reactions, opsonization and labelled (or tagged) antibody tests.
- A reaction between a soluble antigen and a specific antibody resulting to form floccules (or precipitates) is called **precipitation reaction**.
- The interaction between a particulate antigen and a specific antibody resulting in clumping of Ab and Ag is called **agglutination reaction**.
- Agglutination reactions using RBCs are called **hemagglutination reactions.**
- **Complement fixation test** indirectly detect antibodies in serum to antigens by determining the depletion of a fixed amount of complement in the presence of an Ab-Ag reaction.
- In **neutralization reactions** the effect of an antigen, bacterial exotoxin or virus is neutralized on mixing with its specific antibody.

- **Fluorescent-antibody techniques** (immunofluorescence) use antibody labelled (tagged) with fluorescent dyes.
- **Radioimmunoassay** involves the use of a radioisotope to indicate the presence of Ab-Ag reaction.
- **ELISA** techniques use antibodies linked to an enzyme and Ab-Ag reactions are detected by enzyme activity.
- Serum antibodies separated by electrophoresis are identified with an enzyme-linked antibody.

IMPORTANT QUESTIONS

1. Enumerate various antigen-antibody reactions with a brief definition of each.
2. Write short notes on:
   (a) Precipitation reactions.
   (b) Agglutination reactions.
   (c) ELISA.
   (d) Immunofluorescence.
   (e) Western blotting.

MULTIPLE CHOICE QUESTIONS

1. Reaction between a particulate antigen with its antibody is termed:
   (a) Precipitation reaction
   (b) Agglutination reaction
   (c) Complement fixation
   (d) Immunofluorescence.
2. Reaction of soluble antigen with antibody to form lattice-like network is known as:
   (a) Precipitation reaction
   (b) Agglutination reaction
   (c) Specificity
   (d) Complement fixation.
3. Antibody excess in an antigen-antibody reaction is called:
   (a) Postzone effect (b) Prozone effect
   (c) No zone effect (d) None of these.
4. Which of the following test(s) is/are used in the toxin neutralization principle?
   (a) Nagler's reaction (b) Schick test
   (c) Both (a) and (b) (d) None of these.

5. VDRL is an example of:
   (a) Ring test
   (b) Tube agglutination test
   (c) Slide agglutination test
   (d) Immunofluorescence test.
6. Which of the following serological tests is used to detect very small quantities (nanograms) of antigens and antibodies in a sample?
   (a) ELISA
   (b) Radioimmunoassay
   (c) Immunoelectrophoresis
   (d) Viral neutralization.
7. Which of the following is the confirmatory test of the HIV infection?
   (a) Hemagglutination
   (b) Radioimmunoassay
   (c) Coombs' antiglobulin test
   (d) Western blotting.
8. Which test is used to detect antibodies against a pathogen?
   (a) Direct ELISA (b) Indirect ELISA
   (c) Both (a) and (b) (d) None of these.
9. Which of the following tests is used to detect the presence of antibodies in a patient's serum?
   (a) Indirect fluorescent – antibody test
   (b) Direct fluorescent – antibody test.
10. The *direct* ELISA detects antigens and the indirect ELISA detects antibodies. True or False?
11. Fluorescent – antibody techniques use antibodies labelled with fluorescent dyes. True or False?
12. ELISA techniques use antibodies labelled with a dye. True or False?
13. In Western blotting, serum antibodies separated by electrophoresis are identified with an enzyme-linked antibody. True or False?

ANSWERS TO MCQs

1. (b)	**2.** (a)	**3.** (b)	**4.** (c)	**5.** (c)
6. (b)	**7.** (d)	**8.** (b)	**9.** (b)	**10.** (True)
11. (True)	**12.** (False)	**13.** (True).		

77

Hypersensitivity Reactions (Immune Hypersensitivity)

The immune system (or immunity) is an integral part of human protection against disease. The normally protective mechanism can sometimes cause death, mental effects in the host called intolerance, hypersensitivity or hypersensitivity reactions.

A **hypersensitivity reaction** refers to an over-reaction or an appropriate or exaggerated response to an antigen or an allergen that leads to tissue damage, sometimes death.

Allergy is a more common term which is essentially synonymous to hypersensitivity. The reaction occurs in individuals who have been **sensitized** by previous exposure of an antigen. The first exposure leads sensitization to the allergen, but when the individual is exposed to that allergy on further occasions, the hypersensitivity reaction occurs. Hay fever, which results from repeated exposure to plant pollens, is an example of harmful immunic reaction.

CLASSIFICATION OR TYPES OF HYPERSENSITIVITY

A. Traditional classification: Based on the duration between exposure to an antigen or reaction hypersensitivity reactions, has been classified into two types:

1. **Immediate type hypersensitivity**
   - Appears and recedes rapidly.
   - Induced by antigens or haptens by any route.
   - Antibody mediated reaction.
   - Passive transfer possible with serum.
2. **Delayed type hypersensitivity**
   - Appears slowly, but lasts longer.
   - Induced by antigen or hapten intradermally or by skin contact.

- Cell-mediated reaction.
- Transferred possibly work T cells or transfer factor, but not with serum.

B. Gell and Coombs' Classification: Robert Coombs and **Philip Gell,** British immunologists in 1963, classified hypersensitivity reactions (allergic reactions) into four patho/physiological types:

- **Type I (Immediate anaphylactic):** Allergy symptoms appear after a few seconds to minutes (30 minutes)
- **Type II (Cytotoxic):** Reactions appear after minutes to hours (12 hours)
- **Type III (Immune complex-mediated):** Allergic reactions after 3-8 hours.
- **Type IV (Delayed cell-mediated or delayed hypersensitivity):** A long latency of hours to days (24-48 hours)

Types I to III are also termed **humoral reactions** because these are mediated by antibodies, whereas in type IV T-cells are involved.

Autoimmune disorders represent a form of hypersensitivities in which the autoantibodies or T-cells attack self-antigens.

TYPE I HYPERSENSITIVITY

Type I hypersensitivity, also called immediate hypersensitivity, is an allergic reaction provoked by re-exposure to a specific type of antigen (referred to as an allergen) that often occurs within 2 to 30 minutes. Exposure may be by ingestion, inhalation, injection, or direct contact. Pollen allergy, hay fever, food allergy, allergic asthma or sweet itch are common examples of type I.

Anaphylaxis (Gr. *ana* = against phylaxes = protection) means "the opposite of protected" refers to the detrimental effects to the host caused when certain antigens (allergens) combine with IgE antibodies (earlier called **reagin**). These effects are the opposite of **prophylaxis,** the preventive effects generated by an immune response.

There are two forms of anaphylaxis:

- **Localized anaphylaxis (atopy):** Produces shock and breathing difficulties and are sometimes fatal resulting from a sudden extreme drop in blood pressure.
- **Generalized (or systemic) anaphylaxis:** A severe systemic reaction occurs within minutes, leading to symptomatology: such as acute asthma, laryngeal edema, diarrhea, urticaria and shock. It is of two types: **respiratory anaphylaxis** (in which

the airways are constricted) and **anaphylactic shock** (blood pressure is greatly decreased that is sometimes fatal). Classic examples are penicillin allergy and bee sting allergy.

- **Localized anaphylaxis (atopic immune reaction):** It is also called **atopy** (which literally means "out of place") refers to localized allergic reaction to an allergen (antigen) that are ingested (foods) or inhaled (pollen grains). Atopic immune reaction symptom occur first at the site when the allergen enters the body. For example:
    - **Entry through skin:** As *wheal and flare reaction*, characterized by reddened, swelling and itching of the skin (Fig. 77.2).
    - **Inhalation:** Runny nose and watery eye, inflammation of the respiratory tract mucous membrane.
    - **Ingestion:** Abdominal pain, diarrhea and inflamed mucous membrane and skin rashes by drugs and foods.

Mechanism of Immediate Hypersensitivity: In the first (or initial) exposure to an allergen (called *sensitization*), allergen binds to B cells and is presented as allergen fragments on the surface of macrophages. These fragments of the allergen activate T_H cells, which activate B cells that develop into plasma cells that produce IgE antibodies. The IgE by its Fc tail becomes bound to basophiles and mast cells in places such as respiratory tract mucosa. In a second or later exposer (i.e., encountering the allergen again), the binding (cross-linking) of two adjacent IgE antibodies to an antigen leads to mast cell **degranulation** i.e., the rapid release of *preformed or primary mediators* (e.g. histamine, serotonin) which cause vasodilation, broncoconstriction, and release of **secondary mediators** (e.g., leukotrienes, prostaglandin) which lead to symptoms of allergies.

ALLERGENS AND SKIN TESTS FOR ALLERGY

Any foreign substance (often a protein) that induces allergic state or reaction (i.e., allergy), type I hypersensitivity in humans is called an **allergen** (or **allergin**). The first exposure produces no visible signs or symptoms. Allergens are introduced into the body through four main routes: The airways (inhalation), the gastrointestinal tract (ingestion), the circulatory system and skin (injection). The mode of introduction of various allergens into the body is as follows:

Routes of entry into the body	Examples of allergens
A. Ingestion	Animal proteins (essentially from milk and eggs), foods (fruits, grains, nuts, seafood), drugs (penicillin, aspirin, hormone)
B. Inhalation	Pollens (from weeds, grasses, trees); household (dust), spores (fungal and bacterial), mites or their feces, face powder, insecticides, herbicides, dander and cocane.
C. Injection	Insect bites and stings (venoms from insects, snakes, spiders), through drug administration (e.g., penicillin cephalosporin, heroin, hormone and vaccines (flu, tetanus toxoid).

Major symptoms produced by various types of allergens are:

- Airborne allergens cause sneezing, runny nose, and itchy, bloodshot eyes of allergic rhinitis (hay fever).
- Allergens in food cause itching or swelling of the lips or throat, crarmps and diarrhea and sometimes urticaria, angioderma and anaphylaxis.
- In contact with the skin, they cause reddening, itching and blistering, called **contact dermatitis** and **atopic dermatitis**.

Skin tests are used to identify an allergen and allergy diagnosis through wheel and flare reaction.

SKIN TESTS FOR ALLERGY DIAGNOSIS

Sensitivity to an allergen (antigen) is determined by skin testing. Skin tests are performed by administering a tiny dose of the suspected allergen by pricking or scratching, punching or injecting the skin. Such testing is usually done on the extremities to keep an hypersensitive reaction away from major organs, usually on the forearms, back or tip of the thighs.

In this test, drops of fluid containing test substances (allergens) are placed on the patient's skin followed by making a needle to allow the substance to penetrate the skin. Reaction is observed, approximately 15 minutes after exposure. A *wheal and flare reaction* (reddening and swelling) at the site of skin inoculation, a hypersensitive reaction, identify the substance as the possible cause of an allergic reaction (Fig. 77.1). *Wheal* stands for a white raised area and *flare* stands for reddened area, in skin test.

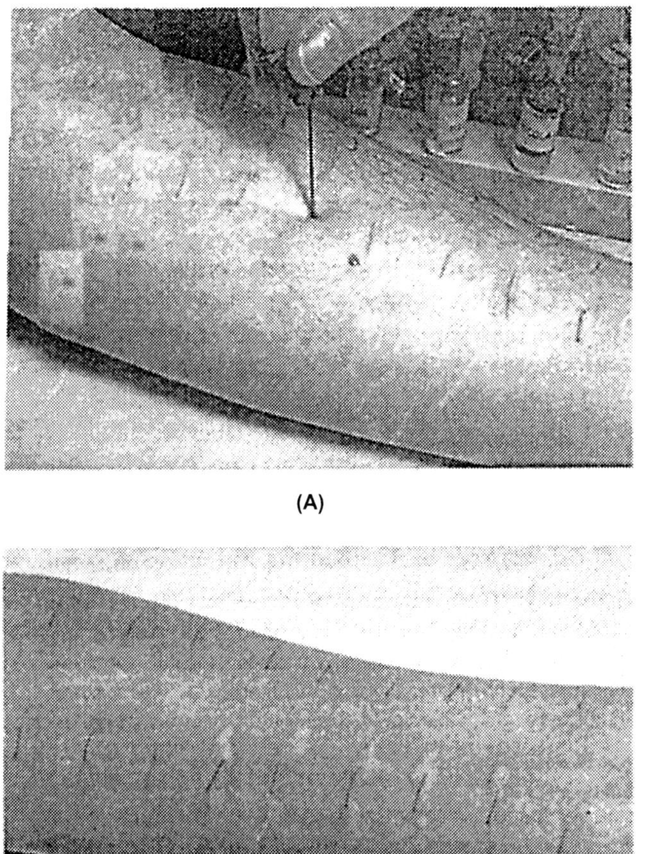

(A)

(B)

Fig. 77.1 Allergy testing. (A) Possible allergens are placed on prongs and introduced under the patient's skin. (B) If an individual is hypersenstitve, a wheal (white raised area) and flare (reddened area) soon becomes visible on the skin. Such testing is usually done on the extremitites to keep any hypersenstitive reaction away from major organs.

Intradermal skin tests involve injection of the allergen into the skin dermis. These test are more sensitive and associated with the risk of death, such is allergies to antibiotics.

Prevention and Treatment of Allergies

Once the responsible antigen has been identified by skin testing, two approaches are used to prevent/treat a person.

- To avoid contact with the specific allergen.
- **Desensitization (hyposensitization)** is the only currently available treatment for allergy. This procedure consists of a series of gradually increasing dosages of the antigen carefully injected beneath the skin, which leads to the formation of blocking (IgG) antibodies against the allergen.

TYPE II (CYTOTOXIC) HYPERSENSITIVITY

Type II hypersensitive reactions (i.e., cytotoxic hypersensitivity reactions) are mediated by IgG and IgM antibodies bound to cell surface antigens or malaria-associated antigens on basement membranes. These antibodies can either activate, complement, resulting in an inflammatory response and lysis of the largest cells, or they can either activate, complement, resulting in an inflammatory response and lysis of the targetted cells, or they can be involved in **antibody-dependent cell – mediated cytotoxicity (ADCC)** with cytotoxic T cells (hence called cytotoxic hypersensitivity).

In some cases, the antigen may be a self-antigen and the reaction is described as an **autoimmune disease** (or **autoimmune disorder**). Examples of type II hypersensitivity are:

- Hemolytic (blood) transfusion reaction (HTR)
- Hemolytic disease of the newborn (HDN) (erythroblastic fetalis)
- Drug-induced hemolytic anemia.

HEMOLYTIC TRANSFUSION REACTION (HTR)

Incompatible blood transfusions lead to the complement-mediated a strong, potentially lethal type II hypersensitivity cytotoxic reaction (HCR) lysis of the donor lower red blood cells resulting in hemolytic anemia.

For instance, if blood from a type A donor is administrated to a person with type B blood, the anti-isohemagglutinin IgM antibodies in the recipient bind to and agglutinate to incoming donor type A RBCs. The bound anti-A antibodies activate the **classical complement cascade**, resulting in the destruction of the donor's RBCs (i.e., massive hemolysis of the transfused RBCs) (Fig. 77.2). Occlusion of blood vessels in the alveoli of lungs and glomeruli of the kidneys can occur from the damaged and distroyed RBCs debris. Within 1 to 24 hours of incompatible transfusion, the patient experiences fever, chills, *itching*, urticaria (hives), dyspnea, hemoglobinuria (hemoglobin in the urine) and low blood pressure (hypotension). In most serious reactions, it can lead to shock, multi-organ failure and death of the patient.

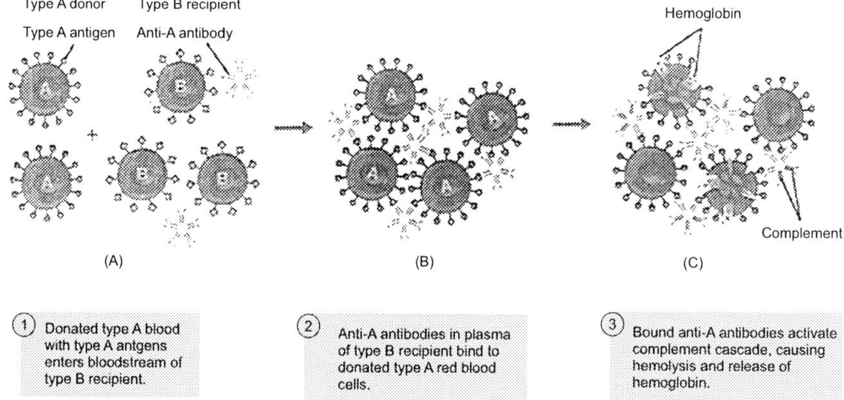

Fig. 77.2 A type II hypersensitivity hemolytic transfusion reaction (HTR) leading to hemolytic anemia. (1) Blood from a type A donor is adminstered to a patient with type B blood. (2) The anti-A isohemagglutinin IgM antibodies in the recipient bind to and agglutinate the incoming donor type A red blood cells. (3) The bound anti-A antibodies activate the classical complement cascade, resulting in the destruction of the donor red blood cells.

Hemolytic Disease of the Newborn (HDN)

Rh factor in compatibility between the mother and fetus can cause HDN due to type 11 hypersensitivity reaction when an Rh^- mother has an Rh^+ fetus, fetal RBCs are produced into mother's circulatory system before or during birth, leading to production of anti-Rh IgG antibodies. These antibodies remain in the mother, and if she becomes pregnant with a second Rh^+ baby, they can cross the placenta and attach to fetal Rh^+ RBCs.

Complement-mediated hemolysis of fetal RBCs results in a lack of sufficient cells for proper oxygenation of the fetus and cause HDN, a potentially lethal condition of the baby (Fig. 77.3). Thousands of deaths occur every year worldwide due to HDN.

HDN can be prevented by administering **human Rho (D) immune globulin** (e.g., RhoGAM) intravenously or intramuscularly onto the mother during the 28th week of pregnancy or within 72 hours of delivery with an Rh^+ fetus (i.e., passive immunization). The RhoGAM binds fetal Rh^+ RBCs that gain access to the mother's bloodstream, preventing activation of her primary immune response.

Drug-induced Throbocytopenia (DITP)

DITP is a skin condition resulting from a low platelet (thrombocytes) count due to drug-induced anti-platelet antibodies caused by drug. Heparin, quinine, sulfonamines, quinidine, diqoxin, penicillin can cause DITP.

TYPE III HYPERSENSITIVITY

Type III hypersensitivity is mediated by the formation of antigen-antibody aggregates, called **immune complexes**, hence also called **immune complex hypersensitivity**. These complexes precipitate and may accumulate in various tissues in the body such as kidneys, joints, vessel, skin and glomeruli. Clinical signs appear within 3 to 8 hours.

Mechanism: Ag-Ab immune complex is formed in the blood when antigen is introduced into a previously sensitized individual. Upon deposition in the tissue, the immune complex activates complement producing allergic reactions, such as fever, itching, rash or hemorrhagic areas, joint pain and acute inflammation.

Two notable examples of type III hypersensitivity reactions:

- **Serum sickness:** It occurs when foreign antigens in sera (e.g. horse serum in vaccine) combine with antibody to form immune complexes which are deposited in various tissues.
- **Arthus reaction:** It is a local immune response seen in the skin to an antigenic substance (usually an injected substance) that causes edema and hemorrhage around the injection site in 4 to 10 hours.

TYPE IV (DELAYED CELL-MEDIATED) HYPERSENSITIVITY

Type IV HS or delayed cell-mediated HS. It is a T-cell mediated reaction that develops 48–72 hours or longer, after exposure to the allergen, hence it is often called **delayed type hypersensitivity**.

Mechanism: T-cells that have become sensitized to a particular antigen secrete cytokines on subsequent contact with the same antigen fragment. Macrophages are attracted and activated by overly produced cytokines and initiate tissue damage, causing inflammation and cell death.

Examples of DHS: Allergic contact dermatitis, tuberculin skin test and granulomatus hypersensitivity) are the common examples of type IV hypersensitivity.

Allergic contact dermatitis (ACD), a common manifestation of the DHS, an inflammatory disease of the skin, is usually caused by haptens that combine with proteins (particularly lysine, an amino acid) in the skin to produce an immune response in some persons. It results from the contact of an offending chemical or antigen with the skin and subsequent T-cell mediated response within 48 hours. Reactions to poison ivy plant, metals (nickel, chromium), cosmetics, textile chemicals, preservatives, drugs (e.g., penicillin) latex in condoms and handgloves used by healthcare workers, are familiar examples of allergies, which usually appear as eczema.

Poison ivy (*Toxicodendron radicans*) plant is the most common cause of ACD and presents as fluid-filled vesicles are caused when the plant comes into contact with the skin. The leaves of ivy contains pentadeca-catechol, a mixture of catechols, which are oils secreted by the plant that dissolve easily in skin oils and penetrate the skin. In the skin, the catechols function as **haptens,** that is, they combine with the skin proteins to become antigenic and provoke an immune response. The first contact with poison ivy sensitizes the susceptible person (the sensitization step which takes 7–10 days by T-cells), and subsequent exposure results in contact dermatitis by his T memory cells (immune response in 1–2 days) (Fig. 77.3).

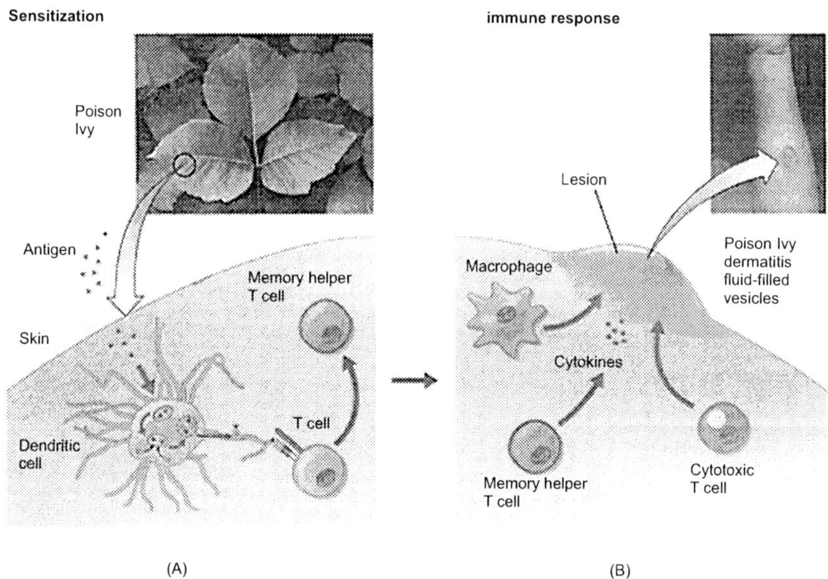

Fig. 77.3 Allergic contact dermatitis, a Type IV hypersensitivity, due to exposure of catechols present in the leaves of poison ivy (***Toxicodendron radicans***), **catechols functioning as hapten antigens**).

TUBERCULIN HYPERSENSITIVITY AND POSITIVE TUBERCULIN SKIN TEST

Tuberculin sensitivity occurs in sensitized individuals (e.g. TB patients or those vaccinated against TB) when they are exposed/injected subcutaneously with **tuberculin** (an antigen lipoprotein derived from the tubercule bacillus *Mycobacterium tuberculosis*, the causative agent of

TB). They cause **skin induration**, a raised, hard, red region of the skin. Similar antigens from several pathogens (e.g., *Mycobacterium leprae*, the cause of leprosy; *Leishmania tropica*, the cause of leishmaniasis) can cause a similar reaction in sensitized individuals. **Tuberculin** in skin test (i.e. the Mantoux reaction) is a familiar example of the classic DTH.

Tuberculin skin test: It is also called **TB skin test** and **Mantoux tuberculin skin test (TST)**. In this test, PPD (a purified protein derivative) from *M. tuberculosis* in injected subcutaneously and observed for the raised area of induration of diameter measurable after 48 to 72 hours of inoculation. An induration of 5 mm or more within 48 hours indicates a positive tubereculin skin reaction, that is, the person had been exposed to the bacterium or had received the BCG vaccine. 2 mm or smaller diameters is a negative test, and 3 to 4 mm are considered doubtful.

GRANULOMATOUS INFLAMMATION/HYPERSENSITIVITY

Granulomatous inflammation is a specific type of chronic inflammatory response that develops due to chronic infections with persistent intracellular organisms or poorly degradable intracellular antigens. It usually occurs when macrophages have engulfed pathogens but have failed to kill or eliminate them, resulting in antigen persistence. Inside the macrophages, the protected pathogens survive and sometimes continue to divide T_H1 cells sensitized to an antigen of the pathogen elicit the hypersensitivity reaction, attracting several cell types to the skin or lung. The result is the development of the **granuloma** (lesions organized into nodules are commonly called granulomas) in the skin (**leproma**) or lung (**tubercle**) 4 weeks or more after exposure to the antigen, an example of most delayed of all kinds of hypersensitivities. Several bacterial (e.g. listeriosis), fungal (*Histoplasma capsulatum*), and helminthic infections show this type of hypersensitivity.

KEY POINTS

- **Hypersensitivity** or **allergy** is an exaggerated antigenic response which occurs only if the person has had on earlier contact with the antigen (allergen).
- **Anaphylaxis** is a life-threatening condition caused when certain antigens combine with IgE antibodies.
- **Atopy** is a localized immediate reaction to an allergen.
- Hypersensitivity types I, II and III are immediate reactions based on **humoral immunity**, and type IV is a delayed reaction based on **cell-mediated immunity**.

- **Hypersensitivity type I reactions** involve the production of IgE antibodies, clinical signs appearing within 30 minutes.
- **Hypersensitivity type II reactions** are mediated by IgG or IgM antibodies and complement, appearance of clinical signs taking 5-12 hours.
- **Hypersensitivity type III reactions** involve IgG antibodies or soluble antigen complexes that cause damaging inflammation in 3 to 8 hours.
- **Hypersensitivity type IV reactions** are due to the proliferation of T-cell and secretion of cytokines in response to antigens.
- A positive tuberculin skin test (Montaux test) or allergic contact dermatitis are examples of type IV hypersensitivities.
- Poison ivy allergic contact dermatitis, an example of Type IV hypersensitivity, develops due to *catechols* or *urushiol*, oil from the plant, which functions as hapten.

IMPORTANT QUESTIONS

1. Define hypersensitivity and its types. What are the main mediators and reaction time for each?
2. Write short notes on:
   (a) Signs and symptoms of localized and systemic anaphylaxis.
   (b) Hemolytic disease of the newborn.
   (c) Tuberculin hypersensitivity and tuberculin skin test.
   (d) Allergic contact dermatitis from poison ivy plant.

MULTIPLE-CHOICE QUESTIONS

1. Which type of hypersensitivity response is evoked by plant pollens?
   (a) Type I (b) Type II
   (c) Type III (d) Type IV.
2. Contact with poison ivy would evoke which type of hypersensitivity response in humans?
   (a) Type I (b) Type II
   (c) Type III (d) Type IV.
3. Which of the following hypersensitivity reactions are T cell-mediated?
   (a) Type I (b) Type II
   (c) Type III (d) Type IV.
4. Hemolytic disease of the newborn belong to which type of hypersensitivity?
   (a) Type I (b) Type II
   (c) Type III (d) Type IV.

5. Which immunoglobulin is responsible for type I hypersensitivity?
   (a) IgG (b) IgA
   (c) IgM (d) IgE.
6. Asthma and hay fever are examples of:
   (a) Atopy (localized anaphylaxis)
   (b) Cytotoxicity
   (c) Delayed hypersensitivity
   (d) All of these.
7. Serum sickness is an example of:
   (a) Type I hypersensitivity
   (b) Type II hypersensitivity
   (c) Type III hypersensitivity
   (d) Type IV hypersensitivity.
8. A positive tuberculin skin test is an example of:
   (a) Type I hypersensitivity
   (b) Type II hypersensitivity
   (c) Type III hypersensitivity
   (d) Type IV hypersensitivity.
9. Allergic contact dermatitis from wearing latex surgical gloves by doctors or nurses is an example of:
   (a) Type I hypersensitivity
   (b) Type II hypersensitivity
   (c) Type III hypersensitivity
   (d) Type IV hypersensitivity.
10. Type III hypersensitivity is also called:
    (a) Cytotoxic hyperactivity
    (b) Immune complex hyperactivity
    (c) Immediate hyperactivity
    (d) Cell-mediated delayed hyperactivity.
11. All of the following hypersensitivity reactions are humoral immunity based immediate reactions EXCEPT:
    (a) Type I hypersensitivity
    (b) Type II hypersensitivity
    (c) Type III hypersensitivity
    (d) Type IV hypersensitivity.

ANSWERS TO MCQs

1. (a)	**2.** (d)	**3.** (d)	**4.** (b)	**5.** (d)
6. (a)	**7.** (c)	**8.** (d)	**9.** (d)	**10.** (b)
11. (d).				

78

Autoimmunity and Autoimmune Diseases

Autoimmunity refers to the state in which the immune system of an organism reacts against the body's own normal components, healthy cells, tissues or organs, producing disease or functional changes. The antibodies and T lymphocytes act against the normal components called **autoantigens** or **self-antigens** of a person. The antibodies and T lymphocytes that recognize the autoantigens are called **autoantibodies** and **autoreactive T cells**, respectively. Autoimmunity is very common but does not necessarily mean autoimmune disease.

Autoimmune disease or **autoimmune disorder** is defined as a pathological and/or functional damage of an organ/tissue/cell due to autoreactive autoantibodies (B lymphocytes) and autoreactive T cells (T lymphocytes) due to the failure of one's own immune system which damages its own tissues. Autoimmune diseases can affect any organ and any one, but women are at greater risk. Fatigue, dizziness, low-grade fever, muscle aches, swelling, and redness are the early symptoms shared by autoimmune diseases. Currently more than 50 different autoimmune diseases/ disorders exist worldwide. They are known to affect 5% of the population in the developed world. Autoimmune diseases are more common in women than men, and they are among the top 10 causes of death in females. These diseases often start during childhood and they often run in families.

HISTORY

Consideration on autoimmunity began, as did immunology itself, around the year 1900, i.e., early 20th century, first with **Paul Ehrlich** doctorine of "*horror autotoxins*" then interpreted as "autoimmunity cannot happen". After a gap of over 35 years, **Erik Waaler**, a Norwegian in 1940 described the first autoantibodies in rheumatoid factor (RF) directed against serum-gamma-globulins, and redescribed by **Herry M Rose** and colleagues in 1948. By the 1950s the modern understanding of autoantibodies and autoimmune diseases started to spread with the work of **Henry G. Kunkel,** an American physician, who made detailed studies on two autoimmune diseases, rheumatoid arthritis and lupus erythematosus, at Rockfeller Hospital. He demonstrated that certain antibodies in the blood of rheumatoid patients reacted with other antibodies, as if they were antigens and were termed the **rheumatoid factor**. The resulting complexes, found in the synovial fluid of joints, causing joint inflammation, the major symptom of rheumatoid arthritis.

MECHANISMS OF AUTOIMMUNITY

The process by which hypersensitivity to self develops is called **autoimmunization**. Exact cause of autoimmunity is unknown. A variety of mechanisms have been proposed for induction of autoimmunity or autoimmune disorders. These include:

1. **Genetic factors:** Certain individuals are genetically suscepitible to developing autoimmune diseases. This susceptibility is associated with multiple genes plus other risk factors. For example PTPN22 has been associated with multiple autoimmune diseases (e.g., Type I diabetes, rheumatoid arthritis, systemic lupus erythematosus, psoriatic arthritis and many more).
2. **Infectious diseases of parasites:** Strong association has been observed with several microbes and autoimmune diseases (e.g. coxsackievirus with. diabetes type I).
3. **Chemical agents and drugs:** Most strinking example is the drug-induced lupus erythematosus.
4. **Cigerette smoking:** Incidence and severity of rheumatoid arthritis is associated with smoking which is related to abnormal citrullination of proteins in the body.
5. **Antigenic or molecular mimicry:** Antigenic memory (the fortuitous similarity between self antigens and foreign antigens of a pathogen is the basis of the **cross reacting antigens** theory of autoimmunity. One such example is Rheumatic fever caused by *Streptococcus pyogenes* that develop rheumatic heart disease later in life. Immune system of such persons have the heart valve tissues as similar to streptococcal antigen that attack the heart valves.
6. **Forbidden clones:** During embryonic life, clones of cells that have immunological reactivity with self-antigens are estimated. Such clones are termed **forbidden clones**. Their persistence or development in later life of an individual by somatic mutation can lead to autoimmunity.

7. **No antigens or attered antigens:** Physical, chemical and biological (i.e., envirornmental) factors can cause antigenic alternation in cells or tissues of an organism. Such altered or neoantigens may elicit an immune response.
8. **Sympathetic nervous system damage:** The number of regulatory T cells decreases in the body while the sympathetic nervous system is damaged and leads to autoimmunity.

MAJOR AUTOIMMUNE DISEASES/DISORDERS

Autoimmune diseases are classified into two classes:

- **Organ-specific autoimmune diseases:** Any disease in which an immune response is directed towards antigens in a single organ. Common examples are: Addison's disease, Gravel's diseases, myasthenia gravis, diabetes type I, Hastimoto's thyroidis, ulcerative colitis, psoriasis.
- **Systemic (disseminated) autoimmune diseases:** Any autoimmune disease in which the immune system attacks self-antigens in several organs. Common examples include: rheumatiod arthritis, systemic lupus erythematosus, Sjögren's syndrome, multiple sclerosis (disseminated sclorisis).

RHEUMATOID ARTHRITIS (RA)

RA is a chronic inflammatory autoimmune disease that affects connective tissues through antibody. It affects mainly joints. It is characterized by inflammation and destruction of cartilage in the joints often causing deformation in the fingers (Fig. 78.1). Redness, warmth, soreness and stiffness are associated with inflammation. In many cases, joint inflammation or destruction are so severe that they result in misshapen digits. RA results when immune complexes of IgM, IgG and complement (autoantibodies, called **rheumatoid factors**) deposited in the joints, causing inflammation or thickening of the synovial membranes (the sacs holding the fluid that lubricates the joints) cause irreversible damage to the joint capsule and the articular (joint) cartilage as these structures are replaced by scan-like extra growth of tissues called **pannus**. It is three times as common in women than men and afflicts 1% of the adult population in the developed nations.

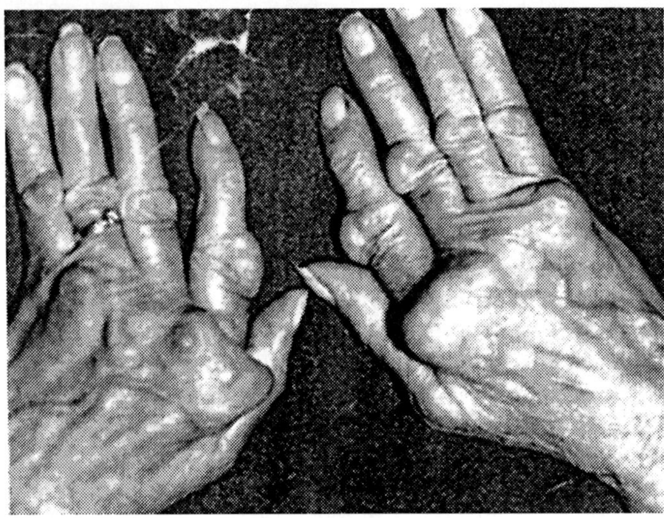

Fig. 78.1 Rheumatoid arthritis. Joint inflammation is typical in people suffering from rheumatoid arthritis. In many cases, joint inflammation and destruction are so severe that they result in misshapen digits.

Diagnosis is made by blood testing to search for IgM and IgG autoantibodies, collectively called rheumatoid factor (RE). Aspirin and ibuprofen are administered (to relieve pain), corticosteroids (e.g., prednisolone) can also be used.

LUPUS OR SYSTEMIC LUPUS ERYTHEMATOUS (SLE)

SLE is an autoimmune chronic inflammatory disease that can last for years or life long. In this disease autoantibodies (IgG, IgM or IgA) complexes are made which are anti-DNA and damages various healthy tissues. These complexes are deposited between the dermis and epidermis and in blood vessels, joints, glomeruli of the kidney and the central nervous system affecting joints, skin, kidneys, brain, heart and lungs. Rate of SLE varies between the countries for 20 to 70 per one lakh, women are affected 9 time more than men. In India, more than 10 lakh cases occur every year. Common symptoms of SLE are painful and swollen joints, feeling tired, fever, chest pain, swollen lymph nodes, mouth ulcers, hair loss and a butterfly-shaped red rash, which is most commonly seen on the face (Fig. 78.2). Often there are periods of illness (called **flares**) and periods of **remission** (when there are few symptoms) in SLB. **Lupus** is Latin for "wolf" the disease was so named in the 13th century as the rash was thought to appear like a wolf's bite. **Erythematisus** is derived from the reddened skin rash (erythematose) (Fig. 78.2).

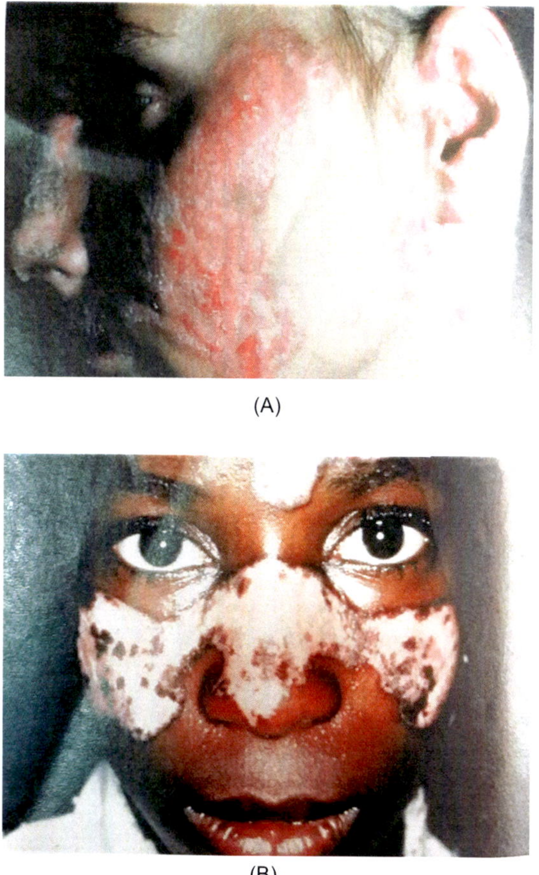

(A)

(B)

Fig. 78.2 Systemic lupus erythematosus. The characterisitic butterfly-shaped rash appears red in fair-skinned people, but white in dark-skined people.

Diagnosis of SLE is based on the clinical symptoms and blood tests.

Treatment: There is no cure for SLE. Treatment includes antipyretics to control fever, corticosteroids to reduce inflammation and immunosuppressant drugs to prevent or decrease future autoimmune reactions.

MYASTHENIA GRAVIS (MG)

Myasthenia gravis (MG) (from the Greek and Latin words meaning "**severe muscular weakness**") is an autoimmune disease which results from antibodies that block or destroy *nicrotinic acetylcholine receptors (AChR)* at the junction between the nerve and muscle and prevents nerve impulses from triggering muscle contraction. The most commonly affected muscles are those of the eye, face and swallowing.

It can result in double vision, drooping eyelids, trouble walking, speech and facial movements. Onset can be sudden. Those affected often have a large thymus or develop a thymoma.

MG is a rare disease that affects 5 to 200 per million people. Every year, it is nearly diagnosed in 3 to 30 per million people. MG most commonly occurs in women under the age of 40 and in men above 60 years of age.

Diagnosis is made by blood tests for specific antibodies, the edrophonium test and nerve conduction studies.

Treatment: Treated with drugs that include *acetylcholine sterase inhibitors* (e.g., neostigmine, pyridestigmine). The surgical removal of the thymus is used to treat a patient.

PSORIASIS/PSORIASIS ARTHRITIS

Psoriasis is a long-lasting, noncontagious, autoimmune, skin disease characterized by red (purple on dark skin), itchy, scaly patches of skin. These vary in severity from small localized patches to complete body coverage. Injury to the skin can trigger psoriatic skin changes at that spot, which is termed the **Koebner phenomenon**. Up to 30% patients develop **psoriasis arthritis**, characterized by swelling, stiffness and pain in the joints.

The word **psoriasis** comes from Greek meaning "itching candition" or 'being itchy' from *psora* 'itch' and *lasis*, 'action', condition.

The disease affects 2–4% of the population, equally affecting men and women. The disease may begin at any age, but typically starts in adulthood.

Psoriasis results when immune system reacts to skin cells. It is generally considered to be a genetic disease that is triggered by environmental factors.

Psoriasis is diagnosed based on the typical itchy-red patches of the thickened skin. It is a lifelong noncurable disease. Treatment consists of topical steroid creams, vitamin D cream, UV light or use of immunosuppersive drugs (e.g. methotrexate).

MULTIPLE SCLEROSIS

Multiple sclerosis (**MS**, also called **encephalomyelitis disseminata and dissesminated sclerosis**) a long-lasting (choronic), and one of the most common autoimmune diseases, affecting the brain and spinal cord (CNS). The immune system attacks the **myelin sheaths**, the protective covering of neurons, disrupting the communication between the brain and body. Major MS symptoms include double vision, blindness in one eye, muscle weakness and trouble with sensation or coordination. Genetic and environmental factors being triggered by the Epstein-Bars virus infection are the proposed causes.

The name MS is derived from numerous ***glial scars*** (or sclerae–essential plaques or lesions) that develop on the white matter of the brain and spinal cord. It was first described in 1868 by **Jean-Martin Charcot,** a French neurologist. Every year more than 2 million people are affected globally, the number of women affected is twice to men.

Diagnosis: Clinical symptoms, MRI of the brain and spines and testing of CSF for oligoclonal bands 5 of IgG on electrophoresis.

Treatment: There is no known case for MS. Physiotherapy and administration of anti-inflammatory, immunosuppressive drugs, steroids and herbal medicines are used to treat the patients.

Ocrelizumab is the latest medication to treat the RRMS (relaping remitting multiple sclerosis).

DIABETES

Diabetes mellitus (or **diabetes**) refers to disorder of carbohydrate metabolism characterized by impaired ability of the body to produce or respond to insulin and thereby maintain proper levels of sugar (glucose) in the blood. The name is derived from symptoms: **diabetes**, from the Greek *diabainein,* meaning to pass through, describes the copious urination and *mellitus* for the Latin meaning "sweetened with honey" refers to sugar in the urine. Other symptoms of diabetes include itching, hunger, weight loss and weakness.

There are three major forms of the disease.

Type 1 diabetes (earlier referred to as **insulin-dependent diabetes mellitus, IDMM** and **juvenile diabetes**) results from failure of the pancreas to produce enough insulin due to loss of beta cells which is caused by an autoimmune response. This disease usually arises in childhood, accounting for 5 to 10% of cases of diabetes. The hormone insulin is responsible for regulating blood sugar levels in the body. The high blood sugar levels called **hyperglycemia** can lead to damage of blood vessels as well as organs like the heart, kidneys, eyes, nerves. Polyuria and polydipsia (excessive thirst), weakness, fatigue, weight loss and increased appetite (polyphagia) are the common symptoms observed in the patients. Diabetics are more prone to infections (e.g. vaginal and urinary tract infections), and an infection may be presenting manifestation of diabetes. In general 2–5% of children whose mother or father has type 1 diabetes also develop type 1 diabetes (i.e., a genetic disorder).

- **Type 2 diabetes** is strongly associated with **obesity** and is a result of **insulin resistance,** a condition in which cells fail to respond to insulin properly.
- **Gestational diabetes:** It occurs when pregnant women without a history of diabetes develop high blood sugar levels.

Diagnosis: The diagnosis of diabetes is based on the presence of blood glucose concentrations equal to or (greater than 126 mg per dL (7.0 mmol per litre) after an overnight fast (i.e., fasting) or the presence of blood glucose concentration greater that 200 mg/ dL (11.1 mmol/litre). 2 hours after eating, during the day, sugar levels tend to be at their lowest just before meals.

Increased thirst, and urination and elevated blood sugar level are physical symptoms of diabetes.

People with fasting glucose values between 100 and 125 mg per dL (6.1 to 6.9 mmol per litre) are diagnosed as **prediabetes**, as normal fasting blood glucose levels are less than 100 mg per dL (6.1 mmol per litre)

A glycosylated hemoglobin called **hemoglobin subtype A1C (HbA 1c)** is particularly useful in monitoring hyperglycemia and the **efficiency** of diabetes treatments.

Management of diabetes

Type 1 diabetes must be managed with insulin injection.

Type 2 diabetes can be prevented by managing a healthy diet, regular physical excercise, a normal body weight, avoiding use of tobacco. It may be treated with oral medications, with or without insulin. Metformin, glyipizide or glimepiride are used to treat type 2 diabetes.

GRAVES' DISEASE

Graves' disease (also known as **toxic diffuse goiter**) is an autoimmune disease that causes hyper-thyrodism, or overactive thyroid, characterized by butterfly-shaped gland in the lower neck. It results from an antibody, called **thyroid-stimulating immunoglobulin (TSI)** (that has a similar effect to thyroid stimulating hormone, TSH), that causes the thyroid gland to produce excess thyroid hormone. The disease is named after **Robert Graves**, an Irish surgeon, who in 1835 described a case of goiter with exophthalmos Greaves' disease occurred in about 0.5% of people, women are affected 7.5 times more than men. The disease often starts between the ages of 40 and 60. More than 10 million cases are recorded every year in our country.

Symptoms of hyperthyroidism are anxiety, a fast heartbeat, and tremor, weight loss, heat sensitivity, puffy eyes and enlarged thyroid.

Complications result to **Graves' ophthalmopathy**, characterized by eye bulging and staring eyes (**exophthalmos**) or lid retraction in 25% to 80% of the patients.

Diagnosis: Clinical symptoms, especially exophthalmos and nonpitting edema, goiter and hyperthyroidism–overproduction of thyroid hormone T3 and T4.

Treatment: It includes **antithyroid drugs** (carbimazole, methimazole and propylthiouracil), radioiodine (radioactive iodine-131) or **thyroidectomy** (surgical removal of the gland): mild eye cases are treated with lubricant eye drops or nonsteroidal anti-inflammatory drops, and severe cases those threatening vision (corneal exposure or optic nerve compression) are treated with steroids and orbital decompression.

SJÖGREN'S SYNDROME

Sjögren's syndrome (Sjs SS) is an autoimmune disease that affects the body's moisture-producing (lacrimal and salvary) glands. Dry mouth, dry eyes, dry skin, vaginal dryness are the major symptoms. Among 15% of the patients, it may lead to lymphoma. It is one of the most common autoimmune diseases affecting 0.2 to 1.2% of the population globally. Females are affected 10 times more frequently than the males. It is named after **Henrik Sjögren** who described it in 1933.

Diagnosis: By biopsy of moisture producing glands for lymphocytes with them; blood tests for specific antibodies.

Treatment: Artificial tears medications for dry eyes and for dry mouth-chewing gum, sipping water or a saliva substitute are used for SS treatment.

INFLAMMATORY BOWEL DISEASE

Inflammatory bowel disease (**IBD**), the chronic inflammation in the lining of the intestinal wall, results when the immune system responds incorrectly to environmental triggers and causes inflammations of the gastrointestinal tract. Prolonged inflammation results in damage of the GI tract. It is of two types:

- **Crohn's disease:** Inflammation can occur at any part of the GI tract, i.e., from the mouth to anus.
- **Ulcerative colitis:** It occurs in the innermost lining of the large intestine (colon) and the rectum.

Persistent diarrhea, blood stools/rectal bleeding, abdominal pain, fatigue and weight loss are the common symptoms.

Diagnosis: IBD is diagnosed using a combination of endoscopy (for Crohn's disease) or **colonoscopy** (for ulcerative colitis) or MRI (magnetic resonance imaging) or CT (compound tomography), and stool samples test (to make sure that it is not due to infection) or blood tests.

Treatment: Aminosalicyclates, corticosteroids (e.g., prednisolone) and immune modulators are used to treat IBD. Severe IBD may require surgery to remove the damaged portions of the intestine.

CELIAC DISEASE

Celiac disease is also characterized by inflammation of the intestine with similar symptoms to IBD. It is an inflammatory response to **gluten** (a protein found in wheat, rye and other cereals) which is acted upon by this immune system when it is in the GI tract. It is common in the USA where 1% of the people suffer from this disease.

Treatment: Gluten-free diet is recommended for the patients although it usually will be months before the full effects of the new diet will appear.

AUTOIMMUNE VASCULITIS

Vasculitis refers to the inflammation of blood vessels, causing thickening of their walls resulting to reduced blood flow through them, which can result in organ and tissue damage. The condition can be short tremor long-lasting. Fever, headache, fatigue, weight loss, general aches and pains are the common symptoms. Complications include blood clots and blood aneurysms (bulging of blood vessels), vision loss or organ damage and prone to more infections.

Diagnosis: Blood, urine and stool tests to find the cause.

Treatment: Combinations of steroids and immune suppressive agents are used.

KEY POINTS

- **Autoimmunity** refers to an abnormal immune response of an organism against its own healthy cells, tissues, organs due to loss of self-tolerance.
- Reaction of one's own antibodies (i.e. auto-antibodies) or T cells with self-antigens (self-proteins) cause autoimmunity.

- Damage to one's own organs due to the action of the immune system (autoimmunity) is called an **autoimmune disease**.
- **Autoimmunization** refers to the process by which hypersensitivity to 'self' develops.
- Tissue damage from autoimmune disorders can be caused by cytotoxic, immune-complex of cell-mediated hypersensitivity reactions.
- Examples of common organ specific autoimmune diseases include: Graves' disease (blood gland), diabetes type 1 (pancreas), myasthenia gran's (skeletal muscles), ulcerative colitis (colon), Addison's disease (adrenal glands), and soriasis (skin).
- **Example of systemic autoimmune diseases** are rheumatoid arthritis (joints), systemic lupus erythematous (many tissues), Sjögren's syndrome (lacrimal and salivary glands).
- Women are more prone to autoimmune diseases.

IMPORTANT QUESTIONS

1. Write short notes on:
   (a) Define autoimmunity, autoimmune disease and rheumatoid factor.
   (b) Rheumatoid arthritis.
   (c) Myasthenia gravis.
   d) Systemic lupus erythematous.
   (e) Diabetes type 1.
   (f) Graves' disease.
   (g) Organ-specific autoimmune diseases.

MULTIPLE-CHOICE QUESTIONS

1. All are autoimmune diseases EXCEPT:
   (a) Rheumatoid arthritis (b) AIDS
   (c) Type 1 diabetes (d) Psoriasis.
2. Autoimmune diseases strike which group more often?
   (a) Children (b) Women
   (c) Men (d) All of the above.
3. Which tissues, organs or body systems can be affected by autoimmune diseases?
   (a) Joints (b) Skin
   (c) Thyroid (d) All of the above.

4. If you have an autoimmune disease, what happens with the immune system.
   (a) Your immune system makes too many immune cells
   (b) Your immune cells die
   (c) Antibodies from your immune system mistakenly attack tissues in the body
   (d) None of the above.
5. Why are some autoimmune diseases difficult to diagnose?
   (a) Symptoms may be vague
   (b) Symptoms may come and go, making it hard to pin-point the problem
   (c) No specific lab tests exist to confirm a diagnosis
   (d) All of the above.
6. Which of these autoimmune diseases can be cured?
   (a) Lupus
   (b) Multiple sclerosis
   (c) Rheumatoid arthritis
   (d) All of the above.
7. All are organ-specific autoimmune diseases EXCEPT:
   (a) Rheumatoid anthritis
   (b) Myasthenia gravis
   (c) Type 1 diabetes (Juvenile diabetes)
   (d) Hashimoto's thyroditis.
8. Which of the following scientist who made notable contribution in rheumatoid arthritis and lupus, two autoimmune diseases in the 1950s, is called the pioneer in clinical immunology?
   (a) Paul Ehrlich
   (b) Elie Metchnikolf
   (c) Henry G Kunkel
   (d) van Behring and Kitasato.

ANSWERS TO MCQs

1. (b) **2.** (b) **3.** (d) **4.** (c) **5.** (d)
6. (d) **7.** (a) **8.** (c).

79

Vaccines, Sera-Types and Cold Chain Management

WHAT IS A VACCINE?

Vaccines are the substances made of suspension of organisms or fractions of organisms that stimulate the body's own system to protect the individual against the infection or disease. A vaccine typically contains an agent that resembles a disease causing microbe. Vaccines are often made from living but **attenuated** (i.e., weakened) microorganisms, dead organisms, microbe's toxins or one of its surface proteins. Vaccines stimulate the body's immune system to provide specific protection against a disease by inducing the production of specific antibody and other immune mechanisms. The administration of vaccines is called **vaccination**, the most effective and method of preventing, controlling infectious diseases. Vaccines can be **prophylactic** (to prevent or ameliorate the effects of a future infection by a natural or wild pathogen), or **therapeutic** (to fight a disease that has already occurred). The word vaccine is derived from the Latin *vacca*, meaning cow, because of the early use of the live cowpox virus against smallpox by **Edward Jenner**, a British physician in 1798.

TYPES OF VACCINES

There are several approaches for designing/developing a vaccine such as

- Use of a whole microbe (virus or bacterium) approach.
- Use of just the parts of the causative agent that trigger the immune response.
- Use of just the genetic material that provides the instructions for making specific proteins and not the whole virus.

Based on the mode of development of an antigen, the vaccines are broadly classified into 6 types:

1. Live-attenuated vaccines
2. Inactivated vaccines
3. Subunit vaccines
4. Toxoid vaccines
5. Nucleic acid (mRNA) vaccines
6. Viral vector vaccines
7. Conjugant vaccines
8. Plant-derived vaccines

1. Live-Attenuated Vaccines

A live-attenuated vaccine uses a living but weakened version of the microbe (i.e., attenuated microbe), that does not cause any symptoms of infections. These vaccines, especially in case of viruses, provide **life-long immunity**, probably due to replications of viruses in the body therby increasing the original dose and acting as a series of secondary (booster) immunization. Hence, these vaccines do not require booster doses. However, these type of vaccines may not be suitable for people with compromised immune systems.

Examples include:

- MMR (measles, mumps and rubella)
- BCG (tuberculosis)
- Chickenpox
- Smallpox
- Rotavirus
- Yellow fever
- Oral typhoid vaccine (typhoral).

2. Inactivated Vaccines

These vaccines use inactivated or killed microorganism using chemicals (usually formaline or phenol), heat or radiation. These do not offer life-long immunity or do not trigger an immune response that is as strong as that triggered by live-attenuated vaccines, and often require 2-3 repeated doses. However, these are considered safer than live vaccines.

Examples include:

- Inactivated poliovirus (IPV)
- Whole cell pertussis (whooping cough)
- Rabies
- Hepatitis A virus.

3. Subunit Vaccines

These vaccines use only the very specific parts (the subunits) of a virus or bacterium (antigen) that the immune system needs to recognize. The subunits may be proteins or sugars. Vaccines that use sugar molecules, called polysaccharides, from outer layer of a bacterium or virus, are called **polysaccharide vaccines**. Subunit vaccines made using genetic engineering techniques are called **recombinant techniques**. Most of the vaccines on childhood schedule are subunit vaccines.

Examples include:

- Hepatitis B
- Hib (Hemophilus influenza type b)
- Whooping cough (acellular pertussis vaccine)
- Meningococcal
- Pneumococcal
- Shingles.

4. Toxoid Vaccines

These vaccines use **inactivated toxins**, which are directed at the toxins produced by a pathogen which can be considered a subunit of the pathogen, hence also considered under the **subunit vaccines**. They do not offer life-long immunity and need to be topped up over time.

Examples include:

- Diphtheria
- Tetanus
- Botulism.

5. Conjugate Vaccines

These vaccines use the combination of the desired antigen with a protein, a type of subunit protein, that boosts the immune response.

Examples include:

- Hemophilus influenza type b (Hib).

6. Nucleic Acid (mRNA) Vaccines

A nucleic acid or mRNA vaccine just uses a section of the genetic material that codes for a disease-specific antigen (proteins) or not the whole microbe. This type of vaccine delivers a specific set of instructions to our cells, either as DNA or mRNA, for them to make the specific protein that triggers an immune response inside our bodies (for example, **spike protein** which is found on the virus causes COVID-19).

The approach, called the **genetic approach**, is a new way of developing vaccines with several advantages over the others, such as require short manufacturing times and cheep to produce. However, these vaccines require an ultra low temperature for storage due to the fragility of mRNA.

Because of the COVID-19 pandemic, research in this area has progressed very fast and some mRNA vaccines for COVID-19 are getting emergency use authorization (EUA) which means they can now be given to people beyond using them only in clinical trials. COVID-19 vaccines are the first time mRNA vaccines approved for use in humans, end of 2020 (31st Dec 2020) and 2021.

Examples include:

- Pfizer-BioNTech (EUL on 31st Dec. 2020)
- Moderna COVID-19 (mRNA-1273).

7. Viral-Vector Vaccines

These vaccines use the genetic material of the causative virus agent into a different kind of weakened live virus—the **viral vector** that delivers the desired instructions to our cells and provide protection from the intended virus. Examples of the vectors used are adenovirus, influenza virus, measles virus and vesicular stomatitis virus.

Examples include:

- Ebola virus vaccines (RVSV-ZEBOV vaccine and GamEvac – Combi vaccine)
- COVID-19 vaccines
  - J&J Covid-19 vaccine
  - Covishield
  - Sputunik –V

8. Plant-Derived Vaccines

Plant-derived vaccines, also called **plantibodies**, use modified plants (e.g., potato, tobacco, corn, banana) to produce antigenic proteins from pathogenic bacteria or viruses. There could either be used as pills (*edible vaccines*) or applied on mucosal surfaces. These vaccines are considered the 3rd generation technology vaccines.

Medicago, a Canadian company, has taken a lead to produce a vaccine for COVID-19 that uses a virus-like protein (VLP) in tobacco plant and produced COVID-19 vaccine doses in just 19 days. As of 30 November 2020, the vaccine has reached the 2nd phase of clinical trial.

PRINCIPAL VACCINES FOR SPECIFIC DISEASES

The principal vaccines used for individuals at risk of acquiring specific viral and bacterial diseases are described here.

A. Vaccines for Human Bacterial Diseases

- **DPT vaccine** is a combination of three vaccines that develops immunity to three deadly infectious diseases in humans: diphtheria, pertussis (whooping cough) and tetnus. Its components include diphtheria and tetanus toxoids and either killed whole cells of the bacterium that causes pertussis or pertussis antigens. The whole cells or antigens will be depicted as either DTwP or DTaP, where the lower-case *w* indicates whole-cell inactivated pertussis at the lower-case *a* indicates pertussis antigens. In our country, under the Universal Immunization Programme (UIP), DPT is given by intramuscular injection at 16–24 months of age–called DPT first booster and DPT 2nd booster at 5–6 years of age.
- **Meningococcal vaccine:** It is a heat-stable lypholized polysaccharide vaccine prepared from *Neisseria meningitidis*. It provides protection against some or all of the five types of meningococcus: A, B, C, W-135 and Y for two years (85-100% effective). A single dose (subcutaneous) is recommedend for people with substainial risk of infection.
- **Pneumococcal vaccine:** There are two types of pneumococcal vaccines that provide protection against pneumonia, meningitis and sepsis caused by *Streptococcus pneumoniae*.
    - **Polysaccharide pneumococcal vaccine** (PPV-23, pneumovox) is recommended for persons above 65 years of age with specific risk factors.
    - **Conjugate pneumococcal vaccine** (PCV-7, prevnar): The WHO recommends as routine immunization for children, especially those with HIV/AIDS in 3 to 4 doses given by injection either into a muscle or just under the skin.
- **Hemophilus influenza type of vaccine (Hib conjugate):** It is a conjugate vaccine, polysaccharide from ***Hemophilus influenzae*** type b (Hib) conjugated with protein, used as a routine vaccine to prevent diseases like meningitis, pneumonia and epiglottis caused by HIB. Vaccination for all children younger than 5 years in four doses of 2 months, 4th month and 6 month and a booster dose at 12-15 month.

- **BCG vaccine:** The **Bacillus Calmette and Guerin** (BCG), named after its inventors: **Albert Calmette** and **Camella Guerin,** made from a weakened strain of *Mycobacterium tuberculosis,* provides protection against TB (disseminated) and meningitis. Intradermal vaccination at birth or as early as possible till 1 year of age (one dose) is administered.
- **Typhoid vaccines: Three vaccines:** Ty21a (a live, weakened virus oral vaccine), Vi capsular polysaccaharide vaccine (ViPS) and typhoid conjugate vaccine (TCV) are available to prevent typhoid. Ty21a vaccine is given as 3 capsules on alternate days. Vi vaccine is given as a single injection. Vaccination is recommended for those only who are travelling to parts of the world where typhoid is occuring.

B. Vaccines for Viral Diseases

- **MMR vaccine:** The vaccine is a mixture of **live weakened (attenuated viruses)** of three diseases, namely, measles, mumps and rubella (German measles). This vaccine was developed by **Maurice Hilleman** and was licensed for use in the United States by Merck in 1971. Two doses are given to children by injection **First dose** between 9 to 15 months of age and second dose at 15 months to 6 years of age (with at least 4-week gap between the two doses).

  An MR vaccine, without coverage for mumps, is also occasionally used in some countries.

  In the developing countries including India only the **measles vaccine** is given at 9 months, the earlier age when it is likely to be immunogenic in the presence of maternal antibody in the baby.
- **MMRV vaccine:** It is a combination of the attenuated virus MMR (measles, mumps and rubella) vaccine into the addition of the chickenpox vaccine or varicella vaccine (V stands for varicella). It is given to children between one and two years of age either subcutaneously or intramuscularly. It was approved for use in 2005 in the USA as *ProQuad* and marketed by March.
- **Varicella vaccine:** Also called **chickenpox vaccine** is a **live attenuated vaccine** based on the Oka strain of the varicella virus, first became commercially available in 1984 that protects against chickenpox. One to two doses are given to children by injection just under the skin. First dose is given when kids are between 12 and 15 months old and a booster shot at 4 to 6 years of age.

- **Hepatitis B vaccine:** This is a recombinant vaccine based on the hepatitis B surface antigen (HBsAg) gene inserted into *Saccharomyces cerevisiae*, a yeast and allowed the yeast to produce only the noninfectious surface protein, without any danger of introducing actual viral DNA into the final product (i.e., vaccine). It prevents hepatitis B, a liver disease including liver cancer and cirrhosis. It is recommended for all infants within 24 hours of birth, children up to age 18 and adult at high risk (e.g., healthcare workers, homosexual men, injecting drug users and household contacts of hepatitis B carriers). Route of administration is intramuscular (IM).
- **Hepatitis A (Hep A) vaccine:** Mostly a formalin-inactivated virus vaccine (somatic attenuated virus) that prevents hepatitis A disease. It is recommended mostly for travellers to endemic areas and protecting contacts during outbreaks. It is given in two shots: First for children 12 months or older, second dose 6 months later and provides protection for 10 years.
- **Rabies vaccine:** It is a dried or fluid preparation of the rabies fixed virus (i.e., killed) grown in several tissues of the rabbits, sheep, mice or rats.

  It is used to prevent (pre-exposure prophylaxis) and for a period of time after exposure to the rabies virus (i.e., post-exposure, prophylaxis), causing rabies disease characterized by inflammation of the brain. It is commonly caused by a dog bite or a bat bite. Two-site intradermal (ID) vaccines administration is recommended on days 0, 3, 7 and 14 and an additional dose (i.e., 5th) for immune compromised persons. It is recommended veterinarians, for field biologists in contact with wildlife endemic areas; and for people exposed to rabies virus by bites.
- **Smallpox vaccine:** This formulation is based on **live vaccina virus** (not the variola virus that causes smallpox), the first vaccine to be developed against a contagious disease in 1796 by Edward Jenner. WHO in 1980 declared the elimination of smallpox around the globe, hence public doesn't need protection from this disease. It is no longer available to the public.
- **Herpes zoster vaccines.** These vaccines are: attenuated (Zostavax) and recombinant protein subunit (Shingrix) vaccines, used to provide protection from herpes zoster (shingles) caused by the varicella zoster virus, which is also responsible for chickenpox. Shingrix, a newlly discovered vaccine, has been used in many countries since 2017.

Both the vaccines are given in two doses, 2 to 6 months apart, by subcutaneous injection (Zostavax) and intramuscular injection (Shingrix) for adults over 50. Of the two, Shingrix is more effective.

- **Human papillomavirus (HPV) vaccines:** Three HPV vaccines: 9-valent HPV (Gardasil 9), quadrivalent HPV (Gardasil 4) and bivalent HPV vaccine (Cervarix), are protein subunit (antigen) based vaccines, are effective against various types of HPV, which cause cervical cancer in females. These are administered in 2-3 doses intramuscularly to girls around the ages of 9-13 (all females under the age of 26).
- **Polio vaccines:** Two polio vaccines based on **inactivated poliovirus** or a **weakened poliovirus** have been used to prevent poliomyelitis (polio) since 1955. These vaccines have eliminated polio from most of world.
    - **Inactivated polio vaccine (IPV)** was developed in 1952 by **Jonas Salk** at the University of Pittsburgh and mass polio vaccination began in the US. It is given as an intramuscular injection in 4 doses – first 3 doses at an interval of 1-2 months and 4th dose at an interval of 6-12 months after 3rd dose in the leg or arm. It is commonly called **Salk's vaccine**.
    - **Oral poliovirus vaccine (OPV)** was developed by **Albert Sabin** in 1957 that came into commercial use in 1961 (hence called **Sabin's vaccine**). It is administered by mouth (orally). There is mass administration of OPV on a single day to all children, 0-5 years of age, regardless of previous immunization, under the **pulse polio immunization (PPI)**. PPI occurs as two rounds, 4-6 weeks apart during the transmission season of polio between November and February.
- **Influenza vaccines:** Also known as **flu shots** and **flue jabs** are injected vaccines (a trivalent or quadrivalent intramuscular injection) which contain the inactivated form of the influenza virus and **nasally administered vaccine** with attenuated or weakened virus. These vaccines protect against upper/and/or lower respiratory tract infections caused by influenza viruses (A and B). Recommended for chronically ill including children 6 months to 9 years of age need two doses of the injected vaccine, given at least 4 weeks apart, for healthcare workers and others in contact with risk groups (yearly). Healthy persons aged 5–49 years can receive intranasal spray.
- **Caronavirus Disease (COVID-19) vaccines**–Four types of vaccines currently approved to protect against COVID-19

caused by severe acute respiratory syndrome **coronavirus** (SARS-CoV-2) include:

- **Whole virion vaccine: Covaxin** (manufacted by Bharat Biotech). It is based on the weakened or inactivated form of the coronavirus. Two intramuscular doses, at an interval of 28 to 42 days are needed.
- **RNA or mRNA vaccines:** Pfizer–BioNTech and **Moderna** consist of mRNA molecules made in a lab that code specifically for the coronavirus spike protein. Two doses (intramuscular) at an interval of 28 days are needed.
- **Non-replicating viral vector vaccines:** Oxford-AstraZeneca and Serum Institute of India **Covishield** and **Sputink V** (Gamaleya Research Institutes, Russia) based on the introduction of a safe, modified version of the virus, called the **vector**, to deliver genetic code for the antigen (i.e., spike proteins) of the coronavirus. Two intramuscular doses at an interval of 12–16 weeks Covishield and 21 days to 3 months (Sputink V)
- **Protein Subunit vaccines: Novavax (Covavax)** that contains protein nanoparticles with matrix MI adjuvant (i.e., recombinant spike). Two intramuscular doses are given.

COLD-CHAIN MANAGEMENT: STORAGE AND HANDLING OF VACCINES

Vaccines are damaged by exposure to excessive cold, heat and/or light. Their proper storage and handling practices through cold-chain management play an important role in protecting individuals and communities from vaccine-preventable diseases.

Cold chain: A **cold chain** refers to a temperature-controlled supply chain that includes all vaccine related equipment and procedures. The cold chain begins with the cold storage unit at the manufacturing plant, extends to the transport and delivery of vaccine and proper storage at the provider facility, and ends with administration of the vaccine to the patient.

The cold-chain system is necessary because vaccine failure may occur due to failure to store or transport vaccines under strict temperature control and storing of vaccines in their original packing, with lids closed in separate containers to protect them from light.

One common temperature range for a cold chain in pharmaceutical industries is between 2°C to 8°C (36°F and 46°F) which is maintained by a simple refrigerator. Most flu vaccines are stored at this temperature.

Frozen temperature chain, requiring a temperature of–20°C, is required for some vaccines, such as varicella and zoster vaccines.

Deep-freeze cold chain, i.e., ultracold storage, requiring a temperature of –90°C for Ebola vaccine and most of the COVID-19 vaccines (such as Pfizer-BioNTech) produced on mRNA technology need a temperature of –70°C for storage and transportation, i.e., a **colder chain** infrastructure.

Manufacturers, distributors, public health staff, and healthcare providers share responsibility to ensure the vaccine cold chain is maintained from the time vaccines are manufactured until they are delivered.

SERUM, ANTISERUM AND PLASMA

SERUM

Serum and plasma are both liquid components of blood, mainly make up of water. **Serum** (pl. **sera**) is the clear, straw-coloured (or pale-yellow) fluid that is devoid of blood clotting factor and cells. It can also be defined as blood plasma with fibrinogens (or clotting factors), i.e., **plasma-clotting factor**. Besides water, plasma contains electrolytes, hormones, antibodies and proteins, like globulin and albumin and the exogeneous substances (such as drugs or microorganisms). It does not contain leukocytes (WBCs), erythrocytes (RBCs), platelets, and clotting factors. The word is derived from Latin ***serum*** = whey. The study of serum is called **serology**.

Isolation of Serum from Blood

To obtain serum from blood, the blood sample immediately after collection from a person, is allowed to clot (coagulation) in a test tube at room temperature for 15 to 30 minutes. It is then centrifuged to remove the clot and blood cells, and the resulting liquid supernatant is serum (Fig. 79.1).

Major uses of Sera

It is used in numerous diagnostic tests, to test enzymes and other chemicals in blood. DNA testing, Added to cell culture i.e., media to support the growth of white blood cells, patients serum is used to test certain diseases. It is also used in protein electrophoresis.

ANTISERUM

Antiserum (pl. **antisera, antiserums**) refers to blood serum that contains specific antibodies against an infective organism (e.g., becteria

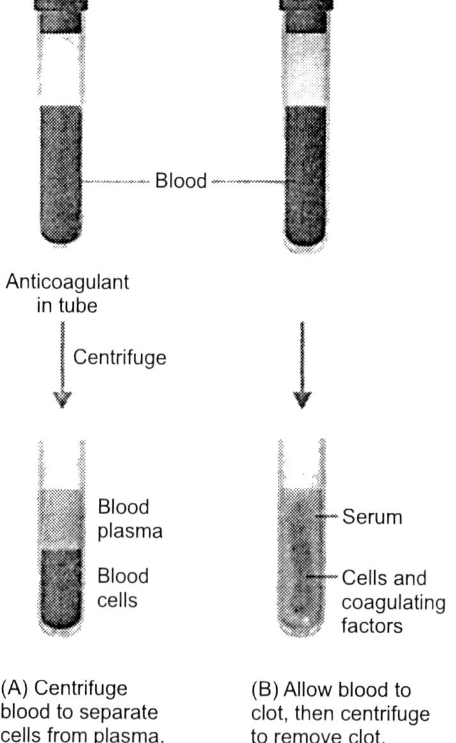

Fig. 79.1 Separation of serum and plasma from a blood sample.

or virus) or poisonous substance (e.g., snake venom) and is used to prevent and treat diseases via blood donation (**plasmaphoresis**). It is produced from blood of humans or animals inoculated with an antigenic material or from those that recovered from a disease when they naturally developed certain antibodies against particular antigens. It may be a **monovalent** (or **specific**) **antiserum** or **polyvalent antiserum**. For example, convalescent serum, passive antibody transfusion from a previous human survivor, used to be the only known effective treatment for **ebola** infection with a high success rate of 7 out of 8 patients surviving.

The treatment of an infectious disease using the serum of animals that have been immunized against the specific organisms and their product is called **serum therapy** or **serotherapy**. This technique was invented in 1891 by **Emil Behrias**, the first Nobel prize winner in medicine, to treat diphtheria by using guinea pigs to produce serum.

Major Uses of Antisera

- Antisera are widely used in diagnostic virology laboratories.

- It is commonly used as antitoxin or antivenous to treat envenomation in humans.
- Modern use of convalescent blood plasma includes the treatment of severe cases of COVID-19 patients, during the early stages of the coronavirus diseases 2019 pandamic, reliable treatment options has not been found.

PLASMA

Plasma or **blood plasma** (referred to as the liquid gold running through our veins) is a transparent and straw-coloured liquid part of the blood before coagulation and free from RBCs, WBCs, platelets and other cellular components. In other words, plasma comprises clotting factor and serum. It is up to 95%, water and makes up around 55% of total human's body blood volume. It contains mostly dissolved proteins (serum albumins, globulins and flurinogen), glucose, salt, lipids, electrolytes, and hormones, CO_2 or O_2 with the density of 1.025 g/ml (1025 kg/m^3). The main functions of plasma in our body are: to deliver oxygen and nutrients to cells and removal of wastes from cellular function, to regulate blood pressure and maintain homeostatis (i.e., temperature) of the body, and in preventing excessive bleeding a the time of injury.

Separation of Plasma from Blood

Plasma is separated from the blood through centrifugation before clotting. In this process, the blood collected from a person is added with an anticoagulant (e.g., EDTA, sodium citrate, heparin) (to prevent the blood from clotting and separate blood components–WBCs or RBCs) in a test tube followed by centrifugation until the blood cells fall to the bottom of the tube (Fig. 79.1). The liquid plasma is then poured or drawn off into another tubes.

Clinical Applications

Albumin has been used since the 1940's as a volume replacement therapy **(blood plasma transfusions)** for blood or fluid loss and for the liver diseases, sepsis, septic shock, therapeutic plasma exchange, burn therapy and renal dialysis. Plasma replacement therapy is mostly used to treat patients missing clotting protein (or coagulation factor, clotting factors), those suffering from Hemophilia A, Hemophilia B, von Willebrand diseae (VWD).

KEY POINTS

- A **vaccine** is a suspension of organisms or fractions of organisms that induces immunity against a specific infectious disease and protects the individual against subsequent infection or disease.
- The **name vaccine** is derived from Latin *vacca*, meaning cow due to the first use of cowpox virus against smallpox.
- **Major types of vaccines** include: inactivated, live attenuated. mRNA, subunit, recombinant, polysaccharide and conjugate; viral vector, toxoid and plant-derived vaccine.
- The vaccines currently in use against COVID-19 belong to **inactivated** (Covaxin), **mRNA** (Pfizer BionTech, Moderna COVID-19), **vactor-based** (Covishield, J&J, COVID-19, Sputunik V) vaccines.
- **Blood serum** is the straw coloured fluid isolated from blood, lacking fibrinogen, and is mostly used for blood typing and diagnostic testing.
- **Plasma** is the transparent, straw coloured liquid part of the blood containing fibrinogen (clotting factor) and mostly used for blood clotting related problems.
- **Antiserum** refers to the blood serum that contains specific antibodies (as antitoxins or aggglutinins) and is used to provide passive immunity to many diseases.
- **Cold chain** is a temperature controlled supply chain from the place of its manufacturing to the place of vaccination.

IMPORTANT QUESTIONS

1. What is a vaccine? Name various types of vaccines. Describe the three vaccines for COVID-19 being used in India.
2. Write notes on:
   (a) Differentiation between the attenuated and inactivated vaccines. Give two examples of each type.
   (b) mRNA vaccines for COVID-19.
   (c) Differentiation between serum, antiserum and plasma.
   (d) Vaccine cold chain.

MULTIPLE-CHOICE QUESTIONS

1. Which of the following statement is *not* true about the live attenuated vaccine?
   (a) Prepared using whole-weakened living virus or bacteria
   (b) It can generate long-term immune response in an individual with a single dose of vaccine

(c) It is stable at normal room temperature
(d) Measles, MMR and oral polio vaccine.

2. Which of the following is NOT the example of a live attenuated vaccine?
   (a) Dipetheria vaccine (b) Measles vaccine
   (c) BCG vaccine (d) Oral polio vaccine.
3. Subunit vaccine is all, EXCEPT:
   (a) A whole purified virus
   (b) A purified part or pieces of the antigen
   (c) An expensive type of vaccine
   (d) A Hepatitis B vaccine.
4. Which of the following types of vaccines were recently approved for use for the COVID-19?
   (a) Live attenuated (b) mRNA vaccine
   (c) Conjugated vaccine (d) Toxoid vaccine.
5. Which of the following types of vaccines did the Moderna, Pfizer, BioNtech companies design for COVID-19?
   (a) mRNA vaccine (b) Vector-borne vaccine
   (c) Toxoid vaccine (d) Subunit vaccine.
6. All are examples of inactivated vaccines EXCEPT:
   (a) Rabies vaccine (b) Flu (influenza)
   (c) Smallpox vaccine (d) Covaxin.
7. All of the following statements are true for serum EXCEPT:
   (a) It is a straw-coloured liquid after blood clotting
   (b) EDTA, an anticoagulant is needed for its isolation
   (c) It is used to test for enzymes and other chemicals in the blood.
   (d) It is the plasma minus the clotting factors.
8. All are true for plasma EXCEPT:
   (a) Whole blood is added with an anticoagulant for its extraction/collection
   (b) Anticoagulated blood is centrifuged to separate blood cells
   (c) Blood plasma is the liquid left after formed elements are removed from unclotted blood
   (d) It is the straw-coloured liquid remaining after blood is allowed to clot.
9. Antiserum is the blood serum that contains specific antibodies.
   (a) True (b) False.

ANSWERS TO MCQs

1. (c) **2.** (a) **3.** (a) **4.** (b) **5.** (a)
6. (c) **7.** (b) **8.** (d) **9.** (a).

80

Immunoprophylaxis (Immunization/Vaccination) and Immunization Schedule

WHAT IS IMMUNOPROPHYLAXIS?

Immunoprophylaxis refers to the prevention of infectious diseases by immunization or other immunological methods. In simple words, it is prevention of disease in an individual by the production of active or passive immunity. Immunological preparations, such as vaccines, immune serums and gamma globulins are used to create immunity in an individual. The word had its origin in 1930s from *immuno* + *prophylaxis* means prevention.

TYPES OF IMMUNOPROPHYLAXIS

Immunoprophylaxis (also called prophylactic immunization) can be achieved by three methods:

- Active immunization (vaccination)
- Passive immunization
- Combined active-passive immunization

ACTIVE IMMUNIZATION

Active immunization, also called **vaccination**, involves the administration (inoculation) of an antigen, i.e., vaccine either orally or intramuscularly. Antibodies are created against the specific infection agents, and the recipient that provides protection against that disease permanently (troughout life) for several years. Vaccination is the most effective method of preventing/eradicating infectious diseases.

Edward Jenner, a British physician, was the first to start a series of inoculation experiments by injection of skin scratches with cowpox virus, which is not a serious pathogen and closely related to the smallpox virus, to protect them against smallpox disease. The inoculation provoked a primary immune response in the recipients, leading to the formation of antibodies and long-term memory cells. Later, when the recipient encountered the smallpox virus, the memory cells were stimulated, producing a rapid, intense secondary immune response. The **cowpox vaccine**–suspension of a live virus that is used to induce immunity against smallpox was soon replaced by a **vaccinia virus vaccine,** a smallpox vaccine. Ten centuries later, i.e., 1979, the smallpox disease was eliminated worldwide by vaccination. Jenner's work gave rise to the words-**vaccine** and **vaccination** (derived from the Latin for cow (*vacca, vaccinus*). Although Jenner did not invent this method, he is often considered the **Father of vaccines** because of his scientific approach that proved the method worked.

Louis Pasteur the noted French microbiologist, furthered the concept with the development of vaccines: **live attenuated cholera vaccine** in 1897 and **inactivated anthrax vaccine** in 1904 in humans. Pasteur's principle of inactivating or killing the infectious agent and then using to produce protective immunity into the host led to the development of several vaccines in the 20th century. These included vaccines that protected against pertussis (1914), diphtheria (1926), and tetanus (1938). These three vaccines were combined in 1948 and named in combination as the DTP vaccine.

Development of the viral tissue culture methods between 1950 and 1985 led to the advent of **Salk (inactivated polio vaccine)** and the **Satin (live attenuated oral polio vaccine) vaccines,** with the eradication of polio around the globe through mass polio immunization program.

With the modern innovative techniques, numerous vaccines have been developed and are in use, as described earlier in chapter 79.

Currently, a lot of emphasis is being laid on technology development for the production of vaccines, keeping in view that it takes less time, low cost, better efficiency and safety of human being. Based on the mode of production and technology, vaccines are classified into the following types: live attenuated vaccines, inactivated (killed) vaccines, subunit vaccines, toxoid vaccines, conjugated vaccines, DNA (or mRNA) vaccines, vector vaccines and plant-derived vaccines (described earlier in chapter 79).

HERD IMMUNITY

Herd immunity (also called **population immunity**, **community immuntity**, **mass immunity**) describes a type of immunity that occurs when most of the population (**herd**) is immune to an infectious disease, outbreaks are limited to sporadic cases because there are not enough susceptible individuals to support the spread of epidermic. Depending on how contagious an infection is, usually 50% to 90% of a population needs immunity before infection rates start to decline.

There are two ways to achieve herd immunity for any disease. A large proportion of the population either gets infected or gets a protective vaccine. Vaccination acts as a sort of immunological barrier in disease spread, slowing or preventing further transmission of the disease to others. The higher the level of immunity the larger the benefit. This is why it is important to get as many people as possible vaccinated.

We would need atleast 70% of the population to be immune to keep the rate of infection down (achieve herd immunity with SARS-CoV-2) without restriction on activities.

Measles, mumps, polio and chickenpox are examples of infectious diseases in which we have achieved herd immunity through vaccination.

CONTACT IMMUNITY

Contact immunity is the property of some vaccines, where a vaccinated individual can counter immunity upon immunized individuals through contact with bodily fluids or excrement. The potential for contact immunity exists primarily on live or alternated vaccines. The most popular example is the **oral polio vaccine (OPV)**. The recently immunized children with OPV shed live virus in their feces for a few days after immunization, an unimmunized person coming into contact usually gained protection from polio through this form of contact immunity.

PASSIVE IMMUNIZATION

Passive immunization (also called **passive immunotherapy** and **passive immunity**) is defined as the administration of purified antibodies (immunoglobulins) or serum containing antibodies to non-immune persons to provide rapid protection. It is used when there is a high risk of infection or insufficient time for the body to develop its own immune response, or to reduce the symptoms of ongoing or immune suppressive diseases.

Passive immunization was first used to treat disease in the late 19th century. In 1890, **Shibasabaro Kitasato** and **Emil von Behring**, were the first to treat diphtheria, a dangerous disease of human that obstructs the throat at airway, by using antibody containing blood derived substance, called **diphtheria antitoxin**. From 1895 onward, attempts were made to treat tetanus, smallpox, babonic plague with antibody containing blood products.

Two types of preparations are available for passive immunization.

1. **Pooled immunoglobulins** (use a mixture of antibodies prepared from pooled normal human serum containing human

immunoglobulins to treat a number of health conditions. The formulations (Flebogamma, Gammagard, Hizentra) can be administered by injection therapy which is called **immunoglobulin therapy**. The effects last a few weeks. It has been used to treat, HIV/AIDS, Kawaski disease, measles, Guillian-Barre' syndrom.

2. **Specific (hyperimmune) immunoglobulin (SIG)** is a formulated preparation made) from sera of patients who are recovering from an infection (convalescent sera) or from a person that has been actively immunized against a specific infection (e.g., hepatitis B, rabies, chickenpox, pertussis) which contain high titre of antibodies. These are useful for prophylaxis in person who have been exposed to these diseases.

COMBINED ACTIVE - PASSIVE IMMUNIZATION

Combined active and passive immunization therapy uses passive immunization with inactivated vaccine products to provide both immediate (but temporary) passive immunity and slowly developing active immunity. Both are given at the same time but at different sites (locations) of the body. Examples include tetanus, diphtheria and rabies.

IMMUNIZATION (VACCINATION) SCHEDULE

Immunization (as **vaccination**) is the process whereby a person is made immune or resistant to an infectious disease, typically by the administration of a vaccine. A **vaccination schedule** is a series of vaccinations, including the timing of all doses, which may be either recommended or compulsory, depending upon the country of residence. Vaccine schedules are developed by government using required and recommended vaccines for a locality while minimizing the number of healthcare system interactions. The WHO monitors vaccination schedules across the world, noting that vaccines are included in each country's program, the coverage rates achieved and various auditing measures.

Immunization program in India: IP was introduced in our country in 1978 as **Expanded Programme of Immunization** by the Ministry of Health and Family Welfare, Govt. of India. It was modified in 1985 as Universal Immunization Programme (UIP). Under this program, Ministry of Health and Family Welfare, provides several vaccines to infants, children and pregnant women as described below:

- **BCG (Bacillus Calmette-Guerin) vaccine:** Intradermal injection in the left upper arm at birth.

- **OPV** (oral polio vaccine): Orally 2 drops – 4 doses (at birth 6, 14 and 14 weeks) and a booser dose at 16-24 months.
- **Hepatitis B vaccine:** Intramuscular injection at anterolateral side of mid thigh at birth within 24 hours, 3 doses of 6, 10 and 14 weeks in combination with DPT and Hib in the form of pentavalent vaccine.
- **Pentavelent vaccine:** Diphtheria, tetanus, pertussis, hemophilia, influenza type b and hepatitis B. Intramuscularly at anterolateral side of mid thigh at 6, 10 and 14 weeks of age.
- **Rotavirus vaccine (RVV):** 5 drops or 2.5 ml of liquid (lyophilized vaccine) is given orally.
- **Pneumococcal conjugate vaccine (PCV):** Intramuscular injection at antero-lateral side of mid-thigh, two doses at 6 and 14 weeks of age, and a booster dose aged 6-12 months.
- **Fractional inactivated poliomyelitis vaccine (fIPV):** Two intrademal injections at right upper arm at 6 and 14 weeks of age.
- **Measles/MR vaccine:** Subcutaneous injection on right upper arm, first dose at 9 to 12 months and second dose at 16–24 months.
- **Japanese encephalitis vaccine:** Two doses 1st 9 to 12 months of age and 2nd dose at 16–24 months of age. Subcutaneous injection on left upper arm (live attenuated) and intramuscular injection in anterolateral of mid-thigh (killed vaccine).
- **Diphtheria, tetanus and pertussis (DPT) booster vaccine:** DPT booster dose at 16–24 months of ages (as intramuscular injection) and second DPT booster dose at 5-6 years of age (as intramuscular injection in left upper arm).
- **Tetanus and adult diphtheria (Td) vaccine:** Td is given as intramuscular injection in upper arm, to adolescent at 10 of 16 years of age.

  Pregnant women:
  - First dose (Td1) early on the pregnancy.
  - Second dose (Td2) after 4 to 6 weeks after first dose.
  - Td-booster is given within 3 years.

The childhood immunization vaccination schedule as per Universal Immunization Programme, for children aged 0–6 years, in India (2021) is given in Table 80.1.

Table 80.1 Latest national baby immunization schedule table 2021 (Vaccine wise)

Vaccine	Age	Dose	Route	Site
Vaccination chart for babies				
BCG	At birth till aged (one)	0.1 mL	Intradermal	Left/upper arm
Hepatitis B (birth dose)	At birth (or within 24 hours)	0.5 mL	Intramuscular	Left-mid thigh anterolateral side
OPV (birth dose)	At birth (or the first 15 days)	2 drops	Oral	–
OPV, 2 and 3	At 6, 10 and 14 weeks	2 drops	Oral	–
IPV	14 weeks	0.5 mL	Intramuscular	Right-mid thigh anterolateral
Pentavalent 1, 2, and 3	At 6, 10 and 14 weeks	0.5 mL	Intramuscular	–
Rotavirus	At 6, 10 and 14 weeks	5 drops	Oral	–
Measles (1st dose)	9 completed months to 12 months (given up to 5 years, if not received at 9-12 months age)	0.5 mL	Subcutaneous	Right/thigh
Vitamin A (first dose)	At 9 months with measles	1 mL (1 lakh units)	Oral	–
DPT 1st booster dose	16–24 months	0.5 mL	Intramuscular	Left-mid thigh anterolateral
OPV booster	16–24 months	2 drops	Oral	–
Measles (2nd dose)	16–24 months	0.5 mL	Subcutaneous	Right upper/ side
Vitamin (2nd to 9th dose)	16 months with DPT/OPV booster, then one dose every 6 months upto the age of 5 years	2 mL	Oral	–
DPT 2nd booster	5–6 years	0.5 mL	Intramuscular	Left upper arm
TT	10 years and 16 years	0.5 mL	Intramuscular	Upper arm

KEY POINTS

- **Immunoprophylaxis** provides specific protection against infectious diseases by stimulating (in vaccination) or agumenting the human's immune system.
- **Vaccination** (or **active immunization**) referes to the oral or intramuscular administration of vaccine for making a person immune or resistant to an infectious disease.
- The term vaccine and vaccination are derived from the Latin for cow (*vacca*).
- Edward Jenner developed the modern practice of vaccination.
- **Herd immunity** results when most of the population is immune to an infectious disease.
- Immunity achieved through contact with bodily fluids of a vaccinated individual with unimmunatory individual is **contact immunity.**
- Vaccines are the safest and most effective means of preventing/controlling infectious diseases.
- **Passive immunization** referes to the transfer of preformed antibodies or sera to an infected person.
- **Immunization (or vaccination) schedule** involves a series of vaccinations including the timing of all doses, to prevent control infectious diseases.
- Vaccines under the Universal Immunization Programme in India 2021 include: BCG, OPV, hepatitis B, pentavalent, rotavirus pneumococcal, fractional inactivated poliomycelitis, measles, Japanese encephalitis, DPT and Td vaccine.
- COVID-19 vaccines include: Covaxin, Pfizer-BioNTech, Moderna, Covishield, Sputnink V and Covavax are being administered to prevent and create herd immunity.

IMPORTANT QUESTIONS

1. Write brief notes on:
   (a) Vaccination.
   (b) Passive immunization.
   (c) Indian Immunization Schedule, 2021.
   (d) Herd and local immunity.
   (e) Name at least five vaccines with their mode of administration that are given to babies below 12 months of age.

MULTIPLE-CHOICE QUESTIONS

1. Active immunization is conferred by:
   (a) Gamma globulins (b) Antitoxins
   (c) Toxoids (d) All of the above.
2. Passive immunization is conferred by:
   (a) Vaccines (b) Toxoids
   (c) Gamma globulins (d) All of the above.
3. All are intramuscular vaccines EXCEPT:
   (a) BCG vaccine
   (b) Pentavalent 1, 2, and 3 vaccine
   (c) DPT vaccine
   (d) Hepatitis B vaccine.
4. Which of the following vaccines is administered at birth:
   (a) MMR vaccine (b) BCG vaccine
   (c) Measles vaccine (d) Tetanus toxoid (TT) vaccine.
5. Type of polio vaccine invented by the scientist Salk:
   (a) Inactivated virus (b) Live attenuatated virus
   (c) Subunit vaccine (d) None of these.
6. How much of the population should be immune to SARS-CoV-2 (COVID-19) to achieve herd immunity:
   (a) 50% (b) 70%
   (c) 90% (d) 100%.
7. Herd immunity has been achieved through vaccination in all these diseases EXCEPT:
   (a) Polio (b) Measles
   (c) TB (d) Chikenpox.
8. Which of the following vaccines is an example of contact immunity:
   (a) Toxoid vaccine (b) Oral polio vaccine
   (c) BCG vaccine (d) Measles vaccine.

ANSWERS TO MCQs

1. (c) **2.** (c) **3.** (a) **4.** (a) **5.** (a)
6. (b) **7.** (c) **8.** (b).

Index

J

K

L

M

P